LIPPINCOTT CERTIFICATION REVIEW

Pediatric Acute Care Nurse Practitioner

LIPPINCOTT CERTIFICATION REVIEW

Pediatric Acute Care Nurse Practitioner

● **Andrea M. Kline-Tilford**, MS, CPNP-AC/PC, FCCM
Pediatric Nurse Practitioner, Children's Hospital of Michigan
Department of Cardiovascular Surgery
Detroit, Michigan

● **Cathy Haut**, DNP, CPNP-AC/PC, CCRN
Specialty Director,
Pediatric Nurse Practitioner Program
University of Maryland School of Nursing, Baltimore, Maryland
Pediatric Nurse Practitioner
Pediatrix Medical Group and Beacon Pediatrics

®.Wolters Kluwer

Philadelphia · Baltimore · New York · London
Buenos Aires · Hong Kong · Sydney · Tokyo

Executive Editor: Shannon W. Magee
Product Development Editor: Maria M. McAvey
Senior Marketing Manager: Mark Wiragh
Editorial Assistant: Kathryn Leyendecker
Production Project Manager: Joan Sinclair
Design Coordinator: Holly Reid McLaughlin
Manufacturing Coordinator: Kathleen Brown
Prepress Vendor: S4Carlisle Publishing Services

9   8   7

Printed in the United States of America

Library of Congress Cataloging-in-Publication Data

Kline-Tilford, Andrea M., author.
  Lippincott certification review : pediatric acute care nurse practitioner / Andrea M. Kline-Tilford, Catherine Haut. — First edition.
    p. ; cm.
Includes bibliographical references and index.
    ISBN 978-1-4963-0856-6 (paperback)
I. Haut, Catherine, author. II. Title.
  [DNLM: 1. Critical Care Nursing—Examination Questions.   2. Pediatric Nursing—Examination Questions.   3. Licensure, Nursing—standards—Examination Questions.   4. Nurse Practitioners—Examination Questions. WY 18.2]
  RC86.9
  616.02'8076—dc23

2015020307

LWW.com

We dedicate this book to all of our expert colleagues who provide tireless care for critically ill children, especially to the memory of two incredible people who were taken from us too soon, Lisa Milonovich and Don Artes. Both epitomized excellence in knowledge and skill in pediatric critical care. Their impact on the lives of acute and critically ill children cannot be measured. We miss you.

Andrea & Cathy

To my incredible husband, Brad, and children, Ella and Graham. Thank you for your unending support in my professional endeavors. Without your love, patience, and late-night giggles, this book would not have been possible.

Andrea M. Kline-Tilford

To my husband, Lou, who has always supported my professional activities, including this book, which has taken many, many hours of our lives to complete, and to our children Melissa and Briana, whose confidence in my success is never-ending.

Cathy Haut

Contributors

Tageldin M. Ahmed, MD, MRCPCH
Assistant Professor of Pediatrics
Division of Critical Care Medicine
Children's Hospital of Michigan
Wayne State University School of Medicine
Detroit, Michigan

Kristen Altdoerffer, MSN, RN, CRNP
Assistant Clinical Professor
Pediatric Nurse Practitioner
Drexel University College of Nursing &
Health Professions
Pediatric Rehabilitation Unit
Children's Hospital of Philadelphia
Philadelphia, Pennsylvania

Sheree H. Allen, DNP, APRN, CPNP-PC/AC
Director
Pediatric Acute Care Nurse Practitioner Program
Vanderbilt University School of Nursing
Nashville, Tennessee

Cheryl N. Bartke, MSN, RN, PNP-BC, CPNC-AC
Critical Care Nurse Practitioner
The Children's Hospital of Philadelphia
Philadelphia, Pennsylvania

Miriam R. Batista, MSN, RN, CCRN, CPN
Nurse Educator
Hospital Education at San Antonio Military
Medical Center
San Antonio, Texas

Caroline Bauer, RN, MSN, CPNP-AC/PC
Pediatric Cardiothoracic Surgery Nurse Practitioner
University of Maryland Medical Center
Pediatric Cardiothoracic Surgery
Baltimore, Maryland

Marcella D. Bono, JD, MSN, RN, CPNP-PC, TNS
Clinical Education Specialist
Trauma Services
St. Louis Children's Hospital
St. Louis, Missouri

Cris A. Bowman-Harvey, MSN, PNP-BC, PC, AC
Pediatric Nurse Practitioner Faculty
Children's Hospital Colorado-Emergency
Denver, Colorado

Carole A. Branch, DNP, RN, PNP-BC
Pulmonary Hypertension/Lung Transplant APN
Transplant Services
St. Louis Children's Hospital
St. Louis, Missouri

Deborah W. Busch, DNP, CPNP
Assistant Professor
Pediatric Nurse Practitioner
University of Maryland
School of Nursing Pediatric Nurse Practitioner Program
Baltimore, Maryland

Alyssa Cavanaugh, PharmD
Pharmacy Practice Resident
Detroit Medical Center
Children's Hospital of Michigan
Detroit, Michigan

Joe D. Cavender, MSN, RN, CPNP-PC
Vice President
Associate Chief Nursing Officer
Children's Medical Center Dallas
Dallas, Texas

Mary C. Caverly, MSN, RN, CPNP
Pediatric Nurse Practitioner
Pediatric Intensive Care Unit
Detroit Medical Center
Children's Hospital of Michigan
Detroit, Michigan

Monika Chauhan, MBBS
Assistant Professor of Pediatrics
Division of Critical Care Medicine
Children's Hospital of Michigan
Wayne State University School of Medicine
Detroit, Michigan

Daniel K. Choi, MD, MS
Instructor of Pediatrics
Attending Physician
Division of Pediatric Hematology/Oncology
University of Illinois at Chicago
College of Medicine
Chicago, Illinois

Myra Cleary, DNP, CPNP-PC
Neurodevelopmental Pediatrics
Childrens National Health System
Washington, District of Columbia

Julie A. Creaden, MSN, APN, CPNP-PC
Administrator
Advanced Practice Nursing
Pediatric Nurse Practitioner
High Acuity Transition Clinic
Ann & Robert H. Lurie Children's Hospital of Chicago
Chicago, Illinois

Laura Crisanti, RN, MSN, CPNP-PC/AC
Pediatric Critical Care Nurse Practitioner
Pediatric Intensive Care Unit
Ann & Robert H. Lurie Children's Hospital of Chicago
Chicago, Illinois

Ruth DeVoogd, MSN, RN, CPNP-AC-PC
Senior Instructor
Advanced Practice Nurse
Breathing Institute
Children's Hospital of Colorado
Aurora, Colorado

Kimberly L. DiMaria, MSN, CPNP-AC, CCRN
Pediatric Nurse Practitioner
Pediatric Intensive Care Unit
Children's Hospital Colorado
Denver, Colorado

Jessica L. Diver, MSN, CPNP-AC, CPHON
Pediatric Nurse Practitioner
Blood and Marrow Transplant
Children's Hospital of Michigan
Detroit, Michigan

Sharron L. Docherty, PHD, PNP (BC AC/PC), FAAN
Associate Professor/School of Nursing
Associate Professor/Department of Pediatrics
School of Medicine/Co-Director
Adapt Center for Cognitive/Affective Symptom Science
Duke University School of Nursing
Durham, North Carolina

Michelle Dokas, RN, MSN, CPNP-AC
Pediatric Nurse Practitioner
Department of Cardiovascular Surgery
Children's Hospital of Michigan
Detroit, Michigan

Karen G. Duderstadt, PHD, RN, CPNP, PCNS, FAAN
UCSF Clinical Professor
UCSF School of Nursing
Department of Family Health Care Nursing
San Francisco, California

Brian Eells, CRNA
Certified Registered Nurse Anesthetist
Department of Anesthesiology
Children's Hospital of Michigan
Detroit, Michigan

Valarie D. Eichler, RN, PNP
Pediatric Nurse Practitioner
Critical Care Services
Children's Medical Center of Dallas
Dallas, Texas

Susan K. Emerson, CPNP
Nurse Practitioner/Pediatric Nursing
Johns Hopkins Children's Center
Baltimore, Maryland

Jessica S. Farber, DNP, CRNP, CPNP-AC, PPCNP-BC
Nurse Practitioner
Pediatric Intensive Care and Pediatric Progressive Care Units
The Children's Hospital of Philadelphia
Philadelphia, Pennsylvania

Richard P. Fernandez, MD
Attending Physician
Cardiothoracic Intensive Care
The Heart Center
Nationwide Children's Hospital
Assistant Professor of Clinical Pediatrics
The Ohio State University
Columbus, Ohio

Kelly Finkbeiner, APN, NP
Pediatric Nurse Practitioner
Pediatric Surgery (General)
Ann & Robert H. Lurie Children's Hospital of Chicago
Chicago, Illinois

Wendy S. Fitzgerald, RN, MSN, PPCNP-BC, CPON
Nurse Practitioner
Oncology Division
Children's National Health System
Washington, District of Columbia

Louise M. Flynn, MSN
Liver Transplant Coordinator
Division of Solid Organ Transplant
Nemours/Alfred I. DuPont Hospital for Children
Wilmington, Delaware

Viswanath Gajula, MD
Fellow
Division of Critical Care Medicine
Children's Hospital of Michigan
Detroit, Michigan

Deiadra J. Garrett, MD
Board Certified
General Surgery
Women's and Children's Hospital
Lafayette, Los Angeles

Erin M. Garth, MSN, RN, PPCNP-BC
Pediatric Nurse Practitioner
Department of Gastroenterology, Hepatology
Children's National Health System
Washington, District of Columbia

Lisa Genualdi, CPNP
Pediatric Nurse Practitioner
Division of Pediatric Critical Care
Ann & Robert H. Lurie Children's Hospital of Chicago
Chicago, Illinois

Terea Giannetta, DNP, RN, CPNP
Associate Professor
California State University
Fresno and Chief Nurse Practitioner
Children's Hospital Central California
Fresno and Madera, California

Michele Goodwin, RN, MSN, CRNP-AC
Nurse Practitioner
Progressive Care Unit
Children's Hospital of Philadelphia
Philadelphia, Pennsylvania

Keshava Gowda, MBBS, MD, FAAP
Pediatric Intensivist
Department of Pediatric Critical Care Medicine
Cleveland Clinic
Cleveland, Ohio

Christina Graham, NP
Nurse Practitioner
Munster Orthopaedic Inst., LLC
Munster, Indiana

Michele Grimason, RN, FNP-BC, PNP-AC
Pediatric Nurse Practitioner
Neuro Critical Care
Ann & Robert H. Lurie Children's Hospital of Chicago
Chicago, Illinois

Christine Guelcher, MS, APRN, PPCNP-BC
Program Coordinator
Hemostasis and Thrombosis Program
Department of Hematology
Children's National Health System
Washington, District of Columbia

Tamara L. Hill, RN, BSN, MSN, CPNP-AC
Pediatric Nurse Practitioner
University of Maryland
Medical Center
Division of Pediatric Nephrology
Baltimore, Maryland

Kristen Hittle, MSN, RN, CPNP-AC, CCRN
Pediatric Nurse Practitioner
Pediatric Intensive Care Unit
Children's Health
Children's Medical Center
Dallas, Texas

Sharon Y. Irving, PHD, RN, CRNP, FCCM
Assistant Professor
University of Pennsylvania/Division of Anesthesiology and
Critical Care Medicine
Department of Nursing/Respiratory Care and
Neurodiagnostic Services
Family and Community Health
University of Pennsylvania/School of Nursing
The Children's Hospital of Philadelphia
Philadelphia, Pennsylvania

Jennifer L. Joiner, MSN CPNP-AC/PC
Lead Nurse Practitioner
Pediatric Nurse Practitioner
Children's Hospital of San Antonio
Pediatric Intensive Care Unit
Clinical Instructor
Baylor College of Medicine
San Antonio, Texas

Brian F. Joy, MD
Assistant Professor of Clinical Pediatrics
Department of Pediatrics
Section of Pediatric Cardiology
Nationwide Children's Hospital
Columbus, Ohio

Jason M. Kane, MD MS, FAAP, FCCM
Assistant Professor of Pediatrics
Attending Physician Pediatric and Cardiac Intensive Care
Rush University Medical Center
Rush Children's Hospital
Chicago, Illinois

Mariam I. Kayle, MSN, RN, CCNS
Research Assistant
Clinical Instructor
Duke University School of Nursing
Durham, North Carolina

Lisa M. Kohr, RN, MSN, CPNP-AC/PC, MPH, FCCM
Pediatric Nurse Practitioner
Cardiac Intensive Care Unit
Children's Hospital of Philadelphia
Philadelphia, Pennsylvania

Shannon Konieczki, RN, MSN, CPNP
Pediatrics Nurse Practitioner
Department of Hematology and Oncology
Children's Hospital of Michigan
Detroit, Michigan

Jill C. Kuester, MSN, CPNP-AC
Pediatric Critical Care Nurse Practitioner
Medical College of Wisconsin-Children's Hospital
of Wisconsin
Milwaukee, Wisconsin

Elizabeth Leachman, CPNP-AC
Nurse Practitioner
Department of Trauma and Burn Surgery
Children's National Medical Center
Washington, District of Columbia

Samantha Lee, MSN, CPNP-AC
Nurse Practitioner
Pediatric Allergy,
 Pulmonary, and Immunology
University of Iowa Children's Hospital
Iowa City, Iowa

Dana L. Lerma, APN, NP
Pediatric Nurse Practitioner
Division of Pediatric Critical Care
Ann & Robert H. Lurie Children's Hospital of Chicago
Chicago, Illinois

Jeanne Little, MSN, NP
Faculty
Department of Women, Children, and Family Nursing
Rush University College of Nursing
Chicago, Illinois

Jennifer Livingston, MSN, RN, CPNP-AC
Pediatric Nurse Practitioner
Pediatric General Surgery
Children's Hospital of Michigan
Detroit, Michigan

Jennifer Manzi, CPNP-PC, AC
Pediatric Nurse Practitioner
Acute Care, Primary Care
Children's Hospital of Wisconsin
Milwaukee, Wisconsin

Kelly K. Marcoux, MSN, APN, CPNP-AC, PPCNP-BC, CCRN
Director, Advanced Practice Nursing
Children's Specialized Hospital
New Brunswick, New Jersey

Jill Marks, CPNP-AC
Pediatric Nurse Practitioner
Pulmonary Department
Children's Hospital of Colorado
Aurora, Colorado

Sarah A. Martin, MS, RN, CCRN, CPNP-AC/PC
Advanced Practice Nurse
Division of Pediatric Surgery
Ann & Robert H. Lurie Children's Hospital of Chicago
Chicago, Illinois

Danielle Mashburn, MPAS
Instructor
Pediatric Critical Care
School of Medicine
University of Colorado
Aurora, Colorado

Carmel A. McComiskey, DNP, CRNP
Director
Nurse Practitioners and Physician Assistants
University of Maryland Medical Center
Baltimore, Maryland

Robin McKinney, MD
Fellow
Division of Critical Care Medicine
Children's Hospital of Michigan
Detroit, Michigan
Detroit, Michigan

Theresa A. Mikhailov, MD, PHD
Associate Professor of Pediatrics
Pediatrics and Medical College of Wisconsin
Milwaukee, Wisconsin

Marisa Mize, DNP, CPNP-AC, PC, CCRN
Pediatric Critical Care Nurse Practitioner
Pediatric Critical Care, Walter Reed National Military
Medical Center
Bethesda, Maryland

Lynn D. Mohr, MS, APRN, PCSN-BC, CPN
Instructor/Program Director Pediatric and Neonatal CNS
Programs
Department of Women, Children, Family Nursing
Rush University College of Nursing
Chicago, Illinois

Leah Molloy, PharmD
Clinical Pharmacist Specialist, Infectious Diseases
Department of Pharmacy Services
Children's Hospital of Michigan
Detroit Medical Center
Detroit, Michigan

Shawna Mudd, DNP, CPNP-AC, PPCNP-BC
Assistant Professor
Senior Nurse Practitioner
Johns Hopkins School of Nursing
Baltimore, Maryland

Melanie Muller, MSN, CPNP-AC
Pediatric Cardiothoracic Surgery Nurse Practitioner
Pediatrics-University of Maryland Medical Center
Baltimore, Maryland

Erin K. Mullaney, MSN, RN, PNP-BC
Pediatric Nurse Practitioner
Palliative Care Program, Children's Healthcare of Atlanta
Atlanta, Georgia

Jessica Hoffman Murphy, MS, RN, CPNP-AC, CPHON
Pediatric Critical Care Nurse Practitioner
Pediatrix Medical Group
Herman and Walter Samuelson Childrens Hospital at Sinai
Baltimore, Maryland

Conni Nevills, MSN, CPNP-AC
Pediatric Nurse Practitioner
Children's Walk-in Clinic Columbia
Columbia, Maryland

Christopher D. Newman, MBA, PA-C
Assistant Professor of Pediatrics
Director of Advanced Practice for the Pediatric
Intensive Care Unit
University of Colorado School of Medicine
Aurora, Colorado

Jan A. Odiaga, DNP, CPNP
Assistant Professor Rush University College of Nursing
Women, Children, and Family Nursing
Chicago, Illinois

Nneka Okoye, MSN, FNP-BC
Nurse Practitioner
Manager
Occupational Health and Safety
Sibley Memorial Hospital
Washington, District of Columbia

Myra L. Popernack, RN, MSN, CPNP
Pediatric Nurse Practitioner
Penn State Hershey Children's Hospital
Department of Pediatrics
Division of Pediatric Rehabilitation and Development
Hershey, Pennsylvania

Elizabeth R. Prentice, DO
Pediatric Critical Care Physician
Helen Devos Children's Hospital
Grand Rapids, Michigan

Elizabeth R. Preze, MSN, CPNP-AC/PC
Director, Cardiac Care Unit
Ann & Robert H. Lurie Children's Hospital of Chicago
Chicago, Illinois

Kristin M. Print, RN, MSN, CCRN, PPCNP-BC, C-NPT
Pediatric Critical Care Nurse Practitioner
Pediatric Intensive Care Unit
The Children's Hospital of Philadelphia
Philadelphia, Pennsylvania

Carmen Rancilio, MSN, RN, CPNP-AC
Pediatric Nurse Practitioner
Department of Pediatric Surgery
Children's Hospital of Michigan
Detroit, Michigan

Elizabeth Rosner, DO
Pediatric Critical Care Physician
Department of Pediatrics Helen Devos Children's Hospital
Grand Rapids, Michigan

Laura T. Russo, RD, CSP, LDN
Registered Dietitian
Clinical Nutrition
Ann & Robert H. Lurie Children's Hospital of Chicago
Chicago, Illinois

Hitesh Sandhu, MBBS, MRCPCH
Assistant Professor
Division of Pediatric Critical Care
Le Bonheur Children's Hospital
Memphis, Tennessee

Preet K. Sandhu, MBBS, MD
Assistant Professor
Department of Radiology
Le Bonheur Children's Hospital
Memphis, Tennessee

Denise C. Schiel, RN, MSN, CPNP-AC
Pediatric Critical Care Nurse Practitioner
Division of Pediatric Critical Care Medicine
Rady Children's Hospital
San Diego, California

Christine A. Schindler, PHD, RN, CPNP-AC/PC, WCC
Clinical Assistant Professor
Marquette University
Milwaukee, Wisconsin

Tonya A. Schneidereith, PHD, CRNP, PPCNP-BC, CPNP-AC
Assistant Professor of Nursing
Stevenson University-Department of Nursing
Stevenson, Maryland

Mary Schucker, MSN, CPNP-PC
Pediatric Nurse Practitioner
Department of Emergency Medicine
Sexual Assault Response Team
The Children's Hospital of Philadelphia
Clinical Faculty Site Coordinator
University of Pennsylvania
Philadelphia, Pennsylvania

Meghan Shackelford, MSN, CRNP-AC
Pediatric Critical Care Nurse Practitioner
Pediatric Critical Care Unit
Johns Hopkins Children's Center
Baltimore, Maryland

Shari Simone, DNP, CPNP-AC, FCCM
Senior Nurse Practitioner Clinical Program Manager
Women & Children's Services
University of Maryland Medical Center
Pediatric Critical Care
Baltimore, Maryland

Lara G. Smith, MSN, RN, CPNP-PC, CPNP-AC
Pediatric Nurse Practitioner
Pediatric Intensive Care Unit
St. Louis Children's Hospital
St. Louis, Missouri

Christopher Sonne, CHEC
Assistant National Director
HSS Emergency Management Services
Denver, Colorodo

Lauren Sorce, RN, MSN, CPNP-AC/PC, FCCM
Pediatric Critical Care Nurse Practitioner
Advanced Practice Nurse Manager Manager
Ann & Robert H. Lurie Children's Hospital of Chicago
Division of Pediatric Critical Care
Chicago, Illinois

Heather Sowinski, DO
Fellow
Department of Cardiology
Children's Hospital of Michigan
Detroit, Michigan

Katie Spillman, RN
Pediatric Intensive Care Unit
University of Maryland
Medical Center
Baltimore, Maryland

David M. Steinhorn, MD, FAAP, FAAHPM
Professor of Pediatrics
Pediatric Critical Care / Pediatric Palliative Care
UC Davis Medical Center
Sacramento, California

Lori Stern, RN, MSN, CPNP-AC
Pediatric Nurse Practitioner
Division of Gastroenterology, Hepatology, and Nutrition
Children's National Health System
Washington, District of Columbia

Kelly A. Swain, RN, MSN, CPNP-AC
Pediatric Critical Care Nurse Practitioner
Pediatric Critical Care Medicine
Duke University Medical Center
Durham, North Carolina

Jill S. Thomas, MSN, CPNP-AC
Pediatric Critical Care Nurse Practitioner
Pediatrics-University of Maryland Medical Center
Baltimore, Maryland

Allison Thompson, MSN, RD, RN, CCRN, CRNP
Pediatric Critical Care Nurse Practitioner-Team Leader
Critical Care Department
The Children's Hospital of Philadelphia
Pediatric Intensive Care Unit
Philadelphia, Pennsylvania

Bradley D. Tilford, MD
Assistant Professor of Pediatrics
Division of Critical Care Medicine
Children's Hospital of Michigan
Wayne State University School of Medicine
Detroit, Michigan

Jacqueline Toia, DNP, RN
Nurse Practitioner
Emergency Department
Ann & Robert H. Lurie Children's Hospital of Chicago
Emergency Department
Chicago, Illinois

Rita Tracewell, MS, CPNP-AC
Pediatric Nurse Practitioner
Pediatric Surgery
University of Maryland Medical Center
Baltimore, Maryland

Megan Trahan, MSN, CPNP-AC
Pediatric Critical Care Nurse Practitioner
Department of Pediatrics
University of Maryland Medical Center
Baltimore, Maryland

Rosanna Tran, PharmD
Pediatric Pharmacist
Children's Hospital of Central California
Fresno, California

Tara Trimarchi, MSN, RN, CRNP
Pediatric Critical Care Nurse Practitioner
Advanced Practice Nurse Manager
Critical Care, Sedation, and Radiology
Children's Hospital of Philadelphia
Lecturer
University of Pennsylvania
Philadelphia, Pennsylvania

Danielle Van Damme, MSN, CPNP-AC
Nurse Practitioner
Department of Hematology/Oncology/Bone Marrow
Transplant
Children's Hospital of Michigan
Detroit, Michigan

Anne Vasiliadis, MSN, CPNP-AC
Nurse Practitioner/Department of Epilepsy,
Neurophysiology, and Critical Care Neurology
Children's National Health System
Washington, District of Columbia
Nurse Practitioner/Division of Pediatric Critical Care
University of Maryland Medical Center
Baltimore, Maryland

Kristi Waddell, APN, NP
Pediatric Nurse Practitioner
Neuro-oncology
Ann & Robert H. Lurie Children's Hospital of Chicago
Chicago, Illinois

Catherine Walsh, RN, MSN, CPNP-AC
Pediatric Nurse Practitioner
Department of General Surgery, Trauma, and Burn
Children's National Health System
Washington, District of Columbia

Katie Ward, DNP, WHNP
Associate Clinical Professor
College of Nursing
University of Utah
Salt Lake City, Utah

Mark D. Weber, RN, MSN, PCCNP
Nurse Practitioner
Division of Pediatric Critical Care Medicine
Duke University School of Medicine
Durham, North Carolina

Mary P. White, MSN, CPNP-PC
Staff Pediatric Nurse Practitioner
Naval Branch Health Clinic Mayport Pediatrics
Mayport, Florida

Megan R. Winkler, MSN, RNC-NIC, CPNP-PC
Duke University School of Nursing
Durham, North Carolina

Barbara Wise, CPNP
Pediatric Nurse Practitioner
National Institutes of Health
Bethesda, Maryland

Katherine Worst, MSN, CPNP
Pediatric Nurse Practitioner
Acute Care, General Surgery, Trauma and Burn Services
Children's National Medical Center
Washington, District of Columbia

Alexandra K. Yockey, RN, BSN, MSN, CPNP-AC
Pediatric Trauma Nurse Practitioner
University of Texas, Pediatric Trauma
Houston, Texas

Tresa E. Zielinski, DNP, APN-NP, PNP-PC
Pediatric Nurse Practitioner
Emergency Department
Ann & Robert H. Lurie Children's Hospital of Chicago
Chicago, Illinois

Foreword

The *Pediatric Acute Care Nurse Practitioner Certification Review* book is a one of a kind resource for graduates of Pediatric Nurse Practitioners—Acute Care (PNP-AC) programs to prepare for certification. Andrea M. Kline-Tilford and Cathy Haut wonderfully use their significant expertise to provide the reader with the information necessary to care for children with acute, critical, and complex chronic illness in a variety of settings. Starting with the needs of the pediatric patient and their family through the test-taking strategies, this book documents important PNP-AC competencies. The robust section on system-based problems highlights the care for a broad range of pediatric patients with life-threatening illness and organ dysfunction and failure. To address the skills needed to work in a complex system, this text also emphasizes important professional issues.

Education of PNP-AC was formalized in the early 1990s. In these early years, we knew the constellation of competencies of the nurse practitioner in pediatric acute care was unique. With the commitment of the Pediatric Nursing Certification Board (PNCB), the first certification exam was offered in 2005. Today PNP-ACs continue to validate their knowledge in a distinct collection of skills to meet the needs of patients.

It seems fitting that the publication of this book occurs during the 10th anniversary of the PNP-AC exam. Through the dedication and commitment of Andrea and Cathy, the *Pediatric Acute Care Nurse Practitioner Certification Review* book is now a reality. Congratulations!

Judy Verger, RN, PhD, CRNP, FCCM

Contents

xviii   Contents

xx   **Contents**

PART ONE

The Pediatric Patient and Family

General Pediatric Considerations, Development, Nutrition, and Sleep

Thermoregulation

Cathy Haut

Background/Definition/Pathophysiology

- Thermoregulation is important in pediatric acute care evaluation and management.
- Hypothermia and hyperthermia can be symptoms of illness or side effects/complications of therapy effects or complications of therapy.
- Maintenance of a normal temperature assists in sustaining normal metabolic rate and hydration, thus decreasing additional demands on the ill child, especially a child with an acute or critical illness.

Heat Loss Concepts

- *Evaporation* of fluids through skin and respiratory tract into the air or environment.
- *Convection* is the transfer of heat from one place to another by the movement of air or fluids.
- *Conduction* is the transfer of heat from one surface to another; body conducts heat to whatever surface it is in contact with.
- *Radiation* is heat generated from the body emitted to the surrounding air or environment.

Physioanatomic thermal considerations in children include the following:
- Larger body surface area to body mass ratio; increased risk for evaporative loss.
- Higher metabolic rates.
- Lower subcutaneous fat stores.
- Additional risks for temperature instability for premature infants:
  - Immature central nervous system: insufficient metabolic response to thermal stress.
  - Low birth weight.
  - Very little subcutaneous fat, immature skin, and decreased brown fat (presence of brown fat facilitates heat production).

Clinical Presentation

- Acute and critically ill infants and children can present with hyperthermia or hypothermia as a symptom or response to illness/disease.
- Temperature alteration can result in tachycardia, tachypnea, irritability, dehydration, acidosis and increased metabolic rate.

Management

- Recognition of febrile or hypothermic states is essential while determining the etiology and correcting to normothermia.
- Maintenance of neutral thermal zones with prevention of heat loss is important for all children, but imperative for preterm infants.

PEARLS
- *Heart rate and respiratory rate/status can be indicators of fever or hypothermia.*
- *Fever is most commonly a symptom of illness and is vital to immune response.*
- *Antipyretics should be used primarily for comfort rather than for fever reduction.*
- *In some conditions (e.g., traumatic brain injury, cerebral anoxia, post–cardiac arrest), hypothermia may be used as a neuroprotective strategy.*

Central Nervous System

Cathy Haut

Background/Definition

- The central nervous system (CNS) develops from the embryonic stage until adolescence.
- Vulnerable periods during the development of the nervous system include illness; environmental and chemical insults predispose infants and young children to potential sensory,

motor, and cognitive dysfunction with possible poor neurodevelopmental outcomes.

- 3% to 8% of infants born in the United States will be affected by a neurodevelopmental disorder such as attention-deficit/hyperactivity disorder (ADHD), autism, developmental delay, or cognitive disability which may be associated with insults to the CNS at a young age.
- The CNS of preterm and very young infants is especially vulnerable to insult.

Anatomy of the Nervous System

- Principal components include CNS and peripheral nervous system.
- CNS comprises the brain and spinal cord:
  - Brain stem:
    - Medulla oblongata: ascending and descending motor function.
    - Pons Varolii: connects midbrain with medulla oblongata and controls breathing.
  - Midbrain:
    - Contains the dorsal rectum, which is the reflex center controlling movement of the eyeballs and head.
  - Diencephalon:
    - Thalamus: interpretation of stimuli, especially pain and temperature.
    - Hypothalamus: autonomic functions related to homeostasis.
  - Cerebrum:
    - Cerebral cortex: frontal, parietal, temporal, and occipital lobes.
    - Controls voluntary actions, speech, senses, thought, and memory.
  - Cerebellum:
    - Controls equilibrium and coordination, muscle movement, and tone.
  - Cranial nerves:
    - Twelve cranial nerves.
    - Cranial nerve function is further explained in the *Neurologic* section.
  - Ventricular system includes four ventricles.
    - Circulates cerebrospinal fluid through the brain, spinal cord, and ventricles.
- Peripheral nervous system:
  - Connects the brain and spinal cord with sensory receptors, muscles, and glands in the limbs and organs.
- Somatic nervous system:
  - Coordinates body movements and receives external stimuli.
- Autonomic nervous system:
  - Controls glands, cardiac muscle, and smooth muscle.

Fluid, Electrolytes, and Nutrition
Cathy Haut

Background and General Concepts

- The balance of maintaining fluid, electrolyte, and nutritional status in an acute or critically ill child is challenging and requires precision in assessment and determination of management.
- Fluid and electrolyte status is affected by disease state, exhibited by dehydration, overhydration, acidosis, alkalosis, or electrolyte derangements.

Fluid and Nutritional Status

- Fluids: 29% extracellular, 19% interstitial, 6% plasma, protein, and lipids, and 45% intracellular.
- Infants are more vulnerable to dehydration.
- Moderate-to-severe dehydration leads to hypovolemic shock.
- Fluids are calculated based on daily needs for healthy children, physiologic state, and insensible losses.
- Despite availability of several methods of calculating nutritional deficits, fluid deficits, and fluid requirements, metabolic response to stress, injury, surgery, or inflammation cannot always be accurately predicted; continuous evaluation is required.
- Accurate evaluation of energy requirements (indirect calorimetry) and provision of fluids, electrolytes, and optimal nutritional support therapy utilizing the appropriate route are important goals of pediatric acute and critical care.
- Malnutrition in hospitalized children is associated with increased physiologic instability and increased resource utilization, with potential poor outcome from critical illness, but recent research indicates that nutritional deficits in early illness do not always result in poor outcomes.
- Both overfeeding and underfeeding hospitalized children can affect outcomes.
- Altered metabolism occurs in hospitalized children based on severity of injury or illness.
- Burns or major trauma affects fluid and electrolyte status and metabolic rates.
- Catecholamines (endogenous and exogenous) result in reduction of insulin secretion and peripheral insulin action and stimulate production of glucagon and adrenocorticotropic hormone, resulting in hyperglycemia, lipid intolerance, and protein catabolism in acutely and critically ill children.
- Hepatic protein synthesis changes during periods of inflammation, resulting in increased production of C-reactive protein (CRP) and reduced production of albumin and prealbumin.

Pathophysiology

- Acute injury markedly alters fluid and energy needs and produces a catabolic response that is proportional to the magnitude, nature, and duration of the injury.
- Increased serum counterregulatory hormone concentrations induce insulin and growth hormone resistance, resulting in the catabolism of endogenous stores of protein, carbohydrate, and fat to provide essential substrate intermediates and energy necessary to support ongoing metabolic stress response.
- See Section 16 for additional information on fluids and electrolytes.

Pediatric Pharmacokinetics and Pharmacodynamics

Alyssa Cavanaugh, Rosanna Tran, & Leah Molloy

Drug Absorption

- Oral absorption is generally slower in neonates and young infants.
- Gastrointestinal tract pH changes over time.
  - Compared to older children and adults, neonates have less acidic gastrointestinal tracts with a relatively high pH (>4).
  - Increased oral bioavailability of acid-labile compounds, such as penicillin G, so may require smaller doses.
  - Decreased oral bioavailability of weak acids, such as phenobarbital, so may require larger doses.
- Enhanced percutaneous absorption during infancy owing to thinner skin, much higher ratio of total body surface area to body mass.
- Intramuscular drug absorption.
  - Despite reduced skeletal muscle blood flow potentially decreasing drug absorption, the greater vascularity of infant skeletal muscle permits equal, if not greater, intramuscular drug absorption.

Drug Distribution

- Neonates and infants have high proportions of total body water.
  - Greater hydration of adipose tissue can yield lower serum concentrations of hydrophilic drugs because they are more liable to distribute into the adipose tissue.
- Circulating plasma proteins.
  - Neonatal albumin has less affinity for weak acids than that of adults and may result in greater free fractions (i.e., not bound to protein) of medications.
  - Ceftriaxone and sulfamethoxazole compete with bilirubin for binding to albumin in neonatal patients.
  - Increased concentrations of free bilirubin increase the risk for kernicterus; thus, these agents are avoided in neonates.
- Metabolism:
  - Phase I enzymes: cytochrome P450 (CYP) enzymes.
    - Different CYP isozymes mature at different rates.
    - Age-dependent variation in CYP-mediated drug metabolism.
      - CYP3A7 peaks shortly after birth and declines to undetectable levels in adults.

- Hours after birth, CYP2E1 increases to a detectable level and CYP2D6 soon after follows suit.
- CYP3A4, 2C9, and 2C19 appear in the first week of life.
- CYP1A2 appears 1 to 3 months after birth.
  - Caffeine and theophylline are substrates for CYP1A2.
  - May need higher doses as CYP1A2 matures.
- Phase II enzymes: glucuronosyltransferase (UGT).
  - Delayed maturation of UGT1A1, the enzyme responsible for conjugating bilirubin, contributes to higher levels of circulating unconjugated, insoluble bilirubin.
  - UGT2B7, responsible for metabolizing morphine in preparation for elimination, is present in infants as young as 24 weeks and increases markedly between 27 and 40 weeks of gestation.
  - Clearance of morphine is correlated with postgestational age, requiring increasing doses to maintain appropriate analgesia as the patient ages, particularly among premature infants.
- Elimination:
  - The processes of glomerular filtration, tubular secretion, and tubular reabsorption determine the efficiency of renal excretion of drugs and their metabolites.
  - These processes may not develop fully for several weeks to 1 year after birth.
- Age-related renal function:
  - The glomerular filtration rate may be as low as 0.6 to 0.8 mL/minute per 1.73 m^2 (0.006–0.008 mL/second/m^2) in preterm neonates and approximately 2 to 4 mL/minute per 1.73 m^2 (0.02–0.04 mL/second/m^2) in term neonates.
  - Creatinine clearance (CrCl) in children may be estimated using the revised Schwartz equation with an age-dependent variable for infants.

Box 1.1 Revised Schwartz Equation
CrCl = [k × height (cm)]/serum creatinine

Age-specific k values are available in some references; typically k = 0.413.
- Additional considerations for pediatric drug dosing:
  - Doses are typically based on weight and body surface area.
  - Higher weight-based doses are often needed in children than in adults to achieve comparable exposures.
    - Voriconazole doses >7 mg/kg are needed for children to achieve similar exposure as adults receiving only 4 mg/kg.
  - Doses given to children should not exceed maximum adult doses—*important for obese pediatric population.*
  - As children clear medications more quickly, shorter dosing intervals are often needed as compared to adults.
- Therapeutic drug monitoring:
  - Some medications have variable dose–exposure relationships and narrow therapeutic indices, necessitating monitoring of serum drug concentrations to guide dosing.
  - Most common examples are vancomycin, aminoglycosides, and antiepileptics.

- Target serum concentrations are patient- and indication-specific; however, typical targets are listed below:
  - Vancomycin: trough 10 to 20 mg/kg.
  - Gentamicin, tobramycin: peak 6 to 12 mg/L, trough <1 mg/L.
  - Phenytoin: steady-state concentration 10 to 20 mg/L.

Normal Childhood Development

Cris A. Bowman-Harvey

Prenatal/Newborn

- Health history:
  - Family health history: chronic and genetic diseases of both maternal and paternal relatives.
  - Pregnancy history: planned or unplanned, number of live births, abortion or miscarriage, health of other children.
- Obstetrics history:
  - Parent ages, maternal health to include hypertension and epilepsy, prenatal care and course, medications (both prescribed and illicit use) during pregnancy, maternal alcohol and cigarette use, and maternal exposures during pregnancy which can include radiation and other environmental substances (including tobacco exposure).
  - Maternal infection history: group B streptococcus status (if known); chlamydia; gonorrhea; hepatitis B; syphilis; HIV.
  - Maternal infection or exposure history and resulting problems with infant: TORCH.
    - Toxoplasmosis: cognitive impairment, learning disabilities, and blindness.
    - Rubella: deafness, blindness, cardiac anomalies, and limb deformities.
    - Cytomegalovirus: Asymptomatic; symptoms present at birth or may appear more than 2 years after birth and include hearing loss, cognitive impairment, learning disabilities.
    - Herpes Simplex Virus (HSV): CNS involvement, skin, eye, and mouth involvement, and liver damage.
  - Maternal Rh and blood-type incompatibilities: RhoGAM administration.
  - Maternal diabetes: large for gestational age (LGA) infants, hypoglycemia, polycythemia.
  - Intrauterine issues and associated conditions:
    - Polyhydramnios can predispose the fetus to umbilical cord prolapse, duodenal atresia, esophageal atresia, intestinal atresia, neuromuscular disorder (e.g., anencephaly), dysplastic kidneys, placental abruption, premature birth, still birth, congenital defect.
    - Oligohydramnios can predispose the fetus to intrauterine growth retardation (IUGR), umbilical cord compression, musculoskeletal abnormalities, and pulmonary hypoplasia.
- Prenatal testing:
  - Ultrasound: size of infant, presence of single or multiple gestations, gross defects.

- α-Fetoprotein measurement: increases as pregnancy progresses to peak during second trimester; good indicator of pregnancy progress; high levels may indicate neural tube defects, multiple gestations, omphalocele, gastroschisis, or nonspecific chromosomal abnormalities.
- Amniocentesis: increased risk of abortion; offers identification of infant's karyotype, enzyme abnormalities, and DNA sampling.
- Chorionic villus sampling: performed at 10 weeks' gestation or later; identification of infant's karyotype, enzyme abnormalities, and DNA sampling; increased risk of amputation of fingers and toes; slight risk of abortion.
- Labor and delivery history:
  - Type of delivery: cesarean section or vaginal birth; position or presentation of newborn (breech); forceps or vacuum delivery; duration of labor; hours of membrane rupture prior to deliver; analgesia or anesthesia.
  - Fever: American Academy of Pediatrics (AAP) Guidelines for prevention of perinatal group B streptococcal (GBS) disease (AAP, 2011), chorioamnionitis.
  - Fetal stress or distress prior to delivery: meconium staining, fetal hypoxia.
- Environmental/Social history:
  - Type, size, and condition of home, heating, and hot water.
  - Number and relationship of people living in the household; demographics including educational level of parents, medical insurance, and income.
  - Health and safety hazards in household, guns, tools, and tobacco exposure.
  - Primary caregiver and care giving arrangements.
- Transition to extra-uterine life:
  - Respiratory system: reabsorption of fetal lung fluid.
  - Sufficient lung surfactant → increased functional residual capacity → decreased inspiratory pressure → alveolar filling → decreased pulmonary vascular resistance → increased blood flow to the lungs.
  - Circulatory system: decreased pulmonary vascular resistance → decreased pressure on the right side of the heart (now lower than left side) → foramen ovale closure. Increased blood oxygen level and decreased pulmonary vascular resistance → ductus arteriosus closure.
- APGAR score:
  - Evaluates heart rate, respiratory effort, muscle tone, reflexes, and color, each parameter on a 3-point scale from 0 to 2, with the highest possible total score of 10.
  - Performed at 1 and 5 minutes of life; sometimes a 10-minute evaluation is warranted.
- Gestational age determination:
  - Maturational assessment of gestational age is based on physical examination to confirm dates and prenatal ultrasound measurement.
  - LGA infant: >90th percentile can result in hypoglycemia, fracture of clavicles, brachial plexus injury, skull injuries, facial palsy, polycythemia.
  - Small for gestational age infant: <10th percentile can result in respiratory distress, perinatal asphyxia, meconium

aspiration, poor feeding, bradycardia, hypoglycemia, hypothermia, polycythemia.
- Prematurity:
  - Classification:
    - Preterm infant: <37 weeks gestation.
    - Late preterm infant: 34 through $36\frac{6}{7}$ = weeks gestation.
    - Very preterm infant: <32 weeks gestation.
    - Low birth weight: <2,500 g.
    - Very low birth weight: <1,500 g.
    - Extremely low birth weight: <1,000 g.
  - Health risks of preterm and low-birth-weight infants:
    - Respiratory distress, apnea of prematurity.
    - Increased susceptibility to infections.
    - Thermoregulation issues.
    - Patent ductus arteriosus (PDA).
    - Necrotizing enterocolitis (NEC), gastroesophageal reflux (GER).
    - Retinopathy of prematurity (ROP).
    - Intraventricular hemorrhage (IVH).
    - Anemia.
    - Hernia/hydrocele/undescended testes.
    - Decreased efficiency conjugating bilirubin, resulting in hyperbilirubinemia.
    - Decreased ability to concentrate urine, resulting in risk of dehydration.
    - Hypocalcemia as a result of decreased levels of parathyroid hormone.
    - Hypoglycemia as a result of decreased glycogen stores.
- Postmaturity: pregnancy >42 weeks of gestation.
  - Health risks associated with postmaturity:
    - Susceptibility to perinatal asphyxia resulting from placental degeneration.
    - Hypoglycemia due to rapid use of glycogen stores.
    - Dry, peeling skin.
    - Decreased amniotic fluid; potential distress during labor.

Newborn

- Pertinent physical examination findings:
  - May lose up to 10% of birth weight in first days of life (beyond 10% requires close monitoring; possible hospital admission).
  - Nutritional needs for growth approximately 100 to 110 kcal/kg/day.
  - Typical weight gain 0.5 to 1 oz/day.
  - Reflexes present at birth: sucking, rooting, asymmetric tonic neck, Moro reflex, grasp.
  - Newborn screening test (blood); also known as metabolic screening.
    - Each state has different screening parameters.
    - Performed before infant is discharged from the hospital, but preferably after infant has been fed for 24 to 36 hours and again at 2 to 3 weeks of life.
    - Commonly tested conditions included in the newborn screening test.
      - Phenylketonuria (PKU): autosomal recessive disorder; inability to break down the amino acid phenylalanine. See Section 9 for more information.
      - Galactosemia (GAL): rare autosomal disorder; deficiency in the enzyme needed to metabolize galactose in milk. See Section 9 for more information.
      - Hypothyroidism: See Section 7 for more information.
      - Hemoglobinopathies: hereditary disorder; sickle cell anemia (several variations) and thalassemia. See Section 10 for more information.
      - Congenital adrenal hyperplasia: autosomal recessive disorder; inborn deficiency of various enzymes necessary for the biosynthesis of cortisol. See Section 7 for more information.
      - Maple syrup urine disease: inherited disorder; inability to metabolize valine, leucine, and isoleucine (amino acids). See Section 9 for more information.
      - Homocystinuria: deficiency of the enzyme cystathionine synthase needed for cystathionine metabolism; results in mental retardation, seizures, behavior disorders, early-onset thromboses, dislocated lenses, and tall, lanky body type. Treatment includes a methionine-restricted diet; cystine supplement and B_6 supplement if responsive.
      - Biotinidase deficiency: inherited metabolic disorder of biotin reuse or recycling. See Section 9 for more information.
      - Toxoplasmosis: infection of the fetus with the protozoan parasite *Toxoplasma gondii*, typically acquired by active infection of the mother during pregnancy. Signs of congenital infection may be present at birth or develop over the first few months of life. Symptoms include CNS abnormalities, enlargement of the liver and spleen, blindness, and mental retardation.
      - Cystic fibrosis (CF): Autosomal recessive disorder that results in an altered transport of chloride ions. See Section 4 for more information.
- Dysmorphology in neonates:
  - Most infants will have some minor malformations or variations of normal; however, primary dysmorphologic concept is that the greater the number of minor malformations, the greater the likelihood that there will be an underlying major malformation—an infant with three or more minor anomalies has an approximately 20% chance of having an underlying associated major malformation.
  - The rule of threes: One minor abnormality can indicate a chance of genetic abnormality. If two minor abnormalities, must look for a third. If three minor abnormalities, there is a 90% chance the child has a syndrome.
  - Minor abnormalities are unusual dysmorphic features commonly located on the face, ears, hair, hands, and feet with no serious medical problems.
- Newborn hearing screening:
  - Universal newborn hearing screening is conducted within 1 month of age.
  - Failed screening, followed by comprehensive audiologic evaluation no later than 3 months of age. Full guidelines available from AAP: www.aap.org.
- Newborn safety:
  - Back-to-sleep campaign.

- All infants sleep on side or back.
- Firm surface in a crib or bassinet.
- No blanket, pillow, bumper pads, wedges/positioners, or soft toys.
- Car seat: rear facing until 2 years of age.

Infant

- First 3 months of age (first 28 days of life is considered neonatal period).
  - Growth:
    - 0.5 to 1 oz per day with 8 to 10 feedings in 24 hours.
    - Weight returns to birth weight by approximately 14 days of life.
    - Height/Length growth is approximately 1 inch per month.
    - Occipitofrontal head circumference growth approximately 2 cm per month.
  - Sleep:
    - Approximately 15 to 16 hours per 24 hours.
  - Hearing:
    - Determined through universal hearing screen guidelines.
  - Gross motor:
    - Moves head side to side, lifts head when prone.
  - Fine motor:
    - Hands closed but will begin to open from fists, palmar grasp.
  - Language:
    - Alert to bells or loud sounds.
    - Strong cry; small throaty sounds when feeding.
  - Socialization/Cognition:
    - Regards face.
- 2 to 6 months of age.
  - Growth:
    - Weight gain approximately 0.5 to 1 oz per day or 5 to 7 oz per week.
    - Birth weight doubles by 4 to 6 months of age.
    - Height growth approximately 1 inch per month.
    - Occipitofrontal circumference grows approximately 2 cm per month until 3 months of age, then 1 cm per month.
  - Posterior fontanel closes by 1 to 3 months of age.
  - Eyes:
    - Fuzzy vision as newborn; increases to several feet away at 4 to 5 months of age.

- Nose:
  - Obligate nose breathers.
- Genitalia: males.
  - Testes present and descended by 6 months of age.
  - If presence of rugae on scrotum, indication that testes descended at some point.
- Musculoskeletal:
  - Hips: no clicks or clunks (i.e., Ortolani and Barlow maneuvers).
  - Hip ultrasound: indicated for infants with unequal buttock skin creases.
- Skin:
  - Mongolian spots: benign congenital birth mark.
  - Café au lait spots: may be faint in infancy and become more noticeable by 2 years of age; associated with neurofibromatosis type 1, McCune–Albright syndrome, tuberous sclerosis, and Fanconi anemia (Tables 1.1 and 1.2).
- 9 to 12 months of age.
  - Growth:
    - Weight gain 3 to 4 oz per week.
      - Birth weight triples at 12 months of age.
    - Height growth is approximately ½ inch per month.
      - At 12 months of age, height is approximately 1.5 times the birth height.
    - Occipitofrontal circumference growth approximately 1 cm per month.
  - Screening:
    - Lead level by 1 year of age; hemoglobin and/or hematocrit (Tables 1.3 and 1.4).
  - Pertinent physical examination findings:
    - Head: anterior fontanel 4 to 5 cm after birth; fontanel closes between 12 and 18 months of age.
    - Eyes: Nasolacrimal duct should be open by 12 months of age.
    - Neurologic: Primitive reflexes disappear by 1 year of age (persistent reflexes may indicate neurologic abnormalities): Moro relfex, rooting, sucking, stepping, palmar grasp, Babinski, asymmetric tonic neck.
  - Anticipatory guidance:
    - Feeding:
      - Exclusive breast-feeding is the preferred method of nutrition for the first 6 months of life.
      - Transition to cup by 12 months of age.

TABLE 1.1 Early Infant Vision and Hearing

Age	Vision	Hearing
2 mo	Follows 30–40 degrees. Focuses on bright light.	Responds to sound. Startle reflex.
4 mo	Peripheral vision to 180 degrees; able to track light during examination. Binocular vision. Doll's eye reflex gone.	Turns head toward sound.
6 mo	Fixates on small objects. Visual accommodation on near objects; able to reach and grasp objects.	Locates objects to side and up and down.

TABLE 1.2   Early Infant Motor and Language Development

Age	Gross Motor	Fine Motor	Language	Social/Cognitive
2 mo	Lifts shoulders when prone. Lifts head when against shoulder. Some head lag, but head becoming stronger.	Brings hand to mouth.	Cooing. Responds to human faces. Begins to smile to stimuli.	Social smile.
4 mo	No head lag when pulled to a sit. Balances head well when upright. Rolls from front to back and back to side. Bears weight when held up.	Reaches for object. Brings object to mouth.	Laughs and squeals. Consonant sounds—N, K, G, P, B	Shows excitement with whole body. Anticipates feeding when sees bottle. Enjoys social interaction. Increased interest in caregiver. Begins to play with toys. Memory span approximately 5 min. Turns head to locate sound.
6 mo	Sits alone or forward on hands. Lifts chest and upper abdomen off table. Bears weight on hands. Sits on chair with straight back. Rolls from back to abdomen.	Transfers object hand to hand. Drops one block when handed another. Eye–hand coordination is improving.	Babbles. Imitates sounds. Begins to make "ma," "da," "ba" sounds.	Holds bottle. Plays "peekaboo". Smiles at self in mirror. Briefly searches for lost object. Adjusts posture to see objects. Begins to respond to name. Begins object permanence. Recognizes parent in different setting or clothing.

TABLE 1.3   Late Infancy Vision and Hearing

Age	Vision	Hearing
9 mo	Eye–hand coordination improving. Can rescue a dropped toy. Prefers yellow and red. Eyes are nearing final color.	Responds to name. Turns head to locate sound in curving arc. Responds to softer sounds.
12 mo	Has depth perception. Can recognize familiar individuals approaching from a distance.	Responds to music.

TABLE 1.4   Late Infancy Motor and Language Development

Age	Gross Motor	Fine Motor	Language	Social/Cognitive
9 mo	Able to get into sitting position. Pulls to stand. Creeps on hands and knees.	Crude pincer grasp. Bangs two blocks together. Can get toy by pulling on string. Reaches for objects and lets them fall.	Says "dada" or "mama," but not specific to person. Responds to simple commands such as "no". Comprehends "no-no" and "bye-bye".	Stranger anxiety at its worst. Waves "bye-bye". Plays "pat-a-cake". Fear of being left alone. Easily frustrated. Depth perception begins.
12 mo	Stands alone. Stoops and stands. Can walk with one hand held. Crawls to get places quickly.	Firm hold on cup. Puts block in cup.	Says "mama" and "dada" specific to person. Says one or two words. Waves "bye-bye". Jabbers.	Mood changes. Cuddles. Imitates others. Searches for hidden toy. Places objects in a container. Knows name.

- Sleep:
  - Back to sleep.
  - Put infant to bed while still awake to learn sleep regimen.
  - Pacifier at bedtime demonstrated to reduce sudden infant death syndrome.
- Immunizations: begin first few days of life and continue throughout lifetime, but are concentrated in the first 2 years. Follow the Centers for Disease Control and Prevention (CDC) annual recommendations.
- Safety/Injury prevention:
  - Falls: stairs, windows.
  - Home proofing, firearm hazards.
  - Burns/hot liquids.
  - Smoke detectors/carbon monoxide detectors.
  - Infant walkers, unsafe unless no wheels.
  - Ingestions/poisonings, choking/suffocation.
  - Appropriate size car seat installed correctly (Table 1.5).

Toddler

- 1 year to 2½ years of age (Tables 1.6 and 1.7).
- Pertinent physical examination findings:
  - Growth:
    - Gains 4 to 6 pounds per year.
    - 1 year of age: triples birth weight.
    - 2.5 years of age: quadruples birth weight.
    - Grows approximately 3 inches per year.
    - Estimated adult height is 2 times 2-year-old height.
  - Head:
    - Circumference increases approximately 1 inch per year.
    - Anterior fontanel closes at 9 to 18 months of age.
  - Mouth:
    - 20 teeth by 2½ years of age.
    - First molars: 10 to 16 months of age.
    - Cuspids (canines): 16 to 20 months of age.
    - Second molars: 20 to 30 months of age.
  - Ears:
    - Hearing loss suggested by absence of communicative speech at 15 months of age.
  - Abdomen is normally protruberant.
  - Genitalia:
    - Males: testicles palpable in scrotum or inguinal canals; foreskin can be retracted (90% by 2 years of age) in uncircumcised males.
  - Musculoskeletal:
    - "In-toeing" due to tibial torsion (tibia slightly internally rotated)—usually resolves by 16 to 18 months of age.
    - "Out-toeing" is a physiologic variant.
    - Genu varum (bowleg) is normal.
    - Pes planus (flatfoot) is normal.
  - Neurologic:
    - Reflexes.
      - Landau (lifts head when suspended in prone position—postural reflex) appears at 3 months of age and disappears by 15 months to 2 years of age.
      - Neck righting (trunk rotates in same direction as head when in supine position) appears at 6 months of age and disappears at 2 years of age.
      - Parachute (extends arms, hands, and fingers when suspended in prone and lowered quickly—postural reflex) appears at 6 to 8 months of age and remains.
      - Babinski: normal up to 2 years of age
  - Screening:
    - Height, weight, head circumference: at all visits.
    - Vision: at all visits by history, risk factors, and examination.
    - Hearing: at all visits by history, risk factors, hearing loss indicators.

TABLE 1.5   Infancy Developmental Red Flags

	0–1 mo	3 mo	6 mo	9 mo	12 mo
Red Flags	Not at birth weight by 2 wk of age. Poor suck or swallow. Sweating or fatigue with feedings. Asymmetrical movements. Hyper- or hypotonia. Hands held fisted only. Irritable. No startle reflex to loud/sudden noise. High-pitched cry. No red reflex.	Poor weight gain. Occulofrontal circumference not increasing. Fussy. Poor suck/swallow. No attempt to raise head. Hyper- or hypotonia. No hand-to-mouth activity. Feeding taking longer than 45 min. Lack of social smile. Does not turn to voice or rattle. No sounds (e.g., "coo"). No tracking.	Has not doubled birth weight. OFC not increasing. Does not sit without support. Head lag. Scissoring. Does not hold rattle or grasp object. No smile. No eye-to-eye contact. No babbling. No response to noise.	Does not sit. Asymmetrical crawl. No self-feeding. No high chair sitting. No solids. Intense or absent stranger anxiety. Does not seek comfort from caregiver. No response to name. No reciprocal vocalization. Lack of toy exploration.	Has not tripled birth weight. Not pulling to stand. Not crawling or mobile. Not attempting to feed or hold cup. Not able to hold toy in each hand or transfer objects. No vocalization. Not imitating speech. Does not point or use gestures. Not saying 2–3 words. Poor eye contact.

TABLE 1.6 Toddler Vision, Hearing, and Physical Development

Age	Vision	Hearing	Physical
1 y	Visual acuity 20/40 to 20/60. Can follow rapidly moving objects. If strabismus is present, visual loss possible.	Knows several words and their meanings. Can control response to sound.	Birth weight tripled. Birth length increased by 50%. Head and chest circumferences equal. Anterior fontanel almost closed. 6–8 deciduous teeth. Babinski reflex gone. Lumbar curve developing.
15–18 mo	Binocular vision develops. Smooth ocular movements. Good eye–hand coordination.	Responds to whisper test.	Anterior fontanel closes. Physiologic control of sphincters develops. Parachute reflex.
2 y	Accommodation well developed.		Has achieved approximately 50% of adult height. Birth weight quadrupled by 30 mo of age. May have neurologic readiness for daytime bowel and bladder control.

TABLE 1.7 Toddler Motor, Language, Social Development

Age	Gross Motor	Fine Motor	Language	Social/Cognitive
12 mo	Cruises well and walks with hand held. May stand alone and walk.	Precise pincer grasp. Bangs two blocks together. Can turn pages in a book. Tries to build 2-block tower.	Says 3–5 words besides "mama" & "dada". Recognizes objects by name. Imitates animal sounds. Understands simple verbal commands. Makes wants known in ways other than crying.	Shows emotions such as anger, fear, affection, jealousy. Starts exploring away from parent. Clings to parent in unfamiliar settings. May have a "security blanket". Plays social games—"pat-a-cake," "so-big". Searches for hidden object in place where first hidden.
15–18 mo	Walks well without help, but loses balance and falls easily. Progresses from creeping up steps to walking up with one hand held. Throws ball overhand. Jumps in place with two feet. Pushes and pulls toys.	Scribbles. Self-feeding skills develop (e.g., cup, spoon). Builds tower of 3–4 blocks. Reaches for, handles, and releases objects well.	Vocabulary of 10 or more words. By 18 mo, uses 2–3-word phrases. Points to common objects. Knows 2–3 body parts.	Imitates. Temper tantrums begin. Awareness of ownership. May become dependent on "transitional" object. Increasing tolerance of parental separation.
2 y	Up and down stairs one step at a time. Runs well with wide stance. Stoops and retrieves object without falling. Kicks ball forward without falling.	Builds tower of 5 or 6 blocks. Draws vertical line and circular strokes. Turns doorknob and unscrews lids.	Vocabulary of at least 20 words. Uses 2-word phrases. Refers to self by name. Verbalizes needs (e.g., food, toileting). Talks a lot. Follows 2-step commands.	Parallel play. Increased attention span. Decreasing temper tantrums. Can dress self with simple clothing. May begin to notice gender differences. Imitates people and events seen in the past. Ritualistic/likes consistency (routine).

- Speech: by history, observation, and Early Language Milestones evaluation.
- Hemoglobin/hematocrit: recommended at 9 to 12 months of age; if abnormal at age 9 months to 1 year, consider recheck at age 2.
- Tuberculosis: assess risk factors, test if at risk or per state guidelines.
- Lead: assess risk factors annually, test if at risk or per state guidelines.
- Toddler anticipatory guidance:
  - Feeding:
    - Drink from cup by 1 year of age.
    - Decreased physiologic nutritional requirements: smaller servings, appropriate amount of time to eat, limit snacks (including juices); two to three healthy snacks a day.
    - Rule of thumb: 1 tbsp of each food for each year of age.
    - Limit juices and calorie-laden beverages.
  - Dental care:
    - Initial visit at age 1 year of life; examinations every 6 months.
    - Fluoride dietary supplementation if deficient level in water supply.
    - Fluoride toothpaste: pea-size amount; twice daily.
  - Behavior:
    - Beginning of negativism may occur as child approaches age 15 months.
    - Balance between attachment to parents and drive for independence.
    - Frustration may occur with too many commands or unrealistic demands, especially when hungry, fatigued, or ill.
    - Biting is a sign of aggression in toddlers, often occurs in children with delayed verbal skills. May be a sign of teething, frustration, and anger.
  - Play and stimulation:
    - Safety of the environment—increased mobility.
    - Communication and sounds are important.
    - Language: name toys, food, animals and their sounds, body parts; encourage reading.
    - Start self-care skills (e.g., removal of clothes, simple household tasks).
    - Solitary play normal; parallel play may begin.
  - Television:
    - Limit to 1 hour or less per day.
  - Language development:
    - Receptive language develops before expressive language.
    - Articulation lags behind vocabulary; may use jargon.
  - Discipline:
    - Provide consistent schedule, importance of routines.
    - Control through behavior modification (e.g., positive reinforcement of good behavior and inattention or "time out" for inappropriate behavior).
    - Set reasonable limits and avoid threats and criticism.
    - Allow child to attempt to problem-solve; simple explanation of unacceptable behavior.
  - Safety:
    - Period of high energy and curiosity with minimal behavioral control.
    - Most common age group for trauma; falls are most frequent mechanism.
    - Poisoning—call 911; poison control—1-800-222-2222.
    - Consistent use of car seat; rear facing until 2 years of age.
    - Drowning hazards (e.g., bucket of water, toilet, bath, pool).
  - Common problems:
    - Guidance for temper tantrums:
      - For prevention, offer child opportunities to make developmentally appropriate choices.
      - Provide safe environment, remain calm, ignore if appropriate, assist child to find acceptable ways to vent anger and frustration.
      - Problematic tantrums: children >5 years of age, >5 tantrums per day, persistent negative mood, destruction of property, harms self or others.
      - Acute illness offers opportunity for child to regress and react to stressful situation.
  - Potty training:
    - Can begin at 2 to 2.5 years of age.
    - Requires myelinization of pyramidal tracts and conditioned reflex sphincter control, which occurs by 12 to 18 months of age.
    - Must have cognitive ability to follow directions.
    - Acute or chronic illness can affect readiness to train and contribute to regression or enuresis.
  - Child maltreatment:
    - Increased risk with males, excessively fussy infants, slow-to-develop and handicapped children.
    - More frequent when nonrelatives live in house.
    - Children of parents who were themselves abused as children or who are highly stressed, abuse alcohol or drugs, or have psychological conditions are at increased risk.
    - See Section 12 for more information on child maltreatment (Table 1.8).
- Screening: modified checklist for autism in toddlers (M-CHAT).
  - Nine items pertaining to social relatedness and communication, useful for well-child screening.
- Preschool age: 3 to 5 years of age.
  - Growth:
    - Weight: 4 to 6 pounds per year and body mass index (BMI) measurement starts at age 2 years.
    - Height: 2.5 to 3 inches per year.
  - Preschool development: See Table 1.9.
  - Pertinent physical examination findings:
    - Vision:
      - 20/40 vision at 4 years of age; 20/30 vision at 5 years of age.
    - Mouth/throat:
      - All deciduous teeth present.
      - Tonsils are large until 9 to 10 years of age and then usually regress.

TABLE 1.8	Toddler Developmental Red Flags	
12 mo	**15–18 mo**	**2 y**
Does not respond or interact with child-appropriate interactive games. Does not imitate sounds. Does not say 2 or 3 words such as "bye-bye," "mama," or "dada". Not pulling up to a standing position. Does not make wants known in ways other than crying. Parents have rigid or overly cautious responses to toddler.	Does not feed self with spoon. Does not imitate speech or vocalize jargon. Does not move about to explore. Does not engage in eye contact. Does not spontaneously squat when picking up objects.	Poor motor coordination, not running, climbing, exploring vigorously. Use of self-stimulative behaviors such as rocking or head banging for extensive periods of time. Not naming a few familiar objects or using a few 2 or 3 word phrases. Not noticing animals, cars, trucks, trains. Not beginning to play symbolically with housekeeping items, toys, or cars. Inability to initiate play or random play. Avoids eye contact. Not walking upstairs. Previously learned language disappearing.

TABLE 1.9	Preschool Motor, Language, Social Development			
Age	**Gross Motor**	**Fine Motor**	**Language**	**Social/Cognitive**
3 y	Climbs stairs alternating feet. Jumps in place. Kicks ball. Rides tricycle.	Builds tower of 8–10 blocks. Wiggles thumb.	Vocabulary 300+ words. 80% intelligible. Names pictures. Says 3-word sentence.	Uses spoon well. Puts on shirt. Mastering self-care skills. Simple household tasks. Knows own gender and others. Many fears including the dark and going to bed. Increased ability to share. Understands concepts of tomorrow and yesterday.
4 y	Balances on each foot. Hops/jumps on one foot. Throws ball overhand. Rides tricycle or bicycle with training wheels.	Copies circle. Draws person with 3 parts. Builds tower with 10 blocks.	Names colors. Sings songs. Gives first and last name. Names one or more colors. Understands prepositional phrases. Talks about day.	Brushes teeth. Dresses self. Can distinguish fantasy from reality. Mood swings. Aware of gender and identifies with same gender parent. Concrete and egocentric.
5 y	Skips. Heel to toe walk. Throws and catches ball. Jumps rope. Walks forward and backward heel to toe.	Copies square, diamond, triangle. Dresses self without help. Draws person with head, body, arms, and legs. Ties shoelaces and laces shoes. Prints some letters.	Counts. Understands opposites. Has vocabulary over 2,000 words. Uses 6–8-word sentences. Can follow 3-part commands. Knows 4 or more colors, coins, days of week, months.	Dresses self without help. Knows own address and phone number. Can count on fingers. Manners improving. Gets along well with parents. Developing sense of conservations of quantity, mass, weight.

- Cardiac:
  - Functional murmur noted in approximately 50% of children.
  - Sinus arrhythmias common in children.
- Abdomen:
  - Protuberant and flattens as child gets older and taller.
- Genitalia:
  - Male: Tanner 1, cremasteric reflex, foreskin easily retracted.
  - Females: Tanner 1, labial adhesions can be common.
- Musculoskeletal:
  - In-toeing due to femoral anteversion usually resolved by 8 years of age.
  - Genu valgum—knock knees.
- Anticipatory guidance:
  - Feeding:
    - Encourage fruit and vegetables and good eating habits young.
  - Elimination:
    - Daytime control average at 28 months of age.
    - Nighttime control average at 33 months of age.
  - Behavior:
    - Imaginary friends, creative imaginative play.
    - Do not understand the concept of lying until about 6 years of age.
    - Plays well by self and associative play.
  - Safety:
    - Household and street safety, water, stranger, and fire safety.
    - Car seat safety based on state regulations.
    - Potential for toxic ingestions.
    - Magical thinking; child may feel he/she can do anything.
    - Learning address, telephone number (Table 1.10).

School-Age Child

- 6 to 12 years of age.
  - Development: See Table 1.11.

- Pertinent physical examination findings:
  - Growth:
    - Gains 4 to 6 pounds per year.
    - Achieves 75% to 90% of adult weight between 10 and 11 years of age.
    - Grows 2 to 3 inches per year.
    - Achieves 50% to 75% of adult height by 10 to 11 years of age.
    - Females usually begin growth spurt at approximately 9 years of age, reach peak height velocity (PHV) between 11.5 and 12 years of age and most growth occurs before menarche; after menarche girls rarely grow more than 2 to 3 inches. Those who start growing early reach PHV and their final height earlier.
    - Body mass index (BMI):
      - Weight in kilograms divided by height in meter squared.
      - Standardized percentiles for age and gender.
      - ≥85% at risk of overweight; ≥95% overweight/obese.
  - Head:
    - Full-adult-size brain is attained by 12 years of age, but the myelinization process continues until early adulthood when the frontal lobe (responsible for problem-solving and decision making) and the cerebral cortex (responsible for intelligence) are fully developed.
  - Eyes:
    - Evaluate for history of squinting and photophobia, having to sit close to the blackboard/whiteboard in school or TV to see; poor school performance.
    - Visual acuity testing using Snellen chart 20/20 expected in both eyes at 7 years of age.
  - Mouth:
    - Start losing deciduous teeth at approximately 6 to 7 years of age.
    - Permanent teeth erupt in the same order in which primary teeth erupt and are usually developed by 12 years of age.
  - Chest:
    - Functional (innocent) murmurs in 50% of children: Pulmonary ejection murmur, Still's murmur, and venous hum are most common; sinus arrhythmia is common.

TABLE 1.10	**Preschool Developmental Red Flags**	
3 y	**4 y**	**5 y**
Problems with toilet training.	Withdrawn or acts out.	Hair or eyelash pulling.
Unable to calm self.	Stool holding.	Unable to copy triangle.
Unable to build tower of 10 blocks.	Unable to copy square.	Unable to draw person with a body.
Not able to dress self some.	Unable to button clothing.	Difficulty sharing.
No pretend play.	Unable to play games or follow rules.	Cruel to animals.
Unable to give name.	Fire starting.	Fire starting.
No plurals.	Severe shyness.	Bullying.
Unintelligible speech.	Cannot understand language.	Withdrawal or sadness.
Unable to balance for 1s.	Limited vocabulary.	Speech not 100% understandable.
In-toeing, causing tripping or problems with running.	Unable to balance for 4s.	Difficulty hopping or skipping.
	Unable to count 3 items.	Unable to count to 10.
		Does not know colors.
		Cannot follow 3-step commands.

TABLE 1.11 School-Age Motor, Language, Social Development

Age	Gross Motor	Fine Motor	Language	Social/Cognitive
6–9 y	Increased muscle strength and coordination. Running, jumping, climbing, hopping, skipping, tandem walking, alternating foot patterns, overhand throwing are practiced and perfected. Rides a bike. Swims. Participates in individual and group sports.	Prints. Progresses to cursive writing and drawing detailed pictures. Self-care skills are improved. Eye–hand coordination improves. Ability to play a musical instrument emerges.	Language becomes very descriptive, stories elaborate. Mastery of articulation may not be achieved until 7 or 8 years old with the sounds of "l" and "th". By 8 years of age, begins to understand and tell jokes. Concrete thinking predominates—understands concrete better than abstract phenomena. Develops concepts of time and money. Understands concepts of space, cause and effect, conservation, and reversibility. Moves from very mechanical reading to more fluid, enjoyable reading.	Able to share and cooperate with others. Understands meanings in social situations and interprets the social cues of others. Develops a sense of self-worth by developing new skills. Enjoys games and group play; clubs and organizations; begins to enjoy competition. Capable of being more socialized and well-behaved. Very interested in peers, especially those of the same sex. Understands right from wrong; learns to follow rules; learns responsibility.
10–12 y	Match sport to physical and emotional development.	Writing skills improve. Fine motor with more focus: Sewing, painting.	Uses connecting words (e.g., if, now, otherwise, anyway). Tells and writes stories in an order that makes sense. Gives their opinion. Understands words that describe personalities.	Peer group becomes source of support, guidance, and self-esteem. More selective in friendships and may have a "best friend". Know how people feel by what they see and hear. Change how they talk based on the situation. Household chores and meeting own needs.

- Genitalia:
  - Delayed puberty is diagnosed as no secondary sex changes (e.g., breast budding; penis or testicle growth) at 13 years of age in females and 14 years of age in males.
- Males:
  - Testicle development begins at 9 to 10 years of age; penile growth starts 1 year after testicular growth.
  - Pubic hair appears at approximately 12 years of age.
- Females:
  - Pubic hair appears at 8 to 13 years of age, vaginal secretions increase.
  - Hips broaden.
- Musculoskeletal:
  - Knee pain and/or limp may indicate slipped capital epiphysis.
- Skin:
  - Increase in body odor; persistent dandruff; may be infected with tinea capitis or head lice.

- Neurologic:
  - Dominance of left- or right-sidedness emerges.
- Screening:
  - Height, weight, BMI, blood pressure: at all visits.
  - Vision: at all visits by history, examination, and visual acuity with well care.
  - Hearing: at all visits by history, examination, and audiometry with well care.
  - Scoliosis: annually starting at age 10 years.
  - Hemoglobin/hematocrit: as needed based on dietary history and risk factors.
  - Tuberculosis: assess risk factors annually, purified protein derivative test if at risk.
  - Screening laboratory tests if elevated BMI; begin at 10 years of age or at onset of obesity.
  - Cholesterol: recommendation that 9- to 11-year-olds should have lipid screening.
- Immunizations:
  - Follow CDC annual recommendations for vaccines.

- Anticipatory guidance:
  - Nutrition and physical activity:
    - Encourage 60 minutes of physical activity each day.
    - Child should be learning basic food groups and how to differentiate nutritious foods from junk foods; family should aim for one meal eaten together each day.
- Dental care:
  - Deciduous tooth eruption onward.
  - Dental visit at least every 6 months; fluoride treatments; teeth sealants once molars erupted.
- Sexuality:
  - Increased curiosity about sexuality and sex.
  - Establish open communication with child on sexual issues, including hygiene and body changes; also begin discussion on contraceptives, sexually transmitted infections (STIs), and HIV.
- Behavior:
  - Expanded horizons and influence of people outside the family on the child from teachers, peers, organized sports and activities.
  - Peers become more important and parents less important across this period.
  - Lying: School-age children are working on differentiating fantasies from reality; may use untruths to avoid unpleasant outcomes.
- Screen time:
  - Limit to 1 to 2 hours per day of appropriate programs.
- Safety:
  - Motor vehicle accidents are the most frequent cause of death, followed by pedestrian accidents, drowning, fires, and falls.
  - Responsibility for own safety is given to child as he or she proves reliable, but parental supervision continues to be necessary.
  - Discuss prevention and emergency plans.
- Bicycle safety or anything on wheels:
  - Helmets and other equipment: knee and elbow pads or wrist guards; "rules of the road."

- Swimming:
  - Always with adult supervision.
- Motor vehicles:
  - Booster seats (per state law) placed in the back seat, optimally in the middle.
  - Utilize booster seat from age 4 years to at least 8 years of age or until the child reaches 80 pounds and is 4 feet 9 inches tall.
  - Backseat until age 13 years of age.
- Fire safety:
  - When to dial 911.
  - Exit plan for the house.
  - Proper use of matches.
- Gun safety:
  - Firearm(s) and ammunition must be stored separately and locked securely.
- Stranger safety:
  - Teach child how to behave with strangers.
  - Role-play situations with strangers, using a creative variety of situations (Table 1.12).

Adolescent/Young Adult

- Adolescence: 12 to 21 years of age
  - Pertinent physical examination findings:
    - Growth:
      - Female growth spurt is approximately 2 years prior to males.
      - Females typically grow approximately 8 inches between 10 and 14 years of age.
      - Males typically grow 11 inches between 12 and 16 years of age.
      - PHV occurs at approximately 12 years of age for females.
      - PHV occurs at approximately 14 years of age for males.
    - Eye/Vision:
      - 20/20

TABLE 1.12 School-Age Red Flags	
6–9 y	**10–12 y**
Poor school adjustment and not working up to capability. Using aggressive behavior to gain attention. Accident prone or frequent illnesses. Problems with peer group. Difficulty learning. Unable to state special quality about self; flat affect, depression, withdrawal. Cruelty to animals.	Regressive patterns of overdependence on family, shyness, passivity, or aggression. Use of food as a way of getting attention and satisfaction. Using illness as a means to avoid challenges. Inability to make and maintain friends. Antisocial behavior; not using language to express ideas and feelings. Poor school performance. Risk-taking behaviors: smoking, alcohol, sex. Cruelty to animals. Flat affect, depression, withdrawal. Defiant, rebellious attitude.

- Oral:
  - Permanent teeth complete development.
  - Wisdom teeth erupt at approximately 18 years of age.
- Chest:
  - Gynecomastia in 30% to 50% of boys; normal; provide reassurance.
- Genitalia:
  - See Table 1.13.
  - First pelvic examination at age 21 years or 3 years after becoming sexually active.
- Skin:
  - Acne, body odor, tinea pedis.
- General principles of sexual development:
  - Breast development typically precedes pubic hair by 6 months.
  - Average age of menarche 12.5 years.
  - Testicular development precedes pubic hair by 6 months in the majority of boys.
- Left testicle hangs lower than the right.
- Spermarche average is 13.5 to 14.5 years; nocturnal emission at 14.5 years of age or Tanner III (Tables 1.13 and 1.14).
- Screening:
  - Height, weight, BMI, blood pressure, vision, hearing.
  - Hemoglobin, if indicated.
  - Tuberculosis testing, if indicated.
  - Lipid screening, if at risk and per guidelines.
  - STI, substance use, mental health screening.
  - Scoliosis.
  - **HEADSSS** screening tool:
    H—home environment, *E*—employment and education, *A*—activities, *D*—drugs, *S*—sexuality and sexual activity, *S*—suicide and depression, *S*—safety.
- Anticipatory guidance:
  - Nutrition/Feeding: healthy eating habits, need for iron, calcium, vitamins B and D; exercise and athletics.

TABLE 1.13 Tanner Stages

	Female		Male	
Stage	Breasts	Pubic Hair	Testicles	Pubic Hair
I	None	None	None	None
II	Breast budding, areola enlarges	Sparse downy straight and located near labia	Enlargement of scrotum and testes. Scrotal skin reddens	Sparse growth of downy hair at base of penis
III	Enlargement of breasts and areola	Hair is coarser, darker, and curlier. Spreads to pubic bone	Further growth of testes and scrotum. Penis begins to elongate	Hair darker, coarser, and curlier. Extends to pubic bone
IV	Projection or areola to form secondary mound	Adult in appearance. Does not spread to thighs	Penis increases in length and width. Skin darkens and rugae appear	Adult in appearance but not to thighs
V	Increase in breast size and adult contour	Adult appearance and to thighs	Adult shape and appearance	Adult appearance and to thighs

TABLE 1.14 Socialization/Cognition in Adolescence

Age	12–16 y	17–21 y
Social/Cognition	Limited ability to think abstractly. Daydreams. Difficulty keeping interest in schoolwork. Develops sense of humor. Narcissistic. Wide mood swings. Peer group very important. Close friends with peers of same sex. Greatest period of parent/child conflict. Express anger outwardly.	Abstract thinking improves. Enjoys intellectual abilities. Worries about schoolwork. Strong creativity. Emotions becoming more stable and constant. Self-esteem more stable. Push for independence. Less conflict with parents/caregivers. Close relationships with opposite sex. Life goals begin.

- Oral health: Dental visit every 6 months, brush/floss 2 times per day; orthodontal work as needed.
- Sexual health: First pelvic examination at age 21 years or 3 years after becoming sexually active.
- Safety:
  - Invincible or feel like nothing will ever happen to them. Need help realizing it can.
  - Impulsive and aggressive behavior occurs to stressful situation.
  - Awareness of suicidal ideation and behavior; depression more frequent.
- Red flags in adolescence:
  - Change in pattern of sleeping, eating, friendships, or school.
  - Change in personality; showing no interest, agitation, anger, carelessness.
  - Increasing attitude of discouragement or disgust, low self-esteem.
  - No support system.
  - Suicidal thoughts or calls for help.
  - Substance abuse with drugs, tobacco, or alcohol.

Developmental Theories

- See Table 1.15.

Developmental Issues during Acute Illness

Terea Giannetta

Acute Care Developmental Issues

Background

- Healthy children accomplish developmental milestones in a consistent pattern.
- Hospitalization and illness can pose risks to the typical advances in development.

- Acute care situations make a child vulnerable to the stressors of the situation and failure to successfully move through a given developmental stage.
- Developmental regression in some milestones may occur (e.g., potty training).
- Communication is essential for helping the child cope with new situations.
- Child life specialists can assist in preparing children for tests, interviews, or procedures.
- Health care providers can assist in support of the child in maintaining developmental level and in experiencing hospitalizations, tests, and procedures at their individual developmental level.

PEARLS

- *Limit explanations to what the child will see, hear, taste, smell, and feel.*
- *Use the child's own words and phrases, as appropriate.*

Siblings and Families

Background

- Family-centered care assures the health and well-being of children and their families through a respectful family–professional partnership.
- Family-centered care is strongly supported by research and many health care organizations.
- The health care provider must be able to negotiate between the family culture and perspectives and the needs of the health care team while recognizing that the family has the ultimate decision-making power.
- Developmental concerns for the siblings are central to providing care to the patient and family.

Definitions

- Structural family data: family composition, extended family, and social aspects such as ethnicity and spirituality.
- Developmental family: stages of the family's life cycle.
- Functional family: routines of daily living.

TABLE 1.15	**Developmental Stages: Classic Theories**			
Age	Erickson	Freud	Piaget	Kohlberg
Infancy	Trust vs. mistrust	Oral	Sensorimotor	Not applicable
Toddlerhood	Autonomy vs. shame and doubt	Anal	Sensorimotor	Preconventional: Avoid punishment/obtain rewards
Preschool	Initiative vs. guilt	Phallic/Oedipal	Preoperational	Conventional: Conformity
School-age	Industry vs. inferiority	Latency	Concrete operations	Conventional: Law and order
Adolescence	Identity vs. confusion	Genital	Formal operations	Postconventional: Moral principles

Developmental Concerns around Death and Grief in the Health Care Setting

Background

- The most powerful tool for health care providers when dealing with end-of-life issues is communication.
- If no communication exists, then there is no avenue for exploring or ameliorating child or parental fears.
- Tasks of grieving:
  - Acknowledging the reality of the death.
  - "Feeling the feelings" of loss.
  - Keeping the loved one's memory alive.
  - Adjusting to life without the presence of the loved one.
  - Finding meaning to the experience.
  - Moving on without forgetting.

Nutrition Assessment and Planning

Laura T. Russo

Definition

- Nutrition assessment discerns the somatic nutrition stores using anthropometrics, biochemical indices (specifically, visceral protein stores), evaluation of malnutrition using clinical manifestations of the skin, hair, nails, lips, tongue, and through obtaining a diet history.
- Nutrition needs, or energy needs, can be determined via actual measurement of energy expenditure through indirect calorimetry. If indirect calorimetry is not available or feasible, predictive energy equations may be used.
- Clinical assessment of nutrition:
  - Anthropometrics:
    - Weight and length (<2 years old)/height (>2 years old).
    - Head circumference (up to 3 years old).
    - Skin fold measures.
    - Plot anthropometrics on respective growth curve options.
      - World Health Organization (WHO) for 0–2 years old = CDC; National Center for Health Statistics (NCHS) for 0 to 36 months of age and 2 to 20 years old.
  - Interpretation of nutrition status:

- Underweight:
  - Ages 0–2 years: WHO curve: <3rd% for weight to length; CDC NCHS curve: <5th% for weight to length.
  - Ages 2–20 years: <5th% for BMI.
- Healthy weight:
  - Ages 0–2 years: WHO curve: 3rd to 97th% for weight to length; CDC NCHS curve: 5th to 94.9th%; ages 2–20 years: 5% to 84.9% for BMI.
- Overweight/Obesity:
  - Ages 0–2 years: WHO curve: >97th% for weight to length; CDC NCHS curve: ≥95th% for weight to length.
  - Ages 2–20 years: ≥85th% to 94% for BMI = overweight; ≥95th% for BMI = obese.
- Malnutrition classifications:
  - Acute malnutrition per Waterlow criteria based on weight.
  - Equation: Actual weight/IBW (ideal body weight) × 100 = % IBW.
    - Mild malnutrition = 81th% to 90th% of IBW; moderate malnutrition = 70% to 80% of IBW; severe malnutrition = <70% of IBW.
  - Calculate IBW by
    - Using growth curve for length or height for age.
    - Determine the age that the actual length/height plotted at 50% corresponds.
    - Once the age to which the length or height for age corresponds is determined, then use that age to determine where that age meets with 50% for weight for age on the growth curve to determine IBW.
    - Chronic malnutrition per Waterlow criteria based on length/height.
    - Equation: Actual height/ideal height for age = (height at 50% curve) × 100.
      - Mild malnutrition = 90th% to 95th%; moderate malnutrition = 85% to 89%; severe malnutrition = <85th%.
  - Skin fold measures:
    - More sensitive than weight to determine somatic protein and adipose stores.
    - Not appropriate for patients with peripheral edema.
    - Requirements:
      - Calipers, tape measure, training in accurate measurement.

Diagnostic Evaluation

- Assessment of visceral protein stores.
- Albumin (half-life = 20 days): not as sensitive if level is being affected by fluid status or liver function.
- Prealbumin (half-life = 2–3 days): more sensitive than albumin; however, can be falsely elevated by impaired renal function or steroids.
- Transferrin (half-life = 7–10 days): affected by anemia, inflammation, and liver disease.
- CRP (half-life = 8–12 hours): acute-phase reactant protein, which is increased during infection or inflammation. Prealbumin level is inversely related to CRP level.

- Nitrogen balance study: can be used to assess protein stores if in positive or negative nitrogen balance per protein in (from dietary sources) versus protein out (via urine, stool, or sweat losses).

$$\text{Equation} = \frac{\text{Protein intake (g/day)}}{6.25} - \frac{\text{Urinary urea (24 hours)}}{2.14} + \ldots 4$$

Clinical Evaluation

- Evaluate skin, hair, nails, face, neck, eyes, mouth, abdomen, and urine.
- Diet: adequacy of dietary intake with a 24-hour diet recall or a 3-day food record; review meal patterns, variety, quantity, preparation technique, and appetite.
- Chewing or swallowing difficulties.
- Presence of nausea/vomiting, diarrhea/constipation.
- Availability/access to food due to socioeconomic situation.
- Special diet/restrictions/allergies; cultural practices.
- Drug–nutrient interactions: Certain medications may inhibit or enhance absorption of nutrients.

Pathophysiology

- Critical illness phases:
  - Acute phase:
    - Duration may be 6 to 8 hours after onset of illness or trauma.
    - Characteristics
      - Fever, tachycardia, hypoglycemia.
    - Growth is inhibited and energy diverted toward stress response/injury.
  - Ebb phase
    - Duration varies.
    - Characteristics:
      - Increased catecholamines, glucagon, and cortisol, resulting in hyperglycemia.
      - Increased growth hormone, cytokine production, and free fatty acids, resulting in hypertriglyceridemia; increased antidiuretic hormone; gluconeogenesis; decreased insulin level and insulin-like growth factor-1.
      - Acute decrease in metabolic rate.
  - Flow phase: catabolic and anabolic.
    - Catabolic flow phase:
      - Duration varies.
      - Characteristics:
        - Hypermetabolism due to endogenous catabolism of fat, carbohydrate, and protein stores; active inflammatory processes; hyperglycemia and glucose intolerance; lipolysis; negative nitrogen balance.
    - Anabolic flow phase:
      - Duration varies.
      - Characteristics:
        - Restoration of tissue composition and depleted energy reserves; reestablish a positive nitrogen balance.
- Management.
  - Ebb phase:
    - Nutrition regimen: Mode and amount of nutrition support depends on acute clinical status.

- Provide calories with caution; an excess amount of nutrients may be deleterious.
- Note an increased amount of calories will not reverse or impair the metabolic and hormonal changes related to the acute stress response.
- Flow phase:
  - Nutrition regimen: Mode and amount of nutrition support depends on acute clinical status.
    - Address basal energy needs until metabolic and hormonal alterations subside.
    - Protein is the one nutrient that should be increased (as possible per liver and kidney status) to promote positive balance.
    - Protein is pulled from muscle, connective tissue, and gut if inactive as substrate for gluconeogenesis and production of acute-phase reactant proteins.
    - There is a concomitant decrease in albumin and prealbumin synthesis.
- Anabolic flow phase:
  - Nutrition regimen: Mode and amount of nutrition support depends on acute clinical status, and amount of nutrient provision should be increased to promote nutrition repletion.
    - Increase calories and continue to augment protein as convalescence/recuperation is reached to enable resumption of growth.
  - Calculation of nutrition needs:
    - Components of energy expenditure: Basal metabolic rate, energy from thermogenesis, energy for activity, energy for growth, energy for healing process.
      - Critically ill patients are not active or growing.
    - Considerations for determining energy needs
      - Phase, severity, and duration of illness, respiratory status (level and mode of support), sedation, analgesia, muscle relaxant, injury or stress factors (fever, sepsis, wounds, burns), cardiac failure, and postoperative state.
    - Baseline calorie needs (especially if chronically ill).
    - Measured energy expenditure: Indirect calorimetry/metabolic cart study is the gold standard.
      - Study performed by a trained respiratory therapist.
      - FiO_2 delivered must be <0.6; cannot be leaks around endotracheal tube or tracheostomy, or result in skewed results.
      - May be minimal weight requirement per calorimeter device used.
      - Limitations: generally unable to obtain a measurement when patients are requiring ECMO, high-frequency oscillation, high-flow nasal cannula, noninvasive positive pressure ventilation, or nasal cannula.
    - Predictive energy equations:
      - Many equations readily available, but concern about overestimation of energy requirements.

- Only equation designed for critically ill child is the White equation, which is complicated (based on age, weight, weight for age z-score, body temperature, number of days after intensive care admission, and primary reason for admission).
- Use equations that estimate resting energy expenditure during acute, ebb, and catabolic flow phases of illness (e.g., WHO, Schofield).
- Resting energy expenditure (REE): See Table 1.16.
  - Stress and injury must be considered when evaluating REE.
    - Fever = 12% increase above REE for every degree above 37° C.
    - Sepsis = 40% increase above REE.
    - Cardiac condition or surgery = 25% increase above REE.
  - Energy needs may increase toward patient's usual baseline calorie needs as the acute illness resolves and patient clinical status improves.
- Protein needs
  - Protein needs during acute illness are usually more than when healthy.
  - Increased protein provision can help to promote a positive nitrogen balance (16% of protein molecule is nitrogen) (Tables 1.17 and 1.18).
- Importance of energy balance:
  - Goal is to meet nutritional needs of patient without underfeeding or overfeeding.
- Concerns for overfeeding and underfeeding
  - Overfeeding is associated with increased carbon dioxide (CO_2) production, which can affect dependence on ventilator, promote fatty infiltration of liver, and provide additional stress on organ systems.
  - Underfeeding is associated with impaired healing of wounds, compromised immune response to infection, decreased gut function, decreased respiratory muscle function, and increased morbidity and mortality.

TABLE 1.16	Predictive Equation for Estimating Resting Energy Expenditure*
Age	REE (kcal/kg/d)
0–36 mo	55
4–6 y	45
7–10 y	40
11–18 y	25 (females) 30 (males)
19–24 y	25

*REE = Basal metabolic needs × Factor for thermogenesis.

TABLE 1.17	Protein Needs for Age per Recommended Dietary Allowances
Age	Protein (g/kg/d)
0–6 mo	2.2
6–12 mo	1.6
1–3 y	1.2
4–6 y	1.1
7–10 y	1
14–18 male/female	0.9 male/0.8 female

TABLE 1.18	Protein Recommendations during Critical Illness
Age	Protein (g/kg/d)
Low-birth-weight infant	3–4
Full-term infant	2–3
Older children	1.5

- Nutrition: enteral and parenteral:
  - Enteral nutrition: preferred method:
    - Advantages:
      - More physiologic than parenteral nutrition; maintains mucosal integrity/barrier; less costly than parenteral nutrition with less complications.
    - Gastric feeds are more physiologic and preferred choice; however, may be associated with higher risk of aspiration.
    - Jejunal feeds may be indicated if patient has gastroparesis, gastric dysmotility, pancreatitis, intolerance to gastric feeds, and/or increased risk of aspiration/reflux.
    - Jejunal feeds must be given as continuous feeding to avoid dumping syndrome (if tolerated, may be able to compress feeding interval to less than 24 hours).
    - Continuous or bolus feeding methods are options; however, they are based on clinical status of patient.
    - No evidence-based benefit of gastric over jejunal feeds.
  - Formula selection:
    - Age category specific: infant (preterm, term), pediatric, older pediatric/adult (Table 1.19).
  - Calorie calculations:
    - Calories from enteral/formula feedings.

Box 1.2 Calculation of Caloric Intake from Enteral Feedings

Step 1: Calculate the total daily intake (e.g., mL/hour × 24 hours).

Example: 4 kg infant receiving 16 mL/hour of feeding.

Daily intake 16 × 24 = 384 mL in a day

Step 2: Determine the number of ounces per day.

1 oz = 30 mL

Example (continued) 384 mL/30 = 12.8 oz/day

Step 3: Multiply the number of ounces by the caloric density of the formula (e.g., 20; 24, 30 cal/oz).

Example (continued) 12.8 oz × 24 cal/oz = 307.2

Step 4: Divide by the weight (kg). Result is the kcal/kg/day.

307.2 calories ÷ 4 kg = 76.8 kcal/kg/day

- Calorie calculations: intravenous solutions.
- Calculation of calories from dextrose.

Box 1.3 Calculation of Calories from Intravenous Dextrose

Step 1: Multiply total volume (in mL) of the dextrose solution administered in a day (24 hours) by the dextrose concentration. This determines the number of grams of dextrose provided in a day.

Step 2: Multiply the number of grams of dextrose by 3.4 (there are 3.4. kcal/g dextrose) to determine how many kcals are provided by dextrose in 1 day.

Example: D10 IV solution infusing at 12 mL/hour × 24 hours

12 mL/hour × 24 hours = 288 mL/day of the solution

288 mL (total volume in 24 hours) × 0.10 (dextrose concentration; derived from 10 g dextrose in 100 mL or 0.10) = 28.8 g of dextrose/day

28.8 g of dextrose × 3.4 kcal/g = 97.92 kcal/day from dextrose

- Calculation of calories from protein.

Box 1.4 Calculation of Calories from Intravenous Protein

Step 1: Multiply the total volume (in mL) of amino acid solution administered in a day (24 hours) by the amino acid concentration.

Step 2: Multiply the number of protein grams by 4 (4 calories/gram of protein).

Example: 288 mL (total volume of the IV solution administered over 24 hours) of 2% amino acids solution (2 g/100 mL or 0.02).

288 mL × 2 g/100 mL = 5.76 g, OR

288 mL × 0.02 = 5.76 g

5.76 × 4 = 23.04 calories from protein

- Calculation of calories from lipids.

Box 1.5 Calculation of Calories from Intravenous Lipids

Background: 10% lipid solution has 1.1 kcal per mL.

20% lipid solution has 2 kcal per mL.

Step 1: Determine the lipid concentration being administered (e.g., 10%, 20%).

Step 2: Calculate the total volume of lipids administered per day (24 hours).

Step 3: Multiply the total daily lipid volume by the appropriate kcal for that solution (e.g., 1.1, 2).

Example: 4 mL/hour of 10% intralipids

4 mL × 24 hours = 96 mL/day of 10% lipid solution

96 mL × 1.1 kcal = 105.6 kcal/day from intralipids

Total caloric intake is determined by calculating all of the calories a patient is receiving. Include calories from enteral feedings (e.g., milk, formula, supplements), IV fluids, TPN (dextrose, protein, and intralipids), and PO intake.

- Nutrition: parenteral.
  - Indications:
    - When unable to feed enterally or meet nutrition needs solely by enteral mode.
  - Intravenous access requirements/limitations:
    - Central line: dextrose concentration limit up to 30%; protein concentration limit up to 6% of total volume.
    - Peripheral line: dextrose concentration limit up to 12.5%; protein concentration limit up to 3% of total volume.
  - Inclusion of macronutrients:
    - Carbohydrate: dextrose solution; calorie density: 3.4 kcal/g; recommended calorie distribution of 40% to 60% of total calories.
    - Protein: Amino acid solutions vary in amounts of specific amino acids that may be appropriate in specific age categories and/or clinical conditions; calorie density: 4 kcal/gram; recommended calorie distribution of 8% to 15% of total calories.
    - Intravenous fat emulsions (IVFEs): 20% IVFE available in the United States contain soybean or soybean and safflower oil, egg yolk phospholipids, and glycerin; 10% IVFE available; however, no longer recommended due to clearance of phospholipids; calorie density: 2 kcal/mL or 10 kcal/g; recommended calorie distribution of 25% to 40% of total calories.
      - Essential fatty acid deficiency (EFAD) may be prevented by providing 0.5 grams of fat/kg/day.
  - Inclusion of micronutrients:
    - Vitamins:
      - Fat-soluble: A, D, E, and K; water-soluble: B_1, B_2, B_3, B_5, B_6, B_{12}, C, biotin, and folic acid: available as multivitamin formulation.

TABLE 1.19   Formula Indications and Contraindications

Type of Formula	Use	Contraindications
Breast milk.	Ideal for most situations.	Mother with HIV (controversial). Maternal medications that are not compatible with breast-feeding. Galactosemia.
Preterm formula.	Hospitalized NICU. Nearing discharge or post hospital discharge.	
Infant standard milk protein base OR Infant milk protein base with hydrolyzed whey.	Healthy term infant. Term infant as alternate to standard formula.	
Infant milk protein base with added rice starch.	May be helpful for infants with GERD.	
Infant milk protein base, lactose-free.	Term infant with lactose intolerance or lactase deficiency.	
Infant or pediatric milk protein base with high medium-chain triglyceride/low long-chain triglyceride.	Term infant with chylothorax, severe long-chain fat malabsorption, fatty acid oxidation defects, or other lymphatic anomalies. Pediatric formula for child with same problems.	
Milk protein base with low electrolyte content.	Term infant with renal impairment.	
Intact nutrient, soy base.	Term infant, vegetarian option, infant with galactosemia, sensitivity to milk protein base formula.	
Term infant, casein hydrolysate base.	Term infant with milk protein intolerance or allergy or impaired digestive or absorptive processes.	
Term infant, amino acid base.	Term infant with severe cow milk allergy or severely impaired digestive and/or absorptive problems.	
Pediatric standard intact nutrient milk protein base with or without fiber. Or with intact nutrient soy protein base.	Child >1 y of age if no compromised GI function or no milk protein allergy. Preference for soy protein or vegetarian diet.	
Pediatric and older pediatric semi-elemental base. Or elemental base.	Compromised GI function. Compromised GI function and/or milk and/or soy protein allergy.	
Pediatric and older pediatric calorie dense.	Volume sensitivity or fluid restriction.	
Condition specific or specialty formula.	Wide variety of other conditions, or impaired organ function, bariatric, etc.	

GI, gastrointestinal; GERD, gastroesophageal reflux disease; NICU, neonatal intensive care unit.

- Single vitamin solutions may also be available, including vitamin A, D, K, B_1, B_6, B_{12}, C, and folic acid.
- Inclusion of minerals/trace elements:
  - Minerals: sodium, potassium, chloride, calcium, phosphorus, magnesium, and acetate.
    - Individually tailored per biochemical indices/clinical status.
  - Trace elements: zinc, copper, chromium, manganese, and selenium.
    - Neonatal and pediatric formulations contain zinc, copper, chromium, and manganese but not selenium.
  - Carbohydrate: determined by glucose infusion rate (GIR).

Box 1.6 Glucose Infusion Rate Equation

$$\text{GIR equation} = \frac{\text{g/kg/day of glucose} \times 1,000}{1,440 \text{ min/day}}$$

- Term infants: starting GIR = 6 to 8 mg/kg/day, advance by 2 to 3 mg/kg/day; final goal = 10 to 14 mg/kg/day.
- Children: starting GIR = 4 to 6 mg/kg/day, advance by 1 to 2 mg/kg/day; final goal = 8 to 10 mg/kg/day.
- Adolescents: starting GIR = 2 to 3 mg/kg/day, advance by 1 to 2 mg/kg/day; final goal = 5 to 6 mg/kg/day.
  - Protein:
    - Starting and advancing concentrations as per individual acute clinical status.
    - Final concentrations:
      - Preterm infants: 3 to 4 g/kg/day.
      - Term infants: 2 to 3 g/kg/day.
      - Children: 1.5 to 2 g/kg/day.
      - Adolescents: 0.8 to 2 g/kg/day.
  - Fat:
    - Starting concentration = 1 g/kg/day, except adolescents (0.5 g/kg/day).
    - Advancing concentration = 0.5 g/kg/day.
    - Final concentration: preterm, term infants, and children—3 to 4 g/kg/day; adolescents—up to 0.15 g/kg/hour.
- Laboratory monitoring for patients receiving parenteral nutrition.
  - Electrolytes, magnesium, phosphorus, kidney function, liver function, and albumin; triglycerides are monitored with lipid infusion.
  - Check laboratory studies 1 to 3 times per week with exception of albumin and liver function tests which can be obtained every 2 to 3 weeks, or as indicated per acute clinical status changes.
  - Prealbumin and nitrogen studies may be evaluated intermittently to provide information about nutritional adequacy and the patient's response to the nutritional support.

- Cycling parenteral nutrition (parenteral nutrition for <24 hour period).
  - Transition to shorter duration of administration occurs gradually (e.g., "ramping up").
  - Used in patients who are on long-term parenteral nutrition.
  - Provides time away from continuous tethering to IV pump.
  - Physiologic benefits include a period of "fasting," allowing the body time to mobilize fat, resulting in less fatty infiltration in the liver.
  - Electrolytes must be stable prior to cycling parenteral nutrition.
- Complications of nutritional support:
  - Patients who are malnourished or with prolonged poor nutritional intake are at risk for refeeding syndrome.
  - Aggressive nutrition support in malnourished patients can cause hypophosphatemia, hypokalemia, hypomagnesemia, and altered glucose metabolism.
  - If concern about patient's nutritional state, initiate nutritional support at lower rate/content and advance slowly while monitoring electrolytes and other clinical signs/symptoms.
  - Gastrointestinal symptoms of intolerance/concern include nausea, vomiting, diarrhea, and constipation.

PEARLS
- *Energy imbalances during acute critical illness are a concern. Overfeeding and underfeeding have serious consequences.*
- *Providing more calories is not necessarily better during acute critical illness; however, more protein has been deemed to be beneficial.*
- *Nutrition evaluation during acute critical illness is challenging. A helpful tool is to obtain CRP and prealbumin levels from the same blood drawn to determine the acute protein status. The CRP and prealbumin have an inverse relationship. If the CRP level is elevated, the prealbumin level will be negatively affected and will not serve as a good marker of nutrition status. If the CRP level is within normal limits, the prealbumin level will reflect nutrition status per acute protein stores.*

Sleep

Cathy Haut

Background/Definition

- Sleep is a basic physiologic function; contributes to normal growth and development patterns.
- Many children from infancy to adolescence have sleep disorders resulting from both physiologic and psychological origins.

- Psychological disorders affecting sleep include posttraumatic stress disorder (PTSD), attention-deficit/hyperactivity disorder (ADHD), mood disorders, anxiety, and depression.
- Parasomnias refer to sleep terrors, sleep walking, and sleep talking which are relatively rare psychological disorders.
- Enuresis and obstructive sleep apnea are often physiologic and may cause sleep disruption.
- Hospitalized children incur additional disruptions in sleep related to discomfort, an unfamiliar environment, and a 24-hour surveillance and therapy.
- Children hospitalized in intensive care units have additional risk factors for disruption of the normal sleep–wake cycle which can lead to delirium, impaired immunity, catabolism, and respiratory compromise. Pain, chaotic environment, medications, and invasive medical interventions contribute to sleep disturbances.
- Mechanically ventilated children in the PICU receive escalating doses of sedatives and analgesics to assist in maintaining intubation and "sleep," but these centrally acting medications contribute to longer periods of ventilation, dependence, and potential for withdrawal symptoms.
- Sleep disruption, especially in hospitalized young infants and children, can result in poor neurodevelopmental and neurocognitive outcomes.
- Additional research is needed to document the outcomes of sleep deprivation in hospitalized children and children who spend long lengths of stay in the PICU.

Pathophysiology

- Sleep needs in children change as neurologic maturation occurs.
- Newborns sleep up to 18 hours per day in irregular patterns and is separated into REM and non-REM sleep. Sleep patterns become more regular over the first year of life and stabilize over the first 5 years of life.
- Healthy children between the ages of 3 and 12 need an average of 9 to 10 hours of sleep at night, which is a different type of sleep from that of adults, considered "slow wave."

Management

- Obvious adjustments in the hospitalized child's environment, including limiting stimulation, limiting unnecessary patient arousals, and sufficient pain management.
- Involvement of family and familiar rituals in the bedtime process may also be helpful in securing successful sleep.
- Assessment of the need for centrally active medications on a shift-by-shift basis has also shown benefit in limiting the length of intubation and ventilation.
- Continued evaluation and documentation of sleep and sleep quality in hospitalized children.

1. A 4-year-old newly diagnosed with leukemia is being admitted to the hospital from the clinic. The single parent has the 7-year-old and 3-year-old siblings with her at the visit. Developmentally appropriate care can be provided to the siblings through which of the following actions?
   a. Provide the 7-year-old with a detailed explanation of all the processes and procedures that will be followed for her sibling.
   b. Identify a family member or staff person (e.g., child life specialist, if possible) who can distract the 3-year-old while the parent is attending to the admission of the patient.
   c. Involve the siblings in the care of the patient so they get a full "hand's on" experience.
   d. Provide the same medical play activities for both siblings so they can experience the patient's situation fully.

Answer: **B**

Although a 7-year-old has reached the "age of reason," detailed explanations of things they are not familiar with is not helpful. Providing brief explanations to their direct questions will give them better support. The 3-year-old is not yet able to separate from the parent, so may be very clinging as the parent is distracted with the patient's needs. A trained child life specialist will be able to distract the child and allow the parent to support the patient. An unfamiliar environment may make the parent even more anxious and thus relieving the siblings from any responsibilities other than being able to ask questions is best.

2. An 8-year-old is in need of a head CT which will take only a few minutes and the health care provider does not think that the time frame warrants the need for sedation. Which of the following will *best* prepare the child for the experience?
   a. Tell him just to be brave and that it will take only about 15 minutes of him lying still for the test.
   b. "Let's practice lying still for 15 minutes now and I will have your teddy bear lie still also."
   c. "I know you can do this because you are such a big boy!"
   d. "You will lie still on a table but there will be people right outside the room if you need anything."

Answer: **B**

Modeling and rehearsing will allow him to understand what is needed of him during the test. He is too young to understand the time mechanism without relationship to actual events. Assuring him that he is a big boy does not acknowledge or let him express his feelings. Telling him that people will be right outside the room may leave him with a sense of abandonment.

The next three questions pertain to the following scenario:
An 18-month-old girl with a history of cerebral palsy, feeding difficulties, milk protein allergy, and poor growth presents with respiratory distress, increased thick secretions, and congestion for 1 week, vomiting 4 to 5 times per day and poor tolerance of feeds. The patient eventually requires intubation and ventilation within the first 24 hours of admission.
Anthropometrics:
Weight: 8 kg (<3rd% on WHO curve)
Length: 80 cm (3–15th% on WHO curve)
Weight/length: <3rd% on WHO curve
IBW: 10.1 kg
She is currently NPO and on maintenance IV fluids, with continuous infusions of sedation and medications.

3. What parameters indicate that this patient is at nutritional risk?
   a. Underweight, moderate acute malnutrition per Waterlow criteria, impaired dietary intake prior to admission.
   b. Underweight, severe acute malnutrition per Waterlow criteria, impaired dietary intake prior to admission.
   c. Underweight, no acute malnutrition present, impaired dietary intake prior to admission.
   d. Low weight/length, mild acute malnutrition per Waterlow criteria, impaired dietary intake prior to admission.

Answer: **A**

This child is underweight as indicated per weight/length = <3rd%.
Moderate acute malnutrition present = 79% of IBW per Waterlow criteria.
Vomiting 4 to 5 times per day indicates impaired dietary intake.

4. What mode of enteral nutrition support would be most appropriate and with what type of formula?
   a. NJ tube with a semi-elemental pediatric formula.
   b. NG tube with a standard, intact nutrient milk protein base pediatric formula.
   c. NG with an elemental pediatric formula.
   d. NJ with a standard, intact nutrient milk protein base pediatric formula.

Answer: **C**

NG tube feedings would be the preferred choice as they are more physiologic and there is no history of aspiration or reflux, nor is this a current concern. A pediatric formula is the age-appropriate choice, and an elemental formula is indicated because the patient has a milk protein allergy.

5. If this child is in the early phases of illness, how many calories and grams of protein per day may be appropriate to provide at this time and at what rate would you start continuous NG tube feeds?
a. 320 calories and 12 g of protein per day, initial NG rate of 8 to 16 mL/hour.
b. 200 calories and 6.4 g of protein per day, initial NG rate of 4 to 8 mL/hour.
c. 440 calories and 16 to 24 g of protein per day, initial NG rate of 8 to 16 mL/hour.
d. 440 calories and 16 to 24 g of protein per day, initial NG rate of 4 to 8 mL/hour.

Answer: **D**

It is important to provide calories near REE during early phases of illness, which is 55 kcal/kg/day based on the patient's age. Protein amount during critical illness per age is 2 to 3 g/kg/day. The recommended initial rate for critically ill, malnourished pediatric patient is 0.5 to 1 mL/kg/hour.

6. A 4-year-old child admitted for pneumonia becomes upset after knowing she is to receive an injection of ceftriaxone. Considering the developmental level, which of the following is the best communication approach by the nurse practitioner?
a. Immediately prior to administration, give information about the medication, including where and how it will be given.
b. Explain that the hurting lasts only a few minutes and it will be quick. Then administer the injection.
c. Ask the mother to step outside and have a nurse assist with the administration.
d. Give the child a syringe to hold, a simple explanation, reassurance, and administer the injection.

Answer: **D**

The nurse practitioner should understand that the child is frightened; therefore, asking the parent to step out of the room would further increase the child's anxiety. The first two options would not allow for the child to interact with the equipment, which is important as most preschoolers desire concrete vocabulary and interaction with medical equipment. Allowing the child to hold and touch the equipment while offering an explanation is the best option.

7. Calculate the creatinine clearance for a 13-year-old girl who weighs 52 kg and is 155 cm tall, with an SCr of 0.8 mg/dL.
a. 60 mL/minute
b. 70 mL/minute
c. 80 mL/minute
d. 90 mL/minute

Answer: **C**

Using the equation $CrCl = \frac{[k \times height]}{Scr}$, where k = 0.413, height = 155 cm, and SCr = 0.8 mg/dL, $CrCl = \frac{[0413 \times 155]}{0.8}$ = 80 mL/minute.

8. Which of the following is a consequence of the greater proportion of total body water seen in infants and neonates compared to older children?
a. Both groups have higher serum concentrations of hydrophilic drugs.
b. They have lower serum concentrations of hydrophilic drugs.
c. They have higher serum concentrations of lipophilic drugs.
d. They have lower serum concentrations of lipophilic drugs.

Answer: **B**

The greater hydration of adipose tissue in neonates and infants can yield lower serum concentrations of hydrophilic drugs because they are more liable to distribute into the adipose tissue.

9. An infant born at 28 weeks' gestation who is now 9 weeks old is admitted to the PICU for suspected sepsis and hypovolemic shock. What is the most important management to prevent increased metabolic demands?
a. Allow the mother to breast-feed the infant ad lib.
b. Oxygenation and prevention of cold stress.
c. Oxygenation and administration of a fluid bolus.
d. Keep the infant NPO and administer IV fluids at 2× maintenance.

Answer: **B**

Maintaining a normal neutrothermal environment is the most effective way to prevent adding additional stress on this infant or increasing the metabolic rate or metabolic demands.

Recommended Readings

American Academy of Pediatrics. (2010). *A compendium of evidence-based research for pediatric practice* (10th ed.). Elk Grove Village, IL: American Academy of Pediatrics.

American Academy of Pediatrics. (2007). Principles and guidelines for early hearing detection and intervention programs. *Pediatrics, 120*(4), 898–921. doi:10.1542/peds.2007-2333

American Academy of Pediatrics and Committee on Infectious Diseases and Committee on Fetus and Newborn. (2011). Recommendations for the prevention of perinatal group B streptococcal (GBS) disease. *Pediatrics, 128*(3), 1–6.

Barlow, S. E., & Expert Committee. (2007). Expert Committee recommendations regarding the prevention, assessment, and treatment of child and adolescent overweight and obesity: summary report. *Pediatrics, 120*(suppl 4), S164–S192.

Burns, C. E., Dunn, A. M., Brady, M. A., Starr, N. B., & Blosser, C. G. (2013). *Pediatric primary care* (5th ed.). St. Louis, MO: Saunders Elsevier.

Chwals, R. J. (2007). Energy metabolism and appropriate energy repletion in children. In S. S. Baker, R. D. Baker, & A. M. Davis (Eds.), *Pediatric nutrition support* (pp. 65–82). Burlington, MA: Jones & Bartlett.

de la Vega, R., & Miro, J. (2013). The assessment of sleep in pediatric chronic pain sufferers. *Sleep Medicine Reviews, 17*, 185–192.

Feigelman, S. (2011). Growth, development, and behavior. In R. M. Kliegman, B. Stanton, J. St. Geme, N. F. Schor, & R. E. Behrman (Eds.), *Nelson textbook of pediatrics* (19th ed.). Philadelphia, PA: Saunders Elsevier.

Kleinman, R. E (Ed.). (2009). *Pediatric nutrition handbook* (6th ed.). Elk Grove Village, IL: American Academy of Pediatrics.

Kudchadkar, S. R., Aljohani, O. A., & Punjabi, N. M. (2014). Sleep of critically ill children in the pediatric intensive care unit: A systematic review. *Sleep Medicine Reviews, 18*(2), 103–110.

Lauer, B. J., & Spector, N. D. (2011). Hyperbilirubinemia in the newborn. *Pediatrics Reviews, 32*(8), 341–348.

Leonberg, B (Ed.), & Pediatric Nutrition Practice Group. (2012). *Pediatric nutrition care manual*. Chicago, IL: Academy of Nutrition and Dietetics.

Mehta, N. M., Compher, C., & A.S.P.E.N. Board of Directors. (2009). A.S.P.E.N. Clinical guidelines: Nutrition support of the critically ill child. *Journal of Parenteral and Enteral Nutrition, 33*(3), 260–278.

Newborn Screening Authoring Committee. (2008). Newborn screening expands: recommendations for pediatricians and medical homes–Implications for the system. *Pediatrics, 121*(1), 192–217. doi:10.1542/peds.2007-3021.

Robbins, S.T., & Meyers, R. M. (2011). *Infant feedings: Guidelines for preparation of human milk and formula in health care facilities* (2nd ed.). Chicago, IL: American Dietetic Association.

Vanek, V. W., Seidner, D. L., Allen, P., Bistrian, B., Collier, S., Gura, K., . . . A.S.P.E.N. Board of Directors. (2012). A.S.P.E.N. position paper: Clinical role for alternative intravenous fat emulsions. *Nutrition in Clinical Practice, 27*(2), 150–192.

Vanek, V. W., Matarese, L. E., Robinson, M., Sacks, G. S., Young, L. S., Kochevar, M. . . . A.S.P.E.N. Board of Directors. (2011). A.S.P.E.N. position paper: Parenteral nutrition glutamine supplementation. *Nutrition in Clinical Practice, 26*(4), 479–494.

Vanek, V. W., Borum, P., Buchman, A., Fessler, T. A., Howard, L., Jeejeebhoy, K., . . . A.S.P.E.N. Board of Directors. (2012). A.S.P.E.N. position paper: Recommendations for changes in commercially available parenteral multivitamin and multi-trace elements products. *Nutrition in Clinical Practice, 27*, 440–491.

World Health Organization. (1985). Energy and protein requirements: Report of a joint FAO/WHO/UNU Expert Consultation. *World Health Organization Technical Report Series, 724*, 1206.

Wiecha, J., & Pollard, T. (2004). The interdisciplinary eHealth team: Chronic care for the future. *Journal of Medical Internet Research, 6*(3), e22. doi:102196/jmir.6.3.e22

Communication, Family-Centered Care, Transitional Care, and Health Care Home

Communicating with Acutely Ill Children at Different Ages

Megan R. Winkler, Mariam I. Kayle, and Sharron L. Docherty

Background

- Communication is a complex process of information exchange within the context of relationships.
- Communication promotes information transfer and also provides opportunities to develop relationships and establish rapport between the child/family and health care provider (HCP).
- Communication is the most common "procedure" in health care; yet HCPs frequently acquire this skill through trial and error rather than through formal training.
- Careful attention to the selection of words, tone of voice, facial expressions, and body language is necessary to ensure effective communication with children and families.
- Good communication can foster a trusting therapeutic relationship between the child/family and the HCP.
- Poor communication can result in negative consequences including patient/family emotional distress, distancing between patient/family and HCP, and compromised patient outcomes.

Communicating with Acutely Ill Children: An Individualized Approach

- Acutely ill children attempt to make sense of their illness using any information available.
- HCPs must involve children in discussions about their health and illness, and provide information that children can understand and process.
- There is broad consensus across research and practice that it is important to involve children, regardless of age, in discussions about their illness and care plans. The appropriate timing and approach for these discussions is less clear.
- The use of chronologic age and/or the child's stage of development as a marker for timing and content of discussions can

be problematic because of the variability in cognitive development within particular ages and stages.
- Communication should be based on the cognitive developmental capabilities (to know and understand) and affective needs (to feel known and understood) of the individual child and his/her readiness for such a discussion. This individualized approach also includes assessment of potential vulnerabilities, experiences with the illness, readiness for information, and relationships with parents and/or caregivers.
- Conceptual models of communication:
  - Child transitional communication model:
    - Based on an ethnographic study involving school-age and adolescent children; emphasizes an individualized approach to communication.
    - HCPs regard children as either passive bystanders or active participants in the communication process. While younger children may more commonly assume the role of passive bystanders and adolescents assume the role of active participants, a child may oscillate between the two roles depending upon their immediate needs and preferences.
    - HCPs require flexibility in their interactions with children, individualizing communication approaches based on the needs of the child.
  - Communication roles model:
    - Children 4 to 12 years of age reside in the "background" of communication between parent and HCP until they reach adolescence.
    - During adolescence, children gain independence, responsibility, and autonomy and become more foreground communicators.
    - Age ranges should not be interpreted as fixed entities, and HCPs should involve children along with parents in discussions about their care, pacing communication to meet the child's needs.
- Developmental concepts of health, illness, and death:
  - Chronological age and developmental stage may serve as a rough guide for understanding the child's conceptions of health, illness, and death. However, HCPs are cautioned against relying solely on those stages in their communication with children (Table 2.1).

TABLE 2.1	Broad Guide to Developmental Concepts of Health, Illness, and Death	
Age Range	**Concepts of Health, Illness, & Death**	**Application**
Early childhood (3–5 yr).	Lack concept of "forever."	Preparation for procedures/hospitalization few hours ahead.
	Experience time as more compacted.	Allow them to touch & examine objects.
	See death as temporary.	Provide concrete simple terms, and explain what you are doing during the procedure.
	Magical egocentric thinking.	Praise frequently.
	Rely on what they see.	Dispel responsibility & guilt.
	Interpret words literally.	Address fear; avoid hiding hands behind your back.
	Need less information/fewer details.	Parental presence may help decrease anxiety.
	Feel they are responsible for what is happening.	Preparation for procedures/hospitalization few hours ahead.
	May experience fear of what they do not know.	
Middle childhood (6–12 y).	Developing logic and reasoning skills.	Preparation for procedures/hospitalization up to 1 wk ahead.
	Awareness of illness and death.	Need to know what will take place and why it is being done.
	Early middle childhood: Tend to personify illness and death (e.g., skeleton, monster).	Use positive reinforcement and provide praise.
	Later middle childhood: See death as more final but not personal.	Walk them through the procedure and explain what you are doing and why.
	Understand death as final.	Allow questions.
	Interest in the physical process of death.	Let them know when the procedure is done.
	Understand how the body works.	Explain how equipment works.
	Heightened perception of body integrity.	Be sensitive to privacy needs.
	Concrete thinking.	Parental presence may help decrease anxiety.
	Rules and rituals are important.	
	Need more information.	
	May experience fear of what they do not know.	
Adolescence (12–18 y).	Well-developed reasoning skills and beginning of abstract thinking.	Full involvement in care planning is important.
	Physical appearance is very important.	Explain what you are doing and why.
	Have likely experienced death of pet or relative.	Discuss unrealized plans for school, relationships.
	Appreciate universality of death.	Respect privacy and opinions.
	May feel distanced from death.	Ask if they wish parents to be present.
		Encourage peer visitation.

- Factors that influence the child's readiness to engage in discussions about their health and illness:
  - Past experience with illness (e.g., traumatic procedures, illness, or death in family members or friends).
  - Family cohesion, support, and emotional resources.
  - Cultural values and ethnicity.
- Creative approaches to assess the child's readiness for discussions about health and illness include using storybooks and analogies.
- HCPs and parents working together to communicate with children about their illness optimizes experience.
- HCPs should consider parental/caregiver preference while acting in the best interest of the child.
- Parents/caregivers often report that young children (<8 years old) are easily frightened, and in cases of an uncertain prognosis, often believe the child should not participate in decision-making discussions.
- Parents/caregivers usually believe that adolescents >16 years of age should be involved in decisions related to their illness, and most parents/caregivers prefer that this age group receive information simultaneously with them.
- Strategies for effective communication with children:
  - Explain medical terms and avoid using confusing words such as "put to sleep" to explain anesthesia or "take blood" to explain collecting blood specimens. Use phrases such as "medicine to help you sleep."
  - Words are important, but modeling and rehearsing are also helpful. Demonstrate procedures by using equipment and dolls whenever possible.
  - Preparing children for procedures:
    - Preparing children for procedures helps separate fantasy from reality, fosters trust, and reduces uncertainty.
    - Children who are more informed about procedures have better treatment outcomes.
    - Best timing for preparation has not been empirically studied.
      - Generally, for younger children, providing preparation as close to the procedure as possible is recommended.
      - For older children, providing preparation up to a week prior to the procedure will allow the child the opportunity to process information and ask questions.
    - When feasible, allowing the child to remain in an upright position may be helpful to reduce anxiety.
    - If family agrees, allow parental/caregiver presence to support and comfort the child.
    - Do not use parents/caregivers to restrain an uncooperative child; holding for comfort is the best technique.
    - Preparation strategies (Mullen & Pate, 2006; Pike & Enright, 2012):
      - Infants: Awaken infant by gently touching them prior to painful procedures.
      - Toddlers: Use simple terminology to explain the procedure immediately prior to the procedure. Be honest. Whenever possible, allow the toddler to manipulate the equipment to reduce anxiety. Provide reassurance and praise. Use a single person to be the patient's coach, as "one voice" minimizes confusion and helps the toddler stay focused on the planned coping strategy. When the procedure is over, use phrases such as "all done."
      - Preschoolers: Use books, dolls, and medical equipment to simulate and prepare the child for the entire sensory experience, focusing on what the child will directly experience and what is expected of the child. Plan with the child "safe time" where no procedures or interventions take place. Allow security object during procedure. Avoid terminology such as "put to sleep" for anesthesia.
      - School-age children: Use books, dolls, and medical equipment to simulate and prepare the child for the entire sensory experience, focusing on what the child will directly experience and what is expected of the child. Preparation can be done over several hours, and even several days, for serious procedures. Ask the child to explain the procedure in his or her own words to verify understanding. Provide/discuss coping strategies with the child to prepare the child to handle the procedure emotionally. Allow choices as much as possible. Provide reassurance and praise during the procedure, and inform the child when the procedure is over.
      - Adolescents: Prepare adolescents as soon as the decision is made for the procedure. Provide facts about the procedure, and encourage the adolescent to ask questions. Promote autonomy and a sense of control by providing the adolescent with choices and asking if he or she wishes parental presence during the procedure.
  - Special considerations:
    - Mechanically ventilated children will be very anxious because of limitations in communication. HCPs should explain to the child why the child cannot speak, and be attentive to nonverbal cues. Use of creative techniques, such as picture boards, to facilitate communication is essential. Ask questions that require "yes" or "no" answers, and ensure that the child knows how to use the call light for help. Parental presence at the child's bedside can help reduce anxiety.
    - Communication with children who are sedated and pharmacologically paralyzed takes special emphasis. Although children may appear to be unresponsive, they still retain the ability to hear and feel. It is important that HCPs explain to the child why he/she cannot move and reassure the child that he/she will not be left alone. Parental presence at the child's bedside can help reduce anxiety.

Communicating with Families

Megan R. Winkler, Mariam I. Kayle, and Sharron L. Docherty

- Parents/caregivers:
  - Child illness and hospitalization disrupt a family's routine.
  - Parental/caregiver roles may shift as only one caregiver/family member may be available to be at hospital while the other(s) remains with children at home or assumes additional home tasks.

- Common reactions experienced by parents/caregivers:
  - Anxiety and fear: Especially when outcomes or reason for hospitalization is unclear.
  - Stress: Related to the perception that the child is in pain or has a poor prognosis, lack of family support, burden of missed work days, additional expenses, and concerns of children who remain at home.
- Strategies to assist parents/caregivers:
  - Provide regular information about the child's condition, treatment, care, and prognosis. Provide a clearly communicated plan of care; encourage parents/caregivers to be part of the care team and connected with providers.
  - Consistent, sensitive, and thorough communication between the HCP and parents/caregivers is crucial, especially in complex medical situations.
  - A designated person on the health care team may be needed in complex situations to establish rapport with the parents/caregivers; a trusting, confidential relationship reduces anxiety and allows involvement in care.
  - A sound understanding of cultural considerations regarding views of health and illness will allow HCPs to attend more fully to the needs of the patient and family.
- Specific communication strategies:
  - Carefully planned statements about the child's condition to the family in critical situations is essential.
  - Avoid vague statements that shield the family from uncertainties and controversies.
  - Avoid derogatory and value-laden terminology such as "brain damage" or "retarded" as these statements can adversely influence how parents/caregivers relate to their child.
  - Definitive statements should be used only when appropriate and necessary.
  - Address parent/caregiver perceptions at the beginning of a discussion: "Tell me what you understand about your child's condition." This provides the opportunity to correct any misconceptions and misinformation and to hear parental concerns.
  - Continue to assess parental interpretations throughout discussions, providing opportunities for clarification, if needed.
  - Communicate in simple language that is understandable to a layperson. Communicating uncertainty by using chance estimates, even for highly educated adults, has the potential to negatively impact understanding and increase risk perceptions.
- Siblings:
  - Many factors influence a sibling's experience, including age, family resources, past experiences with illness, and information received about the ill sibling and illness.
    - Siblings of hospitalized children may experience changes in parental attention.
    - Common reactions observed in siblings may include:
      - Younger children may feel guilt for fighting with or being mean to ill sibling in the past.
      - Fear of becoming ill themselves.
      - Concern that they had a role in the development of their sibling's illness/injury.
      - Nightmares of the sibling's illness or injury.
  - Insecurity, anxiety, and jealousy are common reactions to the change in family roles and routines and the impact of illness on the family.
  - Normative sibling and family challenges will continue and are to be expected (e.g., brothers getting into fights, teasing).
  - Siblings learn about the ill child's condition through clinic visits, observing the child at home, spending time with the child in hospital, and asking questions.
  - Parents tend to determine the appropriate time to share information about the ill child with the sibling based on the sibling's age. Many parents/caregivers feel comfortable to begin these discussions when the sibling is 8 years old, but all children require information and have questions about the sibling and changes in family life.
  - Strategies to improve the sibling's experience:
    - Provide information in developmentally appropriate manner.
    - Visitation:
      - Encourage sibling visitation with preparation of sights and sounds they will experience.
      - Demonstrate ways to talk and touch the ill child.
      - Allow siblings to visit a dying child, which will assist in overcoming any misconceptions as child fantasies are often worse than reality.
      - If visiting the ill child is not possible, encourage siblings to remain in contact through other means (e.g., cards, drawings, e-mails, webcam, etc.).
  - Help parents to establish routines for well siblings.

Communicating Bad News

Megan R. Winkler, Mariam I. Kayle, and Sharron L. Docherty

- Bad news can be defined as any information that is not expected and is perceived as negative or distressful by the patient/family, and may not always pertain to a terminal diagnosis.
- The manner in which bad news is delivered impacts how a family adapts and copes with the child's illness, and influences their acceptance and care of the child.
- Determining when and who to initiate discussions around bad news is difficult to standardize and should be individualized.
- Studies that examined parental satisfaction with communicating bad news found the following issues were important for parents/caregivers:
  - Facilitators of effective communication:
    - Provider availability and attentiveness: Meeting with the provider several times as needed.
    - Honest, comprehensive, and straightforward information was helpful for decision making.
    - Emphasized the need for HCP empathy and compassion when giving information.

- Complexity of vocabulary and pace: Emphasis on layman terms at a rate appropriate for comprehension and time for reflection.
- Balance between parent/caregiver desire for full disclosure with their desire for paced information.
- Hearing bad news from a familiar HCP.
- Follow-up contact with HCP(s) following the death of the child.
- Barriers to effective communication:
  - Provision of false hope and withholding information with the intention of protecting the parents/caregivers elicit a sense of betrayal and lack of trust.
  - Receiving contradictory information from different HCPs.
  - Body language.
- Guiding principles for communicating bad news:
  - Provide privacy and minimize interruptions.
  - Deliver bad news in person with both parents/caregivers present.
  - Limit the number of professionals present to those who have an established rapport with the family. Introduce any new member of the team and the reason they are present.
  - Explore what the patient and family know of the condition and the plan of care, and the reason for the meeting.
  - Provide straightforward, accurate, and honest information using simple terminology, avoiding medical jargon.
  - Demonstrate empathy, acknowledging that feelings experienced by the family are understandable.
  - Pause during delivery of the information, allowing reflection on the information and emotions.
  - Provide time for the family to talk and ask questions.
  - Ensure you understand the patient's/family's response, and expand on information as necessary.
  - Discuss any concerns the family has about sharing this news, and options of using child life specialists to ensure clear communication with children.
  - Discuss therapeutic options and provide referrals/telephone numbers at the end of the meeting.
  - At the close of the meeting, use a final summary plan for the next course of action. Be prepared to set up additional meetings if the patient/family have difficulty comprehending the details.
  - Be prepared to repeat information for patient/family at all subsequent meetings, as memory may be impaired by patients and families under stress.
  - Document meetings and notify the primary care provider (or other key caregivers) of the meeting and the information discussed.

Family-Centered Care Considerations

Miriam R. Batista

Definition of Family-Centered Care within the Hospital Setting

- Family-centered care (FCC) is an approach to health care that not only makes the effort to include the patient in their care,

but also considers the entire family unit. Key concepts in pediatrics include:
  - Family-centered care acknowledges that the family is an important part of the child's life.
  - Definition of the family is not universal and varies based on each unique situation. The family is defined by the patient and his or her caregivers.
  - Benefits of this care model include stronger partnerships between the health team and the family, improved patient outcomes, and increased satisfaction with the care provided.
- Core principles of FCC:
  - The foundation is to form a healthy partnership with the family while caring for the patient.
  - Four core principles that guide the delivery of FCC:
    - Treat the family with dignity and respect.
    - Fully share all pertinent information related to care in a respectful and timely manner.
    - Encourage family participation in care decisions.
    - Utilize a collaborative approach while working with the family unit.
  - Family assessment:
    - Continually assess the family while providing care. The health care team should consider the composition, culture, and routines of the family.
    - Models of care:
      - Friedman Family Assessment Model.
      - Calgary Family Assessment Model.
  - Both of these models offer methods to compile family information from name and address to cultural and religious backgrounds and beliefs.
- Important consideration:
  - Potential stressors related to the hospitalization and illness.
- Ultimately, patients and families must feel educated and empowered in order for patient family-centered care to be successfully implemented in the hospital setting.

Transition of Care

Andrea M. Kline-Tilford

Background

- Many children with chronic illnesses and disabilities are now surviving into adulthood with pharmacologic, surgical, and technologic advances.
- This has resulted in a large number of adolescents that require transition of complex interprofessional care from pediatric to adult HCPs/teams.
- Transition of care is necessary in adolescents with chronic illnesses expected to survive into adulthood.
- Some adolescents will have an uncomplicated transition with one specialty service, and others will require transition of an entire team of specialists for a variety of problems.
- Optimal health care is achieved when individuals receive uninterrupted developmentally appropriate high-quality health care.

Definition

- A deliberate and organized movement from child-centered to adult-centered health care in adolescents with chronic medical conditions.
- "Transition" is distinctly different than "transfer" of care in its multifaceted coordinated approach.

Crucial Steps in Facilitating the Transition

- Identify a HCP with expertise and interest in the challenges in transition of care.
- Design a transition that recognizes the knowledge necessary to manage young adults with specialized health care needs.
- Develop a detailed health history for the transition.
- Initiate a written plan for transition by 14 years of age.
- Acknowledge that additional resources may be needed for the adolescent during the time of transition.
- Ensure accessible and affordable health care coverage during adolescence into adulthood.

Transition Timing

- Establish the time of transition early in the planning process.
- Ideally, occurs between 18 and 21 years of age.
- Document a written plan for transition.
- May be determined by patient readiness or developmental milestone.
- Regular discussion with the patient and family about the transition can promote a coordinated, comfortable, and anticipated transition.
  - Transition should not be a sudden event.

Goals

- Develop an individualized, deliberate process.
- Involve the patient and family in planning.
- Determine goals for self-care.
- Empower the patient within his or her own abilities.
- Provide support for the patient and family during all phases of transition.
- Be available to the adult HCP(s) as a resource or to provide additional information during and after the transition.

Challenges

- Limited availability of adult HCPs prepared to manage young adults with complex chronic conditions.
- Inability to identify an adult primary or specialty HCP to accept transition of care. Often impacted by:
  - Time.
  - Training.
  - Adequate reimbursement for services.
  - Workforce shortages.
- Communication of appropriate medical records (e.g., non-communicating electronic medical records).
- More information on transition of care can be obtained from the National Health Care Transition Center at www.gottransition.org

PEARLS

- *Different families will have different needs during the transition process regardless of the complexity of the transfer.*
- *Recognize the implicit stressors for the patient and family during the time of transition.*
- *Presence of office "transition policy" can facilitate a standardized practice for transitioning all patients to adult providers. Posting the information or providing in brochures can better inform the patient and families about the process.*

Health Care Home

Andrea M. Kline-Tilford

Background

- Health Care home concept was first introduced in the 1960s with the primary aim of developing a centralized location for storing a child's medical record.
- Since that time, the concept of health care home has expanded and has been embraced by HCPs, families, legislators, and insurers.
- It was originally limited to physician-led practices, but is now open to Nurse Practitioners (NPs) in states that allow independent NP practice.
- NPs and Physician Assistants are eligible to be listed as part of a recognized practice if managing their own population of patients.
- The health care home gained recognition for its ability to ensure delivery of quality health care for children with special needs; however, this model has been expanded to serve as a model of care for all individuals.

Definition

- A model of primary care that endorses holistic care for ALL children and their families. Key concepts include:
  - Accessible, continuous health care.
  - Personal HCP (e.g., physician, NP, PA).
  - Whole-person oriented.
  - Comprehensive: Management of acute and chronic health issues (e.g., facile referrals when necessary).
  - Family-centered (e.g., listening, adequate time spent with patient/family).
  - Culturally effective, compassionate (e.g., sensitive to values and customs, interpreter services used when needed).
  - Coordinated (e.g., satisfied with communication between HCPs, satisfied with communication between HCP and specialty services, sufficient assistance in coordinating care).
  - Team based.

Delivery of Whole-Person Care

- Routine and urgent care.
- Motivational and anticipatory guidance:
  - Reinforcement of positive parenting behaviors.

- Behavioral consultation.
- Nutrition counseling.
- Safety education.
- Developmental evaluations.
- Referrals to community resources.
- Oral health services.
- Health promotion.

Quality and Safety Principles and Activities for Health Care Providers

- Advocates achievement of optimal patient-centered outcomes.
- Develops robust partnerships between HCP, patient, families.
- Applies evidence-based practice to guide decision making.
- Participates in quality improvement projects.
- Engages in performance review and improvement plans.
- Patient feedback sought and integrated into decision making.
- Utilizes information technology to support/enhance care delivery.
- Participates in a voluntary health care home recognition process; nongovernmental entity.
- Encourages patients and families to participate in quality improvement activities.

Quality Standards in Health Care

- Developed by national organizations (e.g., National Committee for Quality Assurance, National Quality Forum).
- Recognition as Health care Home if it meets delineated criteria.
  - Whole-person care delivery.
  - Possesses the majority of required health care home–defined elements.

Health Care Home Disparities

- Homes with non-English language as primary language have lower rates of health care home.
- Older children are less likely to have a health care home.
- Large racial and ethnic disparities; non-Hispanic white children are most likely to have a health care home, and Hispanic children are least likely.
- Children living in "safe" neighborhoods are more likely to have a health care home.
- Maternal education beyond high school more likely to have a health care home.
- Insured children are more likely to have a health care home.

1. An 8-week-old infant was admitted to the PICU after being found unresponsive at home. The infant presented to the emergency department (ED) in asystole, but a heart rate was obtained after intubation and 20 minutes of CPR. Ultimately, further neurological testing demonstrated that the infant had suffered a severe anoxic event and brain death testing should be initiated. The team came in to meet the family and discuss care options. Upon entering the room, they found seven people at the bedside: the infant's mother and father, the paternal grandparents, an uncle, the family's rabbi, and a 3-year-old sibling. The best approach of the health care team in this situation is to:
   a. ask everyone but the parents to leave the room so their child's care could be discussed.
   b. ask the parents who they would like to be present for the discussion.
   c. tell the family that the infant is most likely brain dead so testing would begin immediately.
   d. consult neurology and let the family know when they will start the first brain death exam.

Answer: **B**

The definition of family varies in each situation, so it is important to ask who the family would like to be present while making decisions. It is also essential to include parents/caregivers in the decision-making process.

2. The family of a 15-year-old who was admitted in status asthmaticus with pneumonia would like to have a prayer service in the room of their daughter with several clergy members and the extended family. The child is in a semiprivate room, where the rules indicate that there are only two visitors to a bedside at one time. When utilizing the principles of family-centered care, what is the best option for this activity?
   a. Encourage the family to have the prayer service in the hospital chapel without their child present.
   b. Offer a space where the family can meet and pray in private while allowing medical support for the child so that she can attend.
   c. Reassure the family that the child will only be hospitalized briefly, so there is no need to convene the service.
   d. Allow the clergy and immediate family members at the bedside for a short service.

Answer: **B**

Even though brief, the hospitalization of this child is a stress on the family. It is important to support family needs whether cultural or religious during this difficult time.

3. A 6-year-old victim of a motor vehicle accident has died in the intensive care unit. The extended family and siblings have

been at the hospital, but have had limited access due to efforts to stabilize and support the patient. Which approach will provide the BEST support through the grief process for this family?
   a. Identify the family members present and provide a family room where their questions can be answered and they can remain with the loved one as long as needed.
   b. Avoid the use of the word "dead" as this is an absolute term and can be frightening to children.
   c. Children should be shielded from a grieving family member as they are not capable of knowing what is best.
   d. Every child is different, but once the process of grieving starts, the child must be allowed to stay with the family and loved one.

Answer: **A**

Support for the family of a child who died unexpectedly may occur in the patient room or a special room set aside to allow for the individual grieving process needed. Care must be taken to identify the needs of the children and support them developmentally, including allowing them to go to a separate area or room where an attentive adult can attend to them if their immediate family members are unable to give full attention. Language should be honest without providing confusing messages, especially to children. Offering the family an opportunity to ask questions and stay with their deceased child also provides support.

4. A 4-year-old child admitted for pneumonia becomes upset after learning she is to receive an injection of ceftriaxone. Considering developmental level, which of the following is the best communication approach by the nurse practitioner?
   a. Immediately prior to administration, give information about the medication, including where and how it will be given.
   b. Explain that the hurting lasts only a few minutes and it will be quick. Then administer the injection.
   c. Ask the mother to step outside, and have a nurse assist with the administration.
   d. Give the child a syringe to hold, a simple explanation, reassurance, and administer the injection.

Answer: **D**

The nurse practitioner should assess that the child is frightened; therefore, asking the parent to step out of the room would further increase the child's anxiety. The first two options would not allow for the child to interact with the equipment, which is important as most preschoolers desire concrete vocabulary and interaction with medical equipment. Allowing the child to hold and touch the equipment while offering an explanation is the best option.

5. A 13-year-old male has been admitted to the pediatric unit to begin induction therapy for his recent leukemia diagnosis. During the morning assessment, the HCP evaluates Jake's nausea and pain. However, when the HCP asks Jake a question, he shrugs and looks at his mother. Considering Jake's communication, which approach by the HCP is most appropriate?
   a. Continue to push the teen for answers, as during adolescence, children should be active participants in their care.
   b. Address the parents with questions about the child's care.
   c. Realize the child may prefer to be a more passive bystander at this time, and adapt the communication approach to this need.
   d. Expect that this passive communication approach will be used for all subsequent interactions.

Answer: **C**

An individual approach is needed in communicating with all children. It is important for the provider to realize that while adolescents commonly assume a more active role and younger children a more passive role, these are not fixed states. Providers should allow children to fluctuate between passive and active roles based on the immediate needs and preferences for that particular interaction at that particular moment.

6. The ICU team is rounding on a patient with a complex central line infection. This patient has had multiple line infections, requiring many different courses of antibiotics with a new positive culture, indicating a resistant organism. The pharmacist recommends trying two antibiotics together for synergistic effect. The attending physician agrees, and the patient is started on these antibiotics. Of the "12 C's" of teamwork, which is represented in this scenario?
   a. Confronts problems directly.
   b. Consistency.
   c. Conflict management.
   d. Collaboration.

Answer: **D**

A modern interprofessional team is a consistent grouping of people from relevant clinical disciplines, ideally inclusive of the patient, who interact guided by 12 processes that all begin with the letter C to achieve team-defined favorable patient outcomes. In this scenario, the patient is the center of the decision as to which is the best treatment regimen, determined by an interprofessional team.

7. In considering a process to make sure that all children have a health care home, it is important to understand that:
   a. Currently, many disparities exist in providing a health care home for children.
   b. The majority of children are eligible for state health insurance, therefore allowing them the benefit of a health care home.

   c. The nurse practitioner can facilitate entry into a health care home, but cannot manage the process.
   d. Children who are adolescents with disabilities are more likely to have a health care home.

Answer: **A**

Currently, there are many disparities within the provision of a health care home, including the fact that nonwhite children have higher rates of a health care home, children who live in "safe" neighborhoods are more likely to have a health care home, and children who live with parents who have higher education are more likely to have a health care home. The goal of the health care home process is to provide all children with the same opportunities.

8. Which of the following is a key concept for planning transition of care from a pediatric provider to an adult team?
   a. Asking the adolescent if he has considered where he would like his care to be transitioned.
   b. Preparing a written plan for transition of care providers by the age of 14.
   c. Coordinating all documentation, including consults from specialties to have ready, for the move.
   d. Planning for transition at the age of 18 years.

Answer: **B**

There are many steps that will ensure a smooth transition from pediatric to adult providers for a child with complex health care needs. One of the most important steps is to have a written plan for transition in place by the time the child is 14 years old. This allows a long time for the other processes to take shape, such as gathering documentation and having a conference between providers.

9. Two of the four core principles for family-centered care include:
   a. Share all information regarding care and ask family permission for any procedures.
   b. Allow all family members to remain with the patient at all times, and ask them to make all decisions independently.
   c. Treat the family with respect, and encourage family participation in care decisions.
   d. Treat the family with dignity, and ask them to make independent decisions for the patient.

Answer: **C**

There are four core principles for family-centered care. These principles include: treat the family with dignity and respect; fully share all pertinent information related to care in a respectful and timely manner; encourage family participation in care decisions; utilize a collaborative approach while working with the family unit. Family members will need appropriate information to make decisions for their child, so they should not be asked to do this independently.

10. A child with complex health care problems is admitted to the intensive care unit with an acute respiratory illness. The child has never been in the PICU before, and the family is confused and obstructive with care. Different providers attempt to speak with them, but they refuse to sign consent for

(continues on page 38)

important procedures, and the child is critically ill. What is the best approach?

a. Involve familiar care providers, and offer current information in a clear manner, in lay terms, allowing time for questions.

b. Have the attending physician speak to them, offering information that is needed at the moment.

c. Arrange a meeting of all care providers and family members to discuss the projected hospitalization.

d. Engage the hospital ethics committee to assist in making decisions for the child.

Answer: **A**

Communication with patients and families requires skill and purposeful planning. In providing bad news, families have identified some important guidelines, which include a familiar provider giving information, using terminology that the family can understand, and providing an opportunity for them to ask questions. Families ask for empathy and respect when in situations that are extremely stressful and difficult for them. They also need time to review the information provided and to be included in the decision-making process. When a child is critically ill, even though it is frustrating and sometimes not possible to allow additional time for decision making, trying to find the appropriate person to convey the information and allowing the family to have some involvement is very helpful.

Recommended Readings

American Academy of Pediatrics, American Academy of Family Physicians, American College of Physicians, & Transition Clinical Report Authoring Group. (2011). Clinical report—Supporting the health care transition from adolescence to adulthood in the medical home. *Pediatrics, 128,* 182–200.

Ball, J. W., Bindler, R. C., & Cowen, K. J. (2012). The hospitalized child. In J. W. Ball, R. C. Bindler, & K. J. Cowen (Eds.), *Principles of pediatric nursing: Caring for children* (5th ed., pp. 261–289). Upper Saddle River, NJ: Pearson Education.

Bluebond-Langner, M., Belasco, J. B., & DeMesquita Wander, M. (2010). "I want to live, until I don't want to live anymore": Involving children with life-threatening and life-shortening illnesses in decision making about care and treatment. *Nursing Clinics of North America, 45*(3), 329–343. doi:10.1016/j.cnur.2010.03.004

Boyd, J. R. (2001). A process for delivering bad news: Supporting families when a child is diagnosed. *Journal of Neuroscience Nursing, 33*(1), 14–20.

Brady, M., Deloian, B., Jones, D., Keesing, H., Thomas, K. K., Lindeke, L., . . . Shuren, A. (2009). NAPNAP position statement on pediatric health care/medical home: Key issues on delivery, reimbursement, and leadership. *Journal of Pediatric Health Care, 23*(3), 23A–24A.

Eggly, S., Penner, L., Albrecht, T. L., Cline, R. J. W., Foster, T., Naughton, M., . . . Ruckdeschel, J. C. (2006). Discussing bad news in the outpatient oncology clinic: Rethinking current communication guidelines. *Journal of Clinical Oncology, 24*(4), 716–719. doi:10.1200/jco.2005.03.0577

Fisher, M. J., & Broome, M. E. (2011). Parent-provider communication during hospitalization. *Journal of Pediatric Nursing, 26*(1), 58–69. doi:10.1016/j.pedn.2009.12.071

Foresman-Capuzzi, J. (2007). Grief telling: Death of a child in the emergency department. *Journal of Emergency Nursing, 33*(5), 505–508.

Hockenberry, M. J. (2013). Communication and physical assessment of the child. In M. J. Hockenberry & D. Wilson (Eds.), *Essentials of pediatric nursing* (pp. 86–143). St. Louis, MO: Elsevier-Mosby.

Jaaniste, T., Hayes, B., & Von Baeyer, C. L. (2007). Providing children with information about forthcoming medical procedures: A review and synthesis. *Clinical Psychology: Science and Practice, 14*(2), 124–143. doi:10.1111/j.1468-2850.2007.00072.x

Katzmark, L. (2012). Child life: Transition to adulthood. In K. Reuter-Rice & B. Bolick (Eds.), *Pediatric acute care: A guide to interprofessional practice* (pp. 83–84). Burlington, MA: Jones & Bartlett Learning.

Kuziemsky, C. E., Borycki, E. M., Purkis, M. E., Black, F., Boyle, M., Cloutier-Fisher, D., . . . Interprofessional Practices Team. (2009). An interdisciplinary team communication framework and its application to healthcare 'e-teams' systems design. *BMC Medical Informatics and Decision Making, 9,* 43. doi:10.1186/1472-6947-9-43

Lambert, V., Glacken, M., & McCarron, M. (2011). Communication between children and health professionals in a child hospital setting: A child transitional communication model. *Journal of Advanced Nursing, 67*(3), 569–582. doi:10.1111/j.1365-2648.2010.05511.x

Levetown, M., & The Bioethics Committee. (2008). Communicating with children and families: From everyday interactions to skill in conveying distressing information. *Pediatrics, 121*(5), e1441–e1460. doi: 10.1542/peds.2008-0565

Longman, T., Turner, R. M., King, M., & McCaffery, K. J. (2012). The effects of communicating uncertainty in quantitative health risk estimates. *Patient Education and Counseling, 89*(2), 252–259.

McCauley, K., & Irwin, R. S. (2006). Changing the work environment in ICUs to achieve patient-focused care: The time has come. *Chest, 130*(5), 1571–1578. doi:10.1378/chest.130.5.1571

Meert, K. L., Eggly, S., Pollack, M., Anand, K. J. S., Zimmerman, J., Carcillo, J., & Nicholson, C. (2008). Parents' perspectives on physician-parent communication near the time of a child's death in the pediatric intensive care unit. *Pediatric Critical Care Medicine, 9*(1), 2–7.

Moskowitz, J. T., Butensky, E., Harmatz, P., Vichinsky, E., Heyman, M. B., Acree, M., & Folkman, S. (2007). Caregiving time in sickle cell disease: Psychological effects in maternal caregivers. *Pediatric Blood & Cancer, 48*(1), 64–71.

Mullen, J. E., & Pate, F. D. (2006). Caring for critically ill children and their families. In M. C. Slota (Ed.), *Core curriculum for pediatric critical care nurses* (2nd ed., pp. 1–39). St. Louis, MO: Elsevier.

Pike, M., & Enright, K. (2012). Child life: Developmental considerations. In K. Reuter-Rice & B. Bolick. (Eds.), *Pediatric acute care: A guide to interprofessional practice* (pp. 49–57). Burlington, MA: Jones & Bartlett Learning.

Pirie, A. (2012). Pediatric palliative care communication: Resources for the clinical nurse specialist. *Clinical Nurse Specialist: The Journal for Advanced Nursing Practice, 26*(4), 212–215.

Price, J., McNeilly, P., & Surgenor, M. (2006). Breaking bad news to parents: The children's nurse's role. *International Journal of Palliative Nursing, 12*(3), 115–120.

Strickland, B. B., Jones, J. R., Ghandour, R. M., Kogan, M. D., & Newacheck, P. W. (2011). The medical home: Health care access and impact for children and youth in the United States. *Pediatrics, 127,* 604–611.

Zawistowski, C. A. (2012). Communicating bad news. In K. Reuter-Rice & B. Bolik (Eds.), *Pediatric acute care: A guide to interprofessional practice* (pp. 64–66). Burlington, MA: Jones & Bartlett Learning.

Zwaanswijk, M., Tates, K., van Dulmen, S., Hoogerbrugge, P. M., Kamps, W. A., Beishuizen, A., & Bensing, J. M. (2011). Communicating with child patients in pediatriconcology consultations: A vignette study on child patients', parents', and survivors' communication preferences. *Psycho-Oncology, 20*(3), 269–277. doi:10.1002/pon.1721

PART TWO

System-Based Problems

Pulmonary Disorders

Apnea
Katie Ward

Background/Definition

- Cessation of airflow through the respiratory tract for 20 seconds or longer *or* shorter respiratory pause associated with bradycardia or cyanosis significant enough to cause arterial hypoxemia and hypercapnia.

Types

- Central.
  - Disruption of afferent (cessation of output) or efferent (inability of peripheral nerves or respiratory muscles to receive input) signals of the central respiratory center.
  - Inappropriate response to hypercapnia and hypoxemia.
- Obstructive.
  - Reduced airway patency secondary to some form of obstruction causing poor or no air movement through passage.
  - Usually results in significant respiratory effort that is ineffective.

Etiology

- Central: immaturity of the respiratory center (premature infants), head trauma, toxin-mediated.
- Obstructive: obstructive sleep apnea (OSA), mucopolysaccharidosis, craniofacial anomalies, obesity, adenoid or tonsillar hypertrophy, aspirated foreign body, vocal cord paralysis.
- Mixed: obstructive and central.

Pathophysiology

- Within the transition from awake to nonrapid eye movement (NREM) sleep.
  - Reduced amplitude in the electrical activity of medullary inspiratory neurons, diaphragm, and abductor muscles.
  - Accompanied by mild hypoventilation and increased airway resistance.
  - Exaggerated pattern is noted in children with apnea disorders.

Clinical Presentation

- At time of evaluation, patient may appear clinically well.
- History may include poor sleep patterns, fatigue, daytime sleepiness, or difficulty concentrating.
- Examination during apneic episode: no respiratory effort, breath sounds, or chest wall movement; potential hypoxia, cyanosis, and bradycardia.

Diagnostic Evaluation

- Polysomnography.
- Echocardiography and/or electrocardiography (EKG) to evaluate for cardiac sequelae.

Management

- If adenotonsillar hypertrophy, referral to an otolaryngologist for possible adenotonsillectomy.
- If obese, weight management, including nutrition, exercise, and behavioral elements.
- Noninvasive positive pressure ventilation (NIPPV): continuous positive airway pressure (CPAP) or bilevel positive airway pressure (BiPAP).

PEARL

- *Always consider an acute life-threatening event in a young infant presenting with apnea*

Acute Respiratory Distress Syndrome
Katie Ward

Background

- Result of lung injury, specifically to the alveolar capillary barrier (alveolar epithelium, capillary endothelium), which is vital in maintaining lung fluid balance.

Diagnostic Criteria

- Acute onset.
- Bilateral infiltrates on chest radiograph (see Figure 3.1).

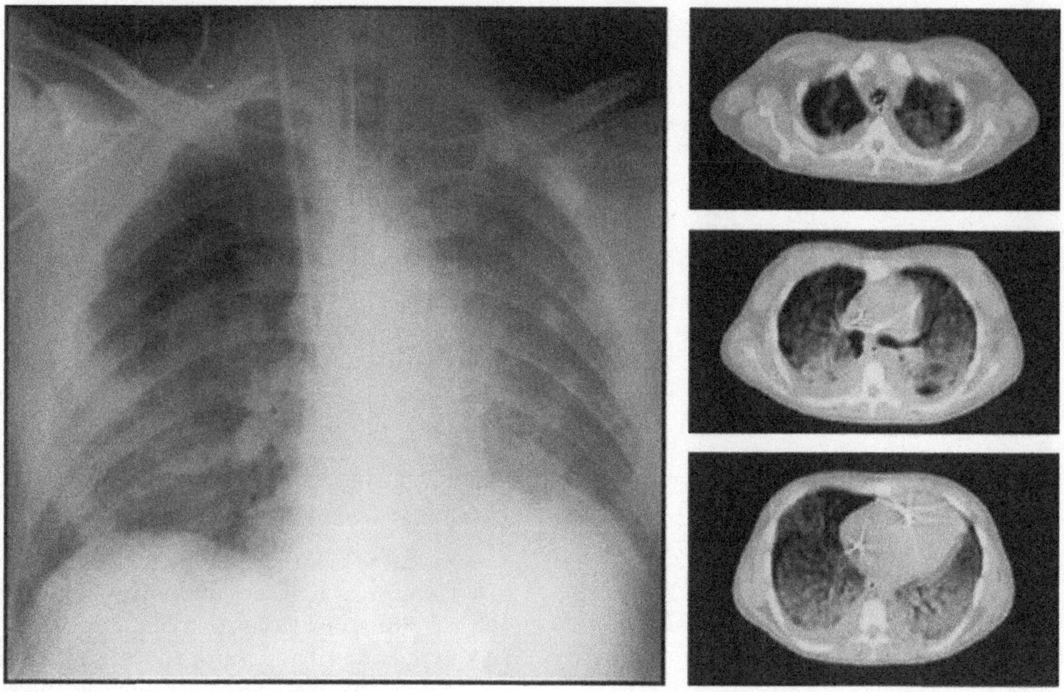

FIGURE 3.1 • **ARDS Radiographic Images**. Nonuniform parenchymal involvement in ARDS. Anterior–posterior chest X-ray and CT scans corresponding to lung apex, hilum, and base from a patient with sepsis and ARDS. Images are taken with the patient in supine position, at a PEEP of 5 cm H_2O. The CT scans illustrate the influence of the gravitational axis on the pattern of alveolar consolidation in ARDS: Nondependent regions are aerated, while dependent regions remain consolidated.

- Pao_2/Fio_2 ratio of <200.
- Noncardiogenic origin: pulmonary artery wedge pressure <18 mmHg or absence of clinical evidence of left atrial hypertension.

Etiology

- Direct lung injury as a result of pneumonia, aspiration, pulmonary contusion, pulmonary embolism, submersion injury, or inhalational injury.
- Indirect lung injury as a result of sepsis, shock, burn injury, pancreatitis, exposure to cardiopulmonary bypass, transfusion-related acute lung injury (TRALI), or cardiopulmonary arrest.

Pathophysiology

- Exudative phase: Injury to the alveolar capillary barrier causes disruption of fluid balance, leading to capillary permeability and pulmonary edema, in turn leading to a disruption of gas exchange and resulting in decreased pulmonary compliance and arterial hypoxemia.
- Acute inflammatory response: follows with adherence of neutrophils to damaged epithelium and resultant release of proinflammatory cytokines (TNF-α, interleukins).
- Proliferative phase: Resolution of ARDS begins.
- Chronic/fibrotic phase: If complete resolution does not occur after phase 1, it may progress to fibrosing alveolitis, persistent hypoxemia, increased alveolar dead space, decreased pulmonary compliance, and pulmonary hypertension, which may lead to right ventricular (RV) failure.

Clinical Presentation

- Tachypnea, labored breathing.
- Hypoxia, labored breathing.
- Hypocarbia followed by hypercarbia.
- Rales/crackles, decreased breath sounds.

Diagnostic Evaluation

- Chest radiography: bilateral infiltrates.
- Arterial blood gas (ABG): Pao_2/Fio_2 ratio <200.
- Complete blood count (CBC): evaluation for infectious process as well as hemoglobin level to calculate arterial oxygen content.
- ECHO: evaluation for cardiogenic etiology of pulmonary disease.
- Bronchoalveolar lavage (BAL): neutrophil activation, culture for infectious origin.
- Oxygen index calculation ([Fio_2 × MAP]/Pao_2): If >20, consider high-frequency oscillatory ventilation (HFOV); if >40, consider extracorporeal membrane oxygenation (ECMO).

Management

- Supplemental O_2
- Noninvasive ventilation (CPAP, BiPAP): may reduce intubation; Recent studies have included high flow nasal cannula (HFNC) as an additional modality to provide oxygenation prior to intubation or for management.
- Intubation and ventilation.

- High positive end-expiratory pressure (PEEP) to achieve Fio_2 <0.5–0.6, low tidal volume (7–8 mL/kg); avoid peak inspiratory pressure (PIP) >30 cm H_2O.
- Permissive hypercapnia (unless contraindicated).
- Escalation of symptoms.
  - Titrate PEEP upward.
- HFOV.
  - Smaller tidal volume.
  - Higher mean airway pressures.
  - Limited PIPs.

Additional management strategies may include the following:
- Surfactant.
  - Reduces alveolar surface tension.
  - Dosing: 50 to 100 mg/kg administered 1 to 2 times within 12 to 48 hours of initiation of mechanical ventilation.
- Nitric oxide.
  - Results in capillary and pulmonary dilation.
  - Dose: 20–80 ppm continuous inhalation.
  - Requires methemoglobin level monitoring.
- Conservative fluid management.
- Neuromuscular blockade.
- Bronchoscopy.
- Corticosteroid administration.
  - No evidence in pediatrics.
  - Typically initiated 7 to 10 days into course of ARDS.
- If oxygen index is not improving on conventional ventilator or HFOV, consider ECMO.

PEARLS
- *ARDS is a clinical syndrome with multiple etiologies*
- *Management focuses on lung-protective strategies*

Air Leak Syndromes
Katie Ward

Background/Definition

- Any condition in which air is present within a thoracic space that is otherwise normally closed.
- Defined by the location/space where air has abnormally infiltrated.
  - Pneumothorax: air in pleural space.
  - Pneumomediastinum: air in mediastinum.
  - Pneumopericardium: air in the pericardial space.
  - Subcutaneous and interstitial emphysema.

Etiology

- Spontaneous.
- Trauma.
- Underlying lung disease.
- Ventilator-induced.

Pathophysiology

- Normally, pressure gradients within thoracic cavity maintain alveolar ventilation and lung expansion in areas throughout the thoracic cavity where air does not normally exist.
- Disturbances of normal thoracic barriers cause disruption of pressure gradients with movement of gas from areas of high pressure to areas of lower pressure for the purpose of equalizing pressures.
  - Le Chatelier's principle of chemical equilibrium: If a dynamic equilibrium is disturbed by changing the conditions, the position of equilibrium moves to counteract the change.

Clinical Presentation

- Depends on the location of air.
- Pneumothorax.
  - Chest pain, dyspnea, tachycardia.
  - Ipsilateral hyperresonance to percussion, decreased air entry, decreased vocal fremitus.
  - Hypoxia: increased PIP on mechanical ventilation.
  - Tension pneumothorax: tracheal deviation (contralateral), hypotension, tachycardia, cyanosis—*medical emergency*.
- Pneumomediastinum.
  - Chest pain, dyspnea, neck pain, subcutaneous emphysema, Hamman's sign (i.e., crunching sound noted over the precordium space that is noted concurrent with heart tones rather than respirations; represents the sound of the heart beating against an air-filled space).
- Pneumopericardium.
  - Tachycardia, tachypnea, mill wheel murmur, muffled heart sounds, hypotension.

Diagnostic Evaluation

- Chest radiography.
  - Pneumothorax: thin line where lung is separated from chest wall.
  - Tension pneumothorax: shift of the mediastinum to the contralateral side (see Figure 3.2).

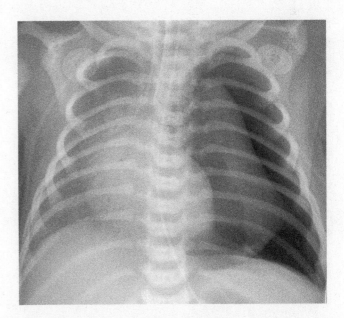

FIGURE 3.2 • **Tension Pneumothorax Chest Radiograph.** Left tension pneumothorax produces collapse of the left lung and mediastinal shift to the right.

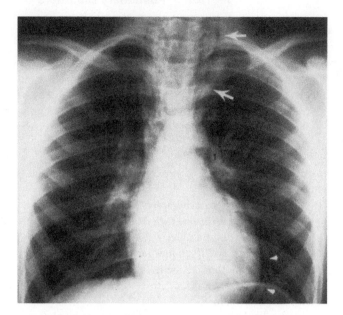

FIGURE 3.3 • **Pneumomediastinum Chest Radiograph**. Asthmatic child with pneumomediastinum with air surrounding the small triangular thymus gland, extending as linear sheaths into the neck and superior mediastinum (upper arrows) and extending along the lower left cardiac edge (lower arrows).

- Pneumomediastinum: radiolucent streaks in mediastinum (see Figure 3.3).
- Pneumopericardium: air in pericardial sac and "halo" sign (see Figure 3.4).
- EKG.
  - Pneumopericardium: ST-segment elevations and low voltage.

Management

- Depends on clinical symptomatology and patient's clinical status.
- Goal is to remove pathologic air and restore normal pressure gradient.
- Needle decompression.
  - May require thoracostomy tube placement; most common in pneumothorax.
- Limiting PIP, if requiring mechanical ventilation.
- Surgical evacuation is rare.
- Observation.

PEARLS

- *Pneumomediastinum may be associated with subcutaneous emphysema on clinical examination*
- *Pneumomediastinum and pneumopericardium typically do not require intervention unless associated with marked cardiopulmonary compromise*

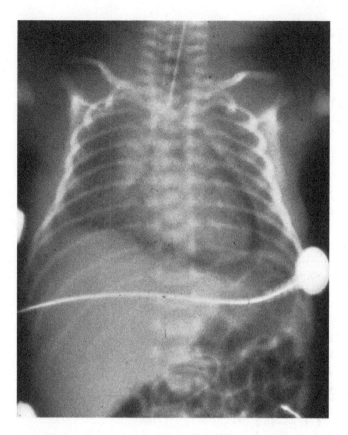

FIGURE 3.4 • **Pneumopericardium Chest Radiograph**. In this chest X-ray, air can be seen within the pericardial sac surrounding the heart (pneumopericardium), and in the right hemithorax.

Pneumothorax

Anne Vasiliadis

Definition

- A pneumothorax is an abnormal collection of air between the visceral and parietal pleura in the thoracic cage.
- Traumatic pneumothorax.
  - Caused by blunt, crush, or penetrating trauma to the chest.
- Iatrogenic.
  - Caused by injury from a diagnostic or therapeutic procedure, or as a consequence of mechanical ventilation.
- Spontaneous.
  - Primary spontaneous: occurs in patients with no underlying lung disease.
  - Secondary spontaneous: occurs as a complication of underlying lung disease such as asthma, cystic fibrosis (CF), connective tissue disorders, infections, malignancies, and interstitial lung disease.

Etiology

- Spontaneous pneumothorax is very rare but more common in males.

Risk Factors

- Tall, thin males aged 10 to 30 years.
- Smoking.
- Underlying lung disease or connective tissue disorder.

Pathophysiology

- Acute increase in transpulmonary pressure that causes alveolar overdistention and rupture.
- Defects in visceral pleura, generally caused by underlying lung disease.
- Catamenial pneumothorax.
  - Spontaneous pneumothorax triggered by menstruation and thought to be associated with thoracic endometriosis.

Clinical Presentation

- History: typically no inciting event for spontaneous pneumothorax.
- Patient may report symptoms occurring after a maneuver that increases intrathoracic pressure, including Valsalva maneuver or other type of straining.
- Patients with traumatic pneumothorax will generally report a history of blunt injury such as a trauma or fall.

Symptoms

- May be asymptomatic.
- Pleuritic chest pain (e.g., sharp and worse with inspiration) and dyspnea.
- Chest pain usually resolves or changes to a dull pain within 1 to 3 days despite the persistence of the pneumothorax.

Physical Examination

- Ipsilateral hyperresonance to percussion, decreased air entry, and decreased vocal fremitus.

Clinical Findings

- Hypoxia, which can be acute.
- Tachycardia.
- Increased PIP or decreased expired tidal volume on mechanical ventilator.
- Tension pneumothorax.
  - May result in tracheal deviation, decreased cardiac output leading to hypotension, tachycardia, and hypoxemia.
  - *Medical emergency* requiring immediate intervention.

Diagnostic Evaluation

- Diagnosis typically confirmed with a posterior–anterior chest radiograph.
  - A lateral decubitus film may be needed if suspicion is high, but PA film is normal.
- CT may help identify underlying blebs/bullae or very small pneumothoraces not detected by radiography.
- There are multiple equations for calculating size of pneumothorax in adults, but these methods are not accurate in the pediatric population.
- Laboratory evaluation: ABG may reveal decreased Pao_2.

Management

- Treatment is determined by type and size of pneumothorax and the clinical condition of the patient.
- Observation.
  - Stable patients may only require observation with pulse oximetry and cardiorespiratory monitoring.
  - During observation, patient should receive 100% oxygen delivered via face mask to "wash out" nitrogen from pleural space.
- Needle aspiration: Air is aspirated via a temporary needle inserted at the second intercostal space at the midclavicular line.
- Thoracostomy tube: Catheter is placed in the pleural space at fourth, fifth, or sixth intercostal space at the midaxillary line and connected to water seal or suction.
- Surgical intervention: video-assisted thoracoscopic surgery (VATS) and/or pleurodesis.

PEARLS

- *Conservative and noninvasive treatment options should be considered first in the clinically stable patient*
- *Tension pneumothorax is diagnosed by clinical findings and is considered a medical emergency*

Asthma

Megan Trahan

Definition

- A chronic disorder that results in airway inflammation.
- Characterized by episodes of cough, wheeze, dyspnea, and chest tightness.
- Associated with airflow obstruction.
- Status asthmaticus results from progressively worsening bronchospasm and airflow obstruction that is unresponsive to conventional therapy for asthma.

Etiology/Types

- Triggers.
  - Extrinsic: allergic/immunologic factors.
  - Intrinsic: Infectious process, very common trigger for status asthmaticus.
  - Exercise-induced bronchospasm.
- Severity classification.
  - Intermittent asthma.
    - Symptoms (difficulty breathing, wheezing, chest tightness, and coughing).
      - Occur fewer than 2 days per week.
      - Do not interfere with normal activities.
      - Nighttime symptoms occur fewer than 2 days per month.
  - Mild persistent asthma.

- Symptoms occur more than 2 days a week, but do not occur every day; they interfere with daily activities.
- Nighttime symptoms occur 3 to 4 times per month.
- Lung function tests are normal when there are no symptoms.
- Lung function tests are ≥80% of the expected value and may vary slightly (peak expiratory flow [PEF] varies 20%–30%) from morning to afternoon.
- Moderate persistent asthma.
  - Symptoms occur daily and interfere with daily activities.
  - Inhaled short-acting asthma medication is used daily.
  - Nighttime symptoms occur more than 1 time per week, but do not happen daily.
  - Lung function tests are abnormal (e.g., >60% and <80% of the expected value); PEF varies more than 30% from morning to afternoon.
- Severe persistent asthma.
  - Symptoms occur every day and severely limit daily physical activities.
  - Nighttime symptoms occur often, sometimes every night.
  - Lung function tests are abnormal (≤60% of expected value); PEF varies >30% from morning to afternoon.
- Acute asthma exacerbation.
  - Mild symptoms: Tachypnea without accessory muscle use.
    - Heart rate is <100 beats per minute.
    - Pulsus paradoxus is not present.
    - Auscultation of chest reveals moderate wheezing, which is often end-expiratory.
    - Oxygen saturation in room air is >95%.
  - Moderate symptoms: Tachypnea and accessory muscles use are common.
    - Loud expiratory wheeze with suprasternal retractions present.
    - Pulsus paradoxus may be present (e.g., 10–20 mmHg).
    - Oxygen saturation in room air is 91% to 95%.
  - Severe symptoms.
    - Tachypnea; respiratory rate >30 breaths per minute, based on age and activity.
    - Accessory muscles use with suprasternal retractions common.
    - Heart rate >120 beats per minute.

- Wheezing; biphasic (e.g., expiratory and inspiratory); usually loud.
- Pulsus paradoxus, common (e.g., 20–40 mmHg).
- Oxygen saturation <91% in room air.

Pathophysiology

- Processes of asthma: triad.
  - Bronchoconstriction.
  - Airway hyperresponsiveness.
  - Airway inflammation.
- Phases of asthma exacerbation.
  - Initial phase: Mast cells, eosinophils, T lymphocytes, macrophages, neutrophils, and epithelial cells initiate inflammatory process.
  - Mast cells cause histamine release, resulting in mucosal edema, mucous production, and bronchospasm.
  - Late phase: Infiltration and congestion of airways leads to obstruction and respiratory insufficiency.
  - Alterations in epithelium, smooth muscle, and bronchial blood vessels may lead to airway remodeling.

Clinical Presentation

- Common symptoms include wheezing, shortness of breath, chest or abdominal pain, and cough which is often at night.
- Symptomatology is often related to trigger.
  - Viral trigger: fever, rhinorrhea, sick contact exposure.
  - IgE-mediated trigger: strong patient or family history of atopy/allergies (Table 3.1).
- Other signs and symptoms.
  - Forced or prolonged expiratory phase.
  - Hypoxia related to ventilation/perfusion (V/Q) mismatch.
  - Pulsus paradoxus, especially when severe asthma exacerbation is combined with hypovolemia.

Diagnostic Evaluation

- Laboratory.
  - ABG (not required in mild/moderate exacerbations).
    - Hypoxemia and hypocarbia with early or mild asthma exacerbation (e.g., respiratory alkalosis).
    - Worsening air trapping results in an inability to clear carbon dioxide, leading to normal or elevated $Paco_2$ (e.g., respiratory acidosis).
  - Serum lactate level; elevated.

TABLE 3.1	Asthma Presentation by Severity		
Mild	**Moderate**	**Severe**	**Impending Respiratory Failure**
Exertional dyspnea Slight tachypnea No retractions No increased work of breathing.	Dyspnea at rest, some difficulty with phonation, tachypnea, loud expiratory wheezing, retractions, accessory muscle use, mild tachycardia, pulsus paradoxus of 10–25 mmHg, PEF 40%–69%, Spo_2 90%–95%.	Dyspnea at rest, tripod position, difficulty with phonation, agitation, tachypnea, inspiratory and expiratory wheezing, retractions and accessory muscle use, tachycardia, pulsus paradoxus of 20–40 mmHg, PEF <40%, Spo_2 <90.	Drowsy or confused, paradoxical thoracoabdominal movement, "silent chest" with absence of wheezing, bradycardia, no pulsus paradoxus secondary to muscle fatigue.

- Electrolyte panel.
  - Evaluates Degree of dehydration and acidosis.
  - Hypokalemia; intracellular shifts of potassium are associated with β-agonist therapy.
  - Magnesium level; in anticipation of magnesium sulfate therapy.
- Imaging: chest radiography.
  - Not required for all children with asthma.
  - Evaluates for suspected pneumonia, pneumothorax and other air leak syndromes, cardiomegaly, pulmonary edema.
  - Common findings:
    - Hyperinflation with flattened diaphragms.
    - Peribronchial thickening.
    - Narrowed cardiac silhouette.

Acute Management

- Initial interventions.
  - Supplemental oxygen—*first priority*.
  - IV fluids.
    - Increased insensible losses with tachypnea.
    - Avoid overhydration; risk for pulmonary edema.
  - β-agonists (e.g., albuterol, levalbuterol).
    - Sympathomimetic medication, result in bronchial smooth muscle relaxation.
    - Intermittent dosing with inhaled nebulization (usually three doses in the first hour) or metered-dose inhaler.
    - Continuous nebulization for refractory asthma exacerbation; typically 10 to 20 mg/hour.
  - Corticosteroids target underlying airway inflammation.
    - IV formulation recommended in severe exacerbations or with high doses of β-agonist; a 3- to 5-day course typically recommended.
    - Taper dosing is recommended for steroid therapy >5 days.
  - Anticholinergics (e.g., ipratropium bromide).
    - Promotes bronchodilation without affecting mucociliary clearance.
    - Used most frequently in the emergency department to prevent hospitalization; data limited on inpatient use.
- Admission criteria.
  - Symptoms after observation for 60 minutes.
  - Oxygen requirement.
  - Short-acting β-agonist required more than every 2 to 3 hours.
  - Prior ICU admissions.

Adjunct Therapies

- Magnesium sulfate is classified as bronchodilator which inhibits calcium-mediated smooth muscle contraction.
  - Usually given as a rapid bolus (over 30 minutes) or as a continuous infusion.
  - Most common adverse reaction is hypotension.
  - Cardiac dysrhythmias noted with very high magnesium levels (10–12 mg/dL).
- Terbutaline and epinephrine are β-agonists delivered through intravenous or subcutaneous route.

- Terbutaline.
  - Administered as a bolus with or without infusion.
  - Monitor EKG and cardiac enzymes for myocardial ischemia.
- Methylxanthines (e.g., theophylline, aminophylline).
  - Promote bronchial smooth muscle relaxation by unknown mechanism.
  - Used for patients with status asthmaticus refractory to steroids and inhaled/IV β-agonists.
  - Narrow therapeutic window; monitor drug levels.
    - Therapeutic level 10 to 20 mcg/mL.
  - High side-effect profile (e.g., nausea, vomiting, abdominal discomfort, arrhythmias, seizures).
- Antimicrobials.
  - Common coinfections include pneumonia or acute sinusitis.
  - Macrolides have anti-inflammatory properties, although studies do not recommend empiric macrolide use.
- Helium–oxygen mixture (Heliox): inhaled (no definitive evidence that this works).
  - Helium: low-density gas that reduces airflow resistance and allows laminar flow.
  - Enhances inhaled β-agonist delivery.
  - Mixtures include 60/40 (i.e., 60% helium, 40% oxygen), 70/30, and 80/20.
  - Can also be entrained into ventilator or noninvasive ventilator circuits.
    - Lowers peak airway pressures, facilitates weaning, but limited use if severe hypoxemia.
- Noninvasive mechanical ventilation: includes CPAP and BiPAP.
  - Used for hypoxemia or increased work of breathing.
  - Reduces work of breathing and dyspnea.
  - Limited by patient cooperation.
- High-flow nasal cannula can be used as a noninvasive method of respiratory support.
- Mechanical ventilation (used in cases refractory to other therapies).
  - Increased risk for barotrauma, air leak syndromes, nosocomial infection, pulmonary edema, circulatory dysfunction, steroid/muscle relaxant–associated myopathy, and death.
  - Anticipate hypotension with onset of positive pressure ventilation (PPV) related to dehydration combined with the effects of PPV on preload.
  - Allow permissive hypercapnia, long expiratory phase with slow ventilator rates.
- ECMO or inhaled anesthesia may be considered in extreme cases.

Chronic Management

- Controllers: stepwise therapy; based on National Heart, Lung, and Blood guidelines.
- β-agonist: monitor usage; >2 canisters per month requires reevaluation.
- Asthma Action Plan: details when to use medications, call providers, and seek emergency care. Provided to each patient on every encounter.
- Identify and avoid triggers; consider allergy evaluation.

- *Assess risk factors for asthma severity*
  - *Previous PICU admissions*
  - *History of respiratory failure requiring mechanical ventilation*
  - *Previous sudden deterioration*
- *For acute exacerbation, primary intervention is oxygen, followed by inhaled β-agonists*
- *For respiratory acidosis, lowering the ventilator rate will prolong the exhalation phase and facilitate carbon dioxide removal in acute status asthmaticus*
- *Follow National Institute of Health guidelines: National Heart, Lung, and Blood Institute, National Asthma Education and Prevention Program, 2007, Expert Panel 3: Guidelines for the diagnosis and management of asthma*
- *Every child should have Asthma Action Plan, required by Joint Commission for hospital discharge, and includes environmental controls, algorithm for use of long-term and rescue medications, medication regimens and rescue medications, and steps to take when treatment is not effective/emergent care*

Bronchiolitis
Danielle Mashburn

Background/Definition
- Viral infection of bronchiolar epithelium usually occurs in children <2 years of age.
- Typical pathogens include respiratory syncytial virus (RSV), adenovirus, influenza, parainfluenza, and human metapneumovirus (hMPV).

Etiology
- Risk factors for severe disease include:
  - Prematurity, infants <6 months of age, underlying cardiopulmonary disease, and immunodeficiency.

Pathophysiology
- Usually begins as upper respiratory tract infection that spreads to lower respiratory tract (bronchioles) within the first few days of illness.
- Characterized by submucosal edema, increased mucus production, and increased airway resistance/wheezing.
- Bronchiolar changes cause airway obstruction leading to:
  - Air trapping resulting in hyperinflation.
  - V/Q mismatch resulting in hypoxemia.

Clinical Presentation
- Upper respiratory tract symptoms (e.g., rhinorrhea, congestion, low-grade fever).

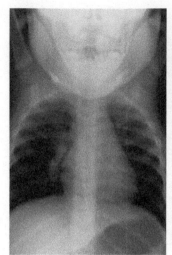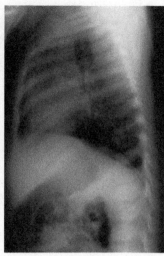

FIGURE 3.5 • **Bronchiolitis Chest Radiographs**. Chest radiographs of 6-month-old infant with hMPV bronchiolitis, showing hyperinflation and diffuse perihilar infiltrates.

- Lower respiratory tract symptoms (cough, tachypnea, dyspnea, decreased oral intake).
- Physical examination findings: hypoxia, respiratory distress, diffuse crackles/rhonchi, expiratory wheeze, prolonged expiratory phase, irritability.

Diagnostic Evaluation
- Majority of cases can be diagnosed based on history and physical examination.
- Laboratory testing, if indicated (or if needed for isolation purposes).
  - Respiratory viral culture or polymerase chain reaction.
  - Blood gas analysis: moderate/severe cases.
- Chest radiography.
  - Patchy atelectasis, peribronchial thickening, perihilar prominence, airspace disease, hyperinflation (see Figure 3.5).

Management
- Supportive therapy is mainstay.
  - Oxygen supplementation, rehydration, secretion clearance.
  - Routine use of corticosteroids, racemic epinephrine, and bronchodilators is *not* recommended.
- In severe cases, patient may require initiation of:
  - High-flow nasal cannula therapy, NIPPV or mechanical ventilation.

Chronic Lung Disease (Bronchopulmonary Dysplasia)
Danielle Mashburn

Definition
- A form of chronic lung disease occurring in premature infants.

- The result of acute respiratory disease that originates in the neonatal period.

Risk Factors

- Prematurity, intrauterine growth restriction, extremely low birth weight, family history of lung disease, ventilator-associated volutrauma or barotrauma, oxygen toxicity, increased pulmonary blood flow, infection.

Pathophysiology

- Preterm birth leads to an arrest of normal development of lung airways and vasculature.
  - Dysfunction of terminal respiratory units.
  - Higher elastic recoil.
- Postnatal injury results in disordered repair of the underdeveloped lung tissue.
  - Causes of postnatal injury include oxygen toxicity, ventilator-associated trauma, infection.
  - Mediators of epithelial lung injury cause chronic inflammation and fibrosis.

Clinical Presentation

- Premature infant born with severe respiratory distress syndrome.
  - Tachypnea, retractions, scattered rales, hypoxemia, periods of apnea, cyanosis, hypercarbia, increased anterior–posterior chest diameter.
- Long-standing oxygen requirement (>28 days postnatally), chronic diuretic and bronchodilator dependence.

Diagnostic Evaluation

- Chest radiography.
  - Initial findings: pulmonary edema, atelectasis, hyperinflation.

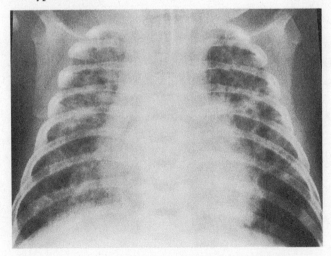

FIGURE 3.6 • **Bronchopulmonary Dysplasia Chest Radiograph.** This 2-month-old child was treated with mechanical ventilation during the first days of life for hyaline membrane disease. The chest radiograph shows generalized overaeration and course modularity with multiple cyst-like areas throughout both lung fields.

- Chronic findings: hyperexpansion (air trapping), areas of focal hyperlucency (cystic changes), linear stranding (fibrosis) (see Figure 3.6).
- Blood gas analysis: evaluates the ability to oxygenate and ventilate.
  - Respiratory acidosis usually present.
- ECHO: evaluates for congenital heart disease (CHD) as cause of respiratory distress.
- Otolaryngology evaluation: to exclude anatomic airway abnormalities.

Management

- Therapies to avoid preterm birth.
- Supportive care.
  - Goal: Promote neonatal growth while supporting respiratory needs and minimizing further injury through:
    - Lung-protective ventilator strategies or use of NIPPV as able.
    - Maintaining functional residual capacity by using optimal PEEP levels.
    - Judicious use of diuretic and bronchodilators.
    - Use of antibiotics until pulmonary infection excluded.
    - Prevent gastroesophageal reflux disease.
    - Nutritional support: may require nasogastric or gastrostomy tube feedings.
- Use of steroids remains controversial and is not currently recommended (Table 3.2).

Congenital Central Hypoventilation Syndrome

Danielle Mashburn

Definition

- Inadequate respiratory drive as a result of a genetic defect in the autonomic nervous system's control of breathing.

Etiology

- Mutation of PHOX2B gene.
  - Gene is essential for embryologic development of the autonomic nervous system in the neural chest.
  - Majority of cases are a result of spontaneous gene mutation.
  - In a small percentage of cases, congenital central hypoventilation syndrome is inherited (autosomal dominant).

Pathophysiology

- PHOX2B gene defect results in an abnormality of integration of chemoreceptors responsible for autonomic control of breathing.
  - Leads to abnormal function of ventilatory muscles and inadequate ventilation.
  - Patients fail to produce an appropriate ventilatory response to hypercarbia and hypoxemia.

TABLE 3.2	Etiology of Pediatric Chronic Lung Disease
Pulmonary diseases	Cystic fibrosis, asthma, bronchopulmonary dysplasia, acute respiratory distress syndrome, bronchiectasis, pulmonary hemorrhage disorders, primary ciliary dyskinesia, alveolar proteinosis, interstitial lung disease.
Congenital defects	Diaphragmatic hernia, pulmonary hypoplasia, tracheoesophageal fistula, esophageal atresia, complete tracheal rings, chest wall deformities, congenital heart disease.
Cardiac diseases	Patent ductus arteriosus, left ventricular heart failure.
Systemic diseases	Collagen vascular diseases, juvenile idiopathic arthritis (newer term), systemic lupus erythematosus, vasculitis, sarcoidosis, storage and metabolic disease, immune deficiency diseases.
Neuromuscular diseases	Spinal muscular atrophy.
Infections	Pneumonia, bronchiolitis, sepsis, lung abscess, or empyema.
Lung injury	Chronic aspiration pneumonitis, gastroesophageal reflux, swallow dysfunction, oxygen toxicity, ventilator-induced lung injury, inhalation.
Thermal	Smoke, toxic chemical, exposure, therapeutic drug, radiation.

Clinical Presentation

- Usually presents in the newborn period.
  - Apnea, respiratory arrest, hypopnea, cyanosis, tachycardia, diaphoresis, lethargy, hypercarbia, hypoxemia.
- Patients who present outside of newborn period.
  - Learning disabilities, growth failure, cor pulmonale.
  - Develop worsening symptoms with sleep.
  - *Do not* show classic signs of respiratory distress (e.g., tachypnea, retractions).
    - Exhibit monotonous respiratory rate and work of breathing despite hypoxemia and hypercarbia.

Diagnostic Evaluation

- Genetic testing for PHOX2B gene mutation.
- Polysomnography.
  - Findings include hypoventilation, hypoxemia, decreased minute ventilation, and frequent arousal.
- Studies to evaluate for underlying metabolic, pulmonary, cardiac, or brainstem disease.
  - ECHO, chest radiography, brain MRI, urine amino and organic acids.

Management

- Normalization of ventilation.
  - Tracheostomy with mechanical ventilation.
  - Chronic NIPPV.
  - Diaphragmatic pacing.
- Supplemental oxygen is not adequate because it does not address hypoventilation.
- Need continuous pulse oximetry and end-tidal CO_2 monitoring.
- Early intervention may improve long-term neurodevelopmental outcome.

Congenital Diaphragmatic Hernia

Danielle Mashburn

Definition

- Congenital defect of diaphragm resulting in herniation of gastrointestinal contents into thoracic cavity.
- Typically occurs on the left side of the chest.

Etiology

- Failure of pleuroperitoneal folds to close at 6 to 8 weeks gestation.

Pathophysiology

- Abdominal viscera herniate through diaphragmatic defect into thoracic cavity.
- The resultant mass effect causes lung hypoplasia.
  - Primarily occurs on ipsilateral side, but contralateral lung can also be hypoplastic.
  - Reduction in pulmonary mass impairs oxygenation and ventilation, resulting in respiratory insufficiency or failure.

Clinical Presentation

- Signs of respiratory failure in immediate newborn period.
  - Hypercarbia, hypoxia.
- Physical examination findings: retractions, tachypnea, grunting, cyanosis, absent breaths, increased chest diameter, sounds on ipsilateral side, heart sounds shifted to contralateral side, scaphoid abdomen, presence of bowel sounds in thorax.

Diagnostic Evaluation

- Antenatal ultrasound.

- Commonly occurs in infants with a history of polyhydramnios.
  - Often diagnosed prior to birth: allows for counseling and postnatal planning.
- Chest radiography.
  - Fluid-filled loops of bowel seen in thoracic cavity.
  - Associated mediastinal shift (see Figure 3.7).
- ECHO.
  - Allows ability to evaluate for cardiac dysfunction and measures systemic and pulmonary pressures.
- Chromosomal evaluation as disorder is frequently associated with anomalies.

Management

- Cardiorespiratory stabilization.
  - Immediate intubation, sedation, and stomach decompression.
  - Bag-mask ventilation should be avoided as this will introduce air into gastrointestinal tract, worsening lung compression.
  - Lung-protective strategies (when stable) and pulmonary hypertension management.
  - Consider ECMO if conventional ventilation fails.
- Delayed surgical intervention to repair defect.
  - Can be considered after hemodynamic stabilization and resolution of pulmonary hypertension.
- Ongoing pulmonary care.
  - Chronic lung disease is common source of morbidity for survivors of congenital diaphragmatic hernia (CDH).

Laryngotracheobronchitis/Croup

Andrea M. Kline-Tilford

Background/Definition

- An infection involving the subglottic airway, larynx, trachea, and bronchi.
- Most common in children 6 months to 3 years of age, affects males > females.
- Peak incidence is late fall.

Etiology/Types

- Most commonly caused by parainfluenza types 1 and 2.
- Less commonly caused by RSV, influenza types A and B, and parainfluenza type 3.
- Infrequently caused by *Mycoplasma pneumoniae*.

Pathophysiology

- Mucosal airway edema from infectious pathogen.
- Subsequent epithelial necrosis.
  - Reduced airway diameter results in increased resistance to airflow and increased work of breathing.
- Poiseuille's law: Resistance = $8 \times$ viscosity $\times$ length$/\pi \times$ radius^4.
- Decreasing airway diameter dramatically increases airway resistance and increases the flow rate—*Venturi effect*.

Clinical Presentation

- Barking cough, hoarseness, stridor which may be on inspiration only or biphasic.

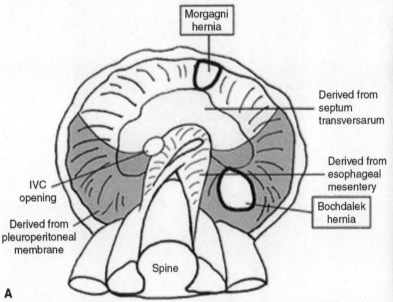

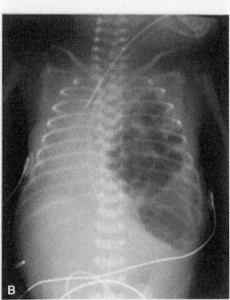

FIGURE 3.7 • **Diaphragmatic Hernia. A:** Abdominal surface of the diaphragm and the derivation of the components during development. The pleuroperitoneal membranes, the septum transversum, and the esophageal mesentery form the diaphragm. A Bochdalek hernia forms when there is a posterolateral defect. Morgagni hernias are less common and are present anteriorly. **B:** Chest radiograph of a child with a congenital posterolateral (Bochdalek) diaphragmatic hernia on the left. The mediastinum is displaced to the right by the intestinal loops present in the left chest.

- Frequently begins 12 to 48 hours after symptoms of a nonspecific respiratory illness.

Diagnostic Evaluation

- Westley croup score (published symptom scoring tool).
  - Provides an objective measure for disease severity.
- Generally diagnosed on history and physical examination.
- Consider lateral neck films.
  - Haziness or narrowing of subglottic area.
  - Distention of hypopharynx.
- Consider chest radiography.
  - Narrowing of subglottic area (e.g., "steeple sign") (see Figure 3.8).
  - Positive findings noted only in approximately 50% of studies.

Management

- Supportive care.
- Humidified or cooled air / gas.
  - Provides soothing vasoconstriction of airway tissue.
- Steroids: dexamethasone 0.6 mg/kg IV/IM.
- Oxygen and additional respiratory support/maneuvers, as needed.
- Consider nebulized epinephrine solution.
  - Results in vasoconstriction of mucosal vasculature.

- Antipyretics, if febrile, and consider IV fluid administration.
- Consider heliox administration.
  - Increases laminar flow of gas, improves airway mechanics, and reduces respiratory workload.
- Consult otolaryngology if patient fails to improve with standard medical therapy.

PEARLS

- *Symptoms typically more prominent at night, peak in 48 hours and can last up to 1 week*
- *Accounts for up to 90% of infectious airway obstruction*

Cystic Fibrosis
Ruth DeVoogd

Background/Definition

- An inherited chronic disease affecting multiple body systems, primarily the lungs and pancreas.
- Most common in Caucasians.
- Life expectancy is increasing; median life expectancy approximately 37 years.

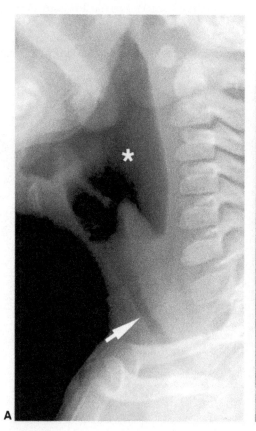
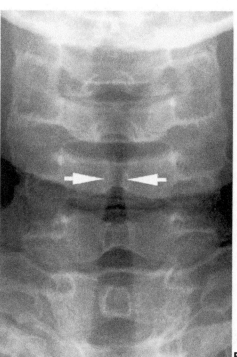

FIGURE 3.8 • **Steeple Sign**. Viral croup in an 18-month-old boy. **A:** Lateral view of the neck shows marked subglottic tracheal narrowing (arrow) and distension of the hypopharynx (*). **B:** Frontal view in another patient shows narrowing of the subglottic trachea (arrows).

Etiology/Types

- Autosomal recessive disorder.
- Over 1,500 gene mutations identified which cause CF; some mutations cause more mild disease.

Pathophysiology

- Defective gene makes an abnormal protein, which impairs movement of salt and water across the epithelial cell wall in the exocrine glands, leading to thick sticky secretions.
- Body systems affected include:
  - Lungs.
    - Sticky mucus traps bacteria in the airways and causes a cycle of infection and inflammation, leading to airways destruction and eventually respiratory failure and death.
  - Pancreas.
    - Sticky mucus blocks the pancreatic ducts, impairing the excretion of pancreatic enzymes and bicarbonate (which are necessary for digestion of nutrients), in turn leading to malabsorption and malnutrition.
    - Majority of individuals are pancreatic insufficient and require pancreatic enzyme replacement therapy.
    - CF-related diabetes may develop due to impaired insulin production.
    - Pancreatitis may develop in small number of individuals who are pancreatic sufficient.
  - Intestines.
    - Fat and protein malabsorption lead to poor growth and large, oily, foul-smelling stools. Risk for constipation and obstruction.
  - Liver.
    - Thick secretions block bile ducts and may lead to liver damage.
  - Sinuses.
    - Sticky mucus builds up and leads to poor drainage. Sinus disease, infection, and nasal polyps are common.
  - Reproductive tract.
    - 98% of males are infertile due to damage to vas deferens; some females have difficulty getting pregnant due to thick cervical mucus.
  - Sweat glands.
    - Abnormally high levels of sodium and chloride are lost through sweat, leading to increased risk for dehydration.

Clinical Presentation

- Traditional signs: poor growth, large foul-smelling and oily stools, increased appetite, and frequent respiratory infections.
- Since newborn screening for CF provides an early diagnosis, infants may present well-nourished without any respiratory involvement.
- Pulmonary: cough, increased sputum, crackles, wheezing, shortness of breath, hemoptysis, chest pain, and hypoxemia; occasionally pneumothorax.
- Gastrointestinal tract: periumbilical or right lower quadrant (RLQ) pain, constipation, loose stools, flatus, abdominal distention, vomiting. RLQ pain mimics appendicitis; however,

is usually due to constipation or distal intestinal obstruction syndrome (DIOS).
- Weight loss.
- Dehydration: *Hypochloremic* and *hyponatremic* alkalosis.
- Hyperglycemia: If has impaired glucose tolerance or CF-related diabetes.

Diagnostic Evaluation

- Sweat chloride test: noninvasive test. Sweat chloride ≥ 60 mmol/L (>30 mmol/L in infants).
- Genotype: positive for combination of mutations.
- Pulmonary exacerbation: Chest radiography (may or may not show acute process), decline in pulmonary function test (FEV_1), oxygen saturation, sputum or throat culture, high-resolution chest CT scan may be indicated.
- Gastrointestinal complications: abdominal radiography to evaluate for constipation, DIOS, abdominal ultrasound.

Laboratory Testing

- CBC with differential, electrolytes, BUN, creatinine, glucose, liver panel with γ-glutamyl transferase, prothrombin time (PT)/international normalized ratio (INR).
- Hemoglobin A1C if history of CF-related diabetes or weight loss.
- Culture for CF pathogens: expectorated sputum (preferred), throat culture, or BAL.

Management

- Pulmonary exacerbation.
  - Airway clearance (e.g., high-frequency chest wall oscillation [vest therapy], handheld device, intrapulmonary percussive ventilator).
  - Airway hydrators (e.g., Dornase alpha [Pulmozyme], hypertonic saline).
  - Antibiotics to cover typical CF pathogens.
    - *Pseudomonas aeruginosa*: aminoglycosides, antipseudomonal penicillins, β-lactams, cephalosporins (third and fourth generations), and fluoroquinolones.
      - CF patients usually clear aminoglycosides more rapidly, necessitating a higher mg-per-kg dose than normal.
    - *Staphylococcus aureus*: antistaphylococcal penicillins, cephalosporins, TMP/SMX, some fluoroquinolones.
    - Methicillin-resistant *Staphylococcus aureus* (MRSA): TMP/SMX, linezolid, vancomycin, clindamycin.
    - *Burkholderia cepacia* complex: meropenem, *plus* one other (e.g., aminocycline, amikacin, ceftazidime, chloramphenicol, TMP/SMX).
  - Aerosolized antibiotics: tobramycin (Tobi), aztreonam (Cayston).
  - Oral antibiotics: depending on airway culture results and susceptibilities.
- Abdominal pain.
  - DIOS: laxative, polyethylene glycol (Miralax, GoLytely), enema (saline or Gastrografin), stool softener.
  - Acute abdomen: surgery consult to evaluate for severe obstruction, appendicitis, intussusception.

- Hyperglycemia.
  - Monitor blood glucose levels, treat if indicated.
  - Risk in CF-related diabetes is that patient will become hypoglycemic because of the production of insulin.

PEARLS

- *Consider the diagnosis of CF in any patient with poor growth and frequent respiratory infections*
- *Newborn screening is not a diagnostic procedure and may not detect all individuals with CF*
- *If airway culture results are unknown or patient quite ill, treat for Pseudomonas initially while waiting for culture results*
- *Cepacia syndrome, which occurs in patients who culture Burkholderia cepacia complex, is life-threatening. Syndrome involves rapid decline, fever, bacteremia, and necrotizing pneumonia*
- *Appendix is often enlarged in CF, even without appendicitis. An abdominal CT may show this enlargement, but patient may not require surgical intervention*
- *A child who presents with hyponatremia and hypochloremia should always be suspected of having CF*

Foreign Body Aspiration

Andrea M. Kline-Tilford

Background/Definition

- A complete or near complete obstruction of the larynx or trachea with a foreign object.
- Complete airway obstruction can result in immediate asphyxia and death if not immediately dislodged.
- Partial airway obstruction symptoms can vary depending on the size and location of the foreign object.
- Children with underlying neurologic disease are at increased risk of foreign body aspiration (FBA).
- Children/adolescents under the influence of alcohol or drugs are at increased risk for FBA.

Epidemiology

- Common in children, with approximately 160 annual pediatric deaths.
- Accounts for >17,000 emergency department visits in children <14 years of age.

Etiology/Types

- Food items are common in all pediatric age groups.
- Nonfood items more common in older pediatric patients (e.g., pen caps, paperclips).

Pathophysiology

- Aspirated objects passing the level of the carina will lodge in a location determined by the size of the child, characteristics of the object aspirated, underlying anatomy, and position of the child during the aspiration event.

Clinical Presentation

- Acute complete obstruction results in asphyxiation and death.
- Acute noncomplete obstruction.
  - Symptoms can vary based on size and location of partial obstruction, but often include a combination of the following: coughing, gagging, choking, wheezing, respiratory distress.
  - Decreased breath sounds over affected lung (if foreign body is in the bronchial tree position).
- Late noncomplete obstruction.
  - Paroxysmal cough, fever and local inflammation, edema, and granulation tissue formation.
- Three stages in noncomplete obstruction FBA.
  - Initial event.
  - Asymptomatic period.
  - Symptoms of ensuing complications.

Diagnostic Evaluation

- History is most important.
- Chest radiography.
  - Most helpful views include:
    - Posterior–anterior views.
    - Lateral decubitus.
    - Inspiratory and expiratory (may be difficult to obtain in infants and young children).
- Chest fluoroscopy.
- Chest CT scan.
- Bronchoscopy (rigid): may be used to visualize and retrieve the object.

Management

- Prompt diagnosis and management are critical.
- Acute presentation.
  - Back blows/chest compressions (infant).
  - Abdominal thrusts (child).
- Direct visualization and manual retrieval (bronchoscopy).

PEARLS

- *Care with transportation of the child with suspected FBA is important as the object can shift to occlude the airway completely*
- *Caregivers commonly believe that the object has been relieved when coughing resolves*
- *A delay in diagnosis is not uncommon*
- *Symptoms of cough, wheezing, and decreased breath sounds can be similar to common childhood diseases (e.g., asthma, bronchiolitis, and pneumonia)*

Lung Transplantation

Carole A. Branch

Background/Definition

- Surgical procedure to replace diseased lung or lungs when all other therapies have been exhausted.

- Trajectory of illness puts individual at risk of dying without lung transplant.

Etiology

- Most common indications in children 0 to 18 years.
  - CF.
    - Baseline FEV_1 <30% of predicted value.
    - Pao_2 <55 mmHg at rest.
    - Worsening severity of hypercapnia.
      - Female pediatric patient with rapid decline in lung function.
      - Frequent respiratory exacerbations requiring hospitalization and IV therapy with no improvement in lung function.
  - Pulmonary hypertension.
    - New York Heart Association/World health Organization functional class III or IV: rapidly progressive disease, elevated right arterial pressures >15 mmHg, cardiac index <2 L/minute/m², failing medical therapy.
  - Other indications for lung transplantation include surfactant dysfunction syndromes, CHD, chronic lung disease, bronchiolitis obliterans (BO), and pulmonary fibrosis.

Evaluation/Referral

- Referral for transplant is usually made by a pulmonologist.
- Evaluation process.
  - Series of diagnostic tests, procedures, and assessments.
  - Evaluation of support system and ability to follow rigorous therapy, daily monitoring, and reevaluation schedule following transplant.
  - Prescribed medical regimen.
  - Tiered allocation scores (lung allocation score).
  - Age <12 years is listed as Priority I or II based on medical condition.
    - Priority I: Respiratory failure or supplemental O_2 to achieve Fio_2 >50% in order to maintain O_2 levels >90% OR arterial or capillary Pco >50 mmHg or a venous Pco_2 >56 mmHg or pulmonary hypertension.
    - Priority II: All other candidates that do not meet criteria for Priority I.
  - Age >12 years.
    - Score from 0 to 100 calculated: based on evaluation criteria.
    - Higher score receives higher priority, based on age, diagnosis, indicators of disease severity, likelihood of successful transplant.
    - Other factors in listing for transplant include blood type, height weight, and geographical area.
  - Contraindications for lung transplant: absolute or relative.
    - Absolute contraindications include malignancy within past 2 years, immunodeficiency syndrome, hepatitis B or C with liver disease, severe neuromuscular disease, multiorgan system dysfunction.
    - Relative contraindications include pleurodesis, renal insufficiency, markedly abnormal body mass index (BMI), chronic airway infection with specified organisms, severe scoliosis, active collagen disease, mechanical ventilation, among others.

Diagnostic Transplant Evaluation

- Organs matched by height, weight, blood type.
- HLA antibody screening is performed.
  - Specific antibodies can be avoided if recipient has elevated antibody levels.

Postoperative Considerations

- ICU settings with mechanical ventilation and chest tubes for first 24 to 48 hours.
- IV antibiotics to cover previous organisms, donor organisms, and current cultures.
- Pulmonary rehabilitation.
- Immunosuppressive therapy: triple therapy per International Pediatric Lung Transplant Consortium.

Potential Postoperative Complications

- Early complications can include hyperacute rejection, primary graft dysfunction, acute rejection, ectopic atrial tachycardia, airway complications, infection, damage to phrenic nerve resulting in diaphragmatic paralysis.
- Late complications include acute or chronic rejection, bronchiolitis obliterans syndrome (BOS), infection, diabetes, hypertension, kidney failure, posttransplant lymphoproliferative disease, osteoporosis.
- Infection: major cause of morbidity and mortality during the first 6 months after transplant.
  - Prevention: prophylactic antimicrobial against bacterial, fungal, and viral causes. Cytomegalovirus (CMV) is the most commonly encountered serious viral infection.
  - CMV pneumonitis is linked to the development of BO.
  - CMV prophylaxis is used at all transplant centers.
  - Fungal infections: *Candida albicans* and *Aspergillus* are most common.

Rejection

- Acute rejection: Cellular rejection is highest in the first few weeks following transplant.
  - May be difficult to distinguish between rejection and infection.
  - Transbronchial biopsy with BAL surveillance performed on a regular basis based on institutional protocol.
  - Acute rejection graded from A0 (none) to A4 (severe) Grades A2 and higher are treated with high-dose pulse steroids.
  - Refractory acute rejection may be treated with augmentation of immunosuppression with monoclonal or polyclonal T-cell antibodies.
- Chronic rejection/BO.
  - Leading cause of morbidity and late mortality 1 year after lung transplant.
  - Approximately half of all lung transplant patients are diagnosed with BO by 5 years after transplant.
  - BOS is the clinical correlate of BO.
    - Symptoms of BOS: unexplained drop in FEV_1 or the forced expiratory flow (FEF) 25% to 75% on pulmonary function tests (PFTs) which does not respond to bronchodilators, plus dyspnea, wheezing.
    - Treatment: no consistently effective treatment; often consists of augmentation of immunosuppression,

photopheresis, total lymphoid irradiation, azithromycin for anti-inflammatory effect or retransplantation.

- Life expectancy: 1-year survival is close to 85%; median 4.3 years with better outcomes when children are 1 to 10 years of age.

Obstructive Sleep Apnea
Andrea M. Kline-Tilford

Background/Definition

- Intermittent upper airway obstruction during sleep.
- Affects 2% to 3% of school-aged children.
- Peak prevalence 2 to 8 years of age.
- Children with obesity, craniofacial abnormalities, cerebral palsy, and neuromuscular disease are at increased risk for OSA.

Etiology/Types

- Most commonly due to hypertrophy of adenoids and tonsils in relation to airway diameter.
- Also may be due to nasal obstruction, fat deposition in the pharynx, cranial facial abnormalities, or abnormal neuromotor tone.

Pathophysiology

- Obstruction arises from an anatomically narrow upper airway and/or abnormal upper airway neuromotor tone, partially or completely occluding the airway.
- Ineffective gas exchange occurs, resulting in hypoxia or hypercarbia.
- Events are terminated through arousal from stimulation of the central nervous system and respiration is resumed.
- Results in fragmented sleep.

Clinical Presentation

- Varies with age, but typical age is toddler/preschool.
- Loud snoring, gasping, and labored breathing during sleep.
- May also have agitated/mobile sleep.
- Signs of hyperactivity and inattentiveness during wakefulness.
- School-age.
  - Agitated sleep, difficult morning arousal, daytime sleepiness, and learning problems.

Diagnostic Evaluation

- Polysomnogram.
  - Quantifies the number and duration of airway obstructions during sleep.
  - Determines presence of hypoxia and/or hypoventilation during sleep.
  - Identifies sleep fragmentation.
- Additional diagnostic tests to be considered:
  - ABG.
  - EKG.
  - Echocardiography.
  - Lateral neck radiography.

Management

- Referral to otolaryngology for consideration of adenoidectomy/tonsillectomy.
- Monitor postoperatively for hypoxia, persistent oxygen requirement, and postobstructive pulmonary edema.
- Counsel family to monitor for return of symptoms.
- Consider noninvasive ventilation: CPAP or BiPAP.

PEARLS

- *Not all snoring results in OSA*
- *History and physical examination alone are not reliable in distinguishing primary snoring from OSA*
- *OSA should be considered in children evaluated for attention-deficit disorder*
- *Long-term, untreated OSA has been associated with neurocognitive impairment, behavior problems, and cor pulmonale*

Pneumonia
Viswanath Gajula

Background/Definition

- Pneumonia is an infection and inflammation of lower respiratory tract.
- Typically associated with fever, cough, adventitious breath sounds, and alveolar-interstitial changes on chest radiograph.

Etiology

- Community-acquired pneumonia.
  - Most common organisms by age group.
    - Neonate: group B streptococcus, *Escherichia coli*, *Staphylococcus aureus*, herpes simplex virus, *Ureaplasma urealyticum*.
    - Infants up to 1 year of age: RSV is most common cause.
    - 1 to 3 months of age: *Streptococcus pneumoniae*, *Chlamydia trachomatis*, *Bordetella pertussis*, RSV, influenza and parainfluenza virus.
    - 3 months to 5 years of age: viral, *Mycoplasma*, *C. trachomatis*, *Strep. pneumoniae*.
    - >5 years of age: *Strep. pneumoniae*, *Mycoplasma pneumoniae*, *C. trachomatis*.
- Aspiration pneumonia.
  - Most commonly associated with oral anaerobes.
- Health-care–associated or hospital-acquired pneumonia.
  - Most commonly associated with gram-negative bacilli, *Staph. aureus*.
- Opportunistic infections in immunocompromised host.
  - Most commonly associated with *Staph. aureus*, gram-negative bacilli, *Legionella pneumophila*, *Aspergillus*, *Pneumocystis jirovecii*, CMV, herpes simplex virus.

Radiographic Patterns of Pneumonia

- Lobar pneumonia: involving a single lobe or one of lobar segments.

- Bronchopneumonia: involving smaller airways and surrounding interstitium.
- Necrotizing pneumonia: *Staph. aureus, Streptococcus,* commonly.
- Interstitial pneumonia: atypical bacteria, viral.

Pathophysiology

- Inflammatory response to infection includes neutrophil and/or lymphocyte localization, complement activation, and production of toxic free radical species.
- Leads to vasodilation and capillary leak with interstitial edema, epithelial and interstitial damage, with airway obstruction and alveolar filling.

Clinical Signs

- Tachypnea, fever, cough, respiratory distress, grunting in younger children, retractions, and hypoxemia.
- Focal diminished breath sounds, rales (crackles), and tactile fremitus.

Diagnostic Evaluation

- Clinical diagnosis in most cases.
- Clinical presentation often precedes radiographic findings.

Complications

- Parapneumonic effusion, empyema, pulmonary abscess, necrotizing pneumonia.
- Pneumatocele and hyponatremia are possible.

Management

- Antibiotics based on suspected organism and age; tailored to pathogen if specimen obtained.
- Oxygen and other respiratory support maneuvers, as needed.
- Monitor for complications and treatment failures.

Pertussis
Viswanath Gajula

Background/Definition

- Commonly known as whooping cough.
- Caused by *B. pertussis,* which is a nonmotile, aerobic gram-negative coccobacillus.
- Transmitted by aerosol droplets.

Pathophysiology

- Initial exposure, organism-specific adhesion proteins allow adherence to the mucosa of the upper respiratory tract.
- Organisms multiply and progress down the lower respiratory tract to induce cascade of inflammatory processes.
- Mucopurulent exudate leads to airway obstruction, loss of surfactant, pneumonia, and small airway disease.

Presentation

- Commonly in children <5 years of age.
- May be severe in infancy, especially <6 months of age.

- Presentation occurs in three main stages.
  - Initial symptoms (catarrhal stage: 1–2 weeks) can include rhinorrhea and cough. Fever may be mild or absent. Progression to paroxysms of cough.
  - Paroxysmal phase (1–2 weeks): often associated with a "whoop" upon inspiration, followed by a convalescent stage with persistent cough.
  - Disease in infants is often atypical and characterized by shortened or absent catarrhal stage. Gagging, gasping, and/or apnea occur often around feedings and may be life-threatening.
  - Severe pneumonia and hypoxemic respiratory failure may also occur.
  - Classic duration of cough is 6 to 10 weeks, but may be longer in older children and adults.

Diagnostic Evaluation

- Direct fluorescent antibody testing, polymerase chain reaction testing, bacterial culture (confirmatory).
- CBC: lymphocyte-predominant leukocytosis (WBC counts may be elevated to 50–80,000/cm³).
- Chest radiography: Radiographic findings may be absent, or may be suggestive of small airway disease.

Management·

- Antibiotics: Macrolides including azithromycin and erythromycin are the treatment for pertussis. In young infants, azithromycin is recommended as first-line therapy.
- Antibiotic treatment after catarrhal stage does not significantly reduce longevity or severity of disease, except possibly in cases of pneumonia.
- Treatment is most important for preventing spread of disease.

Supportive Care

- Hospitalization of infants with evidence of pneumonia or who are at risk for apnea.
  - Monitor and maintain adequate hydration.
  - Mechanical ventilation may be necessary in infants with significant apnea or with alveolar disease.

PEARLS

- *American Academy of Pediatrics recommends antimicrobial prophylaxis for all exposed close contacts regardless of their immunization status*
- *Suspect pertussis in infants <4 months of age if paroxysmal cough is present*

Pleural and Parapneumonic Effusions
Viswanath Gajula

Background

- Inflammation of pleura secondary to adjacent pneumonia is common and often associated with pleural effusion.

- In early stages, effusion may be transudative, but becomes exudative due to leakage of protein and inflammatory cells.
- *Empyema* is accumulation of pus in the pleural space due to overgrowth of bacteria.

Etiology

- Transudative and exudative pleural effusions.
  - *Transudative*: Serous, acellular fluid collection due to increased hydrostatic pressure across the vascular membrane.
    - Often associated with congestive heart failure, pericarditis, hypoalbuminemia, nephrotic syndrome, peritoneal dialysis.
  - *Exudative*: Due to leakage of protein and inflammatory cells, secondary to inflammatory cascade.
    - Often associated with infectious process, chylothorax, neoplasm, connective tissue disease, immunodeficiency.
- Pathophysiology of parapneumonic effusion—three stages:
  - Exudative stage: fibrinous, uncomplicated fluid; common in the first 24 to 72 hours of effusion.
  - Fibrinopurulent stage: loculated, thick, cellular-rich fibrinous exudates; complicates to bronchopleural fistula or pyopneumothorax if left untreated; usually occurs in 5 to 10 days, may occur sooner.
  - Organizational stage: "parietal peel" formation due to fibroblast overgrowth on the parietal and visceral pleura. May compromise lung function, causes restrictive lung disease; occurs 1 to 4 weeks after the initial presentation.

Clinical Presentation

- Similar to pneumonia or can occur as a complication of pneumonia.
- Pleuritic pain exacerbated by deep breaths and coughing; worsening respiratory distress, persistent fevers, expiratory friction rub, diminished or "distant" breath sounds, and dullness to percussion are suggestive of effusion.

Diagnostic Evaluation

- Chest radiography, anterior–posterior.
  - Blunted costophrenic angle (see Figure 3.9).
- Chest radiography decubitus (affected side positioned down).
  - Evaluates mobility of fluid and layering of fluid.
- Ultrasound or CT of chest.
- Pleural fluid sampling for cellular and microbiological analysis.

Management (Based on Presentation, Severity, and Indications)

- Simple effusions.
  - Medically managed (e.g., antibiotics) under close observation.
    - See section on pneumonia for typical pathogens.
- Complicated effusions and empyema.
  - Procedural or surgical intervention; thoracentesis and thoracostomy tube placement.
  - Antibiotic administration.

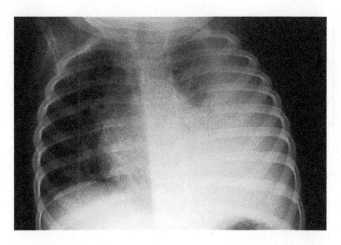

FIGURE 3.9 • **Pleural Effusion Chest Radiograph.** Pneumonia with large pleural effusion. This child presented with bacterial pneumonia and respiratory distress, presumed to be caused in part by the large pleural effusion. In the emergency department, a pleural catheter ("pigtail") was placed for drainage.

- Fibrinolytic therapy (e.g., alteplase, urokinase, streptokinase).
  - May improve drainage, ultimately avoiding further surgical intervention.
- Video-assisted thoracoscopic surgery (VATS) or thoracotomy.
  - VATS is beneficial for the ability of direct visualization of the lung tissue and optimal placement of a thoracostomy tube.
  - Decortication and fibrinolytic therapy may also be performed during the VATS procedure.
- Infectious disease consult may be needed for rare organisms that are captured on culture.
- Children with a history of poor growth or recurrent infection may require consultation with an immunologist; possible underlying immunodeficiency or CF.

Pulmonary Edema
Andrea M. Kline-Tilford

Background/Definition

- A condition resulting in an abnormal accumulation of fluid in the lung tissue and extravascular spaces of the lung.

Etiology/Types

- Cardiogenic.
  - Most commonly caused by left-sided heart failure (e.g., valvular disorders or damage to myocytes from conditions such as infectious myocarditis, hypertension, excessive volume administration, or CHD).

- Abnormalities in cardiac function can lead to blood flow that will "back up" into the pulmonary circulation, leading to alterations in the Starling equation (Table 3.3).
- Noncardiogenic—three categories.
  - Pulmonary (intrinsic).
    - Infectious causes (e.g., pneumonia).
    - Acute respiratory distress syndrome (ARDS).
    - Pulmonary embolism (PE).
  - Neurogenic.
  - Other causes.
- Both cardiogenic and noncardiogenic types will result in fluid accumulation in the interstitial and alveolar spaces.
- Results from any disruption of the Starling forces.

Pathophysiology

- Caused by any decrease in capillary oncotic pressure or interstitial hydrostatic pressure, or any increase in capillary hydrostatic pressure or interstitial oncotic pressure, or any changes in pulmonary capillary permeability.
- Alterations in surfactant and impaired lymphatic drainage may result in pulmonary edema.

Clinical Presentation

- Can include:
  - Tachypnea, dyspnea, increased work of breathing, hypoxia, wheezing, crackles (especially in dependent lungs), paroxysmal nocturnal dyspnea.
  - Cough with frothy sputum (often pink), diaphoresis, orthopnea.
  - Tachycardia, third heart tone/gallop (S_3) (cardiogenic pulmonary edema).
  - Increased pulmonary capillary wedge pressure (if measured).
    - This measurement requires a pulmonary artery catheter (e.g., Swan Ganz catheter) or cardiac catheterization for measurement. Both procedures are associated with high levels of risk.
  - Increased positive end-expiratory pressure (PEEP) and oxygen demands (in intubated patients).

Diagnostic Evaluation

- Often a clinical diagnosis; can be supported with diagnostic studies.
- Chest radiograph.
  - Peribronchial cuffing, perihilar haziness, enlarged cardiac silhouette in some cases.
  - Pleural effusions.
    - Kerley B lines (see Figure 3.10).
    - Represents fluid in the peribronchovascular interstitial space and distended lymphatics.
    - Short parallel lines in the lung periphery.
      - Most frequently noted at the base of the lungs.
  - Pulmonary edema.
    - Butterfly sign (see Figure 3.11).
      - Represents alveolar filling and characterized by patchy infiltrates.
      - Late sign of pulmonary edema.

Clinical Signs

- Hypoxia as a result of increased A-a gradient.
- Laboratory evaluation.
  - Increased brain natriuretic peptide (BNP).
- Elevated pulmonary capillary wedge pressure (i.e., >20 mmHg).
- EKG.
  - Evidence of myocardial infarction, strain, or long-standing cardiac issues.
- Echocardiogram: cardiac function and structure for planning intervention and therapy.

TABLE 3.3	Starling Equation

$$J_v = K_f [(P_c - P_i) - (\pi_c - \pi_i)]$$

J_v = net fluid movement (mL/minute) across a capillary wall and the sum of oncotic and hydrostatic pressures

K_f = water permeability

P_c = capillary hydrostatic pressure

P_i = interstitial hydrostatic pressure

π_c = capillary oncotic pressure

π_i = interstitial oncotic pressure

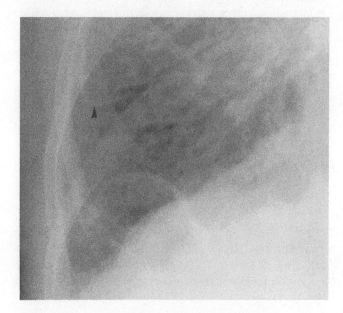

FIGURE 3.10 • **Kerley B Lines Chest Radiograph**. Kerley B lines in interstitial pulmonary edema. These are short opaque lines (arrowhead) seen best along the lateral aspects of the lungs.

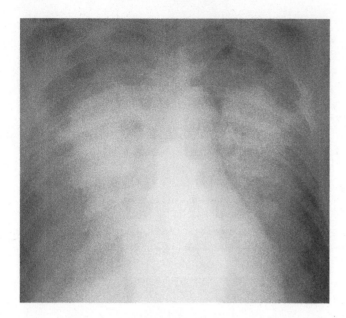

FIGURE 3.11 • **Butterfly Sign Chest Radiograph.**
Classical butterfly pattern of pulmonary edema.

Management

- Oxygen: improves alveolar and arterial oxygenation.
- Noninvasive or invasive ventilation as directed by clinical status.
  - Decreases intrapulmonary shunt by alveolar recruitment.
  - Improves cardiac function.
- In cardiogenic pulmonary edema.
  - Diuretics.
  - Inotropic agents or systemic vasodilators may be needed for afterload reduction in cardiogenic pulmonary edema.

PEARLS
- *Determining the cause will allow a tailored management plan*
- *Initial chest radiographs may be normal*

Pulmonary Embolism
Andrea M. Kline-Tilford

Definition

- Mechanical obstruction of blood flow in a pulmonary blood vessel.
- Can be the result of a primary hematologic problem.

Etiology/Types

- Most often due to a blood clot (thrombus).
- Less commonly due to air, fat, or tumor fragment.

Risk Factors

- Presence of a central venous catheter.
- Congenital heart disease.

- Surgery, trauma, immobility, sepsis, malignancy.
- Necrotizing enterocolitis, peritonitis, nephrotic syndrome.
- Birth asphyxia and oral contraceptive use.
- Two peaks in age: infancy and adolescence.
- Often occurs in conjunction with an underlying medical condition (e.g., CHD, sepsis, hypoxic ischemic events at birth).

Pathophysiology

- Most commonly, a clot breaks off from a large vessel and travels to the pulmonary circulation (thromboembolism).
- Results in V/Q mismatch (e.g., areas of ventilation are no longer being perfused due to the obstruction to blood flow in the pulmonary vessel).
- A sudden decrease in vessel obstruction by <50% may result in an asymptomatic PE.

Clinical Presentation

- Can include:
  - Dyspnea, cough, hypoxia, pallor, hemoptysis.
  - Anxiety/sense of doom, pleuritic chest pain, hepatomegaly.
  - Sudden death.
- Presentation will vary by acuity and severity of the obstruction.
- Symptoms may be masked by underlying pathology.

Physical Examination

- Tachypnea, tachycardia, increased second heart tone.

Diagnostic Evaluation

- Can be difficult to diagnose.
- Radiologic evaluation for PE.
  - Spiral CT scan with venography.
    - >90% sensitivity and specificity in adults (results not yet available in children).
  - V/Q scan.
    - Longer study time.
    - Results difficult to interpret in children with other underlying cardiac or pulmonary disorders.
  - Angiography is the gold standard for diagnosing PE in adults; however, this is invasive and not frequently performed on infants and small children.
  - Doppler ultrasound useful in superficial vessels (e.g., neck or extremity vessels).

Laboratory Evaluation

- See Table 3.4.

Management

- Anticoagulation.
- Fibrinolytics may be needed for severe disease/large thrombi.
- Occasionally, surgical intervention may be needed.
- Symptom relief.
- Consultation with hematology, vascular surgery, pulmonology, and critical care services may be needed.

TABLE 3.4	Laboratory Evaluation for a Child with Pulmonary Embolism

First-Line Evaluation

Complete blood count with differential.

Coagulation studies (e.g., prothrombin time, partial thromboplastin time, fibrinogen, fibrin degradation products [d-dimer]).

Protein C activity.

Protein S activity.

Antithrombin III activity.

Antiphospholipid antibodies (e.g., lupus anticoagulant, anticardiolipin antibodies).

Factor V Leiden.

Prothrombin gene mutation.

Factor VIII activity.

Lipoprotein (a).

Additional studies may be considered if the first-line evaluation is normal and/or in cases of a strong history of thrombosis or recurrent thrombosis.

- Delayed diagnosis may result in severe pulmonary hypertension, right-sided heart failure, or death.

PEARLS
- *Likely underdiagnosed condition which can be associated with significant morbidity and mortality*
- *Often diagnosed at the time of autopsy*
- *Patient and family education must include signs and symptoms of bleeding and recurrence of clot formation*

Pulmonary Contusion
Catherine Walsh

Definition

- Injury to lung parenchyma with edema and hemorrhage without associated pulmonary laceration.

Background

- Most common traumatic chest injury in children.
- Early diagnosis and intervention may improve outcomes.
- Fewer short- and long-term complications in pediatric populations than in adults.

Etiology/Types

- While only 4% to 8% of pediatric trauma patients have thoracic injuries, pulmonary contusions are the most frequently seen.
- Children are more likely to have pulmonary contusions without other chest wall injury (such as rib fractures) due to chest wall compliance.
- Flail chest and scapular fractures are rare in children, but are almost always associated with pulmonary contusions.
- Most commonly seen in children struck by vehicles.
- Seen after blunt chest wall trauma.
- Suspect in patients who have sustained falls, rapid deceleration, or blast injuries.
- Due to severe mechanism of injury, patients frequently sustain damage to other systems.

Pathophysiology

- Lung tissue injury due to hemorrhage, edema, and alveolar collapse.
- Results in poor gas exchange, increased pulmonary vascular resistance, and inflammatory reaction.
- Deceleration at different rates results in shearing of alveolar tissue and hemorrhage.
- Alveolar membrane is disrupted, resulting in increased cell membrane permeability and fluid extravasation.
- Parenchymal damage is caused by overexpansion of intrapulmonary air.
- Pathophysiologic changes worsen in 24 to 48 hours and typically resolve within 7 days.
- Later respiratory impairment may be due to local inflammatory response from sequestered blood, systemic response from associated injuries, and possible nosocomial pneumonia.
- Posttraumatic empyema is rare but has potentially severe sequelae.

Clinical Presentation

- Initial presentation may be subtle.
- Symptoms may include tachypnea, hypoxemia, hypercarbia, hemoptysis, and respiratory distress.
- Additional symptoms: decreased breath sounds, rales, rhonchi, wheezing, and signs of chest wall injury.
- Delayed presentation may occur as symptoms peak approximately 24 to 48 hours after the injury.
- Goal of primary evaluation is to identify potential life-threatening conditions, with a high suspicion given mechanism and type of injury.

Diagnostic Evaluation

- Chest radiography and chest CT are the primary forms of testing to evaluate for consolidation.
- Chest radiography: may not see changes for 4 to 6 hours after injury and may not reflect extent of injury.
  - May include irregular opacification in area of chest wall injury/impact.
  - Enlargement of consolidation on radiograph within the first 24 hours after the injury is likely indicative of increased morbidity.
- May underestimate severity of V/Q mismatch.

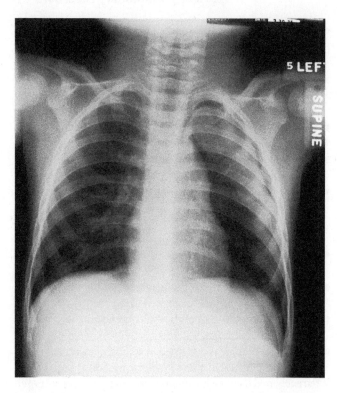

FIGURE 3.12 • **Pulmonary Contusion Chest Radiograph.** This 3-year-old child was an unrestrained passenger in a motor vehicle accident. The patient was tachypneic and had decreased breath sounds on the left side but was otherwise asymptomatic. Chest radiograph revealed a left pneumothorax with a pulmonary contusion.

- Difficult to separate degree of contusion from other conditions, including aspiration and fluid overload (Figure 3.12).
- CT scan of chest.
  - Highly sensitive, but may detect mild and clinically asymptomatic contusions.
  - More accurate in differentiating other causes of consolidation.
  - Subpleural sparing is seen in pulmonary contusions but unlikely with atelectasis or pneumonia.
  - Better able to calculate extent of injury and predict need for ventilator support. (Adult studies demonstrate that individuals with >20% total lung airspace consolidation are at increased risk early intubation and ARDS).
- Ultrasound can be used for unstable patients.

Management

- PRIMARY management is supportive.
- Most children with pulmonary contusions require no intervention.
- Address life-threatening injuries and ensure oxygenation, ventilation, and cardiovascular support.
- Close monitoring; injury evolves over the first 24 to 48 hours.
- Supplemental oxygen for hypoxia.

- Pulmonary toilet, fluid management, and pain control are essential.
- Fluids.
  - Judicious fluid administration.
  - Avoid underresuscitation that may result in hypovolemia and hypoxemia, and overresuscitation possibly resulting in pulmonary edema.
- No benefit of prophylactic antibiotics or corticosteroids.
- Intubation.
  - Most commonly used for patients with extra thoracic injuries.
  - For patients requiring respiratory support, the goal is to maximize oxygenation and minimize secondary lung injury.
  - Use of positive pressure improves alveolar recruitment.
  - Single lung ventilation for unilateral injuries may improve oxygenation and V/Q mismatch.
  - Pain may contribute to hypoventilation, atelectasis, and respiratory deterioration.
- Patients with boney chest wall injury may benefit from regional analgesia.
- Positioning.
  - Frequently change patient position.
  - Prone position and injured lung in dependent position may improve perfusion.
- Complications include:
  - Pneumonia and ARDS.
  - Risk for pneumonia due to blood in alveolar space and decreased pulmonary toilet.
- Appropriate antibiotic coverage for patients with fever with worsening respiratory function.
- Long-term consequences rarely seen in children.

PEARLS
- *Most common thoracic injury in pediatric trauma patients and frequently seen with other injuries to the chest wall and to other organ systems*
- *Primary goal is to identify other life-threatening injuries*
- *Severe pulmonary hemorrhage may be associated with diffuse hemorrhage-related liver damage and massive hilar contusions*
- *Increased morbidity for trauma patients with pulmonary contusions*

Smoke Inhalation

Cathy Haut

Definition/Background

- Lung injury from edema, de-epithelialization of the tracheobronchial region, airway obstruction, and decreased pulmonary compliance as a result of thermal or chemical inhalation.

Etiology/Types

- Leading cause of death due to fires.
- Three types of injuries.
  - Thermal injury to upper airways.
  - Chemical injury to tracheobronchial tree.
  - Systemic toxicity due to carbon monoxide and/or cyanide.

Risk Factors

- Type of fire and materials involved and length of exposure.

Pathophysiology

- Alveolar homeostasis imbalance causing coagulation and fibrolytic activity and massive airway obstruction leading to cast formation, bronchospasm.
- Increase in bronchial circulation and transvascular fluid flux.
- The leading injury in the upper airway, above the vocal cords, is caused by thermal injury where heat destroys the epithelial layer, denatures proteins, and activates the complement cascade, leading to the release of histamine and the formation of xanthine oxidase and the breakdown of purines to uric acid and thereby releases reactive oxygen species.
- In lower airways, nitric oxide formation by endothelial cells is increased by histamine stimulation. Both reactive oxygen and nitrogen species cause an increased permeability of endothelium for proteins, resulting in edema formation. Other chemical releases amplify the inflammatory process, and activation of pulmonary C-fiber receptors causes vasodilation by increasing nitric oxide production, further aggravating edema formation.

Clinical Presentation

- Depends on type and length of exposure.

Physical Examination

- Visible presence of soot, carbonaceous sputum.
- Presence of deep facial burns.
- Work of breathing: tachypnea, hypoxia.
- Hoarse voice, cough.

Diagnostic Evaluation

- Pulse oximetry.
- Chest radiography.
- Carbon monoxide, cyanide levels, and metabolic profile.
- Direct bronchoscopy.

Management

- Airway, breathing, circulation.
- Intubation and ventilation or noninvasive ventilation.
- Intubation is indicated for airway edema, hypoxia, hypoventilation, deep burns to the face or neck, and blistering or edema of the oropharynx, but there are no consensus criteria.
- Anticoagulants, antioxidants, and bronchodilators, especially when administered as an aerosol, can be used as indicated.
- Airway clearance protocol.
- Referral to pulmonology, dermatology, or burn team as indicated.

Complications

- ARDS.
- Pneumonia related to sloughing of damaged tissue, with increased secretions.
- Airway obstruction as a result of edema.

PEARLS

- *Direct bronchoscopy is the diagnostic study of choice*
- *Most children with smoke inhalation injuries do not suffer long-term respiratory sequelae*

Ventilator-Induced Lung Injury

Hitesh Sandhu

Definition/Background

- Lung injury resulting as a consequence of mechanical ventilation, typically at the level of the acinus.
- Often a result of inappropriate ventilation strategies.
- Pathological features resemble acute lung injury (ALI)/ARDS.
- Thought to be partly responsible for ALI/ARDS clinical picture.
- More likely to occur in a lung affected by another pathological process than in normal lung.

Etiology/Types

- Barotrauma is traditionally thought to be the most important cause of ventilator-induced lung injury, due to the use of high inspiratory pressure during mechanical ventilation.
- Volutrauma is thought to be the causative factor which leads to alveolar rupture and tracking of air along the interstitium, causing pneumothorax, pneumomediastinum, and subcutaneous emphysema.
- More likely to occur in the presence of high peak inspiratory pressure, bullae in the lung, or necrotizing pneumonia.
- Due to the use of excessive tidal volumes during mechanical ventilation.

- Physiologic tidal volume in ALI can cause ventilator-induced lung injury as only a small proportion of alveoli receive the entire tidal volume.
- Atelectrauma is due to repeated opening and collapse of alveolus at low lung volumes.
- More likely to occur in the dependent portions of the lungs.
- Shear stress occurs due to friction between the walls of an expanding alveolus and a collapsed alveolus.

Pathophysiology

- Barotrauma, volutrauma, and atelectrauma cause stretching and damage to the alveolar cells and intercellular junctions, leading to cellular edema and alveolar fluid collection.
- The efficacy of the surfactant layer is reduced.
- Results in worsening of the clinical status needing increased ventilator support.
- Multiorgan failure secondary to ALI/ARDS is the most common cause of mortality in these patients.

Diagnostic Evaluation

- Chest radiograph and CT scan look similar to ALI/ARDS.
  - Diffuse alveolar opacity and atelectasis, worse in the dependent portion of the lungs.
- Serial chest radiographies can be used to evaluate for worsening of lung injury.

Management

- Prevention through the use of lung-protective/open-lung strategies.
- General goals same as management of ALI/ARDS.
- Keep alveoli open during all stages of ventilation with the use of appropriate PEEP.
- Incremental increases in PEEP by 2 cm H_2O until there is no significant change in the PaO_2 or by setting PEEP 2 cm above the lower inflection point on the pressure/volume curves.
- Reduce the FiO_2 to less than 0.6.
- High-frequency oscillatory ventilator can be used to achieve the same goals.
- In conventional ventilation, use low tidal volumes of 5 to 6 mL/kg to avoid volutrauma.
- Permissive hypercapnia with steady increase in PaO_2 and decrease in pH and accept lower PaO_2.
- Prolonged mechanical ventilation, inotropic support, chronic ventilation, or tracheostomy may be needed.

PEARL

- *Meeting nutritional requirements of the patient, even to negative fluid balance and physiotherapy may facilitate pulmonary rehabilitation*

Common Diagnostic Testing

Christopher D. Newman

Laboratory Sampling: Blood Gas Interpretation (Arterial, Capillary, and Peripheral Venous)

Background

- Physiologically normal blood pH is between 7.35 and 7.45.
- Derangements that raise or lower blood pH outside of these limits can be divided into two primary processes: metabolic and respiratory.
- The gold standard for evaluating blood pH and the source of the derangement is ABG (Table 3.5).

Source of Laboratory Sample

- Arterial: the gold standard for blood gas interpretation.
  - Sample must be free flowing.
  - pH can be altered by body temperature.
  - Air bubbles can artificially raise the reported PaO_2 if the true value is <158 mmHg or lower the reported value if the true value is >158 mmHg.
  - The sample should be processed as quickly as possible; ongoing consumption of oxygen by red blood cells will alter the results over time.
- Capillary.
  - Often easier to obtain than an arterial sample.
  - Because of source, low PO_2 may not be reliable and the PCO_2 may be slightly elevated.

TABLE 3.5   Definitions in Blood Gas Analysis

Acid: A substance which can donate hydrogen ions.
Base: A substance which can accept hydrogen ions.
pH: The negative logarithm of H^+ ion concentration.
Acidemia: An acid condition of the blood with pH <7.35.
Alkalemia: An alkaline (base) condition of the blood with pH >7.45.
PCO_2: Respiratory component.
HCO_3: Metabolic component.

Balanced: 22–26 mEq/L
Base balance: −2 to +2
Metabolic alkalosis: >26 mEq/L
Base excess: >2 mEq/L
Metabolic acidosis: <22 mEq/L
Base deficit: <2 mEq/L

- Prolonged or vigorous squeezing to obtain the sample can create local cell damage and lysis of red blood cells, which can alter the pH and HCO_3 of the sample.
- Peripheral venous.
  - Should never be obtained using a tourniquet; this can induce a localized lactic acidosis and alter results.
  - Free-flowing samples may more accurately represent the local environment rather than the systemic environment.
  - May provide useful data when no other source is available.
- Central venous.
  - Useful for analysis of pH, Pco_2, HCO_3, and measuring central venous saturation, which may be helpful in determining whether tissue oxygen demand is being met.
  - Not useful for determining oxygenation (Table 3.6).

Step-by-Step Interpretation

- Is the pH acidotic (<7.35), alkalotic (>7.45), or normal (7.35–7.45)?.
  - Acidosis with high pCO_2: *primary respiratory acidosis.*
  - Low pCO_2: compensation for a *primary metabolic acidosis.*
  - Normal pCO_2: either *uncompensated or partially compensated metabolic acidosis.*
  - High HCO_3: *compensation for a respiratory acidosis.*
  - Normal HCO_3: *partial or uncompensated respiratory acidosis.*
  - Low HCO_3: *primary metabolic acidosis.*
- Alkalosis.
  - High HCO_3: *primary metabolic alkalosis.*
  - Low HCO_3: *compensation for a respiratory alkalosis.*
  - Normal HCO_3: *partial or uncompensated respiratory alkalosis.*
  - High pCO_2: *compensation for a primary metabolic alkalosis.*
  - Low pCO_2: *primary respiratory alkalosis.*
  - Normal pCO_2: *partial or uncompensated metabolic alkalosis.*
- Mixed acidosis or alkalosis: If, in the setting of acidosis, the pCO_2 is high while the HCO_3 is low, this may represent a mixed metabolic and respiratory acidosis, such as when a patient

with a primary respiratory infection becomes profoundly dehydrated. Conversely, an alkalosis with both a low pCO_2 and a high HCO_3 may represent a mixed alkalosis, such as when a patient is tachypneic due to neurologic injury, but has also received several doses of a loop diuretic.

Congenital Pulmonary Airway Malformation/Congenital Cystic Adenomatoid Malformation

Preet K. Sandhu

Background

- Benign mass of chest/lung tissue of unknown cause.

Definition

- Congenital hamartomatous lesion.
- Three types based on cyst size radiographically and on pathology.
  - Type I (50%): multiple cysts >2 cm in size or single large cyst.
  - Type II (40%): multiple cysts usually <1.2 cm.
  - Type III (<10%): microscopic cysts (<0.5 cm) appear solid, mediastinal shift from mass effect.
- 95% of cases have single lobe or upper lobe affected, rare in right middle lobe.
- Type II is associated with extralobar sequestration and with renal, cardiac, gastrointestinal, or skeletal abnormalities.
- Also associated malignancy such as embryonal rhabdomyosarcoma, bronchoalveolar carcinoma.

Clinical Presentation

- Respiratory distress, recurrent lung infections.

TABLE 3.6	Comparison of Values by Source		
Component	Arterial	Venous	Capillary
pH	7.35–7.45	7.32–7.42	7.35–7.45
Po$_2$ (mmHg)	70–100	24–48	60–80
Pco$_2$ (mmHg)	35–45	38–52	35–45
HCO$_3$ (mEq/L)	19–25	19–25	19–25
TCO$_2$ mEq/L	19–29	23–33	19–29
SO$_2$ (%)	90–95	40–70	90–95
Base excess/deficit (mEq/L)	−2 to +2	−2 to +2	−2 to +2

Radiographic Findings

- Depend on size and content of cysts.
- Solid or multicystic mass, mass effect with contralateral mediastinal shift. Chest CT will demonstrate a solid or multicystic mass, with variable enhancement after contrast administration.

Chest Radiograph Interpretation

Preet K. Sandhu

Definition/Background

- The most commonly ordered radiographic examination in pediatric patients.
- Normal appearance of neonatal chest is different from that of older children.

Technical factors to be considered in any chest film include the following:

- Lung volume findings.
  - Normal inspiration.
    - Diaphragms are rounded.
    - 6th or 7th anterior rib intersects the diaphragm.

- Lungs are air filled.
- Less than ⅓ heart projects below the diaphragm (Figures 3.13 and 3.14).
- Expiratory film.
  - Suboptimal lung volumes.
  - Criteria of normal inspiration are not met.
  - May lead to misinterpretation of the chest radiograph.
  - Heart may appear enlarged.
  - Vascular congestion, coalescence of vessels at lung bases and hila may lead to pulmonary opacity or hazy lung fields due to influx of blood and poor lung aeration.
- Hyperexpansion.
  - Flattening of the diaphragms and no heart below the diaphragm.
  - On lateral film, diaphragms are vertically oriented and 7th or lower anterior rib crosses the diaphragm.
- Rotation.
  - Normal rotation.
    - Medial ends of the clavicles symmetrically positioned or equidistant from midline (see Figure 3.13).
    - The anterior ends of the ribs are equidistant from the vertebral pedicles, and carina approximates the right pedicles in.

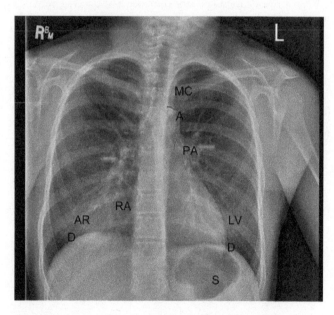

FIGURE 3.13 · Normal Chest Radiograph.
Normal frontal radiograph, shows normal lung volumes with diaphragm (D) rounded and at the level of 6th anterior rib (AR). Proper positioning is evident by medial end of clavicles (MC) being symmetrically positioned and anterior ribs equidistant from the pedicles (long arrow). Cardiomediastinal borders are formed on the left by aortic arch (A), pulmonary artery (PA), left atrial appendage, and left ventricle (LV), and on the right by superior vena cava (short arrow) and right atrium (RA) and inferior vena cava. Block arrows point to the left and right hilum. Stomach (S) in on the left.

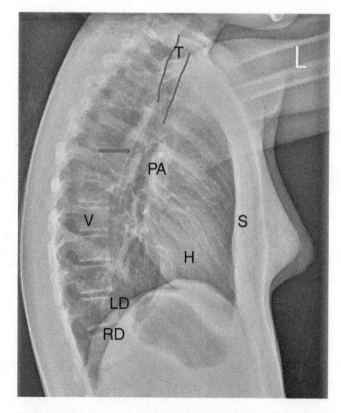

FIGURE 3.14 · Normal Lateral Chest Radiograph. Lateral film of the chest shows trachea (T), vertebral bodies (V), heart (H), right (RD) and left hemidiaphragm (LD), sternum (S), pulmonary artery (PA), and scapulae (arrow).

- Abnormal rotation.
  - Asymmetric aeration (e.g., asymmetric lucency or darkness) or one lung darker than the other suggests an abnormal rotation or other abnormality.
- Exposure.
  - Adequate if the spine and pedicles are seen behind the heart and pulmonary vessels are seen in the peripheral lung.
- Systematic approach to interpretation of a chest film.
- ABCD approach encourages a systematic process to evaluate for abnormal findings.
  - A—Abdomen.
    - Heterotaxy or situs inversus. (Stomach should be on the left side in an anatomically normal radiograph; in the conditions, the stomach is located on the left side.) (See Figure 3.13.).
    - Pneumoperitoneum, portal venous gas (which appears as linear lucencies over the liver shadow and typically represents a perforated abdominal viscus).
    - Calcifications (see Figure 3.15) (a variety of etiologies, including renal calculi, chronic pancreatitis, vascular calcifications).
    - Bowel distension.
  - Air-fluid levels (often the result of a bowel obstruction).
  - Bones and soft tissues.
    - Rib fractures (consider nonaccidental trauma) (see Figure 3.16).
    - Sternum, scapula, arms, vertebral bodies, mandible, and clavicles.
    - Soft tissue evaluation for calcifications, air, swelling, and foreign body.
  - C—Chest: Lungs, pleura, mediastinum, and airway.
    - Chest evaluation includes airway, mediastinum, lungs, pleura, and diaphragm.

- D—Devices.
  - Examples include endotracheal tube, central line, gastric tube, pacemaker, AICD.
- Airway.
  - Visible from oral and nasal pharynges to right and left mainstem bronchi.
  - The walls should be parallel and smooth.
  - Carina approximates the right pedicles.
- Trachea.
  - Observe for tracheal compression, deviation, or indentation.
- Mediastinum.
  - Anterior, middle, and posterior mediastinum and contains heart, great vessels, thymus, trachea, esophagus, nerves, and lymph nodes.
  - Anterior mediastinum is in front of the pericardium, middle mediastinum contains pericardium and its contents, and posterior is behind the pericardium.
  - Right mediastinal border is formed by superior vena cava, right atrium, and inferior vena cava.
  - Left mediastinal border is formed by aortic arch, pulmonary artery, left atrial appendage, left ventricle from above to below.
- Heart.
  - Normally positioned in the left hemithorax.
  - Heart size on frontal film is assessed by cardiothoracic ratio. Cardiothoracic ratio is measured by measuring the cardiac size (maximum extension of the heart to the right of

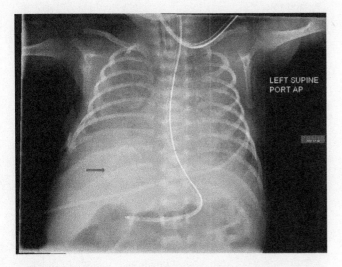

FIGURE 3.15 • **Abdominal Calcification.** Frontal view of the chest shows calcification in the right upper quadrant (arrow) which was not shown to be in the liver on ultrasound.

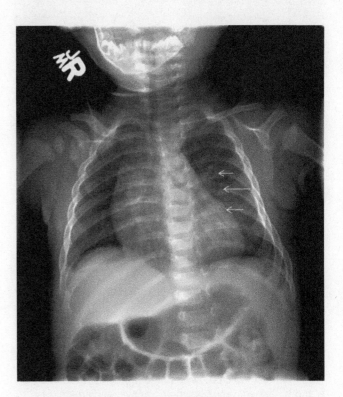

FIGURE 3.16 • **Rib Fractures.** Frontal chest radiograph demonstrates multiple posterior rib fractures on left side (arrows).

midline (a) and to the left of midline (b) and adding them, i.e., a + b) and dividing it by the transverse diameter of the chest [the maximum measurement of the thorax to the inside of the ribs (d)] (see Figure 3.17).

- Upper limit for normal cardiothoracic ratio is 50%.
  - It may exceed 60% in normal neonate.
- Appearance of heart on frontal film in children is affected by thymus and degree of inspiration.
- Lateral film is better for assessment of cardiac size.
- Two methods for assessing cardiomegaly on lateral film:
  1. Draw a line paralleling the anterior wall of trachea and extend it inferiorly toward the diaphragm. The line should not intersect the heart, nor it should be pushed back to hit the spine before the diaphragm.
  2. Second method is a perpendicular line drawn from the carina to the diaphragm; should not intersect the heart.
- Aortic arch.
  - Should be on the left side, but is not always visualized (see Figure 3.13).
  - Position of trachea helps in locating the aortic arch.
  - Normal tracheal bifurcation should approximately be over the right pedicles.
  - Right aortic arch associated with CHD or vascular ring.

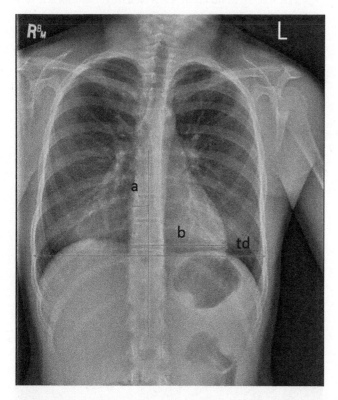

FIGURE 3.17 • Measurement of Cardiac Size. Maximum extension of heart to the right and left of midline, a and b, respectively. Maximum transverse diameter of the heart is a + b, and maximum transverse diameter of thorax is td.

- Lungs.
  - Should be symmetrically aerated.
  - Major fissure separates the upper and lower lobes on both sides, often seen on the lateral film.
  - Minor fissure on the right side separates the upper and middle lobes, and can be noted on the frontal film.
- Hila.
  - Right hilum is mostly lower than the left, but never higher. (See Figure 3.13).
  - Pulmonary vessels are seen branching in the medial two-third of the lung fields, and major bronchi are noted centrally.
  - There should be no other opacity, and lungs should be black with the exception of the pulmonary vessels.
  - A pulmonary opacity can be due to consolidation, atelectasis, mass, or localized fluid collection.
  - Consolidation is due to the replacement of air in the distal air spaces with fluid (e.g., transudate, exudate, blood) or tissue (e.g., lymphoma).
- Air bronchogram.
  - Noted when alveolar air is replaced by fluid, pus, or blood (e.g., pulmonary edema, pneumonia, or pulmonary hemorrhage).
  - Air in the bronchi is seen against the background of airless lung or filled alveoli.
  - Differentiation may not always be possible, but there may be signs of volume loss in atelectasis (discussed later), such as mediastinal shift or displacement of the fissures, though not in cases of pneumonia or pulmonary edema.
- Silhouette sign.
  - Assists in detection and localization of an abnormality.
  - The loss of an anatomical border by an intrathoracic abnormality.
  - Only achieved if the two intrathoracic structures are in contact with each other.
  - Example:
    - An opacity that causes obliteration of the cardiac border will be located anteriorly and lie in the middle lobe on the right.
    - An opacity obliterating the diaphragm would be in the lower lobes along with a lingular segment of the left upper lobe.
- Diaphragm.
  - Normally represented on frontal chest film by a smooth, curved line that is convex upwards (see Figures 3.12 and 3.14).
  - Appearance of diaphragm changes with respiration and patient position.
  - The right hemidiaphragm is slightly higher than the left.
  - Elevation of a single diaphragm may be related to diaphragmatic paralysis, eventration, or other pathologies including pulmonary collapse, abdominal organomegaly or mass, intestinal distension, or subpulmonic effusion.

For determining the area of involvement on a chest radiograph (see Figures 3.18–3.21).

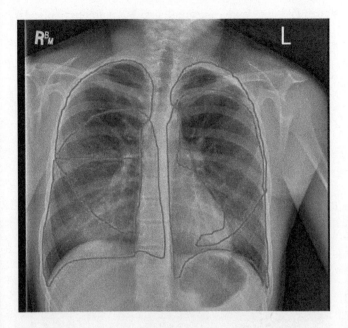

FIGURE 3.18 • **Positioning of Lung Lobes on Chest Radiograph**. Blue lines depict lung lobes.

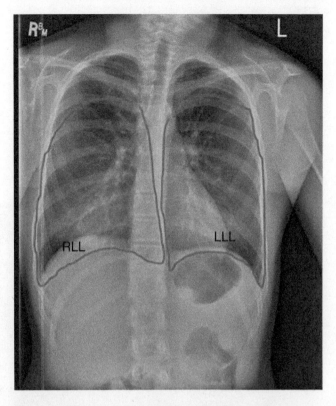

FIGURE 3.20 • **Positioning of Right and Left Lower Lobes**. Right lower lobe (RLL) and left lower lobe (LLL).

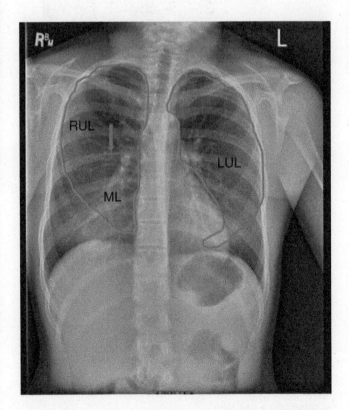

FIGURE 3.19 • **Positioning of Upper and Middle Lobes**. Right upper lobe (RUL), middle lobe (ML), left upper lobe (LUL), and minor fissure (bold arrow).

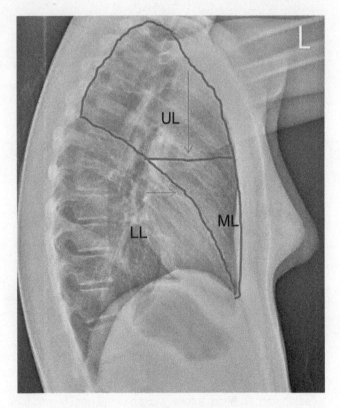

FIGURE 3.21 • **Positioning of Lung Lobes on Lateral View**. Lateral film shows normal anatomy, right upper lobe (UL), lower lobes (LL), middle lobe on right side (ML), minor fissure (long arrow). On the left, lung anterior to major fissure (short arrow) is left upper lobe.

Normal Variants and Special Considerations

- Thymus.
  - Prominent in children until 4 to 5 years of age.
  - Anterior in position.
  - Variable in shape and size and can extend inferiorly to the diaphragm or laterally to the lateral thoracic wall.
  - Wavy in contour, insinuates between anterior ribs.
  - Normal thymus does not cause mass effect or displace adjacent structures such as the trachea (see Figure 3.22).

- Skin folds may mimic pneumothorax but pulmonary vascular markings extend into that space.
- Central cleft in the vertebral bodies is related to unfused post neural arches (spinous processes fuse by 3–5 years).
- Sternal ossification centers may project laterally in rotated patients and may mimic rib fractures.
- Tracheal buckling seen on frontal film is a normal variant due to flexibility and movement of infant's trachea with inspiration and posture (see Figures 3.23–3.38 and Tables 3.7 and 3.8).

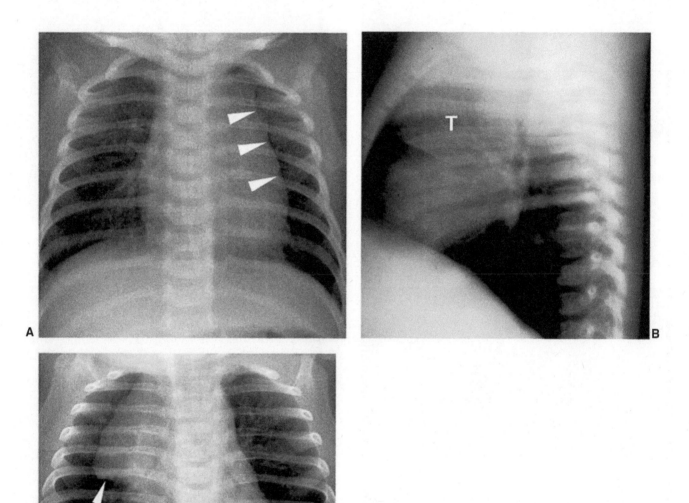

FIGURE 3.22 • **Thymus on Chest Radiograph**. Normal thymus. **(A)** Frontal and **(B)** lateral radiographs show the normal anterior and substernal position of the thymus (T). The thymus in the newborn is often prominent and may mimic a mediastinal mass. The absence of tracheal mass effect or compression helps confirm the diagnosis of normal thymus. Wavy contour of the lateral thymic margin (arrowheads) at each rib end, termed the wave sign, is seen on the frontal radiograph. **C:** Sharp inferior margin of the right thymic lobe (arrow) produces a sail sign.

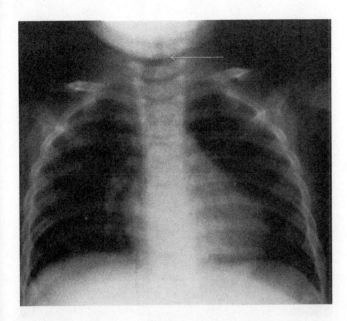

FIGURE 3.23 • **Tracheal Buckling**. Frontal chest radiograph shows normal tracheal buckling.

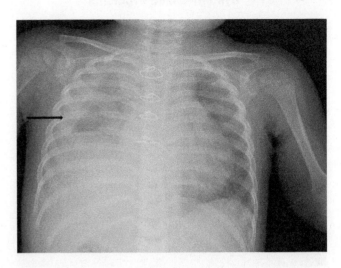

FIGURE 3.24 • **Pleural Effusion**. Frontal film in a postoperative patient shows a right pleural effusion (arrow).

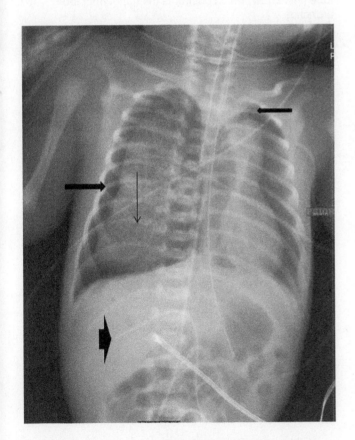

FIGURE 3.25 • **Pneumothorax**. Frontal view of the chest shows bilateral pneumothorax (bold arrows) larger on the right side, pulmonary interstitial emphysema (linear and round lucencies in the collapsed right lung) (long thin arrow), and abnormal position of the umbilical venous catheter in the right portal vein (arrow head).

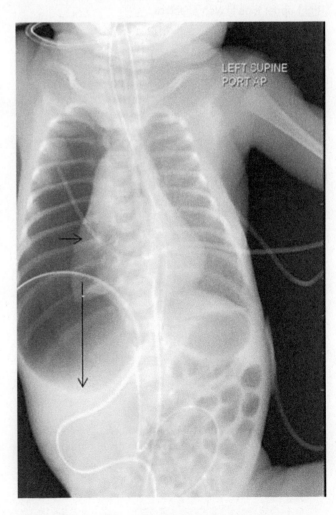

FIGURE 3.26 • **Tension Pneumothorax**. Right-sided tension pneumothorax in an intubated patient. Note the inversion of the right hemidiaphragm (long arrow), collapse of right lung (short arrow), and mediastinal shift to the left.

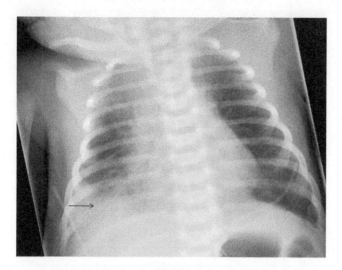

FIGURE 3.27 • **Right Lower Lobe Pneumonia.** Frontal radiograph of the chest shows opacity in the right lower lobe obscuring the right hemidiaphragm (arrow). Right upper lobe is also affected.

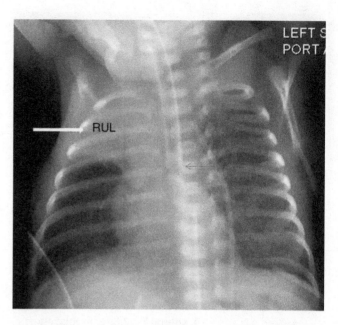

FIGURE 3.29 • **Atelectasis.** The right upper lobe (RUL) is opaque (bold arrow) with concave lower margin. The RUL is collapsed due to a deeply placed endotracheal tube (thin arrow) which obstructs the right upper lobe bronchus.

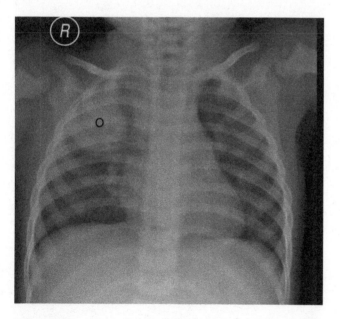

FIGURE 3.28 • **Round Pneumonia.** Frontal view of the chest shows rounded opacity (O) in the right upper lobe.

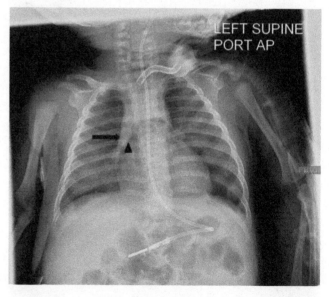

FIGURE 3.30 • **Pneumomediastinum.** Frontal chest film shows air in the mediastinum (triangle) elevating the thymus (arrow).

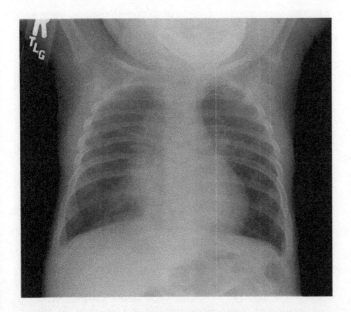

FIGURE 3.31 • **Bronchiolitis**. Chest radiograph of an 8-month-old boy with typical findings of bronchiolitis, including hyperinflation, peribronchial thickening, and scattered opacities representing areas of atelectasis.

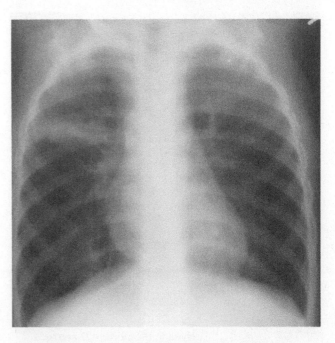

FIGURE 3.33 • **Asthma Exacerbation**. Chest radiograph of a 3-year-old patient obtained during an asthma exacerbation test demonstrates severe hyperinflation, increased anteroposterior diameter of the chest, a depressed diaphragm, and several areas of atelectasis.

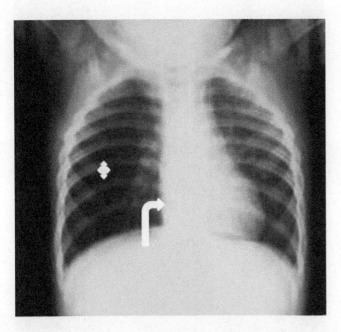

FIGURE 3.32 • **Foreign Body**. Chest radiograph shows hyperinflation (quad arrow) of right lung and mediastinal shift to the left (bent arrow), away from the side of the foreign body.

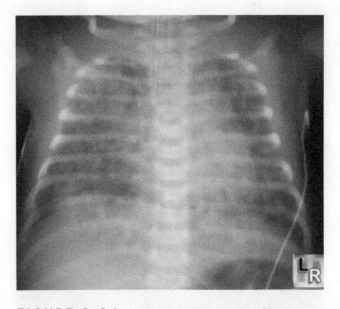

FIGURE 3.34 • **Meconium Aspiration Syndrome**. Meconium aspiration. Frontal radiograph of the chest shows bilateral coarse and heterogenous opacities, worse on the right.

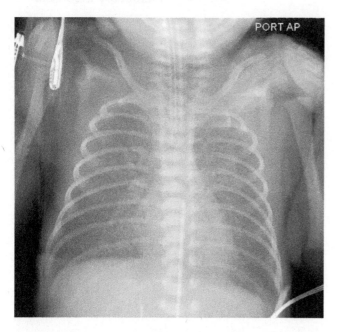

FIGURE 3.35 • **Hyaline Membrane Disease**. Frontal view of the chest shows diffuse reticulonodular opacities in both lung fields that are uniform from medial to lateral aspects of the lung.

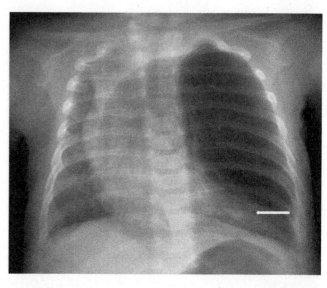

FIGURE 3.37 • **Congenital Lobar Emphysema**. Frontal view of chest shows large cystic lesion of the left upper lobe with compression atelectasis of the adjacent lung (arrow) and rightward mediastinal shift.

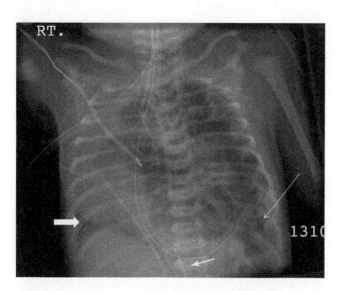

FIGURE 3.36 • **Congenital Diaphragmatic Hernia**. Diaphragmatic hernia on the left with stomach in the chest indicated by the abnormal position of the nasogastric tube (long arrow). Rightward mediastinal shift (block arrow). Also note abnormal position of the umbilical catheter which is coiled back on itself (short arrow).

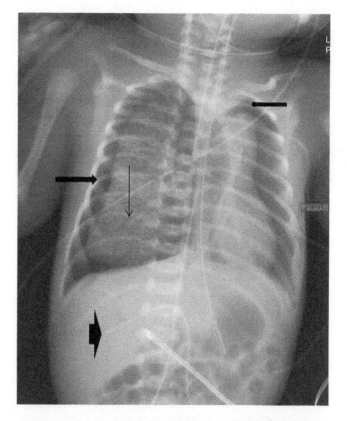

FIGURE 3.38 • **Pneumothorax and Pulmonary Interstitial Emphysema**. Frontal view of the chest shows bilateral pneumothoraces (bold arrows) larger on the right side, pulmonary interstitial emphysema (linear and round lucencies in the collapsed right lung, long thin arrow), and abnormal position of the umbilical venous catheter in the right portal vein (arrow head).

TABLE 3.7	Radiographic Findings of Common General Pediatric Diseases	
Diagnosis	Radiological Findings	Additional Details
Pleural effusion	Homogenous opacity causing blunting of the posterior costophrenic angle on lateral chest radiograph (50 mL of fluid accumulation is required to cause blunting of the costophrenic angle) and lateral costophrenic angle on frontal chest radiograph (200 mL fluid is required to cause blunting of the costoprenic angle). It extends posteriorly, laterally, and superiorly with a concave medial margin (see Figure 3.24) Fluid may accumulate in the fissures and is seen as a linear density along the major and minor fissures on lateral and frontal views.	Large effusion causes contralateral mediastinal shift. Supine film not sensitive for detection of small amount of fluid. Lateral decubitus view (with the affected side down) is used for differentiating loculated versus free-flowing pleural effusion (fluid layers out on decubitus view).
Pneumothorax	Lung and visceral pleura are separated from the chest wall by a radiolucent space with the absence of pulmonary vascular markings (see Figure 3.25).	Expiratory film or decubitus view may be helpful. Supine radiograph view: Air accumulates anteriorly and medially to produce hyper lucent hemithorax and deep sulcus sign (prominent costophrenic sulcus).
Tension pneumothorax	Contralateral mediastinal shift, diaphragmatic depression, and rib cage expansion (see Figure 3.26).	
Pneumonia Bronchopneumonia Acute interstitial pneumonia Round pneumonia	Homogenous or patchy opacity obscuring bronchovascular markings. Air bronchograms are present and lung volume is preserved. Particular attention is needed when evaluating behind the heart and in the region of liver (normally dense areas), silhouette sign may be noted, loss of the right cardiac border in right middle lobe consolidation, obscuration of diaphragms in lower lobe consolidation (see Figure 3.27). Initially segmental involvement, followed by spread to other areas. Can be bilateral. Increased peribronchial markings and small fluffy opacities. Air trapping leading to hyperinflation and irregular aeration. Bronchial wall thickening leading to perihilar streaky/tram-track opacities and ring shadows. Vascular margins become ill-defined. Children have poorly developed collateral air circulation, which prevents lobar spread and leads to spherical spread or round pneumonia (see Figure 3.28). Increased opacity of the collapsed lobe and displacement of fissures (see Figure 3.29). Indirect signs include ipsilateral mediastinal shift, elevation of the hemidiaphragm, displacement of hilum, narrowing of the ipsilateral intercostal spaces, and compensatory hyperinflation of the remaining aerated lung.	Complete lobar consolidation is unusual in children. Upper lobe pneumonia may mimic enlarged thymus and a lateral film is sometimes necessary. As disease progresses, air space involvement from atelectasis, alveolar edema or hemorrhage, or superimposed bacterial infection can lead to patchy opacities. Usually caused by *Strep. pneumoniae*.

(Continued)

TABLE 3.7	Radiographic Findings of Common General Pediatric Diseases (*Continued*)	
Diagnosis	Radiological Findings	Additional Details
Pneumomediastinum	Air in the mediastinal space as a result of a sudden increase in alveolar pressure → alveolar rupture → air dissects into the interstitium → along bronchovascular bundle into the mediastinum. Air then dissects into soft tissue of neck, retropharyngeal area, or rarely into the abdomen, leading to pneumoperitoneum or pneumoretroperitoneum. Chest radiograph: Streaky lucencies in the mediastinum. Air displaces the mediastinal pleura laterally and separates the thymus from cardiac shadow, called the sail sign, or a sliver of air is seen along the left cardiac border or along the great vessels (see Figure 3.30). On lateral view, air outlines the thymus, and retropharyngeal gas is seen in the neck. Continuous diaphragm sign is seen when air dissects between the heart and the diaphragm, so that obscured central diaphragm becomes visible.	Commonly seen in infants with air leak syndrome and children with asthma. Foreign body should always be considered in an infant with pneumomediastinum and no history of trauma. Pneumopericardium may be difficult to distinguish from pneumomediastinum; however, pericardial air has dome-shaped superior margin, and thymus and aortic arch are not outlined by pericardial air as pericardium attaches to heart between the aorta and pulmonary artery. If pneumopericardium is present, pneumomediastinum is always present except in post–cardiac surgery patients.
Bronchiolitis	Chest radiograph demonstrates generalized hyperinflation, and peribronchial cuffing (see Figure 3.31).	Airway obstruction can occur and leads to atelectasis or air-block syndrome with pneumomediastinum or pneumothorax.
Bronchial foreign body	Radio opaque foreign body can be seen in the bronchus or other area along the tracheobronchial tree. Nonradiopaque foreign bodies require a higher index of suspicion and necessitate both inspiratory and expiratory films to make a definite diagnosis. The findings include static lung volume at different phases of respiratory cycle and asymmetric lung volumes. Volume of affected lung can be normal, increased, or decreased. Decubitus views might be needed if satisfactory inspiration–expiration views cannot be obtained. The dependent side is expiratory and should normally lose volume. When air trapping is present due to ball valve mechanism, it remains there. Other findings include atelectasis, pneumonia, or bronchiectasis (see Figure 3.32).	
Asthma	Radiographs are usually normal. Hyperinflation (with flattening of the diaphragm and increase in retrosternal airspace, increase in AP diameter of the chest), peribronchial cuffing which appears as perihilar tramline opacities or ring like shadows, areas of atelectasis, pneumomediastinum, allergic bronchopulmonary aspergillosis (ABPA) and rarely, pneumothorax (see Figure 3.33).	

TABLE 3.7 **Radiographic Findings of Common General Pediatric Diseases (*Continued*)**

Diagnosis	Radiological Findings	Additional Details
Cystic fibrosis	Air trapping, segmental or subsegmental atelectasis, lobar collapse, bronchial wall thickening (perihilar strand-like or tramline opacities or ring shadows). Ill-defined opacities or nodules from mucus plugging, bronchiectasis predominantly in the upper lobes, cyst formation, hilar lymphadenopathy, pulmonary hypertension (with enlargement of central pulmonary arteries and peripheral pruning).	
Sickle cell disease: acute chest crisis	Pulmonary opacity may be secondary to pneumonia, atelectasis, or pulmonary infarction. Other radiographic findings in sickle cell disease include pulmonary edema, pleural effusion, cardiomegaly (due to anemia and high output failure); avascular necrosis of humeral heads, H-shaped vertebrae, and gallstones.	
Nonaccidental trauma or child maltreatment	Acute rib fractures appear as linear lucencies and may be anterior, lateral, or posterior (see Figure 3.16). Acute rib fractures may be missed if the fractures are incomplete or not displaced. Follow-up radiographs in 2 wk will show healing fractures with callus formation.	Chest radiograph plays an important role in identifying cases of child maltreatment. Positive predictive value of a rib fracture for child maltreatment in children <3 y of age is 95%. Posterior rib fractures are more common and most specific for child maltreatment.

TABLE 3.8 **Newborns: Specific Diseases and Radiological Abnormalities**

Diagnosis	Radiographic Findings	Additional Details
Transient tachypnea of the newborn	Normal to increased lung volumes. Diffuse perihilar, symmetric strand opacities, pleural effusion, fluid in fissures. Normal heart size.	
Meconium aspiration syndrome	Increased lung volumes. Heterogenous opacities, particularly in medial 2/3 of lungs. Patchy areas of atelectasis and hyperinflation (see Figure 3.34).	
Persistent pulmonary hypertension of the newborn	No specific findings, chest radiograph to exclude other pathologies. Heart size and pulmonary vascularity are variable.	
Respiratory distress syndrome	Decreased lung volumes, diffuse, bilateral, ground glass appearance or diffuse granular opacities or reticulonodular opacities, and air bronchograms (see Figure 3.35).	Resultant long-term complications include bronchopulmonary dysplasia. Long-term radiographical findings are not unusual.

(Continued)

TABLE 3.8	Newborns: Specific Diseases and Radiological Abnormalities (*Continued*)	
Diagnosis	**Radiographic Findings**	**Additional Details**
Neonatal pneumonia	Streptococcus Group B pneumonia: Low lung volumes, granular opacities, pleural effusion. Other types of pneumonia: increased lung volumes, patchy areas of atelectasis, perihilar strand-like opacities, and pleural effusion.	
Bronchopulmonary dysplasia	Generalized emphysema or hyperinflation, cystic changes or focal lucencies, reticular or linear opacities of fibrosis, and atelectasis.	
Congenital diaphragmatic hernia	The affected side of the chest may be opaque or may contain multiple cystic areas related to gas containing bowel loops. Contralateral mediastinal shift, paucity of abdominal bowel gas, ipsilateral lung is small. Abnormal position of the nasogastric (NG) tube (e.g. tip above the diaphragm); herniating stomach or contralateral deviation of the descending portion of NG tube (see Figure 3.36). Lateral radiograph demonstrates the defect posteriorly. Right-sided hernia often contains liver (soft-tissue density).	
Congenital lobar hyperinflation or congenital lobar emphysema	At birth, the affected lobe may be fluid-filled and appear as an opacity. When fluid clears, the affected lobe becomes hyperexpanded and hyperlucent with compressive atelectasis of the adjacent lung, contralateral mediastinal shift (see Figure 3.37).	
Air leak syndromes	Air appears as small black dots or black lines. Pneumothorax occurs when air enter the pleural cavity. Pneumomediastinum occurs when there is free air or gas in the mediastinum. Pneumopericardium occurs when air collects in the pericardial sac. Pulmonary interstitial emphysema is the presence of air in the interstitium and vascular sheath. Rarely, PIE may be localized causing mass effect, mediastinal shift, and atelectasis of the surrounding lung (see Figure 3.38).	Air leak syndromes include pulmonary interstitial pneumonia, pneumomediastinum, pneumopericardium, pneumothorax, pneumoperitoneum, and air embolism.

Chest Radiograph in Cardiac Imaging

Preet K. Sandhu

Role of Chest Radiography in Cardiac Imaging

- Ancillary diagnostic role in most cardiac pathology.
- Echocardiography is the primary modality for diagnosing CHD in the fetal and neonatal periods.
- Frequently required in the postoperative cardiac surgery patients to evaluate device placement, pulmonary circulation, secondary lung disease, and signs of congestive heart failure.
- Findings noted on a chest radiograph may suggest a cardiac cause for respiratory distress in newborn patients.

- Systematic approach using a chest radiograph includes assessment of heart size, shape and position, pulmonary vasculature, airway and mediastinum, position of the abdominal viscera, and skeletal abnormalities.

Cardiac Size, Shape, and Position

- Cardiac size may be normal or enlarged.
- Frontal view may not be reliable due to large thymus mimicking cardiomegaly.
- Lateral view is more helpful for evaluation of cardiac size.
- On a lateral view, cardiomegaly is suggested if the heart projects posterior to the oblique line drawn down the tracheal columnar over the vertebral bodies.

Pulmonary Vascularity

- Can be normal, increased, or decreased.
- Increased pulmonary vascularity: Pulmonary artery branches appear to be too many and too prominent, and can be visualized in the peripheral one third of the lung.
- Diameter of the interlobar pulmonary artery is more than that of the trachea.

- Decreased vascularity is difficult to assess, despite paucity of pulmonary arterial structures throughout the lung. *All patients with decreased pulmonary vascularity have cyanosis.*

Increased Pulmonary Venous Congestion

- Prominent pulmonary structure but with indistinct and hazy margins compared to arterial structures that are well defined (Tables 3.9 and 3.10 and Figures 3.39–3.53).

TABLE 3.9	**Radiology Findings in Heart Disease**
Diagnosis	**Radiographic Findings**
Situs inversus	Cardiac apex and stomach bubble are on opposite sides; there is nearly a 100% incidence of congenital heart disease (CHD).
Right-sided aortic arch	Normal carina is at the right pedicles. In right-sided aortic arch, the trachea is midline; there may be right-sided indentation on tracheal column and the aortic knob and descending aorta are seen on the right side.
Atrial septal defect	Small and moderate size defects result in a normal chest radiograph. Large defects demonstrate mild cardiomegaly, normal-sized left atrium, enlarged main pulmonary artery, and increased pulmonary artery flow (see Figure 3.39).
Ventricular septal defect (VSD)	Small VSD demonstrate normal chest radiograph. Moderate to large defects demonstrate cardiomegaly with enlargement of right ventricle, left atrium, left ventricle, enlarged pulmonary arteries, and increased pulmonary artery blood flow (see Figure 3.40). Pulmonary hyperinflation.
Patent ductus arteriosus (PDA)	May be normal. Cardiomegaly with increased pulmonary artery blood flow. In preterm infants, if there is increased granularity after first few days of life with increasing heart size, PDA should be suspected (see Figure 3.41).
Tetralogy of Fallot	Boot-shaped heart due to right ventricular hypertrophy, leading to elevation of angulated cardiac apex from diaphragm and concave pulmonary artery segment. Oligemia or decreased pulmonary vascularity (see Figure 3.42).
Vascular rings	Chest radiograph may demonstrate prominent soft tissue on either side of the trachea, bilateral tracheal indentations, or trachea in a midline position. One form of a vascular ring is a double aortic arch (see Figure 3.43). Lateral view may demonstrate anterior and posterior compression of the trachea.
Pulmonary sling	Asymmetric lung aeration, round soft-tissue density between trachea and esophagus on lateral film, posterior impression on distal trachea at the level of carina and anterior impression on the mid esophagus, narrowing of distal trachea which is displaced toward the left.
Right arch with aberrant left subclavian artery	Left subclavian artery arises as the last branch of the aortic arch and passes behind the esophagus with an oblique course; left ductus persists as ligamentum arteriosum and completes the ring.

TABLE 3.10   Radiologic Manifestation of Support Devices

Device	Radiology Findings
Endotracheal tube (ET)	Ideal position is C7–T2 or 1-1.5 cm above the carina (see Figure 3.44). ET moves downward with flexion, upward with extension of the neck, and upward with lateral rotation of the head and neck. Complications: Esophageal intubation (which can be confirmed with lateral view) or abnormal position into right or left mainstem bronchus. Right mainstem bronchus intubation is more common due to its straighter angle/course and will often result in atelectasis of the left lung and the right upper lobe due to blockage of right upper lobe bronchus.
Tracheostomy tube	Appropriate positioning is wth tip between the thoracic inlet and carina (see Figures 3.45 and 3.46).
Enteral feeding tubes	Normally has gentle leftward and anterior curve with tip in the left upper quadrant in the region of stomach (see Figure 3.47).
Nasogastric (NG) tube	Position of NG tube is helpful in diagnosis of esophageal atresia and congenital diaphragmatic hernia (see Figure 3.36).
NJ tube	Normally placed beyond the pylorus, through the duodenum with tip in the third part of duodenum or at the duodenojejunal junction/ligament of Treitz.
Gastrostomy tube	Normal position is in the left upper quadrant, and placement can be confirmed with contrast injection.
Jejunostomy tube	Position can be confirmed with contrast injection and frontal and lateral views are obtained.
Gastrojejunostomy (GJ) tube	Normally placed beyond the pylorus, through the duodenum with tip in the third part of duodenum or at the duodenojejunal junction/ligament of Treitz; placement can be confirmed with contrast injection.
Venous/Arterial access catheters: Central Venous Catheters (CVC) Peripherally inserted central venous catheter (PICC)	Placed in internal or external jugular veins, subclavian vein, or femoral veins. Radiographically visualized with tip in atria or superior vena cava (see Figure 3.48). PICC line inserted into basilic, cephalic, brachial, or femoral vein. Accessed through internal jugular, subclavian or femoral vein. Ideal position is at the right atrial and superior vena cava junction (which is approximately at T6 level) or inferior vena cava-right atrial junction. Complications include malpositioning with tip in the internal jugular, contralateral subclavian axillary, or azygous vein. Catheters that are too short may migrate into the upper system veins and catheters that are too long/deep can cause right atrial wall perforation and/or tamponade. See Figures 3.49 and 3.50. Pneumothorax (most common with subclavian vein access), vessel (venous or arterial) damage/perforation, and arrhythmias are procedural complications. Additional complications (postprocedural) include migration of catheter, thrombosis formation, and infection.
Medi ports	Radiographically visualized on chest radiograph.
ECMO catheters	Venous cannula is usually placed using the right internal jugular approach. Alternative access sites include left internal jugular vein and femoral vein. Tip of the cannula should lie at approximately the 8–9th posterior rib; the expected level of right atrium (see Figure 3.51). Some venous cannulae have radiolucent distal segment and the tip and lies more distally and some cannulae have a radiopaque tip beyond the radiolucent segment. Arterial cannulae are inserted through the right common carotid artery with tip in the innominate artery, at the origin of the common carotid artery which is at the level of posterior 2nd–3rd rib. Venovenous ECMO using double lumen cannula is another alternative. However its use is limited to smaller patients due to smaller lumen size of the cannulae, limiting the volume of exchange. Tip of the venovenous cannula should be within the right atrium.

TABLE 3.10 Radiologic Manifestation of Support Devices (*Continued*)

Device	Radiology Findings
Umbilical venous catheter (UVC)	The single umbilical vein extends from the umbilicus to left portal vein, ascends in anterior midline location until it courses posteriorly through the liver to the left portal vein. Blood moves from the umbilical vein → left portal vein → ductus venosus → inferior vena cava. The umbilical venous catheter follows the same course.
	The preferred location of the umbilical venous catheter tip is at the inferior vena cava–right atrial junction or in the cephalad portion of the inferior vena cava, approximately at the level of T9. Transient portal venous air can be seen immediately after UVC insertion. Complications of insertion include malposition of the tip into the right or left portal vein, or in the right atrium from where it can migrate into the superior vena cava or through a patent foramen ovale or an atrial septal defect into the left atrium. Other complications include thrombus formation along the catheter course, perforation in intrahepatic vasculature wall with hepatic hematoma, or fluid collection (if fluid instilled through an abnormally located catheter), or rarely, perforation of the right or left atrial wall.
	Paired umbilical arteries course posteriorly and inferiorly to enter right and left iliac arteries and then superiorly into a posteriorly positioned aorta.
	Catheter course: Umbilical artery → internal iliac artery → common iliac artery → aorta.
Umbilical artery catheter (UAC)	Umbilical artery catheter dips down into the pelvis to enter the right or left iliac artery and then courses superiorly and posteriorly into the aorta to the left of the spine.
	The umbilical venous catheter follows an anterior and cephalad course in the midline umbilical vein until directed posteriorly in the liver and is noted to the right of the spine (see Figures 3.52 and 3.53).
	There are two optimal positions of the umbilical artery catheter, away from major branch vessel orifices. Major aortic branches arise at the following vertebral levels: celiac artery at T12, superior mesenteric artery at T12–L1, renal arteries at L1–L2, inferior mesenteric artery at L3 and aortic bifurcation at L4 level.
	High catheter position is positioned with the tip of UAC between T6–T10 and a low position with tip below L3 level.
	Complications of UAC placement include malpositioning with tip in one of the major aortic branches such as superior mesenteric or renal artery, or a catheter that has passed through the ductus into pulmonary artery or into the great vessels such as subclavian artery. Other complications include thrombus formation, infection, catheter fragmentation and migration.

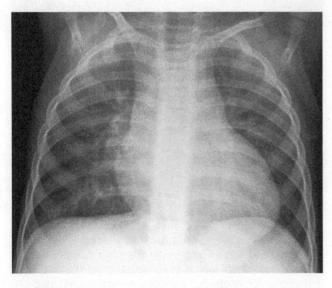

FIGURE 3.39 • **Atrial Septal Defect**. Frontal chest radiograph shows mild cardiomegaly and increased pulmonary vascularity.

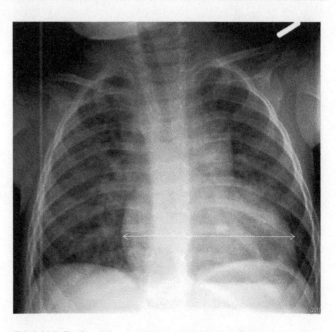

FIGURE 3.40 • **Ventricular Septal Defect**. Ventricular septal defect with left to right shunt. Frontal chest radiograph shows mild cardiomegaly (double arrow) and increased pulmonary vascularity.

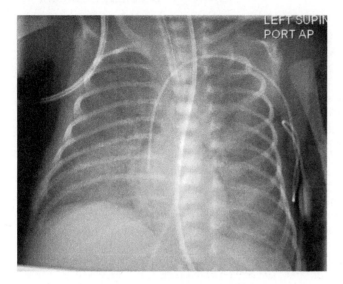

FIGURE 3.41 • **Patent Ductus Arteriosus (PDA)**. Frontal chest radiograph in a premature neonate shows diffuse opacities in both lung fields. The appearance of the lungs was worse when compared to multiple previous radiographs related to PDA and resultant pulmonary plethora.

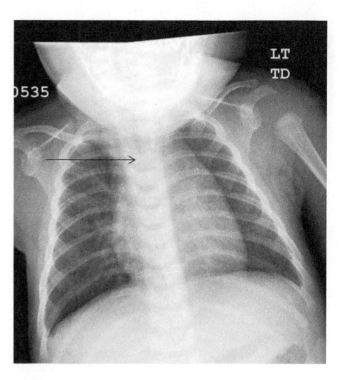

FIGURE 3.43 • **Vascular Rings/Double Aortic Arch**. Frontal view of the chest shows the trachea is midline and there is narrowing of the lower trachea (arrow).

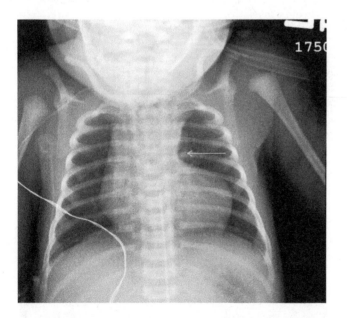

FIGURE 3.42 • **Tetralogy of Fallot**. Frontal view of the chest shows classic "boot"-shaped heart due to right ventricular enlargement, concave pulmonary bay (arrow), and decreased pulmonary vascularity.

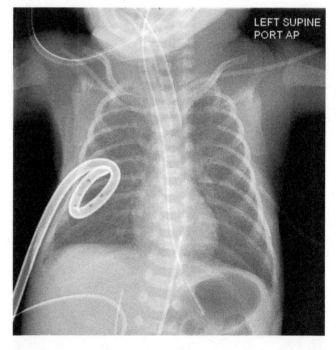

FIGURE 3.44 • **Appropriately Placed Endotracheal Tube**. Frontal view shows normal position of the endotracheal tube with tip between the thoracic inlet and carina. Also note that there is a normally positioned right-sided chest tube.

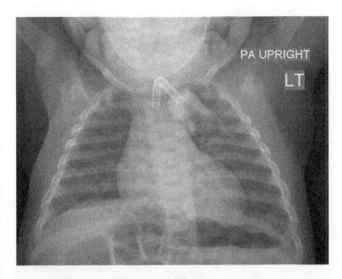

FIGURE 3.45 • **Appropriately Placed Tracheostomy Tube Frontal View**. Frontal view of chest showing normal position of the tracheostomy tube, between the thoracic inlet and carina.

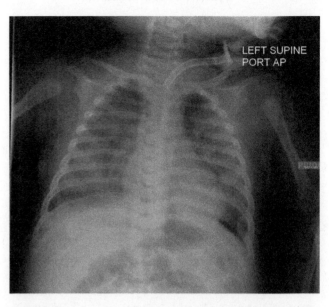

FIGURE 3.47 • **Appropriately Placed Enteral Feeding Tube**. Frontal radiograph of chest shows normal position of the nasogastric tube with gentle leftward curve and tip in left upper quadrant in the region of the stomach. Tracheostomy tube can be seen at the level of the thoracic inlet.

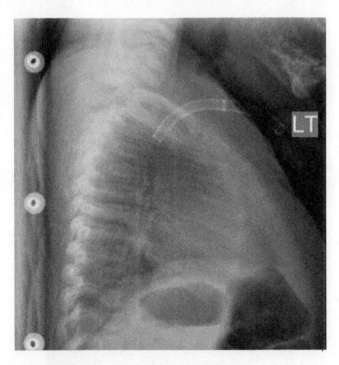

FIGURE 3.46 • **Appropriately Placed Tracheostomy Tube Lateral View**. Lateral view of chest showing appropriately positioned tracheostomy tube between thoracic inlet and carina.

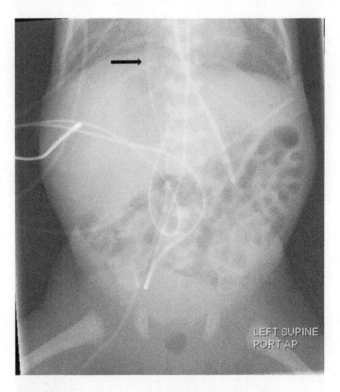

FIGURE 3.48 • **Appropriately Placed Femoral Venous Catheter**. Right femoral venous catheter. Anteroposterior view of the abdomen shows a right-sided femoral line with the tip at the right atrial and inferior vena cava junction (bold arrow).

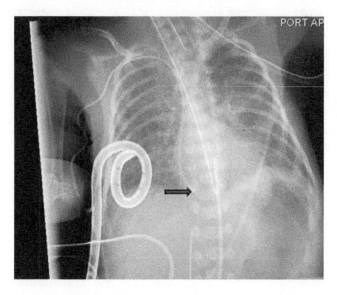

FIGURE 3.49 • **Abnormal Placement of PICC Line**. Abnormal placement of right arm PICC line with the tip deep into the right atrium (arrow) (right-sided pigtail chest tube).

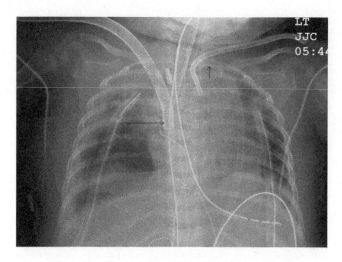

FIGURE 3.51 • **ECMO Cannulae**. Venoarterial ECMO cannulae. Right-sided venous cannula tip in the right atrium (long arrow), and left-sided arterial catheter (short arrow) with tip at the origin of the left common carotid artery.

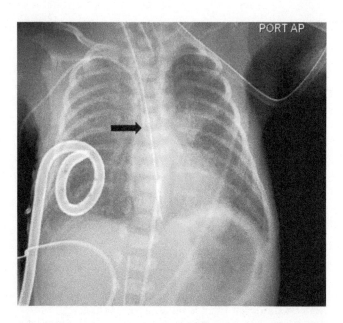

FIGURE 3.50 • **Repositioned/Appropriate PICC Line Placement**.

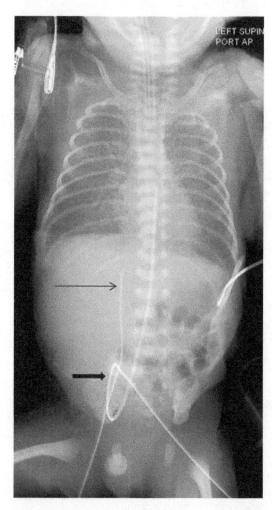

FIGURE 3.52 • **Umbilical Arterial and Venous Catheters Frontal View**. Frontal view of chest and abdomen shows typical course of umbilical arterial catheter (bold arrow) which dips inferiorly before ascending with its tip at T8 level. Umbilical venous catheter (long thin arrow) is seen to ascend with its tip below the diaphragm in the inferior vena cava.

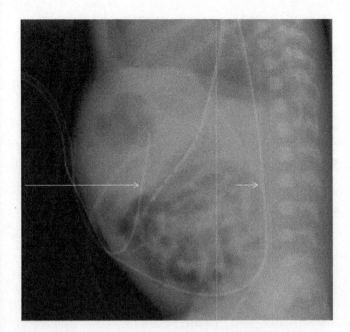

FIGURE 3.53 • **Umbilical Arterial and Venous Catheters Lateral View.** Lateral view shows typical anterior course of the umbilical venous catheter until it is directed posteriorly in the liver (long arrow). The umbilical arterial catheter courses interiorly and ascends posteriorly in the aorta (short arrow).

Bronchoscopy

Jill Marks

Definition

- An invasive procedure in which a trained health-care professional directly visualizes the airway in order to assess structure and functionality.

Indications

- Bronchoscopy is useful for diagnostic, therapeutic, and research purposes.
  - Common indications for bronchoscopy include noisy breathing, (e.g. stridor, chronic wheezing, persistent raiographic abnormalities, congenital abnormality, recurrent pneumonia, retained foreign body).

Types of Bronchoscopy

- Flexible bronchoscopy uses a thin fiber-optic scope.
  - Some scopes may have suction and photography/videography capability.
  - Flexible bronchoscopy may be performed by various trained providers including those working in pulmonology, critical care, anesthesiology, surgery, and emergency medicine.
  - Generally performed via transnasal approach.
  - Can assess dynamic airway events (e.g., tracheomalacia, bronchomalacia) without altering the position, contour, or relationship of the tissues.

- Can be advanced distally into the tracheobronchial tree for evaluation of distal airways.
- Rigid bronchoscopy uses a straight, hollow, rigid metal tube.
  - Should be performed only by a trained otolaryngologist.
  - Allows for airflow in and out of trachea as well as the use of specialized instruments needed for surgical procedures of the airway.
  - Procedure of choice for removal of airway foreign body.
  - Allows for sizing of the airway when evaluating the degree of stenosis.
  - Must be performed in an operating room with use of general anesthesia.
  - Cannot evaluate the distal airways or dynamic airway changes such as bronchomalacia or tracheomalacia.
  - Risks include airway trauma or perforation secondary to rigidity of the bronchoscope.

Relative Contraindications to Bronchoscopy

- At times, bronchoscopy will be indicated with some conditions (e.g., severe mucous plugging causing hypoxemia, part of evaluation in diagnosing etiology of pulmonary hypertension).
- Ability to obtain the same information in a less invasive fashion.
- Untreated bleeding dyscrasias such as thrombocytopenia or clotting dysfunction.
- Profound hypoxemia.
- Moderate-to-severe pulmonary hypertension.

Management of Patient before, during, and after Bronchoscopy

- Unless emergent, preprocedural protocols follow those of impending surgery.
- Postprocedure: Patient will be monitored until awake and stable.
  - Caregivers should be aware that fever for 24 to 48 hours is common after bronchoscopy.
- Complications.
  - Airway trauma resulting in bleeding.
  - Mild and self-limited stridor or hoarseness.
  - Laryngospasm.
  - Hypercapnia and hypoxia.
  - Lower respiratory tract infection.
  - Pneumothorax.

Associated Procedures

- Bronchoalveolar Lavage (BAL).
  - Used to evaluate cell types present in alveoli or as an adjunct to diagnose various lung and systemic diseases and infections.
  - Procedure.
    - Normal saline is instilled into the distal airways via flexible bronchoscope and then suctioned out and sent to the laboratory for further analysis.
  - Criteria for determining a true pathogen include:
    - Presence of a recognized pulmonary pathogen in $>10^4$ colony-forming units/mL and epithelial squamous cells $<1\%$.

- Any bacterial growth considered significant in patients receiving appropriate antibiotic therapy for the isolated pathogen in the previous week.
  - Any positive isolation of *Mycobacterium tuberculosis* or *P. jirovecii*.
  - Isolation of Aspergillus species in any patient with neutropenia or hematologic malignancy.
- Complications: cough, fever, chills, transient infiltrates, bronchospasm, hypoxia, bronchospasm.
- Transbronchial lung biopsy.
  - Used to establish a diagnosis, perform an intervention, or assess transplant rejection.
  - Medication administration.
    - Can administer therapeutic medications into the distal airways (e.g., epinephrine in attempts to control a hemorrhage or dornase alfa as a mucolytic).
  - Stent placement.
  - Balloon dilation of the airway.
  - Laser therapy.

Pulmonary Function Testing

Jill Marks

Background

- Pulmonary function testing (PFT) is useful as an objective measure of lung function in patients with known or suspected lung disease and can be used to exclude or confirm a diagnosis, and assess progression of disease and response to therapy.

Definition

- Provides measures of airflow, lung volumes, gas exchange, response to bronchodilators, and respiratory muscle function.
- Determines presence of obstructive or restrictive lung disease.
- Evaluates respiratory function.
  - Assesses the extent or progression of known pulmonary disease.
  - Provides objective measurement to help determine adequacy of asthma therapy or therapies for other known pulmonary disease.
  - Measures effects of occupational therapy and airway reactivation.
  - Evaluates preoperative risk.
  - Research purposes.

Measurements of PFT

- Peak expiratory flow rate (PEFR).
  - Useful for limited measurement of obstruction in home, primary care, and emergency room settings; useful for those with poor disease perception/symptom recognition.
  - Uses a peak flow meter and is effort dependent.
  - Measures large-airway dysfunction.
  - Values less than 80% of expected or personal best should raise suspicion for obstruction.

- Should be part of a patient's asthma management plan.
- Reference values are available based on patient height.
- Spirometry.
  - Useful for measurement of lung volumes and lung flow.
  - Useful when determining obstructive versus restrictive lung disease.
  - Normal values do not exclude lung disease.
- Usual studies can be performed in children 6 years of age and older.
- Infant PFT can be obtained under sedation by specially trained personnel using forced expiratory procedures.
- Can help determine restrictive versus obstructive lung disease.
- Includes measurements of:
  - Forced vital capacity (FVC).
    - The largest volume of air a person can inhale or exhale.
    - Considered abnormal if less than 80% or predicted.
  - Forced expiratory volume in 1 second (FEV_1).
    - Volume exhaled in the first second.
    - Considered abnormal if less than 80% of predicted.
  - FEV_1/FVC—the ratio between the two.
  - FEF 25 to 75.
    - Measure of flows midway through exhalation.
    - Can provide information about small airways flow.
    - Considered abnormal if <60% of predicted.
  - Flow volume loops.
    - Should be evaluated along with numeric values in order to evaluate reliability of the spirometry studies.
    - There is an inspiratory and an expiratory portion to the loop.
    - Spirometry results are compared to reference values from healthy persons and are based on standing height or arm span, weight, age, gender, and race.
    - Values are given in absolute value and percentage (Table 3.11).

Lung Volume Measurements

- Total lung capacity (TLC).
  - Maximum volume of the lungs with maximum inspiration. Equal to vital capacity + residual volume. Useful in determining obstructive versus restrictive lung disease.
- Residual volume.
  - Measured indirectly and is the volume of air left in the lungs after maximal expiration.
    - Useful in determining restrictive versus obstructive lung disease.
- Functional residual capacity (FRC).
  - Amount of air left in the lung after usual spontaneous expiration.
- Carbon monoxide diffusing capacity (DLCO).
  - Measures carbon monoxide (CO) transfer from inspiration to pulmonary capillary.
  - Will depend on alveolar capillary interface, capillary volume, Hg, and CO/Hg reaction rates.
  - Useful for assessing disease severity related to loss of alveolar surface area over time.

TABLE 3.11 PFT Measurements

Measure	Obstructive Lung Disease	Restrictive Lung Disease
FVC	Normal or increased	Decreased
FRC	Increased	Normal or decreased
TLC	Increased	Decreased
FEV_1	Decreased	Normal or decreased
FEV_1/FVC	Decreased	Normal or decreased
FEF 25–75	Decreased	Normal or decreased

Noninvasive Respiratory Monitoring

Jill Marks

Definition

- Noninvasive respiratory monitoring allows the health-care provider to evaluate oxygenation and ventilation using noninvasive methods.

Pulse Oximetry

- Measures the arterial oxygen saturation via differences in infrared light absorption of oxygenated and nonoxygenated hemoglobin.
- Challenges with the use include inaccuracy at low Sao_2.
- Can give false results secondary to carboxyhemoglobin, methemoglobin, high-intensity ambient light, impaired perfusion, nail polish/artificial nails, IV dyes.

Capnography

- End-tidal CO_2 ($ETCO_2$).
  - Measures ventilation via infrared light absorption or mass spectrometry.
  - Estimates $Paco_2$ and provides information on pulmonary blood flow and dead-space ventilation.
  - Measures ventilation and some devices estimate cardiac output cardiac output.
  - Most commonly used on intubated patients, but can also be measured using special nasal cannula adapters.
- Transcutaneous carbon dioxide (TCO_2).
  - Transcutaneous monitoring technique measures skin-surface Po_2 and Pco_2.
  - Estimates arterial partial pressure of oxygen and carbon dioxide.
  - Locally heats the skin, resulting in hyperperfusion of the area to facilitate measurement—electrochemical measurement.

- Used to assess adequacy of ventilation.
- Can be used to document trends in skin-surface Pco_2.
- This is an indirect measure, and correlation should be completed periodically with another technique (e.g., ABG).
- Contraindications include poor skin integrity and tissue injury at measurement site.

Indirect Calorimetry

Jill Marks

Background

- Nutrition is of vital importance in the clinical management of hospitalized pediatric patients. Malnutrition, defined as deficiency or excess of energy substrates, proteins, or micro-nutrients, can have negative effects on patient recovery and outcomes.

Definition

- Measures oxygen consumed (VO_2) and carbon dioxide produced (VCO_2) and uses these results to calculate resting energy with the Weir equation: REE = [VO_2 (3.941) + VCO_2 (1.11)] × 1440 minutes/day.

Indications

- Encourages optimal nutrition and discourages overfeeding or underfeeding.
- Can be done quickly (as little as 15 minutes) or using a continuous metabolic monitor.
- Should be performed in high-risk patients including but not limited to.
  - Underweight (BMI <5%) or overweight (BMI >85%).
  - Greater than 10% weight gain or loss since admission.
  - Cannot meet prescribed caloric goals.
  - Failure to wean or need to increase ventilator support.
  - Neurologic trauma with evidence of dysautonomia.
  - Oncologic diagnoses.
  - Ventilatory support for >7 days.
  - Suspicion of hypermetabolism (e.g., status epilepticus, hyperthermia, systemic inflammatory response syndrome (SIRS), dysautonomic storms) or hypometabolism (hypothermia, hypothyroidism, intensive care unit stay of more than 4 weeks).

PEARLS

- *Can be cost and/or technology prohibitive*
- *Should not be used during hemodialysis, continuous renal replacement therapy, with oxygen requirement greater than 0.6 or with significant endotracheal tube/tracheostomy tube leak as results will be inaccurate*

1. The parents of a 9-year-old obese boy are concerned that he is falling asleep in school and seems to have decreased energy and attention. He is also reported to snore, especially when in a sound sleep. Which one of the following types of sleep apnea is most likely?
   a. Obstructive
   b. Central
   c. Mixed
   d. Hypoxic

Answer: **A**

Given age and habitus, the most likely explanation is OSA. Central apnea refers to loss of breathing from a primary neurologic problem and mixed apnea would be composed of both central and obstructive. The only method to know whether the child becomes hypoxic during sleep with apnea events is to complete a sleep study with oxygenation saturation monitoring.

2. Which one of the following diagnostic studies is best to obtain for confirming a diagnosis of OSA?
   a. Airway evaluation
   b. Polysomnography
   c. Chest radiography
   d. pH probe

Answer: **B**

Although an airway evaluation may help diagnose adenotonsillar hypertrophy that may contribute to obstructive apnea, a sleep study or polysomnography is the diagnostic test of choice to evaluate for obstructive apnea and the degree of apnea/hypopnea episodes.

3. What are the most appropriate initial management strategies for a child who has definitive OSA?
   a. Nutrition counseling, exercise, noninvasive ventilation for sleep
   b. Nutrition counseling, immediate tonsillectomy, cardiology referral
   c. Exercise, noninvasive ventilation for sleep, chest radiography
   d. Immediate tonsillectomy, cardiology referral, and chest radiography

Answer: **A**

Reduction of body weight would be the first adjustment to managing the sleep apnea along with noninvasive ventilation in the form of CPAP or BiPAP. Adenotonsillectomy would also be a consideration, but after appropriate diagnostic testing and first attempts at weight management.

An 8-year-old weighing 25 kg presents with a 2-day history of cough and respiratory distress, and initially requires supplemental oxygen. He is tachypneic with moderate retractions and has an initial SaO_2 of 88% with bilateral infiltrates present on chest radiograph. He is placed on NIPPV without significant improvement and therefore efforts to intubate him begin. The initial ABG reveals a Pao_2 of 70 mmHg on Fio_2 0.6.

4. The diagnosis of ARDS is made for this child based on which of the following characteristics?
   a. Acute onset, bilateral lung infiltrates, and Pao_2/Fio_2 ratio of 200 to 300
   b. Progressive onset, hyperinflation on chest X-ray, and Pao_2/Fio_2 ratio of <200
   c. Progressive onset, hyperinflation on chest X-ray, and Pao_2/Fio_2 of 200 to 300
   d. Acute onset, bilateral lung infiltrates, and Pao_2/Fio_2 ratio <200

Answer: **D**

The definition of ARDS is based on characteristics of acute onset, bilateral lung infiltrates, noncardiogenic origin, and Pao_2/Fio_2 ratio of <200. ALI has similar characteristics but is defined by a Pao_2/Fio_2 ratio of 200 to 300.

5. Which of the following studies will assist in confirming the diagnosis of ARDS based on the documented criteria?
   a. Complete blood count
   b. Bronchoalveolar lavage
   c. Chest CT
   d. Echocardiogram

Answer: **D**

Determining the etiology of cardiac versus noncardiac origin of ARDS symptoms requires at least an echocardiogram. Placement of a pulmonary artery catheter is an option to obtain more detail, but is quite invasive, and not always available in every critical care setting; so an echocardiography is often done to evaluate for underlying cardiac disease as the cause of pulmonary edema and respiratory distress.

6. Which of the following ventilator settings would be the most appropriate for an 8-year-old who weighs 23 kg with hypoxia in the initial phase of ARDS?
   a. Tidal volume 250, PEEP 10
   b. Tidal volume 175, PEEP 10
   c. Tidal volume 175, PEEP 6
   d. Tidal volume 250, PEEP 6

Answer: **B**

Numerous studies have been done to determine optimal ventilator settings for managing patients with ARDS. Current evidence confirms the incidence of further injury with the use of particular ventilation strategies including high inspiratory pressures; so based on the objective of protecting the lung, low tidal volumes (7–8 mL/kg) and higher PEEP (to keep Fio_2 <0.6) should be considered in the plan of care.

7. Despite optimization of mechanical ventilation settings in the management of the child with ARDS, it is decided to transition to high-frequency oscillatory ventilation for which of the following primary reasons?
   a. Need for higher tidal volumes
   b. Limiting peak inspiratory pressures
   c. Ability to provide lower mean airway pressure
   d. Lowering oxygenation requirements

Answer: B

High-frequency oscillatory ventilation assists in limiting peak inspiratory pressures for the purpose of protecting the lungs and offering a constant distending pressure (MAP), while avoiding overdistention of alveoli.

8. A 17-year-old girl presents to the emergency department after a skiing injury with chief complaint of shortness of breath. Her blood pressure (BP) is 73/35 mmHg and she has unilateral breath sounds. The initial step in management is to:
   a. Intubate the patient
   b. Request a surgery consult for OR management
   c. Perform needle decompression
   d. Obtain a chest radiograph to confirm pneumothorax

Answer: C

Hypotension associated with trauma to the chest indicates high likelihood of a tension pneumothorax, which is a medical emergency requiring immediate intervention with needle decompression. Chest radiography should be ordered at the same time and completed when the patient is stabilized. Surgical consult should also be made for presumed possibility of additional injuries. If the patient is breathing spontaneously, there is no need for intubation at this point.

9. Which of the following radiological findings would be expected in a child with a tension pneumothorax?
   a. Mediastinal shift to ipsilateral side
   b. Mediastinal shift to contralateral side
   c. Halo sign
   d. Hamman sign

Answer: B

Clinical management of the child with a suspected tension pneumothorax includes maintaining oxygenation and determining the need for a needle decompression and/or chest tube insertion. A chest radiograph should be obtained early in the decision-making process to document presence of air. Radiological findings on chest radiograph in the case of a tension pneumothorax include a mediastinal shift to the contralateral side.

10. In the pathophysiology of a tension pneumothorax, the mechanism of injury disrupts the normal thoracic barrier causing normally negative intrathoracic pressure to:
   a. Remain negative but equal to the atmospheric pressure
   b. Become positive but less than the atmospheric pressure
   c. Become positive and equal to the atmospheric pressure
   d. Remain negative and less than the atmospheric pressure

Answer: A

Normally, there is negative intrathoracic pressure compared to the pressure of the atmosphere. When the thoracic barrier is disrupted for any reason, this normal pressure gradient is affected, leading to equalization of intrathoracic pressure compared to atmospheric pressure, thereby drawing air into the pleural space.

11. A 16-month-old is brought to the emergency department with a 3-day history of runny nose and congestion. She has developed a low-grade fever, cough, and increased work of breathing. Which one of the following diagnoses is highest on the differential list?
   a. Bacterial pneumonia
   b. Asthma
   c. Bronchiolitis
   d. Congenital heart disease

Answer: C

A prodrome of upper respiratory tract symptoms followed by lower respiratory tract symptoms and low-grade fever in a child less than 2 years of age makes bronchiolitis the most likely diagnosis.

12. Which one of the following is the most likely causative organism of bronchiolitis in a 4- month-old who was born at 32 weeks gestation?
   a. *Staphylococcus aureus*
   b. Respiratory syncytial virus
   c. *Pseudomonas aeruginosa*
   d. Coronavirus

Answer: B

Bronchiolitis is primarily a viral infection; therefore, bacterial organisms such as *Streptococcus pneumoniae* and *Staph. aureus* are not often causative pathogens in bronchiolitis. A wide range of viruses are responsible for bronchiolitis, with respiratory syncytial virus the most commonly identified.

13. Which one of the following is a common pathophysiologic consequence of bronchiolitis?
   a. Tracheal inflammation
   b. Increased mucus production
   c. Lung hypoexpansion
   d. Focal lobe consolidation

Answer: B

Airway edema, increased mucus production, and increased airway resistance are the hallmarks of the pathophysiologic changes that occur in infants and children diagnosed with bronchiolitis.

(continues on page 90)

14. A 2-month-old infant born at 24 weeks gestation with severe respiratory distress syndrome is unable to wean off ventilator support, but is thriving. What is the most likely diagnosis?
    a. Sepsis
    b. Bronchiolitis
    c. Bronchopulmonary dysplasia
    d. Gastroesophageal reflux

Answer: **C**

A premature infant who develops severe respiratory distress at birth is most likely to be unable to wean off ventilator support as a result of bronchopulmonary dysplasia. Inability to wean off respiratory support is typically a result of arrested development of lung tissue as a consequence of prematurity and the subsequent ventilator-associated lung injury in effort to correct respiratory acidosis.

15. A venous blood gas is performed immediately after the birth of an infant born to a diabetic mother at 35 weeks gestation who has severe respiratory distress. The patient is noted to be tachypneic, tachycardic, cyanotic, with diffuse crackles heard on examination. Which one of the following is most likely to be noted?
    a. Metabolic alkalosis
    b. Respiratory acidosis
    c. Respiratory alkalosis
    d. Metabolic acidosis

Answer: **B**

Infants with severe respiratory distress are often hypoxemic and hypercapneic as a result of underdeveloped lung tissue or an insult to their respiratory or neurologic status during birth process or prior. These abnormalities are seen on blood gas with low pH, elevated CO_2, and normal bicarbonate (initially), meaning the infant has a respiratory acidosis.

16. A key step in the management of an infant with presumed bronchopulmonary dysplasia is:
    a. Use of 100% Fio_2
    b. Low peak inspiratory pressures
    c. Maintaining NPO status
    d. Limiting the use of diuretics

Answer: **B**

Consistently high Fio_2, poor nutrition, and fluid overload all are contraindicated in the management of an infant with BPD. Lung-protective ventilatory strategies (6–8 mL/kg tidal volume, Fio_2 <40%, adequate PEEP), aggressive use of bronchodilators and diuretics, and maintenance of adequate nutrition are supportive and indicated in the management of the infant with chronic lung disease.

17. Which one of the following diagnoses would put an infant at higher risk for the development of bronchopulmonary dysplasia?
    a. Meconium aspiration
    b. Low birth weight with group B streptococcus meningitis
    c. Hydrops fetalis
    d. Low birth weight with severe respiratory distress

Answer: **D**

An infant born with prematurity, extremely low birth weight, and intrauterine growth restriction are all risk factors for the development of bronchopulmonary dysplasia. Term infants born with respiratory distress from a variety of rationales are at some risk of developing chronic lung disease, but not to the extent of those who are preterm or low birth weight.

18. Congenital central hypoventilation syndrome is a result of which of the following genetic abnormalities?
    a. Mutation in CFTR gene
    b. Deletion of chromosome 22q11.2
    c. Extra copy of chromosome 21
    d. Mutation in PHOX2B gene

Answer: **D**

PHOX2B mutation is associated with congenital central hypoventilation syndrome. Cystic fibrosis is associated with a mutation in the CFTR gene. A 22q.11.2 deletion indicates DiGeorge syndrome. An extra copy of chromosome 21 is associated with Down syndrome.

19. A patient diagnosed with congenital central hypoventilation syndrome will likely exhibit which of the following?
    a. Hypercapnia
    b. Hypocapnia
    c. Respiratory distress
    d. Normal neurologic development

Answer: **A**

Patients with congenital central hypoventilation syndrome lack the ability to increase their respiratory drive and therefore will not present with respiratory distress or hypocapnia. Also as a result of their long-standing hypoventilation and hypercapnia, they often have associated developmental disabilities.

20. A newborn infant is found to have congenital central hypoventilation syndrome. Which one of the following is the appropriate management?
    a. Supplemental oxygen
    b. Long-term-assisted ventilation
    c. Immediate neurosurgical intervention
    d. Chest tube placement

Answer: **B**

Patients with congenital central hypoventilation syndrome chronically have inadequate ventilation secondary to a genetic mutation. These patients require some form of assisted ventilation in order to achieve adequate gas exchange. Supplemental oxygen will improve only oxygenation, not ventilation. Unfortunately, the cause is a genetic mutation and therefore neurosurgical intervention is not indicated.

21. Immediately after birth, a neonate is found to have increased work of breathing, absent breath sounds over left lung fields, and a scaphoid abdomen. The most likely diagnosis is:
    a. Meconium aspiration
    b. Congenital diaphragmatic hernia
    c. Transient tachypnea of the newborn
    d. Congenital heart disease

Answer: **B**

The abdomen of the neonate is likely scaphoid as a result of herniation of abdominal contents into thoracic cavity, causing absent breath sounds on the affected side and resultant respiratory distress. CDH is the most likely diagnosis.

22. One of the major physiologic consequences of a CDH is which of the following?
    a. Delay absorption of fetal lung liquid
    b. Insufficient pulmonary surfactant
    c. Pulmonary hypoplasia
    d. Tracheomalacia

Answer: **C**

Pulmonary hypoplasia results from abdominal contents herniating into the chest cavity, which can occur on both sides, but always occurs on the affected side. Pulmonary hypertension is another major physiologic complication of CDH. Both of these problems can contribute to death in the infant.

23. A key step in the resuscitation of a newborn with a CDH is which of the following?
    a. Stomach decompression
    b. Immediate surgical intervention
    c. Thoracentesis
    d. Bag-mask ventilation

Answer: **A**

Stomach decompression and ventilation are the two most important steps in managing an infant with CDH. Bag-mask ventilation should always be avoided and often surgery is delayed until the infant is hemodynamically stable.

24. Which is the most likely causative organism in a child with a barky cough that worsens at night?
    a. *Mycoplasma pneumoniae*
    b. *Streptococcus pneumoniae*
    c. Adenovirus
    d. Parainfluenza type 1

Answer: **D**

The most common cause of laryngotracheobronchitis (croup) is parainfluenza types 1 and 2. Croup can be associated with most viruses, though, to a lower frequency than parainfluenza. It is occasionally associated with mycoplasmal pneumonia.

25. When developing a management plan for a 1-year-old who weighs 12 kg and has rhinorrhea, stridor, and barky cough, which dose of dexamethasone is indicated?
    a. 3 mg
    b. 7 mg
    c. 12 mg
    d. 24 mg

Answer: **B**

One dose of 0.6 mg/kg oral dexamethasone or, in this case, 7.2 mg has been demonstrated to result in faster resolution of croup symptoms and reduce the risk for airway obstruction.

26. When considering administration of heliox to a patient with upper airway obstruction, improved airway dynamics are most likely a result of which of the following?
    a. Steroid enhancing effects
    b. Low gas density
    c. Smooth muscle affinity
    d. Vasoconstriction properties

Answer: **B**

Helium, when combined with oxygen at a ratio of 80% helium to 20% oxygen, has a density 3 times lower than air. This low-density gas can more easily traverse areas of obstruction, delivering oxygen and inhaled medications to the lower airways.

27. A 10-year-old boy with CF is admitted for a pulmonary exacerbation. He is moderately ill and coughing up green sputum. Of the following, which organism is most likely to be present in his airways?
    a. *Pneumocystis (carinii) jirovecii*
    b. *Pseudomonas aeruginosa*
    c. Nontuberculous mycobacterium (NTM)
    d. Burkholderia cepacia complex (Bcc)

Answer: **B**

P. aeruginosa is found in approximately 35% to 40% of children between the ages of 6 to 10 years. *P. jirovecii* is more commonly prevalent in immunocompromised patients, not in those with CF. NTM is identified in 5% to 20% of CF population. Bcc, although potentially very serious, is present in only 2.5% of CF patients.

28. A 13-year-old girl with CF is admitted with a 2-day history of crampy abdominal pain and decreased appetite. Her last bowel movement was the previous day, but it was small. Last menstrual period was 3 weeks before and she denies being sexually active. She is afebrile and interactive with a pain score of 5/10. On examination, she has hypoactive bowel sounds in all four quadrants, no rebound tenderness, and a mass is palpated in the RLQ. CBC and differential are normal. An abdominal radiograph shows mildly distended loops of small

(continues on page 92)

bowel with granular appearance, no free air, and no air-fluid levels. What is the next step?

a. No intervention needed; continue to monitor

b. Oral stool softener (e.g., docusate) twice daily as this is most likely CF constipation

c. Oral polyethylene glycol (PEG) with extra fluid as this is most likely DIOS

d. Place nasogastric (NG) tube to decompress the intestine as this is likely a complete obstruction

Answer: **C**

PEG given orally or by NG tube will provide more rapid results than stool softeners, which can be added later. NG tube placement for decompression is not indicated as this is not a complete obstruction. The patient may be monitored for a longer period, but since she was admitted for pain and there is a risk for complete obstruction, the better option is to initiate therapy immediately.

29. A 15-year-old girl with CF-related diabetes, a history of asthma, and weight loss is admitted for a pulmonary exacerbation. Her home regimen includes long-acting insulin glargine (Lantus) and sliding scale Humalog for hyperglycemia. Prednisone is initiated because of wheezing. Management of potential hyperglycemia includes which of the following:

a. Initiating an oral hyperglycemic agent

b. Initiating a low-dose insulin infusion

c. Frequent monitoring of blood glucose levels

d. Increasing the dose of Lantus

Answer: **C**

Blood glucose levels should be monitored frequently as glucose levels can increase during an exacerbation, with or without steroids, but with the addition of prednisone, there is increased risk of hyperglycemia. Oral hypoglycemic agents are not as effective as insulin and are not recommended in children with CF. An insulin infusion is not indicated as it increases the risk for hypoglycemia. Before considering changing the dose of Lantus, it is necessary to know the patient's current glucose levels. Adding a short-acting insulin may be another option instead of changing the long-acting dose immediately.

30. Which one of the following diagnoses is most likely for a 2-year-old with acute onset respiratory distress, unilateral wheezing, and decreased aeration over the right lung?

a. Partial foreign body obstruction

b. Pulmonary edema

c. Asthma exacerbation

d. Bronchiolitis

Answer: **A**

When an aspirated foreign body passes the carina, it most commonly lodges in the right mainstem bronchus due to the less acute angle at the bifurcation of the mainstem bronchus when compared with the left mainstem bronchus. Placement in the right mainstem bronchus results in decreased aeration and irritation that causes localized wheezing. Asthma and bronchiolitis

frequently result in wheezing; however, they are most commonly associated with bilateral wheezing. Pulmonary edema is more commonly associated with crackles on respiratory examination.

31. A toddler has an acute episode of coughing without any other associated symptoms. He arrives to a small community hospital drooling and positioned with his neck and jaw forward. In addition to planning transport to the closest children's hospital, what is the most important management strategy?

a. Maintaining a calm environment for the child without any stimulation

b. Arranging for immediate surgical intervention

c. Administering dexamethasone at 0.6 mg/kg/dose

d. Planning for urgent intubation and ventilation

Answer: **A**

A young child who acutely develops cough and associated wheezing is most likely to have an airway foreign body which will need to be removed by direct bronchoscopy in the operating room. In order to transport the child without causing the obstruction to move further into the bronchus, it is most important to keep the child calm and minimize noxious stimulation until the child arrives at the appropriate level of care.

32. Absolute contraindication for lung transplantation in a 6-year-old child includes which of the following?

a. Diagnosis of neuroblastoma 2 years ago with failed treatment

b. Diagnosis of asthma 3 years ago which has been well controlled

c. Renal insufficiency with frequent urinary tract infections

d. Recurrent diagnosis of Group A streptococcus pharyngitis

Answer: **A**

The absolute contraindications for lung transplantation include malignancy within the past 2 years, immunodeficiency syndrome, hepatitis B or C with liver disease, severe neuromuscular disease, multiorgan system dysfunction. Relative contraindications include pleurodesis, renal insufficiency, abnormal BMI, chronic airway infection with specific organisms, severe scoliosis, active collagen disease, and mechanical ventilation among other contraindications for lung transplantation.

33. A 16-year-old boy presents to the ED complaining of chest pain that started while he was lifting weights. He is pale and diaphoretic, and his heart rate is 170 beats per minute and SaO_2 is 85% while on 100% non-rebreather face mask. His pulse is thready and breath sounds are inaudible on the right side. What is the first step in managing this patient?

a. Order a STAT chest radiography and ABG

b. Prepare to intubate the patient

c. Prepare to needle decompress the patient's chest

d. Order an EKG and page the cardiologist to evaluate chest pain

Answer: **C**

Tension pneumothorax is a clinical diagnosis made based on the patient's symptoms and the presence of ipsilateral decreased breath sounds, hypoxia, and cardiovascular compromise. Interventions to decompress the pneumothorax should begin immediately before diagnostic tests are performed.

34. An obese 8-year-old who was recently diagnosed with attention-deficit disorder is admitted to the inpatient unit for asthma. At night, he is noted to be snoring loudly and has desaturations to 88% on room air. After his asthma exacerbation has improved, what would be the next step in care?
    a. Refer to an otolaryngologist for a tonsillectomy and adenoidectomy
    b. Consult with PCP to arrange a polysomnography
    c. Adjust inhaled steroids to twice daily dosing
    d. Refer to a pulmonologist for pulmonary function testing

Answer: **B**

Common morbidities of overweight and obese children include OSA, which poses more problems than just snoring. Children who are chronically sleep deprived or experience hypoxia on a regular basis can present with other problems such as school performance and attention-deficit hyperactivity disorder due to their inability to obtain a good night sleep. Chronic effects on cardiac function are another concern with OSA, leading to chronic hypoxia. Most important management is to obtain a formal sleep study to document periods of apnea and then determine appropriate therapy.

35. The most common cardiac complication of OSA is:
    a. Left ventricular hypertrophy
    b. Premature ventricular contractions
    c. Right bundle branch block
    d. Left atrial hypertrophy

Answer: **A**

Children with OSA have chronic hypoxic episodes when they sleep, which result in both respiratory and cardiac complications. An EKG on a child with OSA is very likely to show left ventricular hypertrophy as a result of chronic hypoxia, but if treated with BiPAP or surgery (e.g., tonsillectomy and adenoidectomy), the LVH can resolve.

36. A 2-year-old previously healthy boy, arrives to the ED with fever of 102°F, cough for 2 days, respiratory rate of 60 breaths per minute, with retractions and nasal flaring. Oxygen saturations are 89% breathing room air. Which one of the following organisms is the most likely cause of pneumonia in this child?
    a. *Escherichia coli*
    b. *Listeria monocytogenes*
    c. *Pneumocystis carinii*
    d. *Streptococcus pneumoniae*

Answer: **D**

A previously healthy 2-year-old with community-acquired pneumonia may have either viral or bacterial pneumonia. Of the options presented, *Strep. pneumoniae* is the most common organism responsible for pneumonia in this age group.

37. A febrile 4-year-old with suspected pneumococcal (*streptococcus*) pneumonia has a chest radiograph (Figure 3.54). What is the best therapeutic option for this child based on these results?

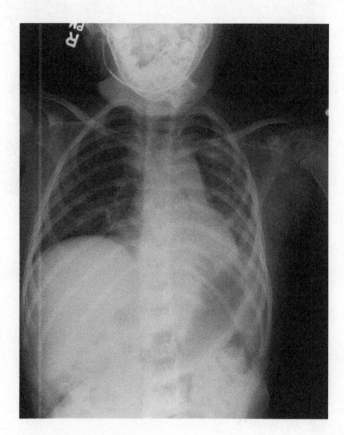

FIGURE 3.54

a. Needle thoracostomy
b. Antibiotic therapy
c. Thoracostomy tube placement + antibiotic therapy
d. Bronchodilator therapy and pulmonary toileting

Answer: **B**

This chest radiograph of a child with suspected pneumococcal pneumonia demonstrates classic left lower lobe alveolar opacities with air bronchograms and alveolar filling. Along with fever, this is most consistent with bacterial pneumonia and should be treated with antibiotics.

38. A 10-year-old boy with cerebral palsy, developmental delay, and hydrocephalus has been managed for 5 days in ICU for aspiration pneumonia. Today, he is noted to be febrile, tachycardic, with increased work of breathing and increased oxygen requirements over the last 24 hours. Examination

(continues on page 94)

demonstrates diminished breath sounds over the right lower chest, coarse transmitted nasopharyngeal sounds throughout the lung fields. Chest radiograph is shown in Figure 3.55.

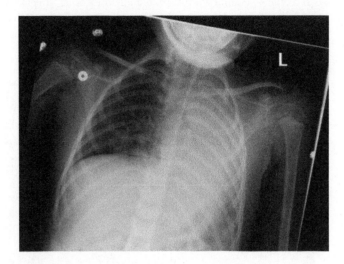

FIGURE 3.55

What is the most appropriate next step in this child's management?
a. Chest CT
b. Chest ultrasound
c. Thoracostomy tube placement for fluid analysis
d. Therapeutic bronchoscopy

Answer: **B**

Ultrasound is an efficient method to determine the presence of a chest pleural effusion and differentiate areas of loculation from fluid. A chest CT can be used to validate or confirm the effusion, but considering radiation exposure and efficiency, it is better to obtain a bedside ultrasound by a competent examiner.

39. A 6-week-old has a 3-day history of rhinorrhea, decreased feeding, and cough for the last 4 days. Vital signs include temperature of 37.4°C, oxygen saturations of 96% on room air, heart rate of 177 beats per minute, respiratory rate of 60 breaths per minute, and normal blood pressure. Auscultation does not reveal an abnormality. Lymphocytosis is noted on the complete blood count. What is the next best step in this patient's management?
a. Oral erythromycin for 14 days as an outpatient with follow-up
b. Oral azithromycin for 5 days as an outpatient with follow-up
c. Admit for bronchodilator therapy and parenteral antibiotic therapy
d. Admit and empirically treat for pertussis pending culture results

Answer: **D**

An infant with classic cough and lymphocytosis most likely has pertussis. Because of the risk of apnea at this age, admission for monitoring is indicated, along with definitive evaluation, monitoring feedings, hydration status, and providing supportive care.

40. When evaluating a chest radiograph of a child with dyspnea and hypoxia, Kerley B lines are noted. Which one of the following is the most likely diagnosis for this child?
a. Asthma
b. Flail chest
c. Pulmonary edema
d. Pulmonary contusion

Answer: **C**

Kerley B lines are thin pulmonary opacities that are the result of interstitial fluid of cellular infiltration in the lungs typically indicating a diagnosis of pulmonary edema.

41. A child is suspected of having a PE. Which one of the following is the greatest risk factor associated with this diagnosis?
a. Renal failure
b. Central venous catheter
c. Implantable cardiac defibrillator
d. Pulmonary edema

Answer: **B**

Children are not typically candidates to develop PE, and a PE often occurs in children who have underlying hematologic or coagulation disorders. A central venous catheter poses a high risk for developing thromboembolism, leading to a pulmonary embolus.

42. After confirmation of the presence of a PE, which one of the following diagnostic tests is indicated?
a. Protein C activity
b. Brain natriuretic hormone
c. Procalcitonin level
d. Vitamin D level

Answer: **A**

Protein C deficiency is the result of a mutation in the PROC gene. Protein C is a protein that is critical in inactivating other proteins that promote clotting. In this rare inherited disorder, the deficiency in protein C leads to the inability to control blood clotting.

43. A 9-year-old, weighing 38 kg, has been brought to the ED after being struck by a car. Injuries include pulmonary contusions with overlying rib fractures on chest radiograph. Patient's heart rate is 100 beats per minute, respiratory rate 20 breaths per minute, oxygen saturation 96% on room air. IVF should be ordered at what rate?
a. 58 mL/hour
b. 78 mL/hour
c. 95 mL/hour
d. 100 mL/hour

Answer: **B**

A child who experienced significant trauma and is hemodynamically stable has a goal therapy to provide adequate tissue perfusion and avoid excess resuscitation. Therefore, the patient should be placed on a weight-based fluid maintenance rate which is equivalent to 78 mL/hour.

44. A 15-year-old pedestrian presents to the ED after being struck on a local road. The patient is tachypneic, has retractions, and has decreased breath sounds on the left side. The first intervention should be to:
    a. Order a STAT chest radiography
    b. Place the patient on his left side
    c. Apply supplemental oxygen
    d. Intubate the patient

Answer: **C**

The primary focus and care for the child who sustains trauma involving the chest should be directed at identifying life-threatening conditions and returning to basic principles of ABSCs. Oxygenation is the first important objective.

45. A 12-year-old was found awake and alert in a house fire once the fire was controlled. The most important indicator that he may have smoke inhalation injury is:
    a. Carbon coloring of his clothing
    b. Cough and low oxygen saturation
    c. Length of time he was exposed to smoke
    d. Abrasions on the face

Answer: **B**

Indications that a patient was exposed to smoke and may have smoke inhalation injury involve physical examination and evaluation. Visible presence of soot on face, neck, or clothing and carbonaceous sputum, the presence of facial burns, hoarse voice, and cough are all indicators that smoke inhalation may have occurred. The most important indicators include work of breathing, and the presence of tachypnea, cough, and hypoxia.

46. An infant who has bronchiolitis with significant apnea events is being ventilated with pressure support mode with settings of Fio_2 of 70%, PIP of 24, PEEP of 5, inspiratory time (IT) of 0.6 seconds, and pressure support of 18, and has ABG values: pH 7.36, pO_2 58 mmHg, pCO_2 43 mmHg, and HCO_3 of 22 mEq/L. Which one of the following setting changes can best assist in improving this blood gas?
    a. Increase the oxygen to 100%
    b. Increase the PEEP to 8
    c. Decrease the IT to 0.5
    d. Increase the PIP to 28

Answer: **B**

This blood gas represents normal values except for a low pO_2. Increasing the oxygen level will assist in improving oxygenation, but instead of increasing to the highest possible oxygen level which may have potential damaging effects for the infant, a better choice is to increase the positive end-expiratory pressure, allowing more time for oxygen to exchange in the alveoli.

47. A 4-year-old, 20-kg child was found unresponsive and hardly breathing, with no apparent inciting event. He is intubated by paramedics and transported to the hospital. He is placed on volume control ventilation with synchronized intermittent mandatory ventilation, tidal volume is 180 mL, pressure support is 10 cm H_2O, PEEP is 5 cm H_2O, and oxygen is 45% with a rate of 20 breaths per minute. On arrival, he is not responsive to pain and is not breathing on his own. The capillary blood gas values are pH 7.56, pO_2 135, pCO_2 24, and HCO_3 25, and base excess is +4. Which one of the following ventilator settings should be adjusted?
    a. Decrease the oxygen to 21%
    b. Decrease the tidal volume to 120 mL
    c. Decrease the tidal volume to 100 mL
    d. Increase the ventilator rate to 30 breaths per minute

Answer: **B**

Interpreting the blood gas involves an understanding that this child has healthy lungs but has a neurologic issue that is preventing appropriate ventilation. He is currently being overventilated as indicated by the high pH and the low pCO_2. Typically, tidal volume is set based on 6 to 8 mL/kg, so the initial setting of 180 mL is too high. Decreasing the tidal volume to 120 mL while making sure that there is adequate chest rise is the first step in managing the ventilator settings. Further changes can be based on blood gas measurements and indications that the child is breathing on his own.

48. A 6-year-old girl has had a cough for 2 weeks which began following an acute "choking episode." She has diminished breath sounds on the right side, and the lateral decubitus chest radiograph demonstrates hyperinflation of the right lung when the patient is positioned with the right side down. The most appropriate next study for this patient would be:
    a. Chest CT
    b. Flexible bronchoscopy
    c. Rigid bronchoscopy
    d. Pulmonary function tests

Answer: **C**

The most appropriate next step in caring for this patient would be rigid bronchoscopy. It is the preferred method of bronchoscopy when there is concern for airway foreign body.

49. A 12-year-old patient with persistent cough and exercise intolerance who has been treated for asthma has an FEV_1 of 63% with an increase to 75% after albuterol. His FVC is 72%. Which one of the following tests would help you determine the category of lung dysfunction (restrictive versus obstructive disease)?
    a. FEV_1:FVC ratio
    b. FEF 25/75
    c. Flow volume loops
    d. Total lung capacity

Answer: **D**

Total lung capacity is a useful study to help categorize restrictive versus obstructive lung disease. It will be increased in obstructive lung disease and decreased in restrictive lung disease.

Recommended Readings

Cairo, J. M. (2012). Effects of positive–pressure ventilation on the pulmonary system. In J. M. Cairo (Ed.), *Pilbeam's mechanical ventilation* (5th ed., pp. 328–332). St Louis, MO: Elsevier Mosby.

Cortez, E., & Ganesan, R. (2012). Pulmonary disorders: Physiology and diagnostics. In K. Reuter-Rice & B. Bolick (Eds.), *Pediatric acute care* (pp. 996–1004). Burlington, MA: Jones & Bartlett Learning.

Cystic Fibrosis Foundation Patient Registry. (2011). *2011 Annual data report*. Retrieved from http://www.cff.org/UploadedFiles/research/ClinicalResearch/2011-Patient-Registry.pdf

Dotson, K., & Johnson, L. (2012). Pediatric spontaneous pneumothorax. *Pediatric Emergency Care, 28*(7), 715–720.

Elliott, E. (2012). Air leak syndromes. In K. Reuter-Rice & B. Bolick (Eds.), *Pediatric acute care* (pp. 1009–1012). Burlington, MA: Jones & Bartlett Learning.

Elliott, E. (2012). Pulmonary edema. In K. Reuter-Rice & B. Bolick (Eds.), *Pediatric acute care*. Burlington, MA. Jones & Bartlett Learning.

Flume, P. A., & Van Devanter, D. R. (2012). State of progress in treating cystic fibrosis respiratory disease. *BMC Medicine, 10*, 86.

Lesser, D. J. (2012). Obstructive sleep apnea syndrome. In K. Reuter-Rice & B. Bolick (Eds.), *Pediatric acute care: A guide for interprofessional practice*. Burlington, MA: Jones & Bartlett Learning.

National Heart, Lung, and Blood Institute (NHLBI). (2007). *National asthma education and prevention program, expert panel report III: Guidelines for the diagnosis and management of asthma*. Retrieved from www.nhlbi.nih.gov/guidelines/asthma/

Paes, B. A., Nagel, K., Sunak, I., Rashish, G., & Chan, A. K., on behalf of the Thrombosis and Hemostasis in Newborns (THiN) Group. (2012). Neonatal and infant pulmonary thromboembolism: A literature review. *Blood Coagulation & Fibrinolysis, 23*, 653–662.

Ricard J. D., Dreyfus, D., Rotta, A. T., & Saumon, G. (2011). Ventilator-induced lung injury. In B. P. Fuhrman & J. J. Zimmerman (Eds.), *Fuhrman and Zimmermans' pediatric critical care* (4th ed., pp. 697–705). Philadelphia, PA: Elsevier Saunders.

Riccioni, M. (2012). Acute respiratory distress syndrome. In K. Reuter-Rice & B. Bolick (Eds.), *Pediatric acute care* (pp. 1005–1009). Burlington, MA: Jones & Bartlett Learning.

Tilford, B. (2011). Ventilator induced lung injury. In B. Bolick & K. Reuter-Rice (Eds.), *Pediatric acute care: A guide for Interprofessional practice* (pp. 1081–1082). Burlington, MA: Jones & Bartlett Learning.

Respiratory Support Modalities

Oxygen Delivery Devices

Donald Artes/Cathy Haut

Discussion

- In order to provide supplemental oxygenation for a child with hypoxia or ineffective ventilation, a variety of oxygen delivery devices are available for use.
- Indications include pathophysiologic hypoxemia, ineffective oxygenation related to neurologic illness or trauma, postanesthesia, and conditions resulting in myocardial ischemia.

Definition

- An oxygen delivery device provides supplemental oxygen through the upper airways to the lungs via either low-flow or high-flow systems.

Types

- Low-flow devices: *Provide oxygen at flow rates that are less than the patient's inspiratory demand.*
  - Nasal cannula: Delivers oxygen concentrations of approximately 24% to 44% at flow rates of 1 to 6 L/minute in adolescents and adults. A humidifier is used if the nasal cannula will be used at higher flows and for longer periods of time.
    - Flow rates as low as 250 mL (0.25 L/min) are used to deliver oxygen in infants.
    - Delivered oxygen concentrations are based on oxygen flow in relation to the patient's minute volume (*tidal volume × rate*) and are therefore difficult to accurately predict in infants and young children.
  - Non-rebreather mask: Delivers oxygen concentrations of approximately 60% to 80% at flow rates of 8 to 10 L/minute.
    - Non-rebreather masks should be used when a child is in respiratory distress, especially when the etiology of the distress is unknown.
- High-flow devices: *Provide oxygen at flow rates that meet or exceed the patient's inspiratory demand.*
  - Venturi mask delivers oxygen concentrations at precisely 24%, 28%, 31%, 35%, 40%, and 50%. This is accomplished by interchanging one of six color-coded adapters.

- Aerosol mask, in conjunction with a jet nebulizer, delivers oxygen concentrations of 28% to 100%. An air entrainment port can be opened and closed to adjust the delivered oxygen concentration. The smaller the opening of the entrainment port, the higher the oxygen concentration and the lower the total flow delivered to the patient (Table 4.1).
- High-flow nasal cannulas: Specific systems that are designed to deliver heated humidified blended oxygen at higher flow rates that may meet or exceed the patient's demand. See additional information under "Noninvasive Ventilation" that follows.

Noninvasive Ventilation

Discussion

- Noninvasive ventilation plays a key role in the support of pediatric patients who once would have required intubation and mechanical ventilation.
- Indications include the need for short-term ventilation, improvement in lung volumes and compliance, and a reduction in oxygen requirements.

Definition

- Noninvasive ventilation is a mechanism of providing ventilatory support without the use of an invasive artificial airway (e.g., endotracheal or tracheostomy tube).

Types

- BiPAP (bilevel positive airway pressure)
  - Allows for the separate regulation of the inspiratory and expiratory positive pressure levels as well as the ability to set a mandatory minimal ventilatory rate.
- CPAP (continuous positive air pressure)
  - Allows for spontaneous ventilation, which provides a constant positive airway pressure throughout the respiratory cycle.
- High-flow nasal cannula
  - Gas delivery using a nasal cannula at gas temperatures near body temperature, allowing for highly saturated water vapor.
  - This highly saturated gas allows for increased flow rates without causing additional discomfort and irritation to the nasal mucosa.

TABLE 4.1	Oxygen Delivery		
Oxygen (%)	Approximate Air/O₂ Ratio	Oxygen Flow Rate (L/minute)	Total Flow to Patient (L/minute)
24	25:1	4	104
28	10:1	4	44
30	8:1	6	54
35	5:1	8	48
40	3:1	10	40
45	2:1	12	36
50	1.7:1	12	33

Note: There may come a point at oxygen concentrations of greater than 50% when the total delivered flow may not meet the patient's demand.

Assessment and Management

- BiPAP/CPAP
  - Finding the appropriate mask fit for a pediatric patient can be challenging because of the variety of pediatric face shapes and sizes.
  - The key to successful noninvasive ventilation is a calm cooperative patient. Slowly increasing the patient's airway pressures to allow for desensitization or the use of small doses of anxiolytics may be required.
  - Heavy doses of sedation and analgesia are contraindicated.
  - Periodic breaks off of the BIPAP/CPAP mask are necessary for proper skin assessment and to reduce the risk of skin breakdown.
  - Skin barrier devices can be applied between the skin and the mask to reduce the risk of skin breakdown.
  - Adequate patient airway protection is necessary to avoid the potential danger of aspiration.
  - Not indicated in patients with conditions that reduce the respiratory drive or in cases of respiratory failure.
  - Care should be taken with patients whose condition interferes with the seal of the mask, such as facial trauma, facial surgery, or the presence of a nasogastric tube.
- High-flow nasal cannula
  - Flow rates are set at 1 to 8 L/minute for infants and young children, although flow rates can be as high as 40 L/minute in older children and adults.
  - Some sources have postulated that the rate of flow may deliver a level of positive pressure similar to CPAP.
- Evaluating patient response
  - Improvement in arterial blood gases (e.g., increase in oxygenation and decrease in carbon dioxide levels).
  - Relief of dyspnea.
  - Improvement in the delivery of medications such as bronchodilators.
- Diagnostic evaluation
  - Consider radiographic imaging while requiring oxygen.

Laryngeal Mask Airway

Brian Eells

Airway Management

Background/Definition

- Inflatable cuff sits in hypopharynx, outside larynx.
- Creates end-to-end tube with trachea, in comparison to standard endotracheal intubation, which is a tube-within-tube.
- Generally considered intermediate to face mask and endotracheal tube.
- Useful as rescue device in difficult airway.
- Does not "secure" the airway like an endotracheal tube.
- Easier blind technique for placement (airway structures not visualized); no laryngoscope needed (Figure 4.1).

Etiology/Types

- Originally designed by Dr. Archie Brain.
  - LMA is LMA North America, now part of Teleflex.

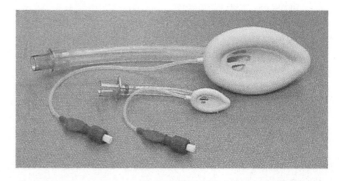

FIGURE 4.1 • **Laryngeal Mask Airway.** The original LMA design: a size 1 and size 6 LMA-Classic. The two bars over the airway aperture prevent the epiglottis from obstructing the LMA barrel.

TABLE 4.2	Standard Sizing for LMA
Mask Size	Patient size
1	<5 kg neonate/infant
1.5	5–10 kg infant
2	10–20 kg infant/child
2.5	20–30 kg child
3	30–50 kg child/small adult
4	50–70 kg normal adult
5	70–100 kg large adult

- Many LMA versions are available (e.g., Classic, Unique, ProSeal).
- Other brands now exist (e.g., i-gel, Ambu Aura-i, Cook air-Q).

LMA Management

- Intact airway reflexes preclude proper placement (e.g., biting, coughing, vomiting) (Table 4.2).
  - LMA size is estimated based on weight (See Table 4.2) and delete (see Table 4.2 at the end of the first bullet)
- Cuff volumes are described by manufacturer.
- Proper inflation usually causes slight upper movement of LMA and slight bulging of anterior neck.
- Risk of ischemia if cuff is overinflated and/or systemic blood pressure is low.
- May cause gastric insufflation if airway pressures exceed gastroesophageal opening pressure (e.g., ~15–25 cm H_2O).

Difficult Airway
Brian Eells

Background/Definition
- Difficulty with mask ventilation, tracheal intubation, or both.

Etiology/Types
- Most assessments and guidelines are based on adult population (e.g., Mallampati classes, ASA's "Practice guidelines for management of the difficult airway") (Figure 4.2).

Associated Underlying Conditions
- Congenital anomalies (e.g., Pierre Robin sequence, Treacher Collins syndrome)
- Tumors (e.g., cystic hygroma)
- Infection (e.g., retropharyngeal abscess, epiglottitis)
- Oral/dental (e.g., severe overbite, wired teeth/jaw, high-arched palate)
- Muscular (e.g., torticollis)
- Skeletal (e.g., ankylosis, cervical fracture)
- Trauma

Clinical Presentation
- Predictors of difficult pediatric laryngoscopy
  - Age <1 year
  - ASA physical status 3 or 4
  - Modified Mallampati class 3 or 4
  - Oromaxillofacial disorder
  - Cardiac dysfunction

Evaluation
- Modified Mallampati classification system:
  - Performed in the sitting position, tongue protruded maximally; no phonation.

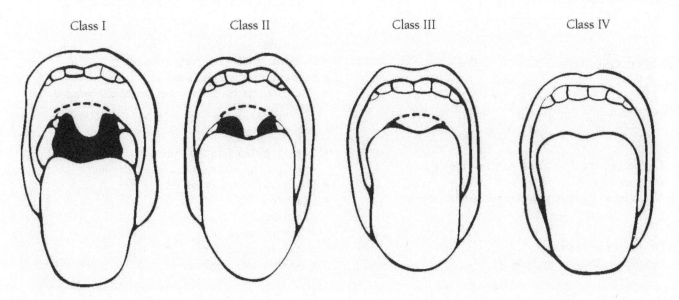

Class I   Class II   Class III   Class IV

FIGURE 4.2 • **Mallampati Scoring.**

- Class I: Faucial pillars, soft and hard palates, uvula visualized.
- Class II: Faucial pillars, soft and hard palates visualized; uvula partially masked by base of tongue.
- Class III: Only soft and hard palates visualized; ± base of uvula.
- Class IV: Only hard palate visualized.
- Thyromental distance
- Head and neck movement (particularly neck extension)
- Upper lip bite test (ULBT)
  - Grade I lower incisors can fully cover the upper lip's mucosa.
  - Grade II lower incisors can touch the upper lip but cannot fully cover the mucosa.
  - Grade III lower incisors fail to bite the upper lip.
- Body mass index
  - Larger body mass index associated with difficult airway.

Management

- Call for help / often need at least two experienced providers.
- Determine best sedation approach: awake, asleep and breathing, or apneic.
- Noninvasive (e.g., standard laryngoscopy) versus invasive (e.g., surgical cricothyrotomy).
- "Difficult airway cart" and oxygen supply
  - Self-inflating manual resuscitator (e.g., Ambu) and face masks of various sizes.
  - Suture for tongue stitch, or nonperforating towel clamps.
  - Multiple laryngoscope blades, handles, and tubes, LMAs, and combitubes.
  - Intubating stylets, bougies, tube changers; light wand.
  - Fiberoptic bronchoscope, rigid bronchoscope.
  - Retrograde intubation kit, percutaneous or surgical cricothyrotomy or tracheostomy.
- The ASA "Difficult Airway Algorithm" is complex.
  - Always have plans A, B, and C (at least).
  - Always have lots of experienced help.

PEARL

- *Early consult with pediatric anesthesia provider facilitates optimal outcomes.*

Tracheostomy

Andrea M. Kline-Tilford & Jason M. Kane

Definition

- Surgical opening through the neck into the larynx to place an artificial airway.
- Allows breathing to bypass the nose and the mouth.

Background

- Provides a stable airway.
- Facilitates pulmonary hygiene.

- Facilitates administration of long-term positive pressure ventilation.

Indications

- Upper airway obstruction: congenital or acquired.
- Long-term ventilation or pulmonary toilet.

Contraindications

- No absolute contraindications.
- Relative contraindication: end-of-life situations.

Procedure

- Most commonly performed in the operating room under general anesthesia.
- Often, stay sutures are placed until the first tracheostomy change; *airway emergency when tracheostomy is inadvertently dislodged prior to removal of stay sutures.*
- Placed during the tracheostomy directly into the laryngeal tissue.
- Gently lifting the sutures up and away from the neck, pulls the trachea closer to the stoma and skin surface, improving visualization of the tracheal tract.
- Facilitates rapid airway recannulation in the event of inadvertent decannulation prior to stoma maturation.

Size

- Diameter
  - Determined by underlying etiology and patient size.
  - Ideally small enough for vocalization or large enough that leak does not result in hypoventilation, especially if requiring positive pressure ventilation.
- Length
  - Too short may result in inadvertent decannulation or creation of a false airway.
  - Too long may result in damage to the carina, stimulation of the vagal response, or intubation of the left or right bronchus.
  - Some patients may require custom-length tracheostomy tubes to bypass areas of tracheal stenosis or malacia.

Management

- Humidified gas delivery.
- Suction tracheostomy tube as needed.
- Soap and water for stoma site.
- Established tracheostomy tubes are usually changed on a weekly basis.

Complications

- Pediatric patients are 2 to 3 times more likely to experience complications from tracheostomy than adults.
- Incidence of complication 5% to 49%.
- Short-term
  - Bleeding
  - Pneumothorax
  - Pneumomediastinum
  - Subcutaneous emphysema

- Tracheoesophageal fistula
- Infection
- Tracheal plugging
- Tracheo-innominate artery fistula
- Intermediate/long-term complications
  - Mucosal injury
  - Ischemia of the tracheal wall
  - Fibrotic changes
  - Stenosis of trachea
  - Tracheal plugging
  - Tracheo-innominate artery fistula

PEARLS

- *Children may be intubated from above in the event of inability to replace the tracheostomy tube or if a false passage has been created. Exception: Presence of a laryngotracheal separation.*
- *In children with cuffed tracheostomy tubes, limit cuff insufflation to reduce the risk of tracheal injury/stenosis.*
- *Life-threatening tracheal bleeding is likely the result of tracheo-innominate artery fistula; associated with a HIGH mortality.*

Endotracheal Tubes and Invasive Ventilation

Jason M. Kane

Invasive Ventilation

Background

- Invasive mechanical ventilation refers to the use of life-support technology that assists with the work of breathing for patients who are unable to effectively do so on their own.
  - Two broad indications for intubation and mechanical ventilation:
    - Failure of oxygenation (hypoxia)
    - Failure of ventilation (hypercarbia)

Types

- Invasive mechanical ventilation is accomplished using an endotracheal tube placed in the trachea and attached to a mechanical ventilator circuit.
- Noninvasive positive pressure ventilation (such as mask BiPAP) results in similar physiology; however, the amount of support provided by noninvasive measures cannot achieve the same pressures compared to invasive ventilation.
- There are multiple manufacturers of mechanical ventilators, all with proprietary modes of ventilation. However, the basic tenets of ventilator function are the same regardless of the brand of ventilator.

Settings

- Ventilator-controlled breaths: A ventilator delivers breath to the patient at a set frequency (rate) prescribed by the clinician.
  - In a pure control mode of ventilation, the ventilator will deliver a full breath at the set rate and if the patient attempts to breathe, the ventilator will deliver an additional full ventilator breath with each patient effort.
- Supported patient-generated breaths
  - The patient may attempt to breathe on his or her own, and there are settings afforded that can assist with patient-generated breaths.
  - Pressure support: A set pressure generated with a spontaneous patient breath effort.
  - Volume support: A set volume generated with a spontaneous patient breath effort.
- Synchronized intermittent mandatory ventilation (SIMV)
  - A set number of full ventilator breaths is delivered to the patient; however, if the patient triggers a breath, the volume of that breath will be determined by the patient effort and the support provided to the patient (if any).
- Positive end-expiratory pressure (PEEP)
  - Amount of pressure delivered to the patient at the end of expiration and in between respirations.
  - Helps to prevent alveolar collapse in between respirations.
- Inspiratory time
  - Amount of time spent on inspiration.
  - Reducing time spent on inspiration increased the time for exhalation.
- Primary methods to increase oxygenation
  - Increase Fio_2.
  - Increase PEEP.
  - Increase pressure control (increased "area under the curve").
  - Increase inspiratory time.
  - In high-frequency oscillatory ventilation, increase mean airway pressure (MAP).
- Primary methods to remove carbon dioxide (CO_2)
  - Increase ventilator rate.
  - Increase tidal volume.
  - Increase pressure control.
  - Increase pressure support.
  - Decrease inspiratory time.

Modes

- Volume-controlled ventilation.
- The delivery of air is a set tidal volume.
- Although the volume of each breath is guaranteed and thus minute ventilation can be guaranteed, there is a risk of barotrauma if lung compliance suddenly decreases.
- Volume control.
- Pressure-regulated volume control.
- Pressure-controlled ventilation.
  - Pressure control.
  - Airway pressure release ventilation.

- Pure spontaneous modes—pressure support (CPAP/pressure support)
  - Patients receive no set frequency of ventilator-delivered breaths.
  - Can result in patient apnea.
- Mixed modes (SIMV)
  - Combines controlled ventilation with spontaneous ventilation.
  - Coordinates mandatory ventilator breaths with patient-generated breaths.
- Alternative modes of ventilation (nonconventional)
  - High-frequency oscillatory ventilation
  - High-frequency jet ventilation

Management

- Ventilator settings should be set to match the needs of the patient, regardless of which particular mode is utilized.
- The basic tenets are to optimize ventilation (clearance of CO_2) and oxygenation (a function of MAP).
  - Ventilation: The clearance of CO_2 from the alveoli is a function of minute ventilation, or the mathematical product of respiratory rate and tidal volume.
  - Oxygenation = MAP. With respect to invasive mechanical ventilation, the MAP can be manipulated by changing minute ventilation, end-expiratory pressure (PEEP), inspiratory time fraction (i-time), or tidal volume. A higher MAP results in improved oxygenation.

Monitoring

- In addition to following clinical examination and pressure/volume parameters, clinicians can use data derived from invasive parameters to gauge efficacy of mechanical ventilation.
  - Arterial blood gas parameters, including Po_2, Pco_2
  - Alveolar–arteriolar oxygen gradient: When the gradient between oxygen in the alveoli and the arterial blood increases, less oxygen diffuses across the alveolar membranes and enters into the systemic circulation. Does not account for changes in the ventilator settings.
  - Oxygenation index
  - Pao_2:Fio_2 ratio (P/F ratio)

Presedation Evaluation

Brian Eells

Background/Definition

- General history (review of medical record).
- Focused history (e.g., fasting status, recent upper respiratory tract infection, significant comorbidities, previous sedation/anesthetics).
- Physical examination; focus on airway and cardiopulmonary status.

- Psychosocial (e.g., Erikson's stages, comfort item/"security blanket").
- Discuss. Plan. Implement. Document.

Types

- Sedation is a continuum (minimal → moderate → deep → general anesthesia).

Pathophysiology

- Sedatives selected on unique pharmacodynamics properties (e.g., maintenance or abolishment of airway tone).

Evaluation

- American Society of Anesthesiologists' physical status classification system:
  - PS 1—Normal healthy patient.
  - PS 2—Patient with mild systemic disease.
  - PS 3—Patient with severe systemic disease.
  - PS 4—Patient with severe systemic disease that is a constant threat to life.
  - PS 5—Moribund patient who is not expected to survive without the operation.
  - PS 6—Declared brain-dead patient whose organs are being removed for donor purposes.
- Modified Mallampati classification system: See "Difficult Airway."

Management

- Cardiopulmonary function may be impaired with sedation.
  - More likely with higher levels of sedation.
  - More likely with significant comorbidities.
  - Sedation provider must be able to "rescue" oversedation.
- Desaturation and laryngospasm are likely if there is current/recent upper respiratory tract infection (Table 4.3).

TABLE 4.3	Fasting Guidelines for Elective Procedures (Minimum Fasting Period)
Substance	**Time**
Clear liquids	2 hr
Breast milk	4 hr
Infant formula	6 hr
Nonhuman milk	6 hr
Light meal: toast and clear fluids	6 hr
Full meal	8 hr or more

Airway Clearance Techniques

Donald Artes

Discussion

- Children are susceptible to airway obstruction primarily with mucus and secretions during a respiratory illness.
- A child's airway is smaller and narrow as compared to that of an older child or adult.
- In order to maintain the highest level of support for the child, airway clearance techniques may be indicated to optimize respiratory status.

Definition

- Airway clearance techniques are used with the primary goal of mobilizing and removing retained secretions, improving pulmonary hygiene, and optimizing oxygenation and ventilation.

Types

- Chest physical therapy
  - The use of postural drainage positions to drain different segments of the lung using gravity.
  - Postural drainage can be augmented with the use of external vibration or percussion to improve mobilization.
- In-exsufflator (cough assist device)
  - The in-exsufflator delivers a set inspiratory pressure, followed by a forced expiratory pressure.
  - This technique attempts to mimic a cough and is often used in pediatric patients with underlying weakness who cannot generate an effective cough.
- Vibratory positive expiratory pressure therapy (Flutter/Acapella)
  - This therapy uses a small disposable handheld device to mobilize secretions.
  - The effect is threefold: first, to vibrate the airways and thus facilitate the movement of mucus; second, to increase endobronchial pressure to avoid air trapping; and third, to accelerate expiratory airflow to facilitate the upward movement of mucus.
- Vest therapy
  - Uses a noninvasive inflatable vest in conjunction with a generator that creates high-frequency chest wall oscillation up to 900 cycles/minute.
  - This oscillation or mini coughs dislodge mucus for the bronchial walls, mobilizing secretions where they can be removed by coughing or suctioning.
  - Unlike chest physical therapy, vest therapy does not require special positioning.
- Intrapulmonary percussive therapy
  - It uses a pneumatic device to deliver small bursts of pressurized gas at rates of 100 to 300 cycles/minute, with peak pressures ranging from 10 to 40 cm H_2O.
  - During the percussive cycle, constant positive airway pressure is maintained in the airway.
  - Often used in conjunction with the administration of bronchodilator therapy.
  - Can be used with natural or artificial airways.
  - More effective than chest physical therapy in treating atelectasis.
- Aerosol therapy
  - A variety of aerosol therapies have been used in the treatment of atelectasis (e.g., α-agonists and nebulized hypertonic saline).
  - Recombinant human DNase (dornase alfa) has been proven to be effective in the treatment of cystic fibrosis.
  - Recombinant human DNase (dornase alfa) has been shown improvements in noncystic fibrosis children with infection-associated atelectasis.

Assessment and Management

- Auscultation.
- Chest X-ray.
- Support ventilation and oxygenation as indicated.

1. The rationale for a child who is experiencing massive bleeding from a tracheostomy is most likely:
   a. Tracheal stenosis.
   b. Pulmonary edema.
   c. Tracheo-innominate artery fistula.
   d. Laryngeal papillomatosis disease.

Answer: **C**

The most common etiology of a massive tracheal bleeding episode in an individual with a tracheostomy is tracheo-innominate artery fistula formation. The brisk bleeding is associated with an artery source and results in mortality as high as 75%.

2. A child has been diagnosed with significant bilateral atelectasis several days postoperatively. The child is immobile and is now requiring oxygen. The most appropriate next intervention is:
   a. Intrapulmonary percussive therapy
   b. Chest physical therapy
   c. In-exsufflator
   d. External percussion

Answer: **A**

Intrapulmonary percussive therapy has been shown to be more effective than chest physical therapy in the treatment of atelectasis.

3. Which statement best describes the process of mucociliary clearance?
   a. It is the primary method of clearing foreign material, bacteria, viruses, and particulate materials from the airway.
   b. It is the process of increasing endobronchial pressure to avoid air trapping.
   c. Mucociliary clearance can be equally effective with or without a cough reflex.
   d. Mucociliary clearance is necessary only in children with cystic fibrosis.

Answer: **A**

Mucociliary clearance is accomplished through many modalities, but is the method of clearing foreign material, bacteria, viruses, and particulate materials from the airway.

4. An infant who was born at 26 weeks' gestation is now 3 months old and is being admitted for bronchiolitis and hypoxia. She has had two episodes of apnea in the emergency department, requiring tactile stimulation and increased oxygen each time. She is breathing between 70 and 100 times per minute and her oxygen saturations vary between 88% and 98%, also depending on her state, alert, or sleeping. What is the most effective oxygen delivery system for this child?
   a. Nasal continuous positive airway pressure (CPAP).
   b. Facial bilevel airway positive pressure.

   c. Non-rebreather mask.
   d. Venturi face mask at 50%.

Answer: **A**

Nasal CPAP improves lung compliance, reducing airway resistance and work of breathing. CPAP improves oxygenation by an increase in functional residual capacity by recruiting alveoli and thereby increasing the surface area for gas exchange. Application of CPAP stretches the pleura and lungs, resulting in stimulation of stretch receptors. This has a beneficial effect on mixed and central apnea.

5. An 8-year-old child admitted for asthma has a respiratory rate of 58 breaths per minute and diminished breath sounds in the bases with scattered wheezing. Oxygen saturation is 90% to 92% on 70% oxygen via an aerosol mask receiving 15 mg of albuterol continuously per hour. The most important rationale for deciding to use noninvasive ventilation with BIPAP/CPAP would be to:
   a. provide ventilatory support with same risk of ventilator-associated pneumonia as intubation.
   b. improve lung compliance and reduce oxygen requirements.
   c. eliminate the risk of upper airway trauma.
   d. eliminate the need for anxiolysis and analgesia when compared to intubation.

Answer: **C**

Benefits of managing patients with noninvasive ventilation include the elimination of the risk of upper airway trauma associated with endotracheal intubation.

6. A 10-year-old child who is being supported with facial CPAP is beginning to show signs of skin breakdown even with the use of barrier devices. In order to give the child breaks off of the mask, which device would be most appropriate?
   a. 50% venture mask.
   b. Non-rebreather mask.
   c. High-flow nasal cannula at 5 L/minute.
   d. High-flow nasal cannula at 20 to 25 L/minute.

Answer: **D**

The high-flow cannula at 20 to 25 L/minute is the most appropriate device while offering time off of facial CPAP/BIPAP. Some sources have postulated that the rate of flow delivered by a high-flow cannula may deliver a level of positive pressure similar to CPAP. While a flow of 5 L/minute via a heated cannula may be considered high flow for an infant or small child, it would not meet the flow demands of a 10-year-old.

7. A 3-month-old infant is admitted to the pediatric intensive care unit with a diagnosis of RSV bronchiolitis and respiratory distress. The infant has not been maintaining acceptable oxygen saturations on a high-flow, heated nasal cannula at 2 L flow. She is breathing 80 times per minute with visible intercostal and substernal retractions. Her chest X-ray is significant for hyperexpansion. What is the next step in oxygenation?
   a. Increase the oxygen liter flow.
   b. Consider using BIPAP.
   c. Obtain a blood gas measurement.
   d. Switch to oxygen by face mask.

Answer: **A**

Heated high-flow oxygen delivery systems include Vapotherm. High-flow therapy is effective for any age child, particularly young children and infants. When lower liter flow is not effective, increasing the flow is appropriate prior to considering a more invasive type of therapy such as BIPAP or CPAP.

8. A 3-year-old with an acute asthma exacerbation has mild hypoxia and is currently receiving albuterol inhalation treatments every 2 hours. In between, her oxygen saturations are 90% to 93% on room air. Which of the following is the most efficient and effective type of oxygen therapy for this child?
   a. High-flow cannula at 4 to 6 L/minute flow.
   b. Bilevel positive airway pressure ventilation.
   c. Nasal cannula at 1 to 2 L/minute flow.
   d. Simple face mask at 40%.

Answer: **C**

Oxygen therapy to provide support for a child with an underlying respiratory illness includes nasal cannula, providing 24% to 44% based on liter flow.

9. A child is brought to the ED via EMS following a motor vehicle collision. His Glasgow coma scale is 12 and he has visible trauma to his chest. The child's respiratory rate is 35 breaths per minute and his oxygen saturation on room air is 89%. Which of the following is the initial mode of oxygen therapy for this child?
   a. Nasal cannula at 3 L flow.
   b. Non-rebreather face mask.
   c. Simple face mask at 40% to 50%.
   d. Intubation and ventilation.

Answer: **B**

Even though the child's Glasgow coma scale is 12 and the child has an oxygen saturation of 89% on room air, there is visible trauma to the chest with a markedly elevated respiratory rate. The child's respiratory rate is 35 breaths per minute and, at this point, does not require intubation and ventilation. Therefore, it is prudent to give high levels of oxygen until the injuries can be adequately assessed.

10. To decrease the risk of aspiration of gastric contents, the laryngeal mask airway should be ventilated with:
    a. low airway pressures.
    b. supplemental heliox to decrease airway resistance.
    c. manual devices only; never mechanical.
    d. the two-person technique.

Answer: **A**

Gastroesophageal opening pressure is around 15 to 25 cm H_2O. If higher airway pressures are needed, gastric insufflation and distention may occur; these are risk factors for regurgitation and aspiration. Consider auscultation over the epigastrium (as commonly done with a nasogastric tube) if concerns that pulmonary ventilation causing secondary gastric insufflation.

11. Which device provides the most secure artificial airway?
    a. Oropharyngeal airway
    b. Face mask
    c. Laryngeal mask airway
    d. Endotracheal tube

Answer: **D**

Endotracheal tube is the "gold standard" for securing an airway.

12. Which of the following diagnoses is most likely to present with a difficult airway?
    a. Marfan syndrome
    b. Turner syndrome
    c. Treacher Collins syndrome
    d. Münchausen syndrome by proxy

Answer: **C**

Treacher Collins syndrome's noneponymous name is mandibulofacial dysostosis. It is characterized by micrognathia. Clearly, Marfan and Turner syndromes *may* have airway findings (high palate and webbed neck, respectively), and as such, neither is the *best* (most likely) answer.

Recommended Readings

American Society of Anesthesiologists. (2003). Practice guidelines for management of the difficult airway. *Anesthesiology, 98*(5), 1269–1277.

American Society of Anesthesiologists. (2009). *Continuum of depth of sedation: Definition of general anesthesia and levels of sedation/analgesia.* Retrieved from www.asahq.org/For-Members/Standards-Guidelines-and-Statements.aspx

American Society of Anesthesiologists. (2010). *Basic standards for preanesthesia care.* Retrieved from www.asahq.org/For-Members/Standards-Guidelines-and-Statements.aspx

American Society of Anesthesiologists. (2011). Practice guidelines for preoperative fasting and the use of pharmacologic agents to reduce the risk of pulmonary aspiration: Application to healthy patients undergoing elective procedures. *Anesthesiology, 114*(3), 495–511.

American Society of Anesthesiologists. (2013). *Physical status classification system.* Retrieved from www.asahq.org/For-Members/Clinical-Information/ASA-Physical-Status-Classification-System.aspx

Eberhart, L. H., Arndt, C., Cierpka, T., Schwanekamp, J., Wulf, H., & Putzke, C. (2005). The reliability and validity of the upper lip bite test compared with the Mallampati classification to predict difficult laryngoscopy: An external prospective evaluation. *Anesthesia & Analgesia, 101*, 284–289.

Heinrich, S., Birkholz, T., Ihmsen, H., Irouschek, A., Ackermann, A., & Schmidt, J. (2012). Incidence and predictors of difficult laryngoscopy in 11.219 pediatric anesthesia procedures. *Pediatric Anesthesia, 22,* 729–736.

Kline, A. & Kane, J. (2012). Ventilation support. In K. Reuter-Rice & B. Bolick (Eds.), *Pediatric acute care: A guide for interprofessional practice.* Burlington, MA. Jones & Bartlett Learning.

Nishisaki, A., Turner, D. A., Brown, C. A. 3rd., Walls, R. M., Nadkarni, V. M., & National Emergency Airway Registry for Children (NEAR4KIDS); Pediatric Acute Lung Injury and Sepsis Investigators (PALISI) Network. (2013).

A National Emergency Airway Registry for Children: Landscape of tracheal intubation in 15 PICUs. *Critical Care Medicine, 41,* 874–885.

Simone, S., & Sorce, L. (2012). Analgesia, paralytics, sedation, and withdrawal. In K. Reuter-Rice & B. Bolick (Eds.), *Pediatric acute care: A guide for interprofessional practice.* Burlington, MA: Jones & Bartlett Learning.

Stojadinovic, B.J. (2012). Rapid-sequence intubation. In K. Reuter-Rice & B. Bolick (Eds.), *Pediatric acute care: A guide for interprofessional practice* (pp. 1301–1304). Burlington, MA: Jones & Bartlett Learning.

Cardiac Disorders

Cardiogenic Shock

Heather Sowinski

Background/Definition

- Inability of the heart to meet the metabolic demands of the body.
  - Cardiac failure, which leads to decreased cardiac output.
  - Systemic vascular resistance and heart rate affect cardiac output.
- Stages of shock include compensated, decompensated, and multisystem organ failure.
  - Compensated shock: signs of poor perfusion; however, blood pressure (BP) is maintained.
  - Decompensated shock: worsening perfusion that leads to organ dysfunction and inability to maintain BP.
  - Multisystem organ failure: Perfusion is affected to the point that end-organ damage occurs. This damage can be irreversible in severe cases.

Etiology/Types

- Multiple types including hypovolemic, distributive, and cardiogenic.
- Caused by a variety of etiologies:
  - Congenital heart disease (CHD): ductal-dependent heart lesions, pulmonary hypertension, and postoperative state.
  - Arrhythmias: unrecognized supraventricular tachycardia, ventricular tachycardia, and bradycardia.
  - Drug toxicity: β-blockers, barbiturates, chemotherapy, radiation, and calcium channel blockers.
  - Cardiomyopathies and myocarditis.
  - Trauma: hemopericardium, pneumopericardium, and tamponade.
  - Metabolic abnormalities: hypocalcemia, hyperkalemia, and acidosis.

Pathophysiology

- Pump failure: Poor systolic function leads to decreased cardiac output and decreased blood flow to the body. Initially, the body is able to increase stroke volume and heart rate to maintain cardiac output.
  - Infants are unable to increase their stroke volume adequately and are dependent on heart rate to maintain cardiac output.
- Once compensatory mechanisms to maintain cardiac output are overwhelmed, the BP will drop, and the state of shock will progress.

Clinical Presentation

- History: increased work of breathing, poor weight gain, difficulty breathing or diaphoresis with feeds, cyanosis, lethargy, and decreased number of urine output/wet diapers wet diapers.
- Physical examination: tachycardia, tachypnea, cyanosis, cool, clammy, pale, or mottled extremities, prolonged capillary refill, decreased peripheral pulses, hepatomegaly, impaired mental status, oliguria, and lactic acidosis.
- Hypotension (a late finding in shock of pediatric patients) in children is defined as a systolic BP <5th percentile for age.
  - <60 mmHg in term neonates (0–28 days of life);
  - <70 mmHg in infants (1–12 months of age);
  - <70 mmHg + (2 × age in years) in children 1 to 10 years of age;
  - <90 mmHg in children ≥10 years of age.
- Patients with ductal-dependent heart lesions may present with hypoxia that is unresponsive to oxygen administration or signs of severe shock. They are dependent on the patent ductus arteriosus to supply pulmonary or systemic blood flow, and as it closes, adequate blood flow to either the lungs or body will not be maintained.

Diagnostic Evaluation

- A clinical diagnosis; however, diagnostic evaluation is needed to determine etiology and aid in management.
- Imaging: chest radiograph, ECG, echocardiogram.
- Laboratory evaluation: complete blood count (CBC) with differential, electrolytes, glucose, calcium, magnesium, BUN, creatinine, blood gas with lactate, AST, ALT, PT, PTT, INR, and toxicology/drug screen.

- Laboratory evaluation can assist in evaluating the degree of organ dysfunction secondary to shock as well as in identifying metabolic derangements that can be corrected with medical management.
- Lactic acidosis develops due to decreased perfusion and development of anaerobic metabolism.

Management

- Constant reassessment after each intervention for a change in BP, perfusion, urine output, and mental status.
- First step in evaluating any patient should include airway, breathing, and circulation (ABCs).
  - Oxygen administration and/or intubation if respiratory compromise is present.
  - Intubation may be needed in severe shock in order to decrease afterload on the heart, thus reducing the workload of the heart.
  - Monitoring should include pulse oximetry, BP, and cardiorespiratory monitoring.
- The second step is cautious fluid administration to increase preload.
  - In forms of shock other than cardiogenic, the patient should receive fluid boluses in increments of 20 mL/kg with an isotonic crystalloid fluid such as normal saline (0.9 NS) or lactated ringers (LR), administered as quickly as possible.
  - Fluid administration must be given cautiously in patients with cardiogenic shock. A large increase in preload may not be tolerated in patients with heart failure and may lead to overdistension of the heart, resulting in decreased cardiac output. This is described by the Frank–Starling Curve (see Figure 5.1).
  - The patient should be given fluid boluses in increments of 5 to 10 mL/kg with reassessment of clinical status after each fluid bolus.
- If there is an inadequate response to fluid administration or the patient develops signs of worsening heart failure, the next step should be inotropic support with vasoactive medications.

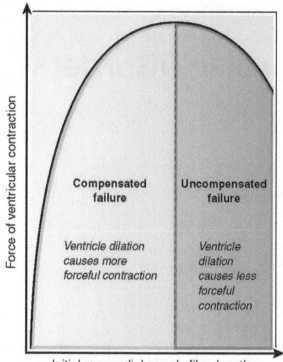

FIGURE 5.1 • **Frank–Starling Curve.** Up to a point (the apex of the curve), cardiac myocytes contract with more force when stretched. Beyond that point, the fibers contract less forcefully.

- Vasoactive medications improve contractility and reduce systemic vascular resistance, making it easier for the failing heart to pump (Table 5.1).
- In infants < 1 month of age, ductal-dependent CHD should be considered.

TABLE 5.1   Common Vasoactive Medications

Dobutamine	Milrinone	Inotropic Agents (Dopamine, Epinephrine, Norepinephrine)
• β-Adrenergic medication. • Increases contractility and promotes vasodilation. • Does not increase heart rate (chronotropic effect) as much as other vasopressor agents (e.g., dopamine and epinephrine). Increased heart rate decreases filling time and can further compromise cardiac output. • Dose: 2–20 mcg/kg/minute.	• Phosphodiesterase enzyme inhibitor. • Reduces systemic vascular resistance (afterload) and increases contractility. • Can cause hypotension; use with caution in hypotensive patients. • Dose: 0.35–0.75 mcg/kg/minute.	• Can be added if insufficient response to first-line therapy. • Use with caution in patients with cardiogenic shock due to the potential to increase systemic vascular resistance and further stress a failing ventricle.

mcg, microgram

- Administration of prostaglandins (PGE_1) at 0.05 to 0.2 mcg/kg/minute is necessary to maintain and/or open the ductus arteriosus.
- Correct metabolic derangements and maintain normothermia.
- Arrhythmias will require specific antiarrhythmic interventions including medications, cardioversion, and/or temporary pacing.
- In case of cardiac tamponade, a pericardiocentesis is indicated to relieve the strain on the cardiac muscle.
- Cardiogenic shock is a clinical diagnosis. Laboratory evaluation and imaging assist in determining underlying etiology and allow correction of metabolic derangements.
- Goal of management is quick recognition and intervention with fluid resuscitation and inotropic support.
- Once an intervention has been initiated, constantly reevaluate for improvement in clinical status or the need to escalate support.

PEARL

- *Recognize and intervene during compensated shock in order to prevent significant morbidity and mortality.*

Cardiac Tamponade

Tageldin M. Ahmed

Background/Definition

- Tamponade means compression.
- Cardiac tamponade is defined as hemodynamically significant heart compression resulting from accumulation of fluid in the pericardial space.
- The terms cardiac tamponade and pericardial tamponade are used interchangeably.

Etiology

- Hemopericardium immediately after cardiac surgery; most common cause.
- Penetrating and sometimes blunt trauma to the chest.
- Viral or bacterial pericarditis.
- Connective tissue diseases (e.g., systemic lupus erythematosus (SLE) and juvenile inflammatory arthritis [JIA]).
- Oncological diseases/malignancies.
- Uremia.

Pathophysiology

- Pericardial sac is composed of fibrous tissue with limited capacity to stretch acutely.
- Rapid accumulation of blood (e.g., trauma or post heart surgery), pus (e.g., infective pericarditis), or inflammatory fluid (e.g., rheumatologic, cancer, uremia) leads to impedance of heart filling during diastole.
- Consequently, a small stroke volume is ejected with each heartbeat.
- Ultimately, obstructive shock develops with loss of cardiac output.
- Cardiac arrest ensues with characteristic pulseless electrical activity (PEA).

Clinical Presentation

- Beck triad (classic):
  - Hypotension—from low cardiac output.
  - Distended neck (jugular) veins—from heart compression.
  - Muffled (distant) heart sounds—from fluid in pericardial space.
- Pulsus paradoxus.
- Narrow pulse pressure.
- Pericardial rub.
- Shock with tachycardia, tachypnea, and depressed mental status.

Diagnostic Evaluation

- Echocardiogram is the diagnostic test of choice, demonstrating:
  - Effusion size and distribution.
  - Impaired diastolic heart filling.
  - Abnormal ventricular wall movement (Figure 5.2).
- Chest radiograph:
  - Enlarged anterior mediastinum.
  - Globular heart shadow (cardiac silhouette).
- ECG:
  - Low-voltage QRS complexes in all leads.
  - Abnormal ST segment.

Management

- Cardiac tamponade is a medical emergency.
- Needle pericardiocentesis is the emergent treatment of choice.
- Fluid resuscitation, oxygen supplementation, and airway control are important adjuncts.
- Further management depends on the etiology of the effusion resulting in tamponade.
- Typically, a pericardial drainage tube (pigtail) or a pericardial window is created to prevent reaccumulation.
- Treat the underlying disease process (e.g., infection).
- Prevention.
  - Postoperative cardiac surgery patients often have mediastinal chest tube.

PEARLS

- *In trauma patients, hypotension refractory to fluid resuscitation should prompt suspicion of tamponade.*
- *Hypotension with distended neck vein should always include tamponade in the differential diagnosis.*

Cardiomyopathy

Caroline Bauer

Definition

- Dilated cardiomyopathy.
  - A dilation of the left or both ventricles with impaired contraction/systolic dysfunction in the absence of an abnormal loading condition (e.g., hypertension, valvular disease, or coronary artery disease).

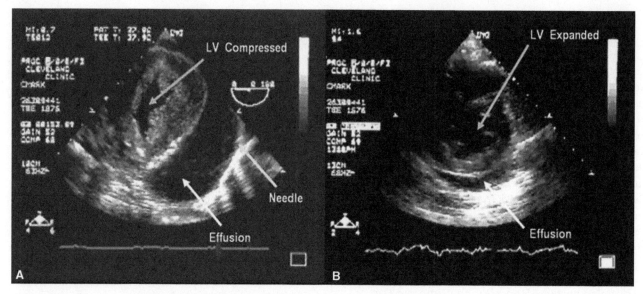

FIGURE 5.2 • **Pericardial Effusion and Tamponade. A:** The pericardial effusion and ventricular compression associated with cardiac tamponade are noted. **B:** Comparison of effusion during the pericardiocentesis and postpericardiocentesis.

- Hypertrophic cardiomyopathy.
  - Hypertrophied, nondilated ventricle in the absence of a hemodynamic disturbance that is capable of producing the existent magnitude of wall thickening (e.g., hypertension, aortic valve stenosis, catecholamine secreting tumors, hyperthyroidism).
- Restrictive cardiomyopathy.
  - Restrictive filling and reduced diastolic volume of either or both ventricles with normal to near normal systolic function and wall thickness.

Etiology

- Dilated cardiomyopathy.
  - Idiopathic in approximately 50% of all pediatric cases.
  - Specific causes include inflammatory, genetic, congenital, viral, metabolic, autoimmune, or toxic etiologies.
- Hypertrophic cardiomyopathy.
  - Idiopathic and familial in approximately 75% of cases.
  - Other etiologies include inborn errors of metabolism (9%), neuromuscular disorders (9%), and malformation syndromes (9%).
- Restrictive cardiomyopathy.
  - One of the most rare forms of cardiomyopathy in children.
  - Almost never has an identifiable cause.
  - Annual incidence is 0.03/100,000 children.

Pathophysiology

- Dilated cardiomyopathy.
  - Ability of the ventricle to pump blood is impaired and cannot maintain adequate cardiac output to meet the body's demand.
  - Over time, the ventricles become progressively stiff and do not fill appropriately.
  - Results in a backup of blood into pulmonary circulation, which causes pulmonary edema, pulmonary hypertension, and atrial enlargement.

- Hypertrophic cardiomyopathy.
  - The ventricles become thick and stiff, leading to impaired filling and the inability to meet the cardiac output demands of the body.
  - Over time, the ventricles become stiffer and can cause obstruction of blood flow out through the aorta.
- Restrictive cardiomyopathy.
  - Leads to decreased filling compliance of the ventricles, causing severely elevated right atrial (RA) pressures and size.
  - The severely enlarged atrium can cause atrial arrhythmias (often difficult to control) as well as significant pulmonary hypertension.

Clinical Presentation

- With all cardiomyopathies, the clinical presentation can vary, but may include:
  - Sudden cardiac death, chest pain (CP)/angina, syncope, palpitations.
  - Dyspnea, exercise intolerance.
  - Absence of symptoms.
  - Patients with severely impaired cardiac function will present with symptoms of heart failure and cardiogenic shock.

Physical Examination

- New nondescript murmur, tachycardia, tachypnea, other signs of reduced cardiac output.
- "Cardiac wheezing" is common with restrictive cardiomyopathy.
  - Patients are often initially misdiagnosed with asthma.

Diagnostic Evaluation

- Chest radiograph.
- ECG (Electrocardiogram).
- Echocardiogram (see Figure 5.3).
- Holter monitor to evaluate for life-threatening arrhythmias.

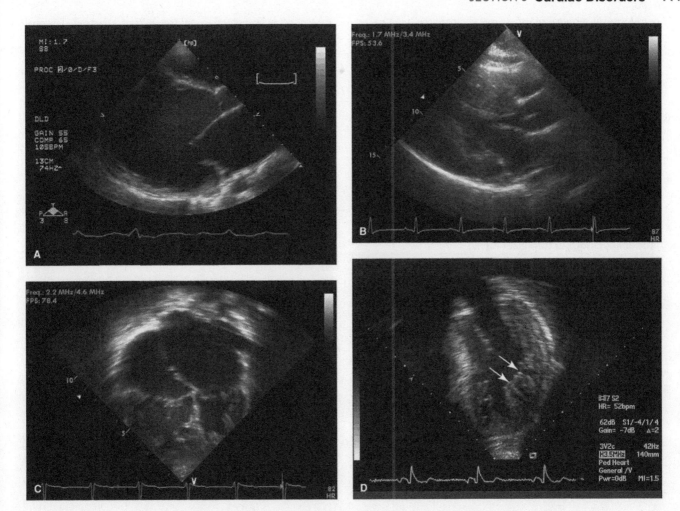

FIGURE 5.3 • **Cardiomyopathy Echocardiogram Findings by Type.** Representative single-frame echocardiograms demonstrating the salient features of the four types of cardiomyopathy seen in pediatric patients. **A:** Dilated cardiomyopathy, parasternal long axis view. Note the dilated left ventricular (LV) chamber and relatively thin LV posterior wall and septum. **B:** Hypertrophic cardiomyopathy, parasternal long axis view. Note the thickened LV posterior wall and septum and the small LV chamber size. **C:** Restrictive cardiomyopathy, apical four-chamber view. Note the markedly dilated right and left atria. **D:** LV noncompaction, apical four-chamber view.

- Complete metabolic profile (CMP), (CMP evaluates for end organ function).
- Other laboratory studies used to determine secondary causes of cardiomyopathy include:
  - Antinuclear antibodies (ANA); genetic/metabolic testing; inflammatory markers (e.g., C-reactive protein, tumor-necrosis-factor-α); viral panels; drug levels.

Management

- Dilated cardiomyopathy.
  - Cardiorespiratory support.
    - Oxygen, ventilation (as indicated by patient clinical status), inotropic support, continuous telemetry.
  - Fluid management.
    - Cautious fluid resuscitation; volume overload can cause pulmonary edema and resultant respiratory failure.
  - Long-term medical therapies.
    - Afterload reducers, diuretics.

- Extracorporeal support.
  - Ventricular assist devices (VAD), extracorporeal membranous oxygenation (ECMO).
- Heart transplantation; may be required for severe cardiac dysfunction.
- Hypertrophic cardiomyopathy.
  - Inotropic support can worsen systolic function and increase obstruction, and should be avoided.
  - β-Blockers: provide rate control and reduce symptoms of CP and palpitations.
  - Calcium channel blockers can be used for angina and to improve diastolic function.
  - Dehydration can worsen obstruction and decrease cardiac output, so should be avoided.
  - Volume status should be carefully monitored to avoid fluid overload, but provide adequate preload to the heart.
  - In failed cases of traditional medical therapy with β-blockers, other treatments include myomectomy

(e.g., surgical removal of excess muscle from the heart), pacemaker implantation, and septal ablation may be considered.

- Asymptomatic individuals should be carefully monitored by a cardiologist; however, may not require any treatment until symptomatic.
- Restrictive cardiomyopathy.
  - No proven therapies currently exist.
  - Anticoagulation is recommended.
    - High risk of sudden embolic events.
  - β-Blockers, angiotensin-converting enzyme inhibitors, diuretics, and pacemakers may be helpful, but none of these therapies are evidence-based.
  - VAD or ECMO may be necessary for cardiopulmonary support or as a bridge to transplantation.
  - The definitive treatment is a heart transplant.
    - Should be considered early as pulmonary hypertension is a contraindication to transplant.
  - Consultations: cardiology, cardiothoracic surgery, genetics, and infectious disease.

PEARL
- *All patients with cardiomyopathy, regardless of type or severity, require restriction from competitive sports.*

Chylothorax

Jennifer L. Joiner

Background

- Disruption of the lymphatic drainage from damage or obstruction that results in an accumulation of pleural chest fluid, leading to chylous pleural effusion with resulting respiratory distress.
- Most commonly found in posttraumatic or postsurgical patients.

Definition

- Accumulation of chyle fluid that is found between the visceral and parietal pleural space.
- Overproduction of chylus fluid overwhelms the resorptive abilities of the lymphatic system.
- When damage or blockage has occurred in lymphatic drainage and a pleural effusion develops.

Etiology/Types

- Postsurgical/traumatic.
- Congenital.
- Spontaneous.
- Oncologic/malignancy.

Clinical Presentation

- Depends on the degree of the effusion.
  - Larger effusions result in tachypnea, hypoxia, increased work of breathing, respiratory distress, or respiratory failure.

- Most often suspected in children with risk factors, demonstrating a pleural effusion on chest radiograph.
- Milky-appearing pleural fluid, if ingesting enteral fat; may be serous if on nonfat nutrition or total parenteral nutrition (TPN).

Diagnostic Evaluation

- Decubitus or lateral chest radiograph (CXR).
- Ultrasound of chest; evaluates presence, size, and location of fluid collection.
- Pleural fluid evaluation (confirmatory).
  - Triglyceride level >110 mg/dL.
  - Presence of chylomicrons.
  - Predominately lymphocytic; white blood cell count (WBC) $>1,000 \times 10^3/\mu L$.

Management

- Larger effusions causing respiratory compromise require a thoracostomy tube and respiratory support.
- Strict dietary fat restriction for 3 to 6 weeks with supplementary fat provided by intralipids or a medium chain transfat (MCT) oil containing formula.
- Diuretics have been used as adjunctive therapy.
- Octreotide has been used in postoperative cardiac patients with mixed results.
- Pleurodesis or ligation of the thoracic duct must be considered in cases refractory to medical management.

PEARL
- *Infants/children with chylothorax should receive feedings with medium chain transfat (MCT).*

Congenital Heart Disease

Julie A. Creaden & Elizabeth R. Preze

Acyanotic Lesions

Patent Ductus Arteriosus (PDA)

Background/Definition

- Vascular communication between the left pulmonary artery (PA) and the descending aorta (Figure 5.4).

Pathophysiology

- Anatomy of PDA can differ if associated with other cardiac lesions.
- Typically, closes within first 12 to 24 hours of life.

Clinical Presentation

- Systolic murmur left sternal border (LSB) (neonates).
- Continuous murmur left upper sternal border (LUSB) (older children).
- Bounding pulses.
- Widened pulse pressure with low diastolic pressure.

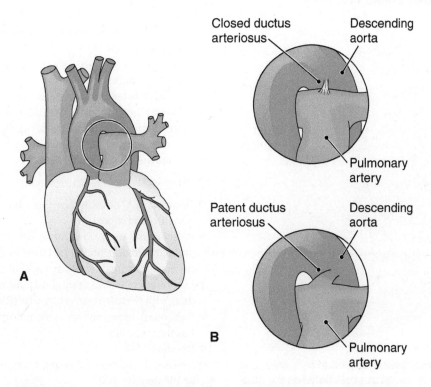

FIGURE 5.4 • **Patent Ductus Arteriosus. A:** Normal. **B:** The ductus arteriosus fails to close.

Diagnostic Evaluation

- Chest radiograph: prominent main PA with increased pulmonary vascular markings (PVM), cardiomegaly.
- Electrocardiography (ECG): left atrial (LA) enlargement and biventricular hypertrophy.
- Echocardiogram (ECHO): usually sufficient for diagnosis.

Management

- Medical management:
  - Nonsteroidal anti-inflammatory drugs (NSAIDS): Indomethacin or a special intravenous (IV) form of ibuprofen has been used to help close a PDA; especially viable alternative for premature infants. Contraindicated in infants with intraventricular hemorrhage (IVH).
- Surgical management: Surgical intervention required if PDA remains open past 3 months of age. Typically performed in the first 6 months of life. Surgical ligation and division through a left thoracotomy incision or via video-assisted thoracoscopic surgery (VATS).
  - Cardiac catheterization intervention: coil embolization used to occlude PDA.
- Postprocedural considerations:
  - Surgical complications: recurrent laryngeal nerve damage, recurrence of patency of PDA, chylothorax, ligation of unintended vessel (e.g., aorta, left PA or left main stem bronchus, bleeding, infection).
  - Postcardiac catheterization complications: coil migration, bleeding, residual shunt.

- Postoperative checklist:
  - Review chest radiograph for common intrathoracic problems.
  - Evaluate pulses to support ligation of PDA rather than nonductus vascular structures (e.g., aorta or LPA).
  - Monitor for bleeding or infection.
- Postcardiac catheterization checklist:
  - Monitor catheter site for bleeding, hematoma, or infection.
  - Monitor distal pulses and perfusion from catheter site.
  - Auscultate for murmurs.
  - Follow postcardiac catheterization protocol (bed rest, keep leg straight) per institutional policy or provider order.
  - Chest radiograph/ECHO to visualize coil placement.

Atrial Septal Defect (ASD)

Background/Definition

- Communication between the atria (see Figure 5.5).
- Three types of ASDs:
  - Ostium secundum: most common type; occurs in the center of the septum.
  - Ostium primum: occurs low in the septum; may involve atrioventricular valve abnormalities and mitral insufficiency.
  - Sinus venosus: occurs high in the septum near the superior vena cava (SVC) and RA junction; can be associated with partial anomalous pulmonary venous return (PAPVR).

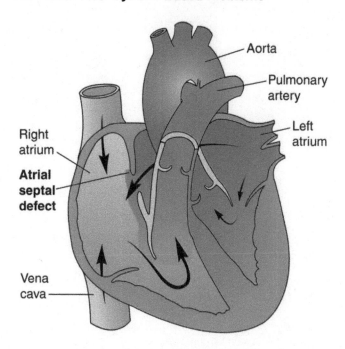

FIGURE 5.5 • **Atrial Septal Defect.** In an atrial septal defect, an abnormal communication exists between the atria, allowing blood to be shunted from the left atrium to the right atrium through the atrial septum.

Pathophysiology

- Left-to-right shunting occurs in ASDs.
- Degree of shunting depends on the size of the ASD.
  - Nonrestrictive: equal pressure in both atria; shunting is determined solely by ventricular compliance.
  - Restrictive: size of the defect is small enough to provide resistance to flow.
- Compliance of the ventricles.
  - Shunting increases with age as ventricle becomes more compliant.

Clinical Presentation

- Physical examination:
  - Systolic ejection murmur LUSB.
  - Widely split S2.

Diagnostic Evaluation

- Chest radiograph: cardiomegaly with increased PVM.
- Electrocardiography: R-axis deviation with right ventricular hypertrophy (RVH) and right bundle branch block (RBBB) pattern.
- Echocardiogram: sufficient for diagnosis; can miss associated PAPVR.
- Cardiac catheterization: not indicated unless suspicion of coexisting lesion or pulmonary hypertension.

Management

- Surgical management:
  - Recommend closure between 3 to 5 years of age.
  - Spontaneous closure of small secundum defects occurs in 87% of infants during the first year of life.

- Mortality in most centers with uncomplicated cases approaches 0%.
  - Repaired using a pericardial or prosthetic patch or direct suture closure.
- Cardiac catheterization intervention.
  - Transcatheter closure commonly used to close ostium secundum ASDs in the cardiac catheterization lab.
    - ASD must be <22 mm in size and have an inferior rim for the device to safely attach.

Postoperative Considerations

- Sinoatrial (SA) node dysfunction: direct trauma or interruption of blood supply.
- Postpericardiotomy syndrome: fever, malaise, lymphocytosis, nausea, vomiting, abdominal pain, pericardial effusion; usually occurs approximately 14 days postop.
- Left ventricular (LV) dysfunction: more common in older children with chronic right ventricular (RV) dilation.
- Pulmonary hypertension: uncommon in children; increases risk for mortality.
- Residual ASD.
- Venous obstruction: following repair of sinus venosus (SVC or PV stenosis) ASD.
- Monitor for signs of pericardial effusion, sinus node dysfunction, and signs of noncompliant left ventricle (older patients).

Postcardiac Catheterization Considerations

- Bleeding and infection from access site.
- Catheter migration/displacement.
- Monitor catheter access site post catheterization, bed rest.

Ventricular Septal Defect (VSD)

Background/Definition

- Communication between the right and left ventricles (see Figure 5.6).
- May occur in isolation or with other associated defects.
- Most common; accounts for approximately 50% of congenital heart defects.
- Four different types of VSDs:
  - Perimembranous: opening in the upper portion of the ventricular septum.
    - Most common type of VSD; *does not usually close on its own.*
  - Outlet type (subarterial): opening in the septum is just below the pulmonary valve in the ventricular septum.
  - Inlet type (canal): opening is just below the AV valves (tricuspid and mitral) in the ventricular septum.
    - Can be associated with atrioventricular canal (AVC) defect.
  - Muscular: an opening in the muscular portion of the lower ventricular septum. Many of these VSDs close spontaneously, and do not require surgery.

Pathophysiology

- Left-to-right shunting at ventricular level.
- Degree of shunting depends on the size of the VSD.
  - Nonrestrictive: no pressure gradient between the ventricles; shunting is determined by pulmonary vascular resistance (PVR).

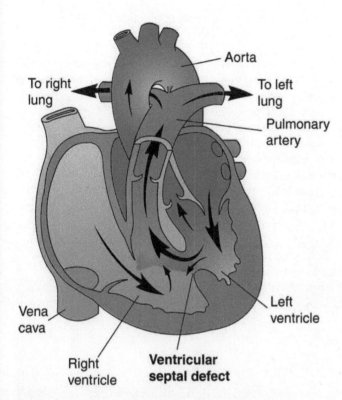

To right lung

Aorta

To left lung

Pulmonary artery

Vena cava

Left ventricle

Right ventricle

Ventricular septal defect

FIGURE 5.6 • **Ventricular Septal Defect.** In a ventricular septal defect, a hole is in the wall of the septum that separates the left and right ventricles. Normally, deoxygenated blood flows through the superior vena cava and inferior vena cava into the right atrium, right ventricle, and pulmonary artery. In a ventricular septal defect, some oxygen-rich blood from the left ventricle flows through the defect and recirculates through the lungs.
Note the thickened LV myocardium and deep trabeculations indicated by the arrows.

- Restrictive: size of the defect is smaller than the aortic root diameter, degree of shunting is determined by the size of the defect.
- PVR (PVR is delayed in neonates with VSDs).

Clinical Presentation

- Physical examination: harsh holosystolic murmur at LSB; may have thrill and/or middiastolic rumble at apex.
- Chest radiograph: enlarged left atrium (LA) with prominent main PA.
- Electrocardiography: biventricular or left ventricular hypertrophy (LVH).
- Echocardiogram: typically sufficient for diagnosis.
- Cardiac catheterization: used to quantify degree of left (L) to right (R) shunt in a moderate-sized defect; may be used if pulmonary hypertension is suspected.

Management

- Medical management:
  - Perimembranous and muscular VSDs can be observed (up to one year of age) as spontaneous closure is possible.
  - Inlet or malaligned septum VSDs will not close spontaneously.

- Once PVR decreases, symptoms of failure to thrive (FTT) and congestive heart failure (CHF) will develop in infants with VSD.
  - Treat symptoms of FTT and CHF until surgery is recommended.
- Surgical management:
  - Timing based on size and location of the defect and degree of FTT and CHF.
  - Typically, surgery is done within the 1st year of life.
  - Mortality <5%; higher in children with multiple muscular VSDs.
- Surgical repair:
  - Requires median sternotomy and cardiopulmonary bypass.
  - Repair of VSD includes: Closure of VSD with prosthetic patch material (Dacron), tanned pericardium (treated with glutaraldehyde), or suture closure; frequent use of pledgeted suture technique; multiple muscular VSDs may require PA banding (difficult to approach surgically).

Postoperative Considerations

- Residual VSD.
- Pulmonary hypertension; delayed closure and large defects are at most risk.
- Heart block (transient or permanent).
- Junctional ectopic tachycardia (JET).
- Monitor for pulmonary hypertension and evaluate for residual VSDs in a timely manner; if signs of low cardiac output, consider residual VSD or additional undiagnosed defect.

Atrioventricular Canal (AVC)

Background/Definition

- Defect resulting from nonfusion of the endocardial cushion.
- Three components: ostium primum ASD; inlet VSD; Abnormal formation of AV valves (see Figure 5.7).
- Three types:
  - Partial: ostium primum defect associated with a cleft in the anterior mitral valve (two separate AV valves); no VSD.
  - Transitional: ostium primum defect with AV valves only partially separated into two valves; has VSD but may be small.
  - Complete: ostium primum defect with large nonrestrictive VSD and a single AV valve; Three subtypes are recognized (Rastelli types A, B, and C).
- Unbalanced AV canal.
  - Hypoplasia of either right or left ventricle.

Pathophysiology

- Partial form: resembles ASD unless severe AV valve regurgitation is present.
- Complete form: resembles VSD with an associated ASD; biatrial and biventricular volume overload; AV valve regurgitation worsens ventricular volume overload.

Clinical Presentation

- Physical examination:
  - Systolic regurgitant murmur at left lower sternal border (LLSB).

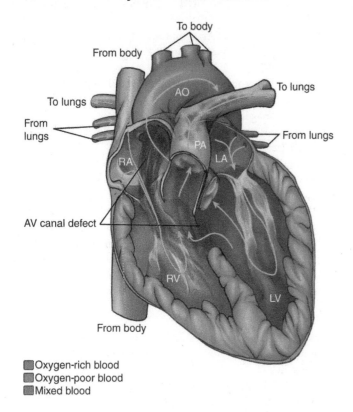

- ☐ Oxygen-rich blood
- ☐ Oxygen-poor blood
- ☐ Mixed blood

FIGURE 5.7 • **Atrioventricular Canal.** Atrioventricular canal defect.

- FTT.
- Respiratory distress.
- CHF.

Diagnostic Evaluation

- Chest radiograph: cardiomegaly with increased pulmonary vascular markings.
- Electrocardiography: left axis deviation, biatrial and biventricular hypertrophy.
- Echocardiogram: used to diagnose and type by closely evaluating AV valves.
- Cardiac catheterization: usually not indicated unless echocardiogram is not sufficient in defining AV valve morphology.

Management

- Surgical management:
  - Partial AV canal: repaired at 1 to 5 years of age; earlier if left AV valve regurgitation is present.
  - Complete AV canal: repaired at 3 to 6 months of age.
- Morbidity/Mortality:
  - Partial AV canal: 5% mortality; If AV valve regurgitation 10%.
  - Complete AV canal: 10% in the first year of life.
- Surgical repair: requires median sternotomy and cardiopulmonary bypass; approach via right atriotomy; one- or two-patch technique may be used.

- PA band: recommended only in specific situations (e.g., severe illness, unbalanced defects).

Postoperative Considerations

- Goals following surgical repair: aim for lower filling pressure; liberal inotropic support; minimize volume loading (exacerbates AV valve regurgitation).
- High incidence of postoperative pulmonary hypertension; correlated with older age at time of surgical repair.
- Low cardiac output.
- Elevated LA pressure.
- Heart block; up to 10% incidence.
- Residual VSD.
- Junctional ectopic tachycardia (JET).
- Following repair, AV valves will never be normal; long-term follow-up is essential.
- Hemodynamic deterioration anytime after repair is considered severe left AV valve regurgitation until proven otherwise.

Cyanotic Lesions

Julie A. Creaden & Elizabeth R. Preze

Tetralogy of Fallot (TOF)

Background/Definition

- VSD.
- Pulmonary stenosis.
- Aortic override of VSD.
- RVH (Figure 5.8).

Pathophysiology

- Dependent on degree of pulmonary stenosis.
- Too much pulmonary blood flow "pink TET."
  - L→R shunt with CHF and pulmonary overcirculation.
- Too little pulmonary blood flow.
  - R→L shunt with hypoxia (SaO$_2$ 70%–80%).
- Balanced circulation.
  - Have mild hypoxia (SaO$_2$ ~ 90%) and are relatively asymptomatic.

Clinical Presentation

- Hypercyanotic (TET) spells:
  - Involves agitation/irritability, profound cyanosis, syncope.
  - Can lead to severe disability and even death.
- Physical examination:
  - Harsh systolic ejection murmur (SEM) at upper sternal border (USB).
  - Cyanosis of lips and nail beds.

Diagnostic Evaluation

- Electrocardiography: right axis deviation with RVH.
- Chest radiograph: *Boot-shaped heart* with either increased or decreased pulmonary blood flow (see Figure 5.9).
- Echocardiogram: Primary diagnostic modality.

Tetralogy of Fallot

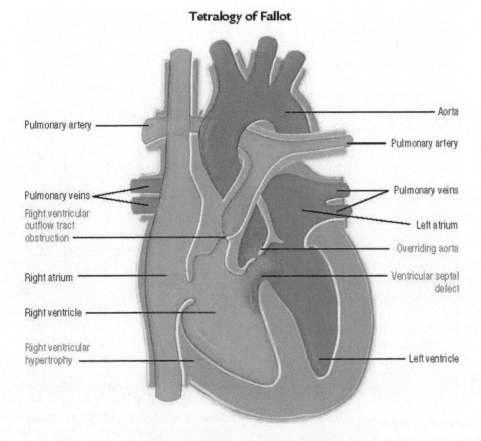

Pulmonary artery

Pulmonary veins

Right ventricular
outflow tract
obstruction

Right atrium

Right ventricle

Right ventricular
hypertrophy

Aorta

Pulmonary artery

Pulmonary veins

Left atrium

Overriding aorta

Ventricular septal
defect

Left ventricle

FIGURE 5.8 • **Tetralogy of Fallot.** Tetralogy of fallot defect.

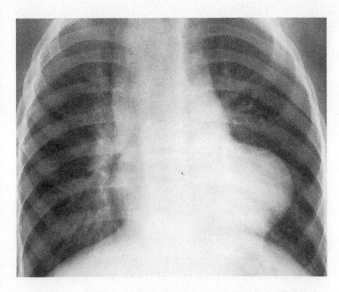

FIGURE 5.9 • **Chest Radiograph TOF.** Tetralogy of Fallot. The upwardly displaced cardiac apex caused by right ventricular hypertrophy and the concave pulmonary artery shadow are characteristic of Tetralogy of Fallot.

Management

- Medical management:
  - Asymptomatic
    - β-blocker agent
    - Neonatal period to 1 year of age

- Symptomatic/TET spells—believed to be caused by infundibular muscle spasms, resulting in right-to-left shunting through the VSD.
  - Treatment includes supplemental oxygen, sedation, volume expansion, knee-chest position.
  - In severe cases, may require phenyl epinephrine, emergency surgery, and/or extra corporeal membrane oxygenation (ECMO).
- Surgical interventions:
  - Blalock–Taussig (BT) shunt made of Gore-Tex (W.L. & Associates, Flagstaff, AZ) connecting the subclavian or carotid artery with the PA to allow blood flow to the branch pulmonary arteries with subsequent complete repair before 1 year of age, or
- Complete repair in the neonatal period.
  - Placement of BT shunt ± CPB (cardiopulmonary bypass), depending on the severity of right ventricular outflow tract (RVOT) obstruction.
  - Complete repair consisting of right atriotomy, closure of VSD, resection of infundibular stenosis, pulmonary arterioplasty, pulmonary valvotomy, or transannular right ventricular outflow tract (RVOT) patch.

Postoperative Complications

- Residual or undiagnosed VSD.
- RVOT obstruction.
- RV dysfunction.
- Electrophysiologic abnormalities.

- Pulmonary regurgitation.
- Shunt occlusion with BT shunt procedure.

Postoperative Checklist

- Evaluate for residual VSD and RVOT obstruction and dysfunction.
- Continuous monitoring of heart rate with evaluation for arrhythmia (e.g., JET, ventricular ectopy).
- Temporary pacemaker available at bedside, in some cases.
- In neonates with BT shunt, consider shunt occlusion with desaturation.

Pulmonary Atresia

Pulmonary atresia with intact ventricular septum.

Background/Definition

- Variable morphology.
- Obstruction of RVOT due to pulmonary valve atresia, intact ventricular septum and variable hypoplasia of right ventricle (RV) and tricuspid valve.
- Patients with small RVs and tricuspid valve annulus may also have coronary artery sinusoids and fistulae.
  - If present, they will greatly determine surgical management strategies (Figure 5.10).

Pathophysiology

- Similar to other single ventricle physiology.
- Desaturation level dependent on size of PDA.
- Atrial level shunting helps preserve cardiac output in the setting of a patent ductus.
- Arterial oxygen saturation serves as a good estimate of pulmonary to systemic blood flow ratio.
  - RV may have very high pressures during systole.

Clinical Presentation

- Progressive cyanosis with ductal closing causing profound hypoxemia, acidosis, and hemodynamic collapse.
- Systolic murmur of ductal flow, single first and second heart sounds.

Diagnostic Evaluation

- Chest radiograph:
  - Normal heart size unless significant tricuspid regurgitation (TR) is present, then right atrium (RA) and RV enlargement are present.
  - Pulmonary vascular markings (PVM) are dependent on size of PDA and PVR.
- Electrocardiogram:
  - Diminished RV force.
  - Dominant LV forces.
- Echocardiography:
  - Sufficient to establish basic diagnosis.
  - RV size and function, tricuspid valve size and function, atrial level shunting and PDA flow are all easily evaluated.
  - Abnormal flow patterns in the RV are suggestive of coronary artery fistulae or sinusoids.

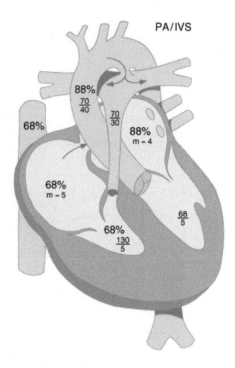

FIGURE 5.10 • **Pulmonary Atresia with Intact Ventricular Septum.** Pulmonary atresia (PA) with intact ventricular septum (IVS) in a neonate with a nonrestrictive patent ductus arteriosus while receiving PGE1. Typical anatomic and hemodynamic findings include (i) hypertrophied, hypoplastic right ventricle; (ii) hypoplastic tricuspid valve and pulmonary annulus; (iii) atresia of the pulmonary valve with no antegrade flow; (iv) suprasystemic RV pressure; (v) pulmonary blood flow through the patent ductus; (vi) right-to-left shunt at the atrial level with systemic desaturation. Many patients have significant coronary abnormalities with sinusoidal or fistulous connections to the hypertensive right ventricle or significant coronary stenoses (not shown). Prostaglandin E1 (PGE1), mean value (m).

- Cardiac catheterization:
  - Should always be performed with echocardiogram to conclusively define coronary anatomy.

Surgical Management

- Because of variable morphology, no single procedure is appropriate for all patients.
- Goals of initial surgery.
  - Provide adequate oxygenation.
  - Provide forward flow across RVOT to encourage RV development; ultimate goal is two-ventricle repair.
- Timing of surgery is in neonatal period.

Surgical Requirements

- Patients with right ventricular dependent coronary circulation (RVDCC)—single ventricle pathway.
  - Palliative BT shunt.
  - Will then go on to have either Glenn and Fontan or a 1½ ventricular repair.

- Patients without RVDCC.
  - Relief of RVOT obstruction with or without a BT shunt.
  - Ultimately, will have a two-ventricle repair.
- Patients with severe RVDCC and evidence of LV dysfunction, ischemia, or arrhythmias, consider for transplantation.
- Z-score (includes echocardiogram measurements and body surface area) of the tricuspid valve size significant in determining risk of biventricular repair success.

Postoperative Complications

- Similar to problems in the management of single ventricle physiology.
- Low cardiac output.
  - Immediate—unrecognized RVDCC with myocardial ischemia.
  - 1 to 3 days postoperative - circular shunt (pulmonary insufficiency [PI], tricuspid insufficiency [TI], ASD).
  - Treatment: Increase PVR and decrease systemic venous return (SVR).
- Hypoxemia; evaluate for:
  - Residual RVOT obstruction, or
  - Severe tricuspid valve (TV) hypoplasia.

Postoperative Checklist

- In shunt-dependent patients, balance circulation.
- Monitor for signs of ischemia with 12-lead ECG and/or echocardiogram.
- Evaluate for signs of low cardiac output and "circular shunting."

Tricuspid Atresia

Background/Definition

- Complete lack of formation of the tricuspid valve with absence of direct connection between the RA and RV (see Figure 5.11).
- Three types based on relationship of great arteries to ventricle.
  - Type I: normally related great arteries.
  - Type II: D-transposition.
  - Type III: L-transposition.

Pathophysiology

- Two subclasses based on amount of pulmonary stenosis and presence of VSD:
  - Too little pulmonary blood flow.
  - Too much pulmonary blood flow.

Clinical Presentation

- Physical Examination.
  - Cyanosis or CHF.
  - 80% will have murmur.
    - Too much pulmonary blood flow.
    - Too little pulmonary blood flow (SaO$_2$ <70%).

Management

- Treatment is tailored to underlying anatomy or pathophysiology.

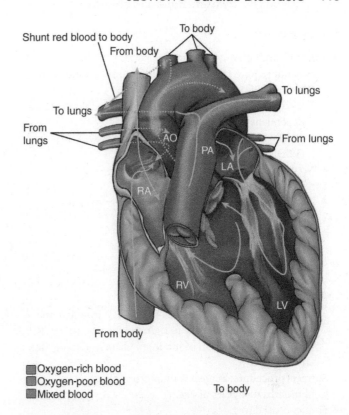

Shunt red blood to body
To body
From body
To lungs
To lungs
From lungs
From lungs
From body

AO
PA
LA
RA
RV
LV
From body

■ Oxygen-rich blood
■ Oxygen-poor blood
■ Mixed blood
To body

FIGURE 5.11 • **Triscuspid Atresia.**

- Intracardiac obstruction.
  - Increase BP or SVR with inotropes.
  - Cardiac catheterization manipulation: Atrial septectomy with restrictive ASD.
- Restrictive ductus arteriosus in ductal-dependent lesions.
  - PGE$_1$ infusion.
- Elevated PVR.
  - Maneuvers to decrease PVR—increase FiO$_2$, hyperventilation, alkalinization, nitric oxide, analgesia/sedation.
- Too much pulmonary blood flow.
  - Digitalis and diuretics.

Diagnostic Evaluation

- Electrocardiogram:
  - RA enlargement, possible first degree heart block.
- Chest radiograph:
  - Cardiomegaly.
  - PVM may be increased or decreased depending on the presence of VSD and degree of pulmonary stenosis.
- Echocardiogram:
  - Sufficient for diagnosis.
  - Can determine basic anatomy.
    - Size and/or presence of an ASD and VSD.
    - Relationship of the great vessels.
    - Degree of pulmonary blood flow.
    - Ventricular function.
- Cardiac catheterization:
  - Indicated when a restrictive atrial septal defect (ASD) is present.
  - If ASD present, balloon septostomy can be performed.

Management

- Surgical Timing:
  - May not require surgical intervention until symptomatic (in 1st year of life).
    - Cyanosis with decreased pulmonary blood flow/ductal-dependent lesion.
    - CHF with increased pulmonary blood flow (PBF) (VSD without PS).
  - No definitive repair, staged approach.
- Surgical procedure: Stage 1.
  - Decreased pulmonary blood flow (most common).
    - BT shunt.
  - Increased pulmonary blood flow.
    - PA band (PAB).
- Surgical procedure: Stage 2 bidirectional Glenn.
  - 4 to 12 months of age.
  - Procedure involves:
    - Disconnecting superior vena cava (SVC) from RA and connecting SVC directly to right pulmonary artery (RPA).
    - Ligation and division of modified Blalock–Taussig Shunt (MBTS).
- Surgical procedure: Stage 3 Fontan procedures.
  - 18 months to 4 years of age.
- Fontan procedures:
  - Lateral tunnel: Inferior vena cava flow is directed into the RPA via a lateral tunnel created through the RA using a Gore-Tex patch.
  - Fenestrations may be placed in the patch to act as a "pop off" until the pulmonary circulation can handle the circulating volume.
- Extracardiac: insertion of a Gore-Tex tube graft connecting the inferior vena cava (IVC) to the underside of the RPA.

Ductal-Dependent Lesions

Julie A. Creaden & Elizabeth R. Preze

Hypoplastic Left Heart Syndrome (HLHS)

Background/Definition

- Most common form of single ventricle physiology.
- Ductal-dependent lesion requiring urgent surgical intervention.
- Characterized by hypoplasia of the LV, and encompasses atresia or critical stenosis of the aortic and/or mitral valves and hypoplasia of the ascending aorta and aortic arch (see Figure 5.12).
- Presents at birth with cyanosis.

Pathophysiology

- Systemic circulation is dependent on the RV via the PDA and mixing of pulmonary and systemic blood at the atrial level.
- Patent foramen ovale is typically present, but can be small and obstructive.

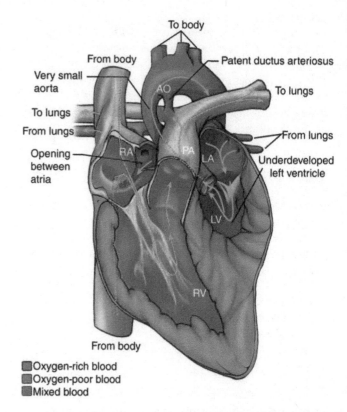

FIGURE 5.12 • **Hypoplastic Left Heart Syndrome.**

- Blood from the pulmonary veins cannot get into the diminutive LV and therefore mixes with systemic venous return in the right atrium.
- The RV pumps mixed blood to both pulmonary and systemic circulations via the PDA.
- Blood is sent to the lungs via the branch pulmonary arteries and the body via the PDA.
- The amount of blood that flows to each circulation is based on the resistance in each circuit.

Physical Examination

- Single S2.
- Soft systolic murmur.

Diagnostic Evaluation

- Electrocardiogram:
  - Right atrial enlargement (RAE).
  - Right ventricular hypertrophy (RVH).
- Chest radiograph:
  - Cardiomegaly and increased PVM.
- Echocardiogram:
  - Determination of cardiac morphology.
  - Evaluation of arch hypoplasia.
  - Diminutive LV with markedly dilated RV with aortic hypoplasia.
  - Determines the size of ASD and/or VSD and the degree of shunting across the septal defect(s).

- Cardiac catheterization:
  - Rarely necessary for diagnosis.
  - Helpful in establishing atrial communication via balloon septostomy.

Management

- Goal is to balance circulations!
  - Excessive pulmonary blood flow (SaO_2 >90%).
    - Results in reduction of systemic blood flow.
    - Despite higher oxygen saturation, tissue perfusion is actually compromised.

Treatment

- Maintain PDA patency with PGE_1 infusion or atrial septostomy (restrictive ASD).
- Maneuvers to increase PVR and decrease SVR.
- Alveolar hypoxia (FiO_2 0.21 or lower using nitrogen blend).
- Permissive hypercarbia (pH 7.30–7.40 with $PaCO_2$ 45–50 mmHg).
- Afterload reduction (e.g., milrinone, nipride).
- Minimize inotropic agents, particularly those with alpha effects.

Surgical Management

- Diagnosis usually occurs in the antenatal or immediate postnatal period and requires timely intervention.
- Stage 1 Norwood procedure.
  - Goals are to:
    - Establish reliable, unobstructed outflow to the systemic circulation, and
    - Balance the systemic and pulmonary circulations.
  - Components:
    - Placement of modified Blalock–Taussig shunt and ligation and division of PDA or Sano modification = placement of 5 mm Gortex shunt from the RV to PA bifurcation.
    - Division of main pulmonary artery (MPA) proximal to bifurcation to the branch pulmonary arteries.
    - Augmentation of the hypoplastic aortic arch with prosthetic material or homograft.
    - Connection of proximal PA to ascending aortic arch.
    - Atrial septectomy.
  - Postoperative management: Stage 1 Norwood.
    - Balance the systemic and pulmonary circulations with SaO_2 75% to 80%.
    - Monitor for pulmonary overcirculation.
      - Elevated O_2 saturations, hypotension, tachycardia, oliguria, metabolic acidosis.
    - Aspirin to avoid shunt thrombosis.
    - Monitor for signs and symptoms of necrotizing enterocolitis (NEC).
  - Postoperative problems: Stage 1 Norwood.
    - Low cardiac output.
      - Globally decreased ventricular output.
      - Elevated Qp:Qs (pulmonary to systemic flow ratio).
      - AV valve regurgitation.

- Cyanosis (SaO_2 <70%).
  - Pulmonary venous desaturation.
  - Systemic venous desaturation.
  - Decreased pulmonary blood flow.
- Elevated oxygen saturations (SaO_2 >90%).
  - Too much pulmonary blood flow.
    - Evaluate for presence of arch obstruction (increases pulmonary blood flow through BT shunt).
- Stage 2 bidirectional Glenn procedure.
  - Usually done between 4 and 6 months of age.
  - Provides reduced volume work on the single ventricle and a predictable Qp:Qs 0.6 to 0.7 with oxygen saturations of approximately 80%.
  - Procedure involves:
    - Disconnecting SVC from RA and connecting SVC directly to RPA.
    - Ligation and division of MBTS or Sano shunt.
  - Postoperative problems: Stage 2 bidirectional Glenn.
    - Headache.
    - Elevated SVC pressure (SVC syndrome).
      - Obstruction at anastomosis.
      - Distal PA distortion.
      - Elevated PVR.
    - Hypoxemia (SaO_2 <75%).
      - Pulmonary venous desaturation.
      - Systemic venous desaturation.
      - Decreased pulmonary blood flow.
    - Hypertension/bradycardia.
- Stage 3 Fontan procedure.
  - Stage 3 usually occurs at 18 months to 4 years of age.
  - Fontan procedure components.
    - Lateral tunnel: Inferior vena cava flow is directed into the RPA via a lateral tunnel created through the RA with a Gore-Tex patch.
    - Fenestrations may be placed in the patch to act as a "pop off" until the pulmonary circulation can handle the circulating volume.
    - Extracardiac: insertion of a Gore-Tex tube graft connecting the IVC to the underside of the RPA.
  - Postoperative management: Stage 3 Fontan.
    - Goal is to optimize cardiac output at lowest central venous pressure (CVP) possible.
    - Low positive end expiratory pressure (PEEP) on mechanical ventilation.
    - Attempt early extubation.
    - Aggressively treat arrhythmias.
      - Junctional ectopic tachycardia (JET) and atrial tachycardia—amiodarone.
      - Pacing; in cases of sinus node dysfunction.
  - Postoperative problems: Stage 3 Fontan.
    - Low cardiac output.
      - Inadequate preload.
      - Elevated PVR.
      - Anatomic systemic venous pathway obstruction.
      - Pump failure.

- Arrhythmias.
- Cyanosis.
- Effusions.
  - Most common cause of prolonged hospitalization.
- Thrombosis.
  - At risk of venous thrombosis and cerebellar nuclei neurons (CNS) complications.
  - Anticoagulation (e.g., warfarin, aspirin).

Transposition of the Great Arteries (TGA)

Complete transposition of the great arteries (D-TGA).

Background/Definition

- Aorta arising from the anatomic RV, and the PA arising from the anatomic left ventricle.
- May have associated VSD (40% of cases).
- Ventricles normally positioned and aorta malposed anteriorly and rightward above the RV, aligned with the RV via the infundibulum (Figure 5.13).

Pathophysiology

- Parallel circulation.
  - The output from each ventricle is recirculated to that ventricle.
  - Results in a deficiency of oxygen supply to the tissues and excessive ventricular workload.
  - Systemic and pulmonary oxygen saturations are dependent on:
    - Intracardiac shunts (PFO, ASD, VSD).
    - Extracardiac shunts (PDA, bronchopulmonary collaterals).

Clinical Presentation

- Physical examination.
  - Soft systolic murmur.
  - Bounding peripheral pulses related to the PDA.
  - Hepatomegaly.
- Hypoxemia.
  - Initial management includes ensuring adequate mixing and maximizing mixed venous oxygen saturation (SVO_2).
  - Ensure adequate mixing.
    - Maintain PDA patency with PGE_1 infusion.
    - If no improvement with PGE1 infusion, consider balloon septostomy.
    - Institute ventilatory maneuvers to decrease PVR and increase PBF.
    - Maximize SVO_2.
      - Decrease O_2 consumption.
      - Improve O_2 delivery.

Diagnostic Evaluation

- Echocardiogram:
  - A posterior great artery diving to the left and right pulmonary arteries arising from the LV along with the aorta arising from the RV confirm the diagnosis.
- Cardiac catheterization:
  - Useful for evaluation of coronary artery anatomy.
  - Enlargement of atrial septum, if needed.

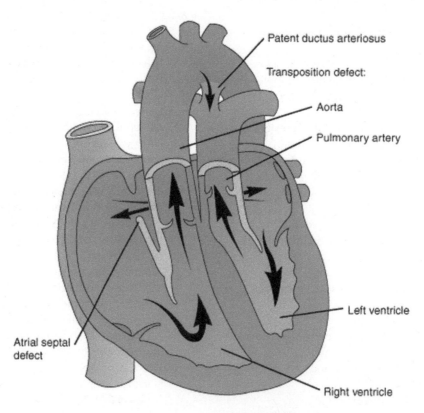

FIGURE 5.13 • **Transposition of Great Arteries.**

Management

- Arterial switch ± VSD closure.
- Timing.
  - Neonatal period.
- Surgical requirements.
  - Cardiopulmonary bypass (CPB) with deep hypothermia and circulatory arrest.
  - Arterial switch.
    - Transection of the great vessels.
    - Translocation of the coronary arteries.
    - Aortic reconstruction.
    - Pulmonary reconstruction.
    - Closure of ASD or VSD.

Postoperative Complications

- Arrhythmias.
- Coronary ischemia.
- LV dysfunction.
  - Coronary ischemia.
  - "Unprepared" LV.
  - Noncompliant LV.

Postoperative checklist

- Evaluate LV function, for arrhythmias, supravalvar aortic stenosis (AS), pulmonary stenosis, residual ASD, or VSD by ECHO.

Total Anomalous Pulmonary Venous Return (TAPVR)

Background/Definition

- Pulmonary veins drain anomalously into a systemic venous structure rather than into the left atrium LA.
- Can be total (all pulmonary veins—TAPVR) or partial anomalous drainage (partial anomalous pulmonary venous return [PAPVR]).
- TAPVR has three main types:
  - Supracardiac.
    - Pulmonary veins drain into the SVC.
  - Intracardiac.
    - Pulmonary veins drain into coronary sinus or RA.
  - Infracardiac.
    - Pulmonary veins drain into a common pulmonary vein→ portal system→IVC via the ductus venosus.

Pathophysiology

- Obstructed.
  - Pulmonary venous hypertension with resultant pulmonary edema.
  - Infracardiac most likely to be obstructive.
- Unobstructed.
  - Right-sided heart failure due to volume overload.

Clinical Presentation

- Dependent on degree of obstruction to pulmonary venous drainage and degree of obstruction to the compensatory right-to-left shunt.

- Obstructed veins will present immediately with hypoxia, severe cyanosis, hypotension, and metabolic acidosis—this is one of the few cardiac surgical emergencies requiring emergent surgical intervention.
- Unobstructive veins may go undetected for a short while, but eventually present with increased work of breathing and notable murmur—loud continuous split S2 together with a systolic ejection murmur over the pulmonary valve.
- Hepatomegaly, venous congestion.

Diagnostic Evaluation

- Chest radiograph:
  - Obstructed: pulmonary edema without cardiomegaly (see Figure 5.14).
  - Unobstructed: increased PVM with cardiomegaly.
- Electrocardiography:
  - RA and RV hypertrophy.
- Echocardiogram:
  - Difficult to diagnose with transthoracic echocardiogram
- Cardiac catheterization:
  - Usually not indicated; avoid with obstructed veins
- MRI/MRA:
  - Becoming more widely used to diagnose TAPVR/PAPVR.

Management

- Surgical intervention—emergent if obstructed.
  - Requires median sternotomy and cardiopulmonary bypass.
  - Includes anastomosing the pulmonary veins to the LA and closure of ASD.

Postoperative Complications

- Low cardiac output.
- Respiratory insufficiency.

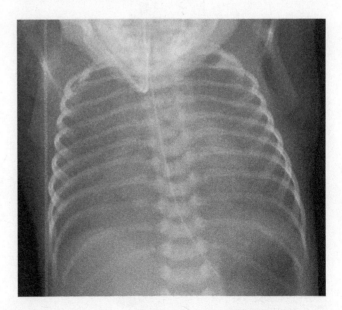

FIGURE 5.14 • Chest Radiograph TAPVR with Obstructed Veins. Chest X-ray demonstrating diffuse interstitial pulmonary edema and a normal cardiac silhouette in a patient with obstructed total anomalous pulmonary venous return.

- Pulmonary hypertension.
- Dysrhythmias.
- Pulmonary vein stenosis; usually appears in the first 6 to 12 months after repair; presents when obstruction is severe; clinical signs are progressive shortness of breath and requires additional surgical intervention.

Postop Checklist

- Monitor for pulmonary hypertension.
  - Suspect pulmonary venous obstruction if present.
  - Be aware of decreased left-sided compliance and avoid aggressive volume.

Truncus Arteriosus (TA)

Background/Definition

- Congenital malformation, which is a single arterial trunk arising from the heart: results from failure of the truncus arteriosus to divide into the aorta and PA.
- Almost always associated with a VSD.
- All conotruncal lesions are associated with 22q11 deletion.
  - Uses site of origin of pulmonary arteries from the truncus to define types
    - Type I to III are true truncus.
    - Type IV more accurately considered pulmonary atresia (Figure 5.15).

Pathophysiology

- Resembles single ventricle physiology.

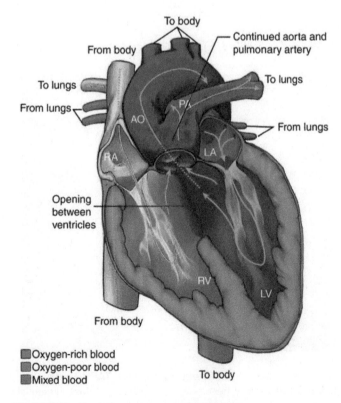

To body
From body
Continued aorta and pulmonary artery
To lungs
From lungs
To lungs
AO
PA
From lungs
RA
LA
Opening between ventricles
RV
LV
From body

☐ Oxygen-rich blood
☐ Oxygen-poor blood
☐ Mixed blood

To body

FIGURE 5.15 • **Truncus Arteriosus.**

- Degree of pulmonary blood flow is dependent on PVR and the degree of pulmonary stenosis.
- In the absence of pulmonary stenosis, the fall in PVR leads to pulmonary overcirculation and symptoms of CHF.
- Congestive heart failure is exacerbated in the presence of truncal valve regurgitation.
- Small PA from the truncus offers resistance to pulmonary blood flow (PBF), resulting in small Qp (pulmonary blood flow) and low oxygen saturation.
- Mild narrowing of PA from the truncus offers mild resistance to pulmonary blood flow, resulting in equal Qp and Qs (pulmonary and systemic blood flow) with acceptable oxygen saturation.
- Normal size PA from the truncus offers no resistance to pulmonary blood flow, resulting in high Qp:Qs and high oxygen saturation. Pulmonary edema and CHF will be present.

Clinical Presentation

- Physical examination:
  - Signs of CHF: tachypnea, hepatomegaly, diaphoresis (e.g., sweating with feeds), FTT, bounding pulses.
  - Harsh systolic murmur with possible ejection click—diastolic murmur present if truncal valve insufficiency or regurgitation.

Diagnostic Evaluation

- Electrocardiography:
  - Normal sinus rhythm (NSR).
  - Biventricular hypertrophy.
- Chest radiograph:
  - Cardiomegaly.
  - Increased pulmonary vascular markings.
  - Absent PA segment.
- Echocardiogram:
  - Provides good information to determine type of truncus arteriosus.
  - Demonstrates origin of coronary arteries, character of the truncal valve and truncal valve insufficiency—usually quadricuspid.
- Computed tomography (CT)/magnetic resonance imaging (MRI) and cardiac catheterization can be helpful in determining coronary anatomy, truncal valve insufficiency, and in measuring PVR.

Management

- Early surgical intervention before decompensated CHF, increased pulmonary vascular resistance, or cardiac cachexia develops; preferably first 2 weeks of life.

Surgical Management

- Median sternotomy with cardiopulmonary bypass.
- Removal of pulmonary trunk with aortic patch at pulmonary trunk removal sites.
- Placement of RV to branch PA conduit to form a pulmonary artery.
- Closure of VSD.
- Truncal valve repair if necessary.

Postoperative Considerations

- Pulmonary hypertensive crisis.
- Low cardiac output.
- Cyanosis.
- Dysrhythmias.
- Neoaortic (truncal) valve stenosis/regurgitation.
- Residual VSD.

Postoperative Checklist

- Pulmonary hypertension:
  - Evaluate for residual VSD and RVOT obstruction.
  - Treat pulmonary hypertension.
- RV dysfunction:
  - Institute appropriate pharmacologic and volume support for the RV.
  - Allow desaturation secondary to shunting at the atrial level.
- Monitor for and treat dysrhythmias, especially JET.

Coarctation of the Aorta (COA)

Background/Definition

- Constriction of the thoracic aorta distal to the left subclavian artery (Figure 5.16).

Pathophysiology/Clinical Presentation

- Neonates:
  - Present in first week of life if blood flow dependent on PDA—ductal closure leads to LV pressure overload and failure with resultant pulmonary edema and circulatory collapse.
    - Presents in shock; tachypnea, tachycardia, decreased or absent lower peripheral pulses, hypotension, hepatomegaly.
- Older children:
  - Present with hypertension on a routine physical examination.
  - Have either hypertension and/or decreased femoral pulses.
  - Diagnosis can be delayed secondary to hypertension evaluation.
  - Often have complaints of headache, leg and stomach cramping, cool extremities, and decreased lower extremities (LE) pulses.

Diagnostic Evaluation

- Chest radiograph: cardiomegaly and signs of CHF
- Electrocardiograph—LV strain pattern
- Echocardiogram—diagnostic in most cases.
  - Demonstrates the anatomic coarctation.
  - Lack of flow in the descending aorta.
  - Coarctation.
  - Size of the transverse arch.
  - Any other cardiac anomalies.
- Cardiac catheterization: can be performed in a stable infant maintained on prostaglandins (PGE) for further delineation of cardiac anatomy.
- CT scan or MRI can be used for the child with a difficult arch to image with echocardiogram.

Management

- Surgical approach.
  - Left thoracotomy for most cases.
    - Resection with (extended) end-to-end anastomosis.
      - Narrowed coarctation section is excised, and direct anastomosis is done with the two segments.
    - Prosthetic interposition graft.
      - Used in patients >10 years of age, or with an associated aneurysm or long segment coarctation.
      - Coarctation is excised and interposition graft placed to connect segments of the transverse and descending aorta.
  - Mediansternotomy is necessary for patients with associated intracardiac anomalies.

Postoperative Considerations

- Paradoxical hypertension.
  - Early (first 48 hours) related to release of the stretch on baroreceptors in the carotid arteries and aortic arch after removal of the coarctation.
  - 48 to 72 hours is related to elevated levels of renin and angiotensin.
- Spinal cord ischemia; paraplegia, rare but serious.
- Residual coarctation—defined as postoperative arm leg BP discrepancy— requires balloon dilation or reoperation.
- Recurrent laryngeal nerve injury.

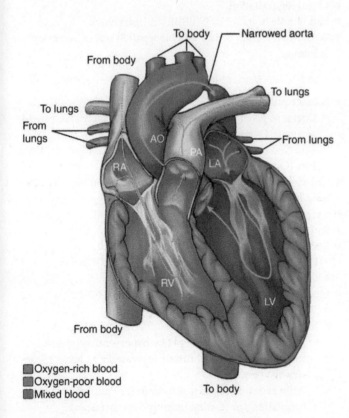

To body — Narrowed aorta
From body
To lungs
To lungs
From lungs
From lungs
AO
PA
RA
LA
RV
LV
From body
To body

■ Oxygen-rich blood
■ Oxygen-poor blood
■ Mixed blood

FIGURE 5.16 • **Coarctation of the Aorta.**

Postoperative Checklist

- Treat hypertension aggressively.
- Evaluate for residual arch obstruction.
- Check four extremity BP and neurological function.

Aortic Stenosis (AS)—Valvar

Background/Definition

- Malformation of the aortic valve that causes obstruction to ejection of blood from the left ventricle LV.
- Infants who present with AS represent a spectrum of anatomic variants from HLHS to thickened aortic valve.
- Older children who present with AS typically have little sequelae.
- Can occur at the valvular level, supravalvar or subvalvar region.

Pathophysiology

- Neonates:
  - Pressure overload of LV with LVH (elevated LV end diastolic pressure [LVEDP]) and eventually pulmonary edema.
  - With critical AS, PDA provides increased cardiac output via R→L shunt.
- Older children:
  - Chronic obstruction leads to LV overload and LVH.
  - With severe hypertrophy, subendocardial tissue ischemia may be noted.
  - Ischemia is further exaggerated by stress/exercise.

Clinical Presentation

- Timing of presentation is related to severity of obstruction.
  - Neonates: shock and signs of circulatory arrest.
  - Infants: Signs of CHF.
  - Older children: systolic murmur radiating to neck and apex; ejection click suggests valvar stenosis rather than supra- or subvalvar narrowing, narrow pulse pressure with normal BP.

Diagnostic Evaluation

- Chest radiograph.
  - Neonates: cardiomegaly with pulmonary edema.
- Electrocardiograph.
  - Older children: LVH with possible ST segment changes.
- Echocardiogram.
  - Sufficient for diagnosis.
  - Must evaluate left-sided cardiac structures.
- Cardiac catheterization.
  - Only indicated with balloon valvuloplasty

Management

- Timing.
  - Neonates.
    - Require immediate intervention.
    - Catheter balloon valvuloplasty or surgical valvotomy is often initial treatment of choice.

- Older infants and children.
  - Require intervention when symptomatic or with high left ventricular LV outflow tract (LVOT) pressure gradient (e.g., LVOT gradient >50 mmHg, anginal pain, or ST segment changes during exercise).
- Surgical procedure.
  - Dependent on anatomy of the valve and other cardiac structures as well as the age of the patient.
    - Stage 1 Norwood.
    - Surgical valvotomy.
  - Older children.
    - Aortic valve replacement.
    - Ross procedure: procedure of replacing the aortic valve with the patient's own pulmonary valve and then using a pulmonary allograft to replace the pulmonary valve; this includes translocation of coronary arteries.
    - Konno procedure: aortic valve replacement with enlargement of LV outflow tract; this includes translocation of coronary arteries.
    - Ross–Konno procedure: uses pulmonary autograft in aortic position and enlargement of the LV outflow tract in addition to placement of pulmonary homograft; this includes translocation of coronary arteries.

Postoperative Considerations

- Ross procedure will require replacement of pulmonary allograft.
- Left ventricular outflow tract (LVOT) stenosis.
- Mitral regurgitation.
- Left bundle branch block (LBBB) or heart block.
- With Ross/Konno or supravalvar repair at risk of coronary ischemia.

Preoperative Management—Single Ventricle Physiology

- Balance pulmonary and systemic circulations.
  - Goal is to provide enough pulmonary circulation to provide adequate O_2 delivery and prevent acidosis.
  - Achieved by maintaining an arterial O_2 saturation of 75% to 80% (Qp:Qs = 1:1).
- Unbalanced circulation results in inadequate pulmonary blood flow, hypoxemia/cyanosis.
- Excessive pulmonary blood flow results in CHF.
- Single ventricle: Goal Qp:Qs = 1:1.
- Excessive pulmonary blood flow: Qp:Qs = 2:1.
  - High saturations >80%.
  - CHF.
- Inadequate pulmonary blood flow: Qp:Qs = 0.7:1.
  - When Qp:Qs is low, SaO_2 drops <70%.
  - Management:
    - Decrease PVR (increase pH by hyperventilation and sodium bicarbonate infusion, increase FiO_2, lower mean airway pressure).
    - Raise systemic vascular resistance (calcium gluconate, maintaining or starting inotropic vasopressors).
    - Prostaglandin (PGE) infusion in ductal-dependent lesions with restrictive PDAs.

- Excessive pulmonary blood flow (SaO_2 >90%).
  - Results in reduction of systemic blood flow.
  - Despite higher oxygen saturation, tissue perfusion is compromised.
  - Treatment includes:
    - Maneuvers to increase PVR and decrease SVR.
      - Alveolar hypoxia (FiO_2 0.21 or lower with nitrogen).
      - Permissive hypercarbia (pH 7.30–7.40 with $PaCO_2$ 45–50 mmHg).
      - Afterload reduction (e.g., milrinone, nipride).
      - Minimize inotropic agents (particularly those with alpha effects).
    - In this setting, patients usually require urgent surgical intervention.

Intraoperative Approach Considerations in Children with CHD

- Palliative versus curative.
- Thoracotomy versus median sternotomy:
  - With or without cardiopulmonary bypass.
  - Deep hypothermic circulatory arrest.
  - Low-flow cerebral perfusion.
- Thoracotomy:
  - Used for procedures including PDA ligation, BT shunt placement, coarctation repair, and PA banding.
  - Entails collapse of one lung during the operation.
  - Postoperative problems specific to this approach include thoracic duct damage, phrenic nerve injury, recurrent laryngeal nerve injury.
- Cardiopulmonary bypass: A mechanical means of circulating and oxygenating blood volume while diverting most of the circulation away from the cardiopulmonary system.
  - Basic components include: pump, oxygenator, reservoir, tubing, and cannulas to carry blood between patient and oxygenator.
    - Most intracardiac repairs also require cardioplegia to arrest the heart.
    - This is achieved by cross-clamping the aorta between the arterial cannulation site and the aortic root where the coronary arteries arise.
    - Cardioplegia cools and protects the myocardium.
- Cardiopulmonary bypass sequelae.
  - Neurologic: emboli (air and/or debris), low cerebral blood flow.
  - Cardiac: ischemia, emboli, direct coronary artery injury.
  - Pulmonary: complement-induced endothelial damage.
  - Renal: elevated antidiuretic hormone (ADH) levels, additional injury due to red blood cell (RBC) hemolysis.
  - Gastrointestinal: emboli.
  - Coagulation: complement activation, platelet consumption, altered platelet aggregation, coagulation factor dilution.
  - Endocrine: elevated growth hormone, elevated insulin, hyperglycemia.
- Cardiopulmonary bypass (CPB) effects on ICU course.

- Rewarming: may require volume infusions to maintain cardiac output.
- Bleeding: due to heparinization during CPB, platelet dysfunction, dilution of coagulation factors.
- Fluid overload: most centers now hemofiltrate at end of CPB to minimize effects of fluid overload.
- Postperfusion syndrome: characterized by a whole-body inflammatory reaction; increased capillary permeability, leukocytosis, fever, peripheral vasoconstriction, hemolysis, bleeding diathesis.
- Deep hypothermic circulatory arrest: facilitates repair of complex lesions, allows for a totally bloodless field and removal of venous cannulae that may obscure visualization of intracardiac structures.
  - Technique: cooling to less than 20°C, removal of bypass cannulas.
- Deep hypothermia and circulatory arrest (DHCA) sequelae: seizures, choreoathetosis.

General Postoperative Management Considerations

- Precise anatomic diagnosis including pathophysiologic effects of defect on cardiovascular system and other organ systems.
- Patient's noncardiac medical and surgical history and preoperative medications.
- Details of the operation.
  - Anesthetic agents used in operating room (OR).
  - Intraoperative complications.

Congestive Heart Failure
Robin McKinney

Definition

- Chronic inability of the heart to generate enough cardiac output to effectively meet the body's metabolic demands.
- Signs and symptoms include edema, respiratory distress, growth failure, hepatomegaly, and exercise intolerance.

Etiology

- Congenital heart lesions or cardiomyopathy.
- Inflammation from infections, genetic factors, toxins, or chemotherapy.

Pathophysiology

- Structural defects or acute damage to the heart leads to decreased ability of cardiac muscle to pump blood adequately.
- Pressure or volume overload leads to decreased cardiac contractility, decreased output, and failure to adequately supply systemic demand.
- *Preload:* The volume needed to fill the heart. As preload increases, cardiac output increases until the preload exceeds the optimum range. When preload exceeds the optimum range, the cardiac output no longer increases, and the body begins to become fluid overloaded.

- *Afterload:* The force against which the heart must pump. Can be increased by fixed obstruction (e.g., AS) or by increasing peripheral vascular resistance.
- Too much preload or afterload from any cause will contribute to the signs and symptoms of heart failure (see Figure 5.1).
- As cardiac function decreases, neurohormonal mechanisms are activated, resulting in compensation; however, they are associated with deleterious effects.
  - Activation of the renin–angiotensin–aldosterone system results in sodium and water retention aimed at increasing circulatory volume and maximizing preload.
  - Sympathetic nervous system activation leads to catecholamine (e.g., norepinephrine) release. Cardiac output is then increased by increased cardiac contractility and vasoconstriction of blood vessels, resulting in improved preload.
  - Long-term sequelae of these compensatory mechanisms lead to volume overload and increased cardiac workload.
- Volume overload contributes to myocardial hypertrophy, which is initially beneficial, but eventually can be a risk for myocardial ischemia, which then leads to decreased contractility.
- Overstretching of cardiac muscle leads to worsening contractility.
- Pulmonary edema results from fluid overload.
- Cardiac remodeling is caused by a catecholamine response and changes in pressure–volume relationship, resulting in myocardium that does not function as well.
- Cycle is progressive with deterioration accelerating over time as initial compensatory mechanisms lead to progressive damage.

Clinical Presentation

- Infants: tachypnea, feeding difficulties (e.g., decreased volume or increased time spent feeding), poor weight gain, excessive perspiration (especially when feeding), and excessive irritability. Wheezing and tachypnea from pulmonary congestion often mistaken for bronchiolitis.
- Children: fatigue, exercise intolerance, anorexia, abdominal pain, dyspnea, and cough.
- Infants and children:
  - Tachycardia, decreased peripheral pulses, delayed capillary refill, and cool extremities.
  - Abdominal pain is a common presenting complaint and may be overlooked or dismissed. Hepatomegaly, ascites can be present with abdominal distension.
  - Edema may be present in dependent portions of the body (e.g., lower extremities in an ambulatory child; body wall and sacrum if nonambulatory).

Diagnostic Evaluation

- Chest radiograph: enlarged cardiac silhouette/cardiomegaly.
  - Exaggerated pulmonary arterial vessels may be present in left-to-right shunts.
  - Pulmonary edema manifests as fluffy perihilar infiltrates.
  - Atelectasis may be present as a result of compression of one of the bronchi or lung lobes by the enlarged heart. This can be mistaken for a retro-cardiac opacity/consolidation, leading to a misdiagnosis of pneumonia.
  - Pleural effusions may be present; usually bilateral.

- Abdominal radiograph: if obtained for complaints of stomach pain, may demonstrate incidental finding of cardiomegaly.
- Electrocardiogram: may indicate LVH, RVH, or an underlying rhythm abnormality responsible for the heart failure.
- Echocardiogram: most useful in evaluating the cardiac structure and function.
- Metabolic acidosis may be present with a large base excess and an elevated lactate.
- Serum B-type natriuretic peptide (BNP) is elevated in response to ventricular wall tension or stretch; useful in trending the response to therapy in heart failure.
- Depending on the degree of dysfunction, other laboratory values may be abnormal:
  - Hyponatremia due to volume overload, elevated creatinine due to underperfusion of the kidneys, elevated transaminases (AST/ALT).

Management

- The initial goal in management of CHF is resuscitation and stabilization.
- In an acute exacerbation or in fulminant failure, it is important to note that many of the outpatient medications can counteract therapies used in the acute setting.
- Therapy should be tailored to the presenting problem and underlying lesion with the goal of maximizing cardiac output.
  - Optimize volume status, judiciously.
  - Augment cardiac contractility.
- If adequate perfusion in the presence of volume overload, diuretics indicated. Furosemide and chlorothiazide are first-line agents.
- Patients with poor perfusion and volume overload require additional support.
  - Afterload reduction: reduces the force the heart is pumping against. This is the most important concept.
  - Vasodilators (e.g., nitroprusside) and diuretics can help with poor perfusion and congestion, but must be used cautiously in the setting of hypotension.
  - Inotropic support with β-agonists such as dopamine or dobutamine can improve cardiac output.
  - Phosphodiesterase inhibitors (e.g., milrinone) are both an inotropic agent and a vasodilator.
  - If inotropic support is needed, discontinue chronic beta-blocker therapy.
- If poor perfusion not associated with fluid overload, fluid resuscitation and inotropic support may be needed.
  - In addition to the β-agonists, epinephrine may be helpful. At low doses, it provides inotropic support and vasodilation, and at higher doses, inotropic support and vasoconstriction.
  - Vasopressin causes peripheral constriction, and while not considered an inotrope, it may improve cardiac output.
  - Calcium increases myocardial contractility; maintain normal ionized calcium levels in the setting of heart failure.
- A variety of medications are used in the outpatient setting for long-term management.
  - Diuretics such as furosemide and chlorothiazide help manage volume overload.

- Aldactone is a potassium-sparing diuretic that has the added benefit of preventing cardiac remodeling.
- β-blockers counteract the long-term effects of sympathetic nervous system activation.
- Angiotensin-converting enzyme inhibitors provide afterload reduction, improving cardiac output.
- Digoxin is used to help improve cardiac contractility.

Endocarditis
Caroline Bauer

Definition

- Infection of the endothelial surface of the heart.
- Can develop on any structure of the heart.

Etiology

- Risk factors:
  - Prosthetic valves.
  - Previous history of endocarditis infection.
  - Complex cyanotic CHD.
  - Surgically placed systemic-to-pulmonary artery shunts.
  - Injection drug use.
  - Indwelling central venous catheters.
- 90% of cases occur in children with heart disease, most commonly in CHD.
  - Incidence is 0.3 per 100,000 children with an overall mortality rate of 11.6%.
  - Most common causative pathogens:
    - Least virulent: α-*hemolytic streptococci*, enterococci, and coagulase-negative *staphylococci*.
    - Most virulent: *Staphylococcus aureus* (accounts for 57% of all cases of endocarditis), *Streptococcus pneumoniae*, β-*hemolytic streptococcus*, and fungal sources such as *Candida* and *Aspergillus*.

Pathophysiology

- Begins with damage to the endocardial cells of the heart.
- Leads to thrombus formation.
  - Pathogens circulating in the bloodstream adhere to the thrombus, and continued deposition of fibrin and platelets occurs, providing a protected environment for organisms to grow and flourish.

Clinical Presentation

- Fever is the most common presenting symptom.
- Fulminate endocarditis:
  - High fever.
  - Hemodynamic instability.
- Subacute presentation:
  - Arthralgias.
  - Myalgias.
  - Headache.
  - Malaise.
  - Relapsing fever.
  - Poor appetite.

- Almost all patients with endocarditis will have a murmur on physical examination.
- Other less common physical examination findings include petechiae, Osler nodes, Janeway lesions, Roth spots, and splinter hemorrhages (see Figures 5.17 and 5.18).

Diagnostic Evaluation

- The modified Duke criteria are the standard approach used to diagnose endocarditis (Table 5.2).
- Criteria for definitive diagnosis of endocarditis:
  - Pathologic evidence of intracardiac or embolized vegetation or intracardiac abscess, OR
  - Two major criteria findings, OR
  - One major and three minor criteria findings, OR
  - Five minor criteria findings.
  - For the possible diagnosis of endocarditis, the following criteria must be met:
    - One major and one minor criteria findings, OR
    - Three minor criteria findings
- Laboratory evaluation.
  - Blood cultures.
    - Three peripheral blood cultures from different locations within a 24-hour period; first culture should be obtained prior to antibiotics.
  - Complete blood count (CBC); may reveal anemia; leukocytosis is uncommon.
  - Urinalysis (UA): may reveal micro- or macrohematuria, suggesting renal embolization of vegetation.
- Diagnostic studies.
  - Echocardiogram.

Management

- Extended-course intravenous (IV) antimicrobials (typically 4–6 weeks) under infectious disease guidance is the mainstay of therapy.

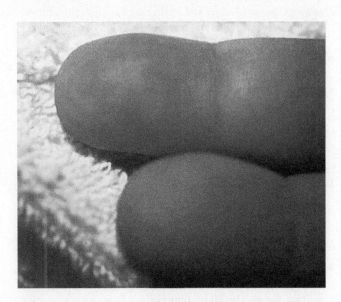

FIGURE 15.17 · **Osler Nodes.** A patient with Osler nodes from Streptococcus viridans bacterial endocarditis.

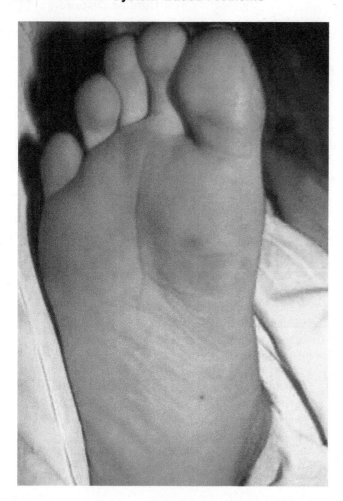

FIGURE 15.18 • **Janeway Lesions.** A Janeway lesion on the sole of an adolescent female with enterococcal endocarditis

TABLE 5.2	Duke Criteria
Major Criteria	
Positive blood culture.	
Positive echocardiogram on two occasions.	
New valvular regurgitation.	
Minor Criteria	
Predisposing heart condition including previous infective endocarditis.	Janeway lesions (painless hemorrhagic lesions on palms and soles).
Injection drug use.	Glomerulonephritis.
Fever.	Osler nodes (painful lesions at fingertips).
Major arterial emboli.	Roth spots (retinal hemorrhages).
Septic pulmonary infarcts.	Positive rheumatoid factor.
Mycotic aneurysm.	Single positive blood culture.
Intracranial hemorrhage. Conjunctival hemorrhage.	Serologic evidence of active infection with an "organism consistent with endocarditis."

Table created by Bauer, C. (content contributor).

- Empiric therapy should be directed at the most common pathogens—*streptococci* and *staphylococcus*—until susceptibilities are available, and then targeted antimicrobial therapy is determined.
- Standard initial antibiotic therapy is penicillin or ampicillin plus vancomycin.
- Surgical referral indications include persistent infection, significant embolic events, new heart block, an abscess that is large or increasing in size, or progressive CHF.

Hypertension

Tresa E. Zielinski

Definition

- Stages:
  - Prehypertension: 120–139/80–89 mmHg.
  - Stage 1: 140–159/90–99 mmHg.
  - Stage 2: 160+/100+ mmHg.

- National High Blood Pressure Education Program (NHBPEP) Working Group on High Blood Pressure in Children and Adolescents.
  - Average systolic BP and/or diastolic BP that is ≥95th percentile for gender, age, and height on ≥3 occasions is hypertension.
  - Hypertension is classified as prehypertensive, stage 1 or stage 2 (see above). All children and adults with a BP above 120/80 mmHg should be classified as prehypertensive.
    - Key differences between stage 1 and stage 2; confirmed stage 1 allows for time for evaluation prior to intervention, while stage 2 requires swift evaluation (referred for evaluation within one week or sooner if symptomatic) and intervention. In symptomatic stage 2 hypertension, immediate intervention is required and prompt referral with a specialist.
  - Stage 1 hypertension is reevaluated on repeat visits; three separate measurements within 1 month.
  - Secondary hypertension is more common in children than in adults. This is hypertension that is not primary in nature, but related to other etiologies (e.g., kidney disease).

- Stage 2 hypertension in children should be investigated more thoroughly than other stages.

Etiology

- Essential hypertension.
  - Unknown etiology: diagnosis of exclusion.
  - Genetic: strong familial association.
- Secondary hypertension:
  - More common in children than adults.
  - 60% to 70% of hypertension in children is secondary to kidney disease. Other causes include: Adrenal gland, medications, obstructive sleep apnea, stress, anxiety, coarctation of the aorta, endocrine causes, pregnancy, metabolic syndrome.

Presentation

- History:
  - Family history (e.g., cardiovascular disease, deafness, endocrine disorders, kidney disease, obstructive sleep apnea).
  - Patient history (e.g., umbilical artery/vein catheterization, CP, diaphoresis, dyspnea on exertion, edema, growth failure, heat/cold intolerance, palpitations, headaches, joint pain/swelling, myalgias, hematuria, recurrent rashes, snoring/sleep disturbances, urinary tract infections (recurrent), weight/appetite changes).
- Physical examination:
  - All children >3 years of age should have BP checked on every health care visit.
  - All children <3 years of age with history of CHD, prematurity, kidney disease, urinary tract infections, malignancy, elevated intracranial pressure, or proteinuria should have BP checked with every health care visit.
  - Physical examination clues to hypertension.
    - Tonsillar hypertrophy (sleep-disordered breathing).
    - Papilledema (intracranial hypertension).
    - Acanthosis nigricans (type 2 diabetes).
    - Murmur (coarctation of aorta).
    - Abdominal mass (kidney tumor, hydronephrosis, polycystic kidney disease).
    - Disparate pulses; upper pulses > lower (coarctation of aorta).
    - Elfin or Moon facies (Williams syndrome, Cushing syndrome).
    - Thyroid enlargement (hyperthyroidism).
      - Muscle weakness (Hyperaldosteronism).
      - Diminished pain response (Familial dysautonomia).
      - Ambiguous genitalia (Adrenal hyperplasia).
      - Advanced puberty (intracranial tumor/pathology).
    - *Most patients are asymptomatic on presentation and may not have a history suggestive of hypertension.*

Plan

- Diagnostic studies.
  - Laboratory evaluation.
    - Should be obtained in anyone with stage 1 hypertension or higher.

- CBC: Anemia is a classic sign of chronic kidney disease.
- Renal function panel: Evaluation of kidney function (i.e., BUN/creatinine) and electrolytes. Hyperphosphotemia and hypocalcemia are commonly noted in kidney disease.
  - Urinalysis.
  - Urine protein/creatinine ratio; consider.
  - Lipid panel.
  - Fasting lipid panel and fasting blood glucose measurement; obese patients.
- Echocardiogram: evaluation for LV hypertrophy (LVH).
- Renal ultrasound: evaluation for kidney scarring, congenital abnormalities, unequal kidney size.
- Retinal examination: Evaluation for retinal vascular changes.
- Nonpharmacologic therapy.
- First-line plan in stage 1 hypertension.
- Lifestyle changes:
  - Weight loss; exercise, dietary modifications.
    - Reduce salt intake: 2.4 g sodium restriction/day.
    - Increase fresh fruit and vegetables.
    - Increase low-fat dairy products.
- Family-based:
  - Avoidance of smoking and alcohol intake.
- Pharmacologic therapy:
  - First-line in stage 2 hypertension.
- General guidelines and classification.
  - ACE (angiotensin-converting enzyme) inhibitors ("-prils"): Dilate blood vessels to decrease resistance.
    - Side effects:
      - Cough.
      - Skin rash (red, itchy).
      - Dizziness/lightheadedness, orthostatic hypotension.
      - Taste impairment (salty or metallic).
      - Edema (lower extremities).
      - Hyperkalemia.
      - Decrease in glomerular filtration rate (GFR).
- Precautions:
  - Not to be used in volume-depleted patients.
  - Not to be used in patients with bilateral renovascular hypertension.
  - Avoid salt substitutions as they contain potassium.
  - Avoid nonsteroidal anti-inflammatory (NSAID) medications.
  - Check BP and kidney function regularly.
  - ARB (angiotensin II receptor blockers) ("-sartan"): angiotensin II receptor blockers decrease chemicals that cause vasoconstriction; decrease intraglomerular pressure through decreasing efferent arteriolar tone.
    - Useful in patients with diabetes, preferred class of medication if ACE inhibitors are not well tolerated because of renoprotective (reduces microalbuminuria) properties.
    - Side effects:
      - Dizziness, orthostatic hypotension (worse with first dose, need to take for a week+ before full effect), muscle cramping, diarrhea.
    - Precautions:
      - Monitor BP and kidney function.

- Calcium channel blockers ("-pine"): dilate blood vessels, decreasing cardiovascular resistance. These agents slow the movement of calcium into cells of the heart and blood vessels. May be the desired class in patients with asthma.
  - Side effects: edema, arrhythmias, fatigue, dizziness.
  - Precautions: monitor heart rate, avoid grapefruit, avoid alcohol, contraindicated in patients with sick sinus syndrome.
- Diuretics: decrease blood volume and excrete sodium.
  - Thiazide-like: most effective in lowering BP (metolazone, hydrochlorothiazide).
    - Can be used as primary therapy.
    - Can enhance the effects of other antihypertensive agents.
    - Requires salt restriction as concurrent therapy.
    - Can infrequently cause hypokalemia, glucose intolerance, adverse lipid effects.
    - Periodic blood chemistries needed.
  - Loop: more powerful; can be helpful in hypertensive emergenices (e.g., furosemide, bumetanide, torsemide).
  - Potassium sparing: can be helpful with CHF; usually prescribed in conjunction with one of the other two types (spironolactone).
  - Side effects: frequent urination, electrolyte imbalance, fatigue or weakness, muscle cramping, dizziness, dehydration, anorexia.
- Vasodilators (e.g., hydralazine, minoxidil).
  - Reserved for patients failing other therapies.
  - Unfavorable side-effect profile.
- Peripheral α_1-antagonists and centrally acting α_2-agonists.
  - May be associated with orthostatic hypotension.
  - α/β-Blockers ("-lol"): β-blockers block the effects of sympathetic nervous system (adrenaline) in the heart.
    - Reduction in heart rate results in a reduction of cardiac output.
    - Use with caution in ambulatory patients.
  - Side effects: β-blockers are contraindicated in children with heart block, asthma, or pregnancy. May reduce the ability of a diabetic patient to identify a hypoglycemic event; use with extreme caution in diabetic patients.
- Hypertensive crisis management:
  - Intravenous (IV) form of antihypertensive medications (e.g., esmolol, labetolol, nicardipine, hydralazine).
  - Fluid management and restriction.
  - Goal is NOT to decrease BP to a normal level, but rather to return BP to a safe level.
  - Overcorrection of hypertension may result in hypoperfusion to end-organ and cerebral ischemia.
    - First 6 to 12 hours, reduce BP no more than 25% to 33% of overall goal reduction. Rest of the correction to occur over subsequent 48 to 72 hours.
    - Monitor for hypertensive encephalopathy; can be further exacerbated by antihypertensive pharmacologic therapy.
  - Treat underlying cause (e.g., intracranial hypertension, pheochromocytoma, collagen vascular disease, glomerulonephritis).
  - Evaluate for end-organ damage.

- Complications of hypertension:
  - Kidney disease.
  - Left ventricular hypertrophy (LVH)/CHF.
  - Seizures.
  - Hypertensive encephalopathy.
  - Obstructive sleep apnea.
  - Cerebrovascular accident.
  - Ongoing hypertension into adulthood; increased risk of cerebrovascular accident, myocardial infarction.

PEARLS
- *Ensure BP has been measured correctly when diagnosing hypertension.*
- *Auscultation is the preferred method of BP measurement unless an arterial line is in situ.*
- *Oscillatory device measurements must be confirmed with auscultation prior to diagnosing hypertension.*

Myocarditis
Caroline Bauer

Definition

Inflammation of the heart muscle with associated cardiac dysfunction.

Etiology

- Estimated incidence is 1 to 10 in 100,000.
- Majority of cases are viral; other causes include bacterial, toxins, hypersensitivity reaction, and systemic disorders.
- Parvovirus B19 and Coxsackie viruses A and B are the most common viral pathogens.

Pathophysiology

Three phases of viral myocarditis have been identified:
- First phase (lasts 0–3 days)—virus enters, disrupts, and kills myocytes; necrotic myocytes trigger immune response that either clears the virus or causes further myocyte damage.
- Second phase (days 4–14)—systematic immune response ensues to attempt to eliminate the virus through more complex mechanisms. Continued necrosis of both healthy and infected myocytes occurs.
- Third phase (days 15–90)—diffuse cell injury progresses to myocardial fibrosis and ventricular dysfunction. During this phase, patients progress from myocarditis to dilated cardiomyopathy.

Clinical Presentation

- Many patients remain asymptomatic.
- Most common symptoms in neonates include vomiting, poor feeding, fever, diaphoresis, irritability, and upper respiratory symptoms.
- Most common symptoms in children include tachypnea, wheezing, and dyspnea.

- Other presenting symptoms include: fever, anorexia, respiratory distress, syncope, lethargy, decreased exercise tolerance, or abdominal or chest pain.
- History of recent viral infection is commonly elicited.
- Physical examination may reveal cardiac findings of resting tachycardia, arrhythmias, mitral regurgitation murmur, laterally displaced point of maximal impulse, gallop, hepatomegaly, jugular venous distension, or decreased pulses and perfusion.

Diagnostic Evaluation

- The definitive test for myocarditis is endomyocardial biopsy. However, owing to the invasive nature of this test, it is reserved for children with new-onset heart failure, hemodynamic significance, or failure to respond to medical therapy.
- Chest radiograph, ECG, echocardiogram, oxygen saturation, and four extremity BP measurements assist in diagnosis.
  - ECG: classically demonstrates sinus tachycardia, low-voltage QRS complexes, and ST-T wave flattening.
  - Chest radiograph: may demonstrate cardiomegaly.
  - Echocardiogram: cannot differentiate myocarditis from other cardiomyopathies; however, will demonstrate decreased function and possible pericardial effusion.
- Cardiac MRI with contrast: becoming an important diagnostic tool and demonstrates edema and scar tissue and should be ordered for any patient with suspected myocarditis.

Laboratory Studies

- Troponin I, CKMB, and C-reactive protein (CRP), brain natriuretic peptide (BNP), monitor over time to estimate myocardial recovery.

Management

- Intravenous immunoglobulin (IVIG) should be administered in the initial phase of myocarditis.
- Supportive therapies should be used if the patient is hemodynamically unstable and may include inotropes, vasopressors, diuretics, and/or mechanical ventilation.
- Prophylactic anticoagulation should be considered in patients with severely impaired ventricular function to prevent an embolic event.

Pericarditis
Caroline Bauer

Definition

Inflammatory process affecting the pericardium.

Etiology

- Kawasaki disease, drug reaction, kidney failure, hypothyroidism, chylopericardium, intrapericardial tumors, malignancy, radiation, cardiac transplantation, congenital pericardial defects, trauma, and idiopathic causes.
- Estimated incidence between 1% and 6% of the population.
- Chronic pericarditis persists longer than 3 months.
- Purulent pericarditis carries a 25% to 75% mortality rate.

Pathophysiology

- The pericardium is composed of two layers—the visceral layer and the parietal layer. In pericarditis, the layers become inflamed and lead to fluid accumulation. Rapid accumulation of fluid can cause hemodynamic instability and cardiac tamponade.

Clinical Presentation

- Precordial CP is the most commonly reported symptom and is typically exacerbated by respiration and movement.
- A pericardial friction rub is almost always present on physical examination.
- Fever is common with acute pericarditis.

Diagnostic Evaluation

- Chest radiograph, ECG, echocardiogram, cardiac enzymes (troponin I and CKMB).
  - ECG reveals diffuse PR segments depression and ST segment elevation.

Management

- Nonsteroidal anti-inflammatory drugs (NSAIDs) are the mainstay of therapy; should be prescribed around the clock.
- Colchicine is used for recurrent or persistent pericarditis lasting >2 weeks.
- Steroid use is controversial, and should be reserved for patients unresponsive to NSAIDs and colchicine.
- Pericardiocentesis should be performed if an effusion is hemodynamically significant.
  - If pericardial fluid is obtained, it should be analyzed for cell count, differential, glucose, protein, triglycerides, gram stain, and culture.

Postcardiotomy Syndrome
Lisa M. Kohr

Background

- The heart is surrounded by the pericardium sac comprised of a fibrous and serous component.
- Normally, the pericardial space contains only a small amount of serous fluid that acts as a lubricant during cardiac movement.

Definition

- Inflammation of pericardial sac due to either damage to the myocardium or surgical cardiotomy with cardiopulmonary bypass.

Etiology/types

- The etiology is unclear.
- Since the majority of children who undergo open heart surgery do not develop postcardiotomy syndrome, the cause is believed to be related to an autoimmune disorder.
- The presence of an either newly acquired or reactivated viral illness (e.g., adenovirus, cytomegalovirus of a dormant organism) may trigger the immunologic response, resulting in the development of postcardiotomy syndrome. A higher

incidence of postoperative pericardial effusion is found during the winter months.

- Postcardiotomy syndrome has also been reported after thoracic trauma, myocardial infarction (Dressler syndrome), epicardial pacemaker placement, and repair of pectus excavatum.

Pathophysiology

- Fluid accumulates in the pericardial sac at a faster rate than it can be reabsorbed.
- If left untreated, the child may progress to develop a hemodynamically significant pericardial effusion and even cardiac tamponade.

Clinical Presentation

- Some patients are asymptomatic; however, if symptoms appear, they generally appear 4 to 6 weeks after open heart surgery.
  - Fever.
  - Malaise.
  - Nausea and vomiting (especially if large effusions are present).
  - Tachycardia.
  - Pleuritic type CP.
  - Shortness of breath.
  - Pericardial friction rub (muffled when tamponade present).
  - Global ST segment change on 12-lead ECG.
  - Pericardial effusion.
  - Occasionally, pleural effusions.
  - Decreased oral intake (infant).
  - Irritability (infant).

Diagnostic Evaluation

- Chest radiograph—enlarged cardiothymic silhouette.
- Laboratory evaluation:
  - CBC: lymphocytosis; eosinophilia may be present.
  - Elevated inflammatory markers (erythrocyte sedimentation rate, CRP).
  - Echocardiogram—fluid collection in the pericardial sac.

Management

- Some data to suggest that anti-inflammatory agents may be beneficial in treating postcardiotomy syndrome including:
  - Aspirin.
  - Nonsteroidal anti-inflammatory agents.
  - Corticosteroids.
- Pericardiocentesis with/without drain placement.

PEARLS
- *ASD closure is the most common surgical procedure associated with postcardiotomy syndrome.*
- *Size is poorly correlated with hemodynamic effects and tamponade.*
- *Symptoms vary with the age of the child, but typically include fever, malaise, nausea, vomiting, and, occasionally, CP.*

Pulmonary Hypertension
Lisa M. Kohr

Background

- Disease of small pulmonary arteries where the vessels are characterized by:
  - High-tone.
    - Caused by an imbalance of nitric oxide, prostacyclin, and endothelin.
  - Structural wall remodeling and reactivity.
    - Occurs when an imbalance of the above vasoactive mediators is sustained for a period of time.
  - Results in decreased surface area from
    - Smooth muscle hyperplasia.
    - Adventitial thickening.
    - At risk for intraluminal obstruction from:
      - Fibroblast proliferation.
      - Thrombosis.
  - Reduced vascular growth.
    - Vasculogenesis.
    - Angiogenesis.
    - Development of systemic-to-pulmonary artery collaterals.

Definition

- Pulmonary hypertension is defined as a mean PA pressure >25 mmHg at rest.
- Pulmonary arterial hypertension (PAH) is defined as a pulmonary arterial wedge pressure >15 mmHg.

Etiology

- Acquired factors causing lung injury.
  - Developmental abnormalities/injury.
  - Hemodynamic stress due to high flow.
  - Hypoxia (intermittent or chronic).
  - Inflammation.
  - Drugs.
  - Infection.
- Genetic factors resulting in lung injury.
  - Genetic mutations.
  - Serotonin transporter mutation.
  - Genetic polymorphisms.

Types

- Revised Clinical Classification of Pulmonary Hypertension (Rosenzweig, 2009).
  - Pulmonary arterial hypertension (PAH).
    - Idiopathic.
    - Heritable.
    - Toxin/drug induced.
    - Persistent pulmonary hypertension of newborn (PPHN).
    - Associated with connective tissue disease, portal hypertension, CHF, CHD.
    - Unknown.

- Pulmonary hypertension due to left-sided heart disease.
  - Systolic dysfunction.
  - Diastolic dysfunction.
  - Valvular disease.
- Pulmonary hypertension due to pulmonary disease or hypoxia.
  - Interstitial lung diseases.
  - Mixed restrictive and obstructive lung disease.
  - Sleep-disordered breathing.
  - Alveolar ventilation disorders.
  - Chronic interface with high altitude.
  - Developmental pulmonary abnormalities.
  - Chronic obstructive pulmonary disease.
- Chronic thromboembolic pulmonary hypertension.
- Pulmonary hypertension with unclear multifactorial mechanisms.

Pathophysiology

- Acute pulmonary vasoconstriction:
  - Not well characterized.
  - Involves endogenous factors that increase smooth muscle cell tone.
  - Observed in patients with abnormal pulmonary vascular beds.
  - Results in alveolar hypoxia and right heart failure.
- Right heart failure:
  - PA hypertension increases RV afterload.
  - Persistently increased RV afterload can lead to RV dilation, hypertrophy, and dysfunction.
  - RV dysfunction can lead to decreased right ventricular output:
    - Tricuspid regurgitation.
    - Decreased LV filling and output.
    - RV ischemia.

Clinical Presentation

- Past medical history:
  - Family history of pulmonary hypertension.
  - History of drug use (e.g., diet pills, contraceptives, methamphetamines).
  - History of CHD/prior cardiac surgery.
  - Place of residence located at high altitude.
- Presenting symptoms:
  - Poor feeding/FTT (infant).
  - Tachypnea.
  - Cyanotic spells.
  - Irritability (infant).
  - Syncope.
  - Dyspnea.
  - CP.
  - Shortness of breath.
  - Decreased exercise tolerance (prolonged feeding time required by infant; child unable to keep up with peers or requires rest periods).

- Seizures.
- Physical examination:
  - Gallop rhythm.
  - Narrow splitting of a loud S2 with an accentuated P2.
  - Soft holosystolic, high-pitched murmur heard best at the lower left sternal border (LLSB) that increases with inspiration or pressure placed on the liver (murmur of tricuspid regurgitation).
  - RV lift due to RV dilation.
  - Early diastolic decrescendo murmur best heard at the 2nd and 3rd intercostal spaces that increases with inspiration (murmur of pulmonary insufficiency).
  - Hepatosplenomegaly.
  - Peripheral edema.
  - Cyanosis.
  - Jugular venous distension.
- Acute pulmonary hypertensive event involves an acute rise in PA pressure with stable arterial BP.
  - Tachycardia.
  - Stable arterial BP.
  - Stable or decreased oxygen saturation.
  - Stable or elevated central venous or RA pressure (CVP/RAP).
  - Stable LA pressure.
  - Decreased cardiac output/SVO_2.
  - Normal serum lactate.
  - Decreased systemic perfusion.
- Pulmonary hypertensive crisis involves an acute rise in PA pressure that equals or exceeds systemic pressures, resulting in systemic hypotension.
  - Initially, tachycardia followed by bradycardia.
  - Decreased arterial BP.
  - Decreased oxygen saturation.
  - Elevated central venous or RA pressure (CVP, RAP).
  - Decreased LA pressure (due to a drop in LA preload).
  - Significantly decreased cardiac output/SVO_2.
  - Decreased serum lactate.
  - Poor systemic perfusion.

Diagnostic Evaluation (to Determine Diagnosis, Degree of Disease, Possible Etiology)

- Chest radiograph: cardiomegaly and enlarged PA segment.
- Electrocardiograph (ECG): RVH and/or ST segment changes.
- Echocardiogram: RVH, tricuspid regurgitation, elevated RV pressure.
  - Evaluate for presence of congenital heart disease/anatomical cause of elevated right ventricular pressure (systemic or suprasystemic pressures).
  - In long-standing pulmonary hypertension, RV dysfunction present.
- Cardiac catheterization: study of choice for diagnosis.
  - Right heart catheterization.

- Determines PA pressures, PVR, cardiac index.
- Evaluate for left-sided heart disease.
  - Evaluate for pulmonary vein stenosis/obstruction and desaturation (if tolerated).
- Angiography.
  - Evaluates cardiopulmonary structures including PA vessels, presence of peripheral pulmonary stenosis, or aortopulmonary collaterals.
- Acute vasodilator testing (evaluates degree of PA hypertension and pulmonary vasoreactivity).
- Laboratory evaluation:
  - Liver function tests; hepatic profile, abdominal ultrasound to evaluate presence of portal pulmonary hypertension. If abnormal, obtain Gastroenterology consult.
  - CBC.
  - Electrolytes including renal function studies.
  - Urinalysis.
  - Basic natriuretic peptide (followed as a marker of worsening heart failure).
  - Human immunodeficiency virus evaluation.
  - Thyroid function tests.
  - Toxicology screen.
  - Hypercoagulable evaluation.
  - Collagen vascular disease evaluation.
    - Antinuclear antibody profile.
    - Rheumatoid factor.
    - Erythrocyte sedimentation rate (ESR).
    - Complement.
  - Chromosome analysis.
- Evaluation of pulmonary disease:
  - Pulmonary function tests with diffusing capacity for carbon monoxide or bronchodilators to exclude obstructive/restrictive lung disease.
  - Polysomnogram (sleep study) to evaluate degree of hypoxemia or diminished ventilatory drive. Evaluates for upper airway obstruction or central hypoventilation.
  - Three 6-minute walk test or cycle ergometry with oximetry.
  - Ventilator/perfusion scan.
  - Chest CT or MRI.
    - Imaging to evaluate the presence of thromboembolic or interstitial lung disease.
- If results of pulmonary tests are normal, consider swallow study or esophageal pH probe study to determine the need for postpyloric feedings.
- If results of pulmonary tests are abnormal, a lung biopsy is recommended to determine the presence of the following: Alveolar capillary dysplasia, pulmonary veno-occlusive disease, pulmonary capillary hemangiomatosis, interstitial lung disease.

Management

- Acute management.
  - Reduce sympathetic stimulation.
    - Maintain normothermia (antipyretics), adequate sedation, and analgesia.

- May require use of muscle relaxants. Premedicate (e.g., sedation, analgesia) prior to noxious stimuli such as endotracheal tube suctioning.
  - Avoid excessively elevated hematocrit.
- Lower PVR:
  - Hyperventilate prior to suctioning, avoid hypoxia.
  - Treat acidosis/avoid hypercarbia.
  - Maintain adequate functional residual capacity.
  - Avoid hypo- or hyperinflation of the lungs.
  - Minimize intrathoracic pressure.
- Administer vasodilating medications.
  - Specific pulmonary vasodilator:
    - Inhaled nitric oxide.
    - Aerosolized iloprost (e.g., prostacyclin analogue).
  - Nonspecific vasodilator:
    - Nitroprusside (works through cyclic GMP system).
    - Milrinone (increases cyclic AMP).
    - Sildenafil (increases cyclic AMP).
    - Isoproterenol (B1 and B2 agonist).
    - Prostacyclin I$_2$ (a prostanoid metabolized from endogenous arachidonic acid through the cyclooxygenase [COX] pathway).
    - Prostaglandin E$_1$ (increases cyclic AMP).
- Chronic management:
  - Antipyretics.
  - Anticoagulation (especially in low cardiac output states).
  - Supplemental oxygen.
  - Cardiac glycosides and diuretics.
    - Management of heart failure.
  - Calcium channel blockade.
  - Targeted therapy based on pulmonary reactivity.
    - Phosphodiesterase type 5 inhibitor (nitric oxide pathway).
      - Sildenafil, Tadalifil.
    - Prostacyclins—therapy of choice for patients with right heart failure or who become clinically worse or are refractory to oral agents.
      - Treprostinil (subcutaneous), Epoprostenol (intravenous), Iloprost (inhaled).
    - Endothelin antagonists:
      - Bosentan, Ambrisentan.
    - Prevention of exacerbation of pulmonary hypertension events:
      - Annual influenza and pneumococcal immunizations.
      - Strict follow-up with pulmonary hypertension specialist/consultants.
    - Monitor for side effects of targeted therapy.
    - Follow pulmonary reactivity.
- Lung transplantation:
  - Worsening of clinical symptoms despite maximal medical therapy.
  - Progressive increase in PA pressures and vascular resistance with lower cardiac output.
  - Palliative care.

PEARLS

- *Patients with diagnosis of an unrestrictive VSD, truncus arteriosus, obstructive pulmonary veins, mitral stenosis, or hypoplastic left heart syndrome with intact atrial septum are at highest risk for postoperative pulmonary hypertension.*
- *Eisenmenger's syndrome occurs when increased flow through an unrepaired left-to- right cardiac shunt leads to irreversible pulmonary vascular changes over time, resulting in pulmonary vascular pressures that exceed systemic pressures and reversal of shunting.*
- *Cardiac catheterization is the study of choice for the diagnosis of pulmonary hypertension.*
- *The acute management of pulmonary hypertension focuses on avoiding factors that stimulate pulmonary vasoconstriction and implementing therapies that lower PVR.*
- *High-risk events for exacerbating pulmonary hypertension include weaning vasodilatory agents such as inhaled nitric oxide, supplemental oxygen, sedation/paralysis, and ventilator support.*
- *Prostacyclin derivatives are the best pulmonary vasodilatory agents for managing patients with pulmonary hypertension and RV failure.*

Rheumatic Fever

Laura Crisanti

Background

- Rheumatic fever is a postinfectious complication of a group A Beta-Hemolytic Streptococcus (GAS) pharyngitis.

Etiology

- Most often affects children aged 5 to 15 years of age.
- Incidence in developed countries is estimated to be <1 case per 100,000 population.

Pathophysiology

- Not been clearly defined.
- Believed to be an autoimmune mediated disease triggered by GAS infection.

Clinical Presentation

- Sudden-onset sore throat, fever, difficulty swallowing, scarlatina rash, nausea, vomiting, abdominal pain, enlarged anterior lymph nodes, tonsillopharyngeal erythema.

Diagnostic Evaluation

- Jones criteria were developed in 1944 to guide diagnosis of acute rheumatic fever.

- Evidence of a streptococcal infection with two major manifestations or one major and two minor manifestations is indicative of acute rheumatic fever.
- Antistreptolysin O titer (ASO); begins to rise within 1 week of infection; continues to rise for 3 to 6 weeks after GAS infection.
- Rapid GAS may be obtained; positive result may reflect colonization rather than current infection.

Box 5.1 Jones Criteria to Guide Diagnosis of Acute Rheumatic Fever

- Major manifestations include:
  - Carditis.
    Suspect in a patient with new apical systolic murmur.
  - Polyarthritis.
    Most frequent major manifestation.
- Occurs in larger joints.
  Symptoms include pain, joint swelling, tenderness. Dramatically responsive to salicylate therapy.
  - Subcutaneous nodules.
    Firm, painless nodules present over extensor surfaces of joints.
- Usually occurs 10 to 28 days after GAS infection.
  - Chorea.
    Purposeless, involuntary rapid movements of trunk and extremities.
- Mainly affects females <20 years of age.
  - Erythema marginatum;
    Occurs in <15% of patients.
- Transient, nonpuritic, nonpainful rash found on trunk and extremities, facial sparing.
- Minor manifestations include:
  - Arthralgia.
  - Fever.
  - Elevated acute phase reactants.
  - Prolonged PR interval (ECG).

- Chest radiograph; evaluation of cardiac silhouette.
- Echocardiogram.
- ECG.
- Blood cultures may be used to evaluate for associated infective endocarditis.
- Sedimentation rate (ESR); C-reactive protein (CRP).

Management

- Single dose of benzathine benzylpenicillin.
- Course of oral penicillin VK or amoxicillin.
- First generation cephalosporin, clindamycin, or a macrolide in the setting of penicillin allergy.
- Anti-inflammatory therapy: aspirin; may require corticosteroids if no improvement of carditis on ASA.
- Long-term prophylactic antibiotics to prevent recurrent exposure to streptococcal antigens.

Long-term Complications

- Valvar complications (e.g., mitral and aortic valve).
- Arrhythmias (e.g., atrial fibrillation).
- Endocarditis.
- Thromboembolism.

Vascular Rings/Slings

Lisa M. Kohr

Background

- Vascular rings result from the abnormal fetal cardiac development of the aortic arch complexes.
- By the 38th day of gestation, normal evolution of the rudimentary aortic arch complexes is complete, resulting in a left aortic arch configuration.

Definition

- Presence of a double aortic arch that encircles the trachea and esophagus, resulting in tracheal compression.

Etiology

- Occurs when specific components of the rudimentary aortic arch complex are not deleted.

Types

- Complete vascular rings.
  - Double aortic arch.
    - Occurs when the right and left 4th arches persist.
  - Right aortic arch with left ligamentum arteriosum.
    - Occurs when the 4th arch involutes.
- Partial vascular rings.
  - Pulmonary artery sling.
    - Occurs when the left PA originates from the right PA instead of the main PA.
  - Innominate artery compression syndrome.
    - Occurs when the innominate artery originates more posteriorly and leftward from the aortic arch.

Pathophysiology

- Complete vascular rings.
  - Double aortic arch.
    - Right and left arches arise from the ascending aorta and form a ring around the trachea and esophagus before joining the descending aorta.
    - The right arch is dominant in 75% of cases, and the left arch in 20% of cases. In 5% of cases, the arches are of equal size.
  - Right aortic arch with left ligamentum arteriosum:
    - Many configurations based on the site of interruption of the left aortic arch and branching pattern off the vessels off the aorta.
    - A right aortic arch with retroesophageal left subclavian artery occurs in 65% of cases.

- The vascular ring involves the subclavian artery originating from the descending aorta, passing to the left behind the esophagus, and completed by the ligamentum arteriosum extending from the descending aorta to the left PA.
  - A right aortic arch with mirror imaging branch occurs in 35% of cases.
    - The vascular ring involves the mirror image branching and the ligamentum arteriosum extending from the descending aorta to the left PA.
- Partial vascular rings.
  - PA sling.
    - The left PA passes around the right main stem bronchus and travels between the trachea and esophagus, forming a sling that compresses the tracheobroncheal tree (see Figure 5.19).
    - Innominate artery compression syndrome; the innominate artery travels to the right, upward, then posteriorly to reach the thoracic outlet, resulting in compression of the anterior portion of the trachea.

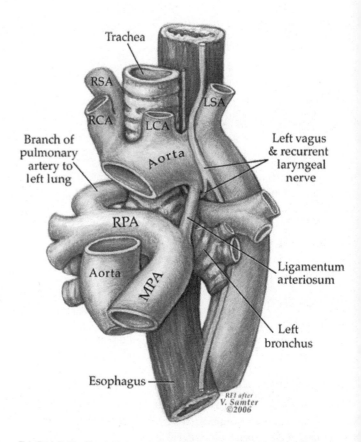

FIGURE 5.19 • **Pulmonary Artery Sling.** The aorta has been cut away to visualize the right pulmonary artery and the anomalous origin of the left pulmonary artery from the right pulmonary artery. The left pulmonary artery courses posterior to the trachea, anterior to the esophagus, and anterior to the descending thoracic aorta on its way to the left lung.

Clinical Presentation

- Most children present with symptoms within the first few months of life:
  - Respiratory distress.
  - Stridor; classic "seal bark."
  - Cough.
  - Apnea that may be precipitated by swallowing a bolus of food.
    - Occurs in 50% of children with innominate artery compression.
  - Dysphagia.
  - Recurrent respiratory illness.
  - Reports of prolonged feeding time due to careful chewing of food.
  - Hyperextended head position to splint trachea for improved breathing.

Diagnostic Evaluation

- Anteroposterior and lateral chest radiograph.
  - Presence of left aortic arch or double aortic arch as determined by the location of aortic arch in relation to the trachea.
    - When the location of the aortic arch is unclear, a double aortic arch should be suspected.
  - A lateral film should evaluate for tracheal narrowing at the level of the aortic arch.
  - Unilateral hyperinflation of the right lung may suggest the presence of a PA sling.
- Barium swallow.
  - Most reliable study for diagnosis of vascular ring when the anatomic abnormality is noted persistently throughout the study.
    - Anteroposterior views, bilateral compressions of the esophagus are consistent with a double aortic arch.
    - A deep extrinsic indentation of the posterior aspect of the trachea is consistent with a double aortic arch or right aortic arch with left ligamentum arteriosum.
    - An oblique indentation angled toward the left shoulder is consistent with a right aortic arch and retroesophageal left subclavian artery.
    - Anterior indentation of the esophagus is consistent with a PA sling.
- Chest CT without contrast.
  - If unable to determine from chest radiograph or barium swallow.
  - The presence of the "four artery sign" noted on images taken cephalad to the aortic arch is suspicious for an aortic arch anomaly.
    - The "four artery sign" consists of the two dorsal subclavian arteries arising from the aortic arch and evenly spaced with the ventral carotid arteries around the trachea. This sign is indicative of a double aortic arch with right arch and aberrant left subclavian artery.
  - Images of the left PA originating from the right pulmonary artery, encircling the trachea, traveling to the left lung hilum anterior to the esophagus and aorta are diagnostic for PA sling.
  - Anterior compression of the trachea by the innominate artery is consistent with the diagnosis of innominate artery compression.
- Bronchoscopy.
  - Bronchoscopy may be obtained before an aortic arch anomaly is suspected in children who present with respiratory distress.
    - Multilevel external compression of the trachea is suspicious for a double aortic arch or right aortic arch with a left ligamentum arteriosum.
    - Pulsatile anterior compression of the trachea just proximal to the vocal cords is consistent with innominate artery compression.
- Echocardiogram.
  - Can be used, but not readily used to diagnose vascular rings due to limited windows.
- MRI.
  - Diagnosis of vascular ring is dependent on the vascular branching pattern, the size of the aortic arch, and narrowing of the airway.
  - Not generally used for diagnosis of vascular rings due to time and sedation required by the study.

Management

- Most children require surgery within 1 year of life.
- Surgical correction is recommended once the diagnosis of a vascular ring or PA sling is made.
  - Surgery for a double aortic arch involves the division of the smaller aortic arch and ligation of the ligamentum arteriosum via a left thoracotomy.
  - Surgery for a right aortic arch with a left ligamentum involves ligation and division of the ligamentum, and, if present, resection of the Kommerell's diverticulum with reimplantation of the left subclavian artery to the left carotid artery via a left thoracotomy.
  - Surgery for a PA sling involves ligation and division of the left PA with reimplantation to the main PA via a median sternotomy on cardiopulmonary bypass.
  - Surgery for innominate artery compression syndrome involves suspension of the innominate artery to the posterior sternum via a right anterolateral thoracotomy.

PEARLS

- *Presenting symptoms generally occur during the first few months of life.*
- *Most children present with respiratory symptoms including the classic seal bark, stridor, and reports of swallowing or feeding problems.*
- *A barium swallow is the most reliable study for diagnosis.*
- *Surgical correction is recommended once the diagnosis is made.*

Syncope
Laura Crisanti

Background

- Syncope is a temporary loss of consciousness and postural tone due to a decrease in cerebral blood flow from systemic hypotension.
- Most common in children >10 years of age.
- Females > males.

Etiology

- Most episodes are benign in nature; however, some are associated with serious cardiovascular disease or other illness.
- Approximately 75% of syncope is due to a vasovagal cause.
  - May be precipitated by dehydration or prolonged standing.
- Approximately 25% is due to seizure, migraines, or cardiac disease; most serious etiologies.

Pathophysiology

- Vasovagal (noncardiac) syncope.
  - Peripheral venous pooling in lower extremities, which leads to decreased ventricular filling and decreased stroke volume.
  - Hypotension leads to cerebral hypoperfusion, causing loss of consciousness and loss of postural tone.
- Neurologic associated syncope (noncardiac).
  - Episodes of seizures or migraines (vasospasm) lead to cerebral hypoperfusion.
- Cardiac syncope.
  - Arrhythmias or cardiac outflow tract obstruction leads to cerebral hypoperfusion.

Clinical Presentation

- Weakness, dizziness, lightheadedness, perspiration, visual disturbances, loss of consciousness.

Diagnostic Evaluation

- ECG: evaluation for arrhythmia or ventricular hypertrophy.
- Holter monitoring: evaluation for cluster episodes of occurrences or palpitations.
- Tilt-table testing: Used for patients experiencing infrequent syncope, unclear history.
- EEG: evaluation for seizures, if suspected.
- ECHO: evaluates for structural heart defect, outflow obstruction.
- Laboratory testing is generally not required.

Management

- Adequate fluid and salt intake.
- Implantable cardiac defibrillator (ICD) in cases of life-threatening arrhythmias.
- Surgery in cases of outflow tract obstruction.
- Pharmacologic management of seizures.
- Avoidance of diuretics such as caffeine.
- Elastic hose to prevent venous pooling.

PEARL
- *Commonly, loss of consciousness > 1 minute is associated with a more severe etiology (e.g., life-threatening arrhythmia).*

Electrocardiogram, Arrhythmias, and Ectopy
Richard P. Fernandez

Electrocardiogram Interpretation

- Introduction:
  - All ECG findings are age-dependent from birth through late adolescence.
  - A consistent, systematic approach will ensure that no details are missed (Table 5.3).
- The standard ECG printout.
  - Standard ECG settings.
    - Paper speed of 25 mm/second.
    - Voltage: 10 mm/mV (Figure 5.20).
- The lead tracings include the following:
  - The standard and augmented limb leads: I, II, III, aVR, aVL, aVF (Figure 5.21).
  - The standard precordial leads: V1, V2, V3, V4, V5, V6 (Figure 5.22).
  - The ECG tracing: waves, intervals, and segments (Figure 5.23).
- Waves are positive or negative deflections from the baseline of the ECG.
- P wave = atrial depolarization.
  - Normal sinus P wave: originates in the sinoatrial node (SA node).
  - Upright in lead II and inverted in lead aVR.
  - Right atrial enlargement (RAE):
    - P wave >2.5 mV (2.5 mm). Typically, this is most easily determined in lead II.
    - Associated with chronic pulmonary hypertension as well as some forms of CHD.
  - Left atrial enlargement (LAE):
    - Age-dependent: P wave duration >0.08 seconds in infants and 0.12 seconds in adolescents. Terminal inversion or deep inversion of the P wave in V1.
    - Associated with mitral stenosis and other left-sided obstructive lesions.
- PR interval = atrial depolarization + physiologic delay of conduction at the atrioventricular node (AV node).
  - The PR interval lengthens slightly over time until it reaches normal adult values.
- Q wave = mostly septal depolarization.
  - Commonly seen in leads II, III, aVF, V5, and V6.
  - The normal Q wave is narrow = 0.015 to 0.02 seconds.
  - The amplitude of the Q wave normally increases until approximately 3 to 5 years of age, then decreases again.
- QRS complex = ventricular depolarization.

TABLE 5.3   Age-Specific ECG Findings (Obtaining Permission)

Age	HR (bpm)	QRS Axis (deg)	PR Interval (s)	QRS Interval (s)	R in V1 (mm)	S in V1 (mm)	R in V6 (mm)	S in V6 (mm)
1st wk	90–160	60–180	0.08–0.15	0.03–0.08	5–26	0–23	0–12	1–10
1–3 wk	100–180	45–160	0.08–0.15	0.03–0.08	3–21	0–16	2–16	1–10
1–2 mo	120–180	30–135	0.08–0.15	0.03–0.08	3–18	0–15	5–21	1–10
3–5 mo	105–185	0–135	0.08–0.15	0.03–0.08	3–20	0–15	6–22	1–10
6–11 mo	110–170	0–135	0.07–0.16	0.03–0.08	2–20	0.5–20	6–23	0–7
1–2 y	90–165	0–110	0.08–0.16	0.03–0.08	2–18	0.5–21	6–23	0–7
3–4 y	70–140	0–110	0.09–0.17	0.04–0.08	1–18	0.5–21	4–24	0–5
5–7 y	65–140	0–110	0.09–0.17	0.04–0.08	0.5–14	0.5–24	4–24	0–4
8–11 y	60–130	(–)15–110	0.09–0.17	0.04–0.09	0–14	0.5–25	4–25	0–4
12–15 y	65–130	(–)15–110	0.09–0.18	0.04–0.09	0–14	0.5–21	4–25	0–4
>16 y	50–120	(–)15–110	0.12–0.20	0.04–0.10	0–14	0.5–23	4–21	0–4

Adapted from Sharieff, G. Q., & Rao, S. O. (2006). The pediatric ECG. *Emergency Medicine Clinics North America*, *24*(1), 195–208, vii–viii.

- The three key components to evaluate when assessing the QRS are the axis, amplitude, and duration.
- Axis represents the mean vector of depolarization. Axis changes with age.
  - Left axis deviation is suggestive of LV volume or pressure overload and LV hypertrophy.
  - Right axis deviation is normal in the newborn period. The axis then shifts leftward over time. In older children, right axis deviation can represent RV volume or pressure overload.
  - "Superior axis" or "extreme right axis deviation" represents marked right axis deviation ($-90°$ to $180°$) and is commonly seen in atrioventricular septal defects.
- Amplitude is an indirect estimate of the mass of depolarizing myocardium. Neonates and infants in the

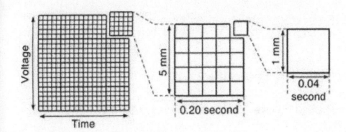

FIGURE 5.20 • **Standard EKG paper.**
Electrocardiographic paper.

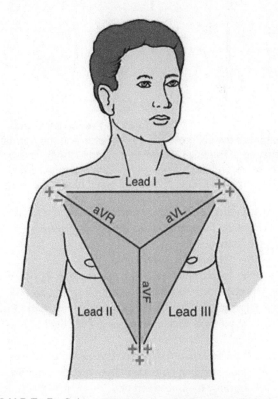

FIGURE 5.21 • **Standard and Augmented Limb Leads.** Frontal plane leads: standard limb leads, I, II, III, plus augmented leads aVR, aVL, and aVF. This allows an examination of electrical conduction across a variety of planes (e.g., left arm to leg, right arm to left arm).

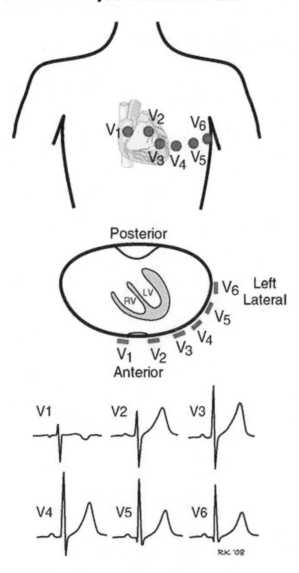

FIGURE 5.22 • **The Standard Precordial Leads.**
Placement of the six precordial chest leads and the normal
appearance of the ECG recording for leads V1–V6. These
electrodes record electrical activity in the horizontal plane,
which is perpendicular to the frontal plane of the limb leads.

first months of life have a predominance of RV forces.
This shifts over time, in the absence of disease, to a LV
predominance.

- Right ventricular hypertrophy (RVH).
  - R wave amplitude >98th percentile in V1 or S wave
    amplitude >98th percentile in V6. Also, an RSR'
    pattern in V1 with the R' being greater than 15 mm
    in infants less than a year or greater than 10 mm in
    children above 1 year.
  - Can be a manifestation of chronic lung diseases,
    long-standing pulmonary hypertension, and RV
    outflow tract obstruction.
- Left ventricular hypertrophy (LVH).
  - R wave amplitude >98th percentile in V5 or V6; or
    S wave amplitude >98th percentile in leads V1 or
    V2. Please refer to Table 5.4 for additional criteria.

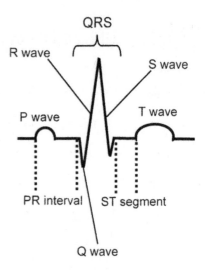

FIGURE 5.23 • **The EKG Tracing.** Figure of wave form.

TABLE 5.4	**Criteria for Chamber Enlargement/Hypertrophy**
Left Ventricular Hypertrophy	
R wave amplitude >98th% in V5 or V6.	Q wave >4 mm in V5 or V6.
R wave <5th% in lead V1 or V2.	Inverted T wave in V6.
S wave amplitude >98th% in V1.	
Right Ventricular Hypertrophy	
R wave >98th% in V1.	RSR' pattern in V1 (R' height >15 mm in infants younger than 1 y; or >10 mm in children >1 y).
S wave >98th% in I or V6.	Q wave in V1 (Normal in 10% of newborns).
Left Atrial Enlargement	
P wave >0.08 s in <12 mo.	Terminal or deeply inverted P wave in V1 or V3R.
P wave >0.1 s in children >12 mo.	Peaked P wave in leads II and V1 that is higher than 3 mm in infants <6 mo.
Right Atrial Enlargement	
Peaked P wave >2.5 mm in infants older than 6 mo of age.	

Adapted from Sharieff, G. Q., & Rao, S. O. (2006). The pediatric ECG.
Emergency Medicine Clinics North America, *24*(1), 195–208, vii–viii.

- Chamber enlargement/hypertrophy is most commonly seen in patients with LV overload (e.g., VSD, PDA) or LV outflow tract obstruction (e.g., AS, hypertension).
- Duration of QRS reflects the time it takes for the ventricular myocardium to depolarize. Normal depolarization results in a narrow QRS complex. Abnormal depolarization results in a widened QRS complex in a pattern of either left or right bundle branch block (LBBB, RBBB).
  - Patterns of Right Bundle Branch Block (RBBB).
    - Left axis deviation.
    - Prolonged QRS >120 msec or 95th percentile.
    - Wide R wave in I, aVL, V5, V6.
    - ST depression and T wave inversion in V4–V6.
  - Patterns of right bundle branch block (RBBB).
    - Right axis deviation.
    - Prolonged QRS to >120 m/second or >95th percentile.
    - RSR' in V1–2 and aVR.
- ST segment.
  - Period from the termination of the S wave to the initial deflection of the T wave.
  - A number of pathological processes can produce abnormalities of this portion of the ECG such as electrolyte abnormalities, inflammation, or ischemia.
- T and U waves.
  - The T wave represents myocardial repolarization.
  - The pattern of T wave deflection changes from birth through adolescence.
- QT interval = Total time required for the completion of the cardiac action potential.
  - Varies little with age, but significantly with heart rate.
  - The most common means of correcting the observed QT duration for heart rate is Bazett's formula (Figure 5.5).
  - In general, the corrected QT interval (QTc) is 410 m/second for most patients with an upper limit of the normal of 450 m/second.

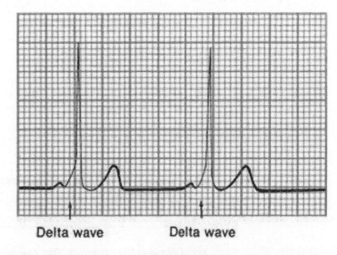

FIGURE 5.24 • **WPW Delta Waves.** WPW syndrome. Current is held up by the normal delay at the AV node but races unimpeded down the bundle of Kent. The EKG shows the short PR interval and delta wave.

BOX 5.2 Bazett's Equation for Correction of the QT Interval for Heart Rate

$$QTc = \frac{Measured\ QT\ Interval}{\sqrt{Preceding\ RR\ Interval}}$$

- Prolongation of QT interval is seen with certain medications, electrolyte abnormalities, and abnormalities of the potassium channels.
- Special waves:
  - Delta wave: In the Wolff–Parkinson–White (WPW) syndrome, early ventricular activation is caused by an accessory pathway between the atrial and ventricular myocardium. It manifests on the ECG as a slurring of the early part of the QRS complex termed the delta wave (Figure 5.24).
    - J wave or Osborn wave: A positive deflection at the terminal portion of the QRS complex that is felt to be pathognomonic for hypothermia (Figure 5.25).

- Determination of rate and rhythm.
  - Determining heart rate:
    - Estimation for regular heart rates: Find a QRS that falls on the thick line between large boxes and counting forward from that complex, "300, 150, 100, 75, 60, 50" until the next QRS complex (Figure 5.26).
    - Estimation for irregular heart rates.
  - Count the number of complexes that occur in 6 seconds (i.e., 30 large boxes), and multiply by 10. On many ECGs, this is facilitated by a series of hatch marks at the bottom of the sheet that mark off 3-second intervals.

Variations of Normal Rhythm

- Sinus rhythm: P waves are upright in lead II and inverted in lead aVR. Each P wave is followed at consistent intervals by a QRS complex, and there is less than 10% variation in the heart rate over the course of the ECG.
- Sinus arrhythmia: normal sinus heart rate varies with respiration, decreasing and increasing slightly with exhalation and inspiration, respectively. In children, this can be more pronounced and is unfortunately termed sinus arrhythmia despite being completely normal (Figure 5.27).
- Sinus tachycardia: heart rate above the upper limit of normal for age, but with normal sinus P waves preceding the QRS complexes. This is a compensatory mechanism and is always secondary to an underlying cause.
- Sinus bradycardia: rhythm originating from the sinus node that is below the lower limit of normal for age. It may be normal in well-conditioned athletes. Vagally mediated sinus bradycardia can be associated with a number of processes, including increased intracranial pressure or airway manipulation. It can also be noted as a side effect of medication, as a result of a toxic ingestion, in cases of myocardial ischemia, and in hypothyroidism.

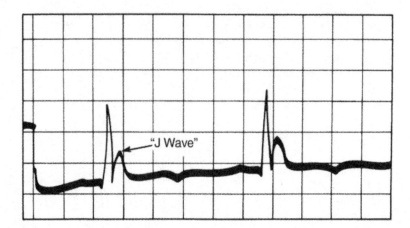

FIGURE 5.25 • **The J Wave in Hypothermia. The J wave is designated by the arrows.** J wave (Osborn wave), pathognomonic of hypothermia. Rounded contour distinguishes it from an RSR' pattern. It may also be confused with a T wave with a short QT interval.

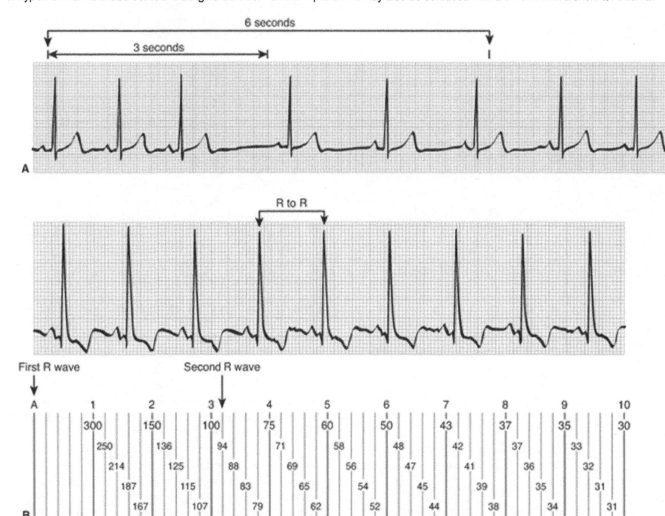

FIGURE 5.26 • **Estimation of Heart Rate. A:** Heart rate determination for an irregular rhythm. Count the number of R-R intervals in a 6-second strip and multiply by 10. In **(A)** there are five complete R-R intervals in a 6-second strip; the heart rate is about 50 beats per minute. **B:** Heart rate determination for a regular rhythm using the rate ruler. Count the number of large and small boxes between R waves on the rhythm strip. In **(B)** there are three large boxes and one small box between the R waves marked on the strip. On the rate ruler, the first R wave is represented by the thick line marked "A." Each large box on the ECG paper is represented by a thick line on the rate ruler and is numbered at the top; each small box on the strip is represented by a thin line on the ruler. The number on the line on the ruler that corresponds to the second R wave on the strip represents the heart rate. In **(B)**, count three large boxes at the top of the ruler and then one small box; the heart rate is 94 beats per minute.

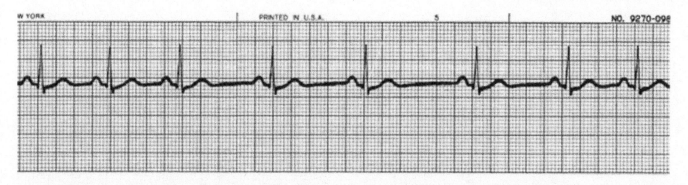

FIGURE 5.27 • **Sinus Arrhythmia.** Sinus arrhythmia in lead II. Note irregular RR and PP intervals.

- Sinus pauses: abrupt prolongations between 2 normal sinus beats—typically, less than 2 seconds. These are common in infants and become less common as children age (Figure 5.28).

Ectopy and Arrhythmias

Richard P. Fernandez

Background

- Cardiac arrhythmias can produce a wide spectrum of clinical presentations.
- Some patients are asymptomatic, but hemodynamic instability and myocardial dysfunction are common manifestations.
- Identification and prompt treatment of cardiac arrhythmia are essential.

Types of Ectopy

- Premature atrial contractions (PACs).
  - Early depolarizations of atrial myocardium.
  - Conducted or nonconducted (blocked PACs). When they are conducted, the result is a narrow QRS complex that looks similar to the normal sinus complex, but with a different P wave morphology.

- In some cases, the P waves will be difficult to discern as they may be buried in the T waves.
- Very common in newborns.
- In older patients, they may be related to electrolyte abnormalities or irritation from central venous catheters in the RA (Figure 5.29).
- Premature ventricular contractions (PVCs).
  - Early depolarizations of the ventricular myocardium.
  - Because the depolarization spreads through the myocardium rather than the conduction system, these tend to be very wide and sometimes with very prominent voltages.
  - Can also be related to myocardial irritation secondary to inflammation, electrolyte abnormalities, or mechanical stimuli.
  - PVCs that occur in a pattern of every other beat is bigeminy; PVCs that occur in a pattern of every third beat is trigemeny (Figure 5.30).
- Supraventricular tachycardia (SVT).
  - Generic term for arrhythmias originating above the level of the His-Purkinje system that require atrial or AV nodal tissue for their initiation and propagation (see Figure 5.31).
- Atrial ectopic tachycardia.
  - An abnormal tachycardia arising from atrial cells outside of the sinus node.

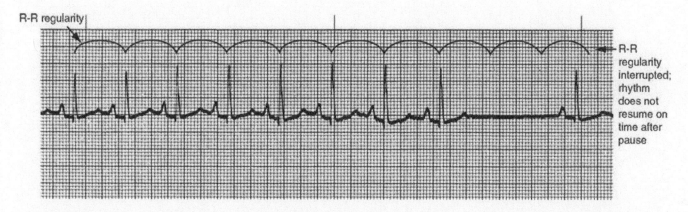

FIGURE 5.28 • **Sinus Pause.** Normal sinus rhythm with sinus arrest. Rhythm: basic rhythm regular, irregular during pause; rate: basic rhythm 94 beats/minute; P waves: normal in basic rhythm, absent during pause; PR interval: 0.16 to 0.18 second in basic rhythm, absent during pause; QRS complex: 0.06 to 0.08 second in basic rhythm, absent during pause.

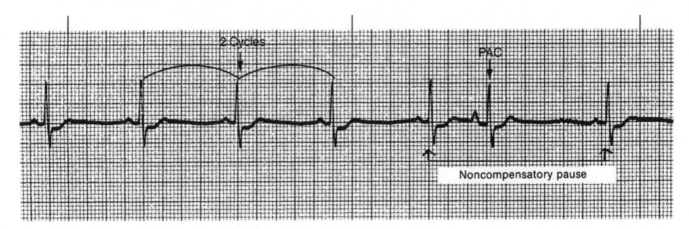

FIGURE 5.29 • **Premature Atrial Contractions.** Normal sinus rhythm with premature atrial contraction (PAC). Rhythm: basic rhythm regular, irregular with PAC; rate: basic rhythm rate 60 beats per minute; P waves: sinus P waves with basic rhythm; premature, abnormal P wave with PAC; PR interval: 0.12 to 0.16 second (basic rhythm); 0.16 second (PAC); QRS complex: 0.08 second (basic rhythm and PAC). Comment: To determine the type of pause after premature beats, measure from the QRS complex before the premature beat to the QRS complex after the premature beat. If the measurement equals two R-R intervals, the pause is compensatory. If the measurement equals less than two R-R intervals, the pause is noncompensatory. ST-segment depression is present.

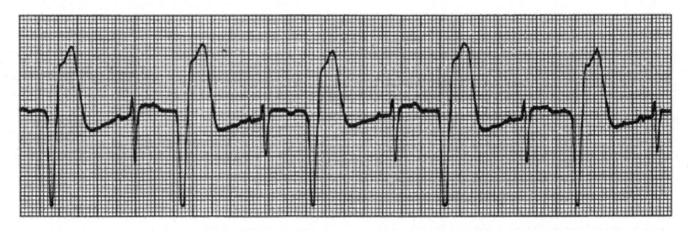

FIGURE 5.30 • **Premature Ventricular Contractions in Bigeminy Pattern.** "Ventricular bigeminy."

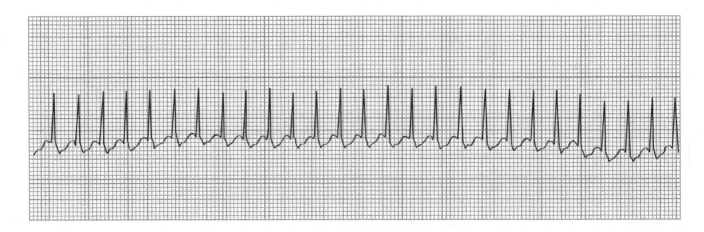

FIGURE 5.31 • **Supraventricular Tachycardia.** Note rate above 220, abnormal P waves, no beat-to-beat variability.

- A 12-lead ECG reveals a narrow complex tachycardia with abnormal P wave morphology and axis.
- Can occur both as a primary abnormality in a structurally normal heart, in relation to elevated catecholamine levels or other metabolic abnormalities, or transiently in patients after heart surgery.
- Treatment is aimed at addressing underlying causes.
- Amiodarone can be used for rate control; for persistent forms, ablation in the electrophysiology lab is the treatment of choice.
- Atrial flutter.
  - In pediatric patients, atrial flutter is typically a narrow, regular, rapid rhythm.
  - Occurs in the setting of structural heart disease, repaired or otherwise.
  - Classic 12-lead ECG findings are "sawtooth" flutter waves that are best seen in lead II or V2.
  - There is variable AV conduction, although usually it is 2:1 conduction.

- Neonatal form can occur in a structurally normal heart and is responsive to both pharmacologic intervention and cardioversion.
- In older patients, when associated with structural heart disease, it is difficult to control medically, and surgical intervention is often required (Figure 5.32).
- Atrial fibrillation.
  - Rarely encountered in childhood and almost exclusively associated with structural heart disease, thyrotoxicosis, or SVT due to an accessory connection.
  - A 12-lead ECG reveals no discernible organized atrial activity. At times, coarse fibrillatory waves can be seen. The QRS complexes are "irregularly irregular" because of variable AV conduction (Figure 5.33).
- Multifocal atrial tachycardia (MAT).
  - Rapid, irregular arrhythmia rare in the pediatric age group.
  - Majority of pediatric patients with MAT present in infancy (approximately 75%), as neonates. Half the patients have structural heart disease.

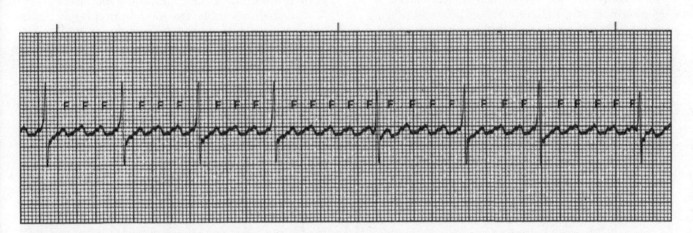

FIGURE 5.32 • **Atrial Flutter.** Atrial flutter with variable AV conduction. Rhythm: irregular rate: atrial: 250 beats per minute; ventricular: 60 beats per minute. Note: If the ventricular rate is irregular, count the number of flutter waves in a 6-second strip and multiply to 10 to obtain atrial rate. P waves: flutter waves before each QRS (varying ratios); PR interval: not measurable; QRS complex: 0.08 second.

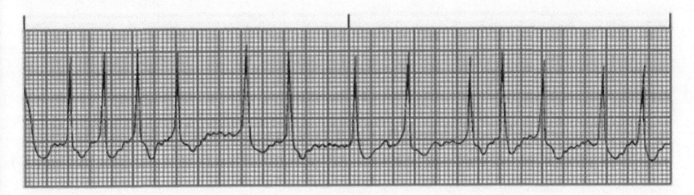

FIGURE 5.33 • **Atrial Fibrillation.** Recognizing atrial fibrillation. The following rhythm strip shows atrial fibrillation: Rhythm: irregular; rate: atrial—indiscernible; ventricular—130 beats per minute P wave: absent, replaced by fine fibrillatory waves; PR interval: indiscernible; QRS complex: 0.08 second; T wave: indiscernible QT interval: unmeasurable

- The 12-lead ECG displays a narrow, irregular tachycardia with at least three different P wave morphologies.
- Treatment is directed at any precipitating events such as hypoxia, acidosis, or digoxin toxicity; spontaneous resolution is very common, pharmacologic intervention is reserved for those patients with incessant tachycardia, hemodynamic instability, or very elevated heart rates.
- Orthodromic reciprocating tachycardia (ORT).
  - Regular, narrow complex tachycardia that accounts for nearly 90% of AV reentry tachycardia in children.
  - Highest incidence is in the first year of life and declines with age.
  - Rhythm is typically referred to as "SVT."
  - Treatment of choice for patients presenting in tachycardia is adenosine; blocks conduction at the AV node and interrupts the arrhythmia circuit.
  - Vagal maneuvers can be attempted while preparing for adenosine administration.
- Ventricular preexcitation and Wolff–Parkinson–White syndrome (WPW).
  - Early activation of the ventricular myocardium through an accessory pathway; resulting early depolarization of a portion of the ventricular myocardium is manifested on the 12-lead ECG as a shortened PR interval and a slurred upstroke of the QRS complex known as the delta wave. (See Figure 5.24—earlier in section.)
  - Wolff–Parkinson–White syndrome is the combination of these ECG findings with clinical SVT.

- AV nodal reentry tachycardia (AVNRT).
  - Type of SVT caused by both fast and slow conduction tissue in the AV node—the so-called fast and slow pathways. The reentry circuit is triggered by a PAC and produces a regular, narrow complex tachycardia on the ECG, similar to that seen in ORT.
  - Age of onset for AVNRT is later than ORT—it is the most common form of SVT in young adults.
  - Treatment of choice for this arrhythmia is intravenous adenosine.
- Junctional ectopic tachycardia (JET).
  - Form of enhanced automaticity that produces a fast, narrow complex tachycardia with variable heart rates.
  - Occurs almost exclusively in the post–cardiac surgery setting.
  - Proposed mechanism is a combination of inflammation and edema in the area of the AV junction, coupled with inotropic medications and metabolic disturbances in the postoperative period.
  - In some patients, the loss of atrial filling during diastole can result in a significant drop in cardiac output. The ECG reveals a narrow complex tachycardia with either AV dissociation or retrograde P waves (Figure 5.34).
  - Treatment is directed at controlling hyperthermia and maintaining normothermia, correcting electrolyte abnormalities aggressively, supplementing magnesium, and reducing exogenous catecholamine infusions as feasible.

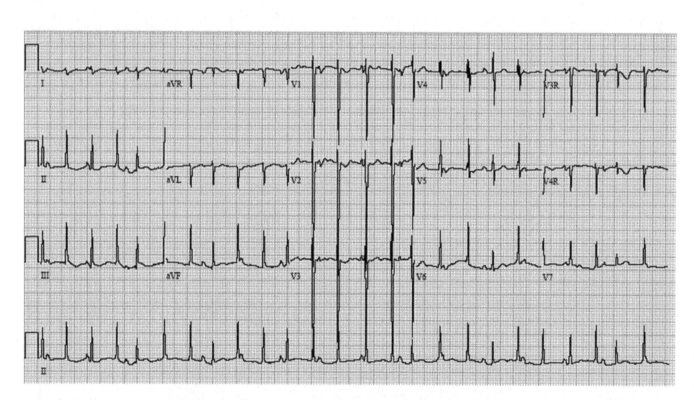

FIGURE 5.34 • **Junctional Ectopic Tachycardia.** ECG showing congenital junctional ectopic tachycardia in a newborn. Note the narrow QRS complex with AV dissociation and a ventricular rate that is faster than the atrial rate.

- If epicardial pacemaker wires are present, dual-chamber pacing at a rate higher than the tachycardia rate may restore AV synchrony.
- If the tachycardia is persistent and there is significant hemodynamic compromise, amiodarone is a first-line pharmacologic agent.
- Ventricular tachycardia (VT).
  - Fast, abnormal, wide complex rhythm originating below the bundle of HIS.
  - While benign forms exist, those encountered in the ICU are almost always pathologic.
  - Can occur after congenital heart surgery as well as in the setting of severe metabolic derangements.
  - 12-lead ECG reveals a wide complex tachycardia with variable rates. Typically, there is AV dissociation.
  - Treatment for hemodynamically unstable VT is synchronized cardioversion (Figure 5.35).
- Ventricular fibrillation (VF).
  - Malignant rhythm that leads to death if not addressed immediately.
- Can be precipitated by metabolic disturbances, ischemia, hypoxia, acidosis, electrolyte abnormalities, and long QT syndrome (LQTS).
- ECG reveals rapid, disorganized, wide complexes of varying sizes.
- Treatment for VF is cardiopulmonary resuscitation and defibrillation.
- Supportive measures include the recommended therapies detailed in the American Heart Association Pediatric Advanced Life Support (PALS) guidelines. If the VF does not respond to initial attempts at defibrillation, a dose of amiodarone is administered (Figure 5.36)
- Torsades de pointes (TDP).
  - Polymorphic VT with a characteristic "spindle-like" appearance on ECG.
  - Often associated with LQTS.
  - Treatment is defibrillation and magnesium IV (Figure 5.37).
- LQTS.
  - Inherited or acquired syndrome of abnormal repolarization and QT prolongation that predisposes to the development of torsades de pointes and sudden cardiac death.

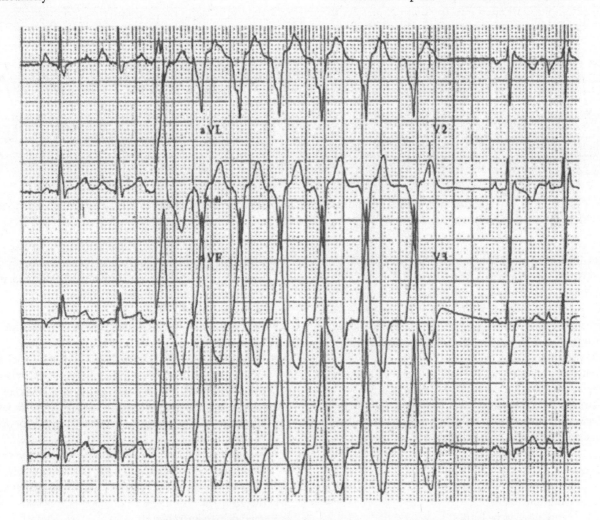

FIGURE 5.35 • **Ventricular Tachycardia.** This rhythm strip demonstrates ventricular tachycardia. There is a sudden onset of a wide QRS tachycardia. No P wave is visible during the tachycardia. The tachycardia ends with a widening of the last two R-R intervals. This is typically seen in the type of ventricular tachycardia called repetitive monomorphic ventricular tachycardia.

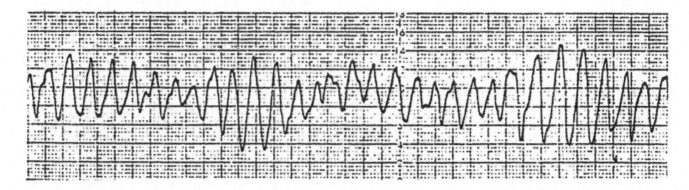

FIGURE 5.36 • **Ventricular Fibrillation.** Ventricular fibrillation (coarse deflections present). Ventricular fibrillation: identifying ECG features; rhythm: none (P wave and QRS are absent); rate: none (P wave and QRS are absent); P waves: wavy, irregular deflection representative of ventricular quivering; deflections may be small (fine ventricular fibrillation) or coarse (coarse ventricular fibrillation); PR interval: Not measurable QRS complex: absent.

FIGURE 5.37 • **Torsades de Pointes.** Torsades de pointes. The widened polymorphic QRS complexes demonstrate a waxing and waning pattern.

- ECG displays relative bradycardia and a corrected QT interval (QTc) longer than 440 milliseconds.
- Acquired forms are most often secondary to medications, especially antibiotics, but can also be precipitated by acute intracranial processes, hypokalemia, hypocalcemia, antifungals, tacrolimus, oral antipsychotics, and tricyclic antidepressants.
- Patients may present with syncope or seizures, although for some, sudden death is the mode of presentation.
- Treatment of LQTS is directed at preventing episodes of torsades de pointes, which includes beta-blockers and implanted defibrillators (Figure 5.38).

Conduction Disorders

- Sick sinus syndrome.
  - Rarely encountered in pediatrics.
  - Almost always seen in patients who have undergone cardiac surgery.
  - Other causes may include digoxin toxicity or myocardial ischemia.

- ECG typically displays marked and persistent bradycardia as well as episodes of atrioventricular (AV) block and, possibly, junctional or ventricular escape rhythms.
- First-degree heart block.
  - Prolongation of the PR interval above the upper limit of normal for age.
  - Prolonged PR interval can be seen in well-conditioned athletes or normal children during sleep; may be related to CHD or result from acquired causes including central nervous system injury, rheumatic carditis, Lyme disease, hyperkalemia/hypokalemia, hypermagnesemia, or drug toxicity.
  - Associated congenital defects include ASD, atrioventricular septal defect, double outlet RV, Ebstein anomaly, and congenitally corrected transposition of the greater arteries (Figure 5.39).
- Second-degree heart block.
  - Two types of second-degree heart block; Type I can be normal children, type II is always pathologic.
  - Mobitz type I.
    - Known as Wenckebach phenomenon.

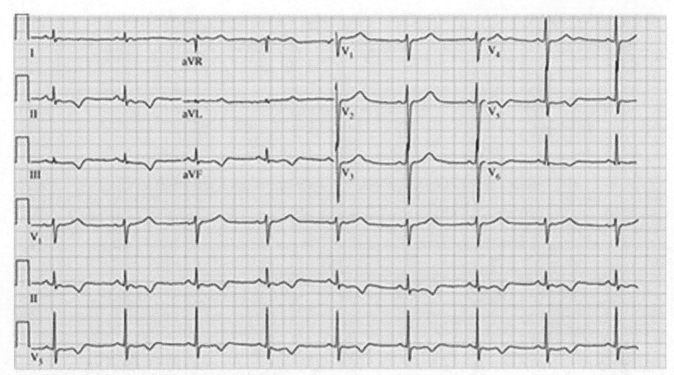

25 mm/s 10 mm/mV 100 Hz 005E 12SL 237 CID: 42

FIGURE 5.38 • **Long QT Syndrome.**

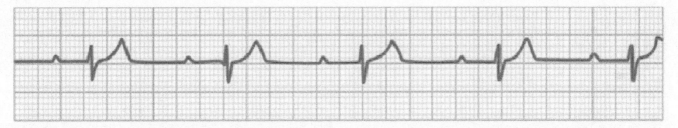

FIGURE 5.39 • **First-Degree Heart Block.** Sustained prolongation of the PR interval with no dropped QRS complexes.

- ECG displays progressive lengthening of the PR interval and then a dropped QRS.
- Seen in normal patients during sleep; not normal during wakefulness and activity (Figure 5.40).
- Mobitz type II.
  - ECG displays intermittently dropped QRS complex in the setting of relatively consistent PR intervals.
  - No progressive lengthening of the PR interval is seen.
  - Increases in heart rate may appear to worsen the block, with AV conduction becoming 2:1 or 3:1.
  - Mobitz type II heart block always requires further evaluation (Figure 5.41).
- Complete heart block (third-degree heart block):
  - No electrical communication between the atria and the ventricles.
  - Acquired or congenital.

- Acquired forms include postoperative myocarditis, Lyme disease, and rheumatic carditis; these forms may be transient and warrant close observation.
- Congenital forms are usually diagnosed prenatally; infant's mother may be asymptomatic, and serum testing is typically positive for autoantibodies (anti-Ro/Anti-La).
- Treatment for both forms is prompt consultation with a pediatric cardiologist along with evaluation of the need for pacemaker implantation (Figure 5.42).
- Pulseless electrical activity (PEA):
  - Organized electrical activity on ECG in the absence of palpable pulses and perfusion.
  - ECG may appear normal at first; with continued absence of perfusion, electrical activity will progress to a terminal rhythm over time with progressive bradycardia and widening of the QRS complex.

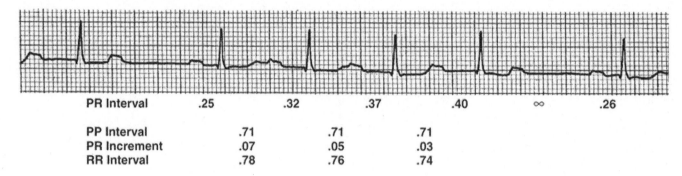

PR Interval	.25	.32	.37	.40	∞	.26
PP Interval	.71	.71	.71			
PR Increment	.07	.05	.03			
RR Interval	.78	.76	.74			

FIGURE 5.40 • **Second-Degree AV Block, Mobitz Type I with Wenckebach Phenomenon.** Mobitz type I second-degree AV block demonstrating the Wenckebach phenomenon (lead II). Beginning with the second QRS complex, which is preceded by a PR interval of 0.25 s, the PR intervals increase progressively until a P wave is completely blocked; this is the typical Wenckebach phenomenon. Because the PR prolongation occurs in decreasing increments, the intervals between successive QRS complexes (RR intervals) shorten before the dropped beat; this causes a slight increase in ventricular rate, called "group beating." The pause that follows the completely blocked P wave allows the AV junction to recover, which accounts for the shortened PR interval of the first cycle after the dropped beat.

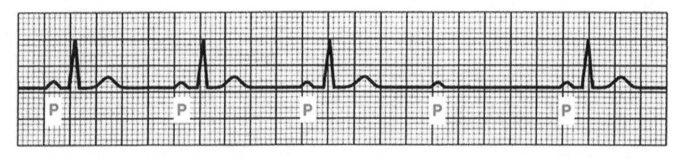

FIGURE 5.41 • **Second-Degree AV Block, Mobitz Type II.** Second-degree AV block: Möbitz type II. A QRS complex is blocked (after the fourth P wave) without gradual lengthening of the preceding PR intervals. While the QRS width in this example is normal, it is often widened in patients with Möbitz type II block.

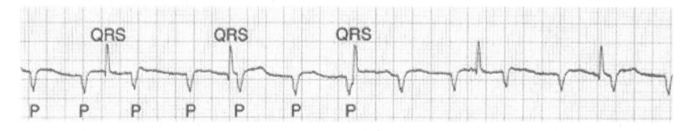

FIGURE 5.42 • **Complete Heart Block.** A rhythm strip demonstrating complete (or third-degree) heart block. The PP interval is equal. The QRS-QRS interval is equal. No consistent association is seen between the P wave and the QRS complex.

- Treatment requires cardiopulmonary resuscitation and ventilatory support.
- Additional treatment is directed at potential underlying causes.

Other Common ECG Abnormalities

Background

- Electrolyte abnormalities can result in ECG changes and arrhythmia.
- Infection and inflammation of the heart muscle and surrounding tissues can result in cardiac arrhythmia.

- Cardiac ischemia, even though unusual in children, can result in typical ECG findings.
- Electrolyte abnormalities can have characteristic ECG findings that can aid in their diagnosis or monitoring.
  - Potassium:
    - Hyperkalemia:
      - ECG findings may not occur at the same serum potassium level for every patient.
      - Typical sequence of progressive ECG changes: Tall, narrow, peaked T waves and shortening of the QT interval → QRS complexes begin to widen; eventual flattening & disappearance of the P wave; PR prolongation and AV

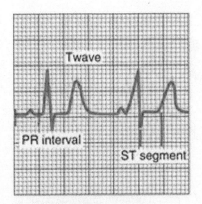

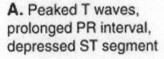

A. Peaked T waves, prolonged PR interval, depressed ST segment

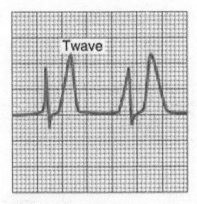

B. Lost P wave

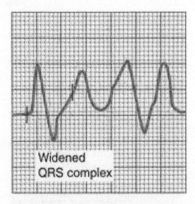

C. Widened QRS complex

FIGURE 5.43 • **Hyperkalemia: ECG Pattern in Various Degrees of Hyperkalemia.** Typical ECG findings indicative of various degrees of hyperkalemia. **A:** When the serum potassium (K^+) level is about 6 to 7 mEq/L, the T waves become peaked, the PR interval is prolonged, and the ST segment is depressed. **B:** At about 8 to 9 mEq/L, the P wave is lost. **C:** At about 10 to 11 mEq/L, the QRS complex widens.

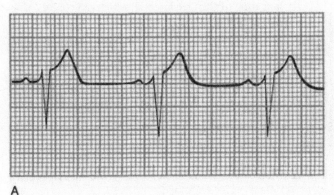

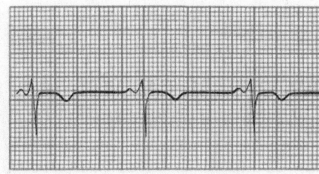

A

B

FIGURE 5.44 • **ST Segment Elevation in a Patient with Acute Pericarditis. A:** Lead V3 shows the ST segment elevation of acute pericarditis. **B:** The same lead several days later shows that the ST segments have returned to baseline and the T waves have inverted. There are no Q waves.

block can also occur → sine-wave pattern transitions into ventricular fibrillation and asystole.

- Hyperkalemia causes narrow, peaked T waves that can progress to prolongation of the PR interval and widening of the QRS and QT interval.
  - A sinusoidal pattern develops, and without intervention, this can lead to ventricular fibrillation and death (Figure 5.43).
- Hypokalemia:
  - ST segment depression and increased prominence of the U wave.
  - If severe, can progress to PR prolongation and QRS widening.
- Calcium:
  - Hypercalcemia produces shortening of the QT interval.
    - Severe hypercalcemia can lead to prolongation of the PR interval and QRS complex, and varying degrees of AV block can be seen.

- Hypocalcemia produces prolongation of the QT interval.
- Pericarditis, pericardial effusion, and myocarditis.
  - Pericarditis.
    - ECG changes in pericarditis are secondary to repolarization abnormalities caused by epicardial inflammation.
      - PR Depression: early and transient phenomenon. Quite specific for the diagnosis of pericarditis. It is seen in all leads (although leads aVR and V1 may display reciprocal elevation instead).
      - ST Elevation: probably the most common finding in acute pericarditis—although it is seen in fewer than 50% of patients. ST elevations are typically less than 5 mm and seen diffusely throughout the limb leads and precordial leads (again, except in aVR and V1, where reciprocal ST depression may be seen) (Figure 5.44).
  - Pericardial effusion.
    - Changes seen are nonspecific.

Lateral	Anterior		Inferior
I	aVR	V1	V4
II	aVL	V2	V5
III	aVF	V3	V6

F I G U R E 5 . 4 5 · **ECG Leads Corresponding to Anatomic Coronary Artery Territories.**

- Sinus tachycardia is the most common finding.
- Can be diffusely diminished voltages in all leads.
- Although rare, electrical alternans —a beat-to-beat alteration in the QRS voltage— can occur, thought to be related to the movement of the heart within a pericardial sac filled with fluid.
- Myocarditis.
  - ECG changes are almost universal.
  - Most common findings are sinus tachycardia with low-voltage QRS complexes throughout the ECG.
  - Other findings include ST segment changes, ventricular hypertrophy, and ectopic beats.
- Myocardial ischemia.
  - Ischemic changes can be differentiated from other changes in the ECG based on history and their distribution in a pattern that follows the anatomic course of the coronary arteries (Figure 5.45).
- T wave changes:
  - Earliest changes are "hyperacute" T waves; taller and more peaked than normal, but difficult to differentiate from normal without comparing with a baseline ECG.
  - T wave inversions are also common in ischemia, but must be differentiated from normal pediatric patterns.
  - T waves may be normally inverted in III, aVR, and V1.
  - Infants and young children may have inversions in V2 & V3 as well.
- ST segment changes.
  - ST segment depression may be subtle initially, but can worsen over time. If there is a high suspicion for ischemia, serial ECGs can be very helpful.
  - ST segment elevation is probably the most well-recognized ECG alteration related to myocardial ischemia.
  - The ST elevation progresses over time from flattening to loss of the concave upstroke of the T wave, then to the convex upward appearance (often referred to a "tombstone" appearance).
  - Pathologic Q Waves signify the transition from ischemia to infarction and necrosis.
  - While Q waves can be normal in some leads, pathologic Q waves are wider and deeper than normal (Figure 5.46).
- ECG abnormalities in CNS disorders.
  - Cerebrovascular disease is associated with ST segment depression, flattening or inversion of the T waves, and prominent U waves.

- QTc prolongation is a very common finding and can be associated with the development of torsades de pointes.
- Findings can be seen in 50% to 90% of patients who have suffered subarachnoid hemorrhages.
- Any form of CNS insult can also be associated with varying degrees of heart block—from PR prolongation to complete heart block. This is typically a transient phenomenon.
- Electrocardiographic changes associated with medications.
  - Numerous drugs employed in the hospital setting result in prolongation of the QTc interval, which can confer a risk of *torsades de pointes.*
  - A complete discussion of these medications is beyond the scope of this review.
  - A list of medications can be found at www.azcert.org

Imaging Studies for Cardiac Diagnoses

Chest radiograph—please see Section 3 for content on chest radiograph imaging and interpretation.

Cardiac Imaging: CT and MRI

Preet K. Sandhu

Background

- Echocardiogram with Doppler is the primary imaging modality for the initial evaluation and follow-up of CHD.
- Further imaging is indicated in complex lesions.
- Digital subtraction angiography (DSA) is performed in such cases to assess the hemodynamics, to evaluate the function of the ventricles and valves. However, DSA is two-dimensional (2-D), with restricted field of view, is more invasive, and exposes the patient to higher radiation dose.
- CT with the advent of multidetector CT (MDCT) offers many advantages over DSA, echocardiography, and MRI.

Advantages of CT Imaging

- Complete assessment of intrathoracic structures including the extracardiac structures, including the lungs and airway that can be affected in cardiac disorders (e.g., tracheal compression from vascular rings, or complete tracheal rings in pulmonary sling).

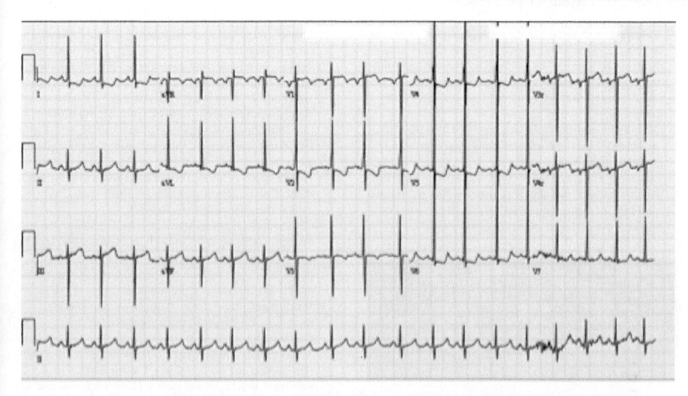

FIGURE 5.46 • **A 12-lead ECG in a 6-Month-Old with Anomalous Left Coronary Artery from the Pulmonary Artery, or ALCAPA with Cardiac Ischemia.** Note the ST segment depression seen in leads I, aVL, and V4–V6, the typical distribution for left lateral ischemia.

- Evaluation of lungs for air trapping using a combination of inspiratory and expiratory CT.
- Fast; requires less sedation and is better tolerated by infants and neonates.
- Allows better monitoring of the patients during the procedure.
- Many support devices including stents and pacemakers are compatible with CT and are contraindicated in MRI.
- MDCT provides excellent multiplanar two-dimensional (2D) and three-dimensional (3D) images, so that the anatomy can be depicted in any imaging plane.

Disadvantages of CT Imaging

- Requires radiation and especially higher doses with electrocardiography (ECG) gated CT.
- Functional MR and echocardiography are preferred over gated CT for functional evaluation.

Contrast-Enhanced CT Angiography (CTA)

- Can provide excellent imaging of the airways and vasculature.
- Indications:
  - Complete evaluation of pulmonary arteries and veins, which cannot be assessed with echocardiography.
  - Evaluation of PA stent for stenosis.
  - Assessment of number, size, and course of arteries, as well as postoperative effects on coronary arteries; coronary artery aneurysm in Kawasaki disease.
  - Assessment of aortic arch anomalies such as double aortic arch, right aortic arch with aberrant left subclavian artery,

coarctation of aorta, pericardial calcification in constrictive pericarditis, assessment of arterial supply, and venous drainage in pulmonary sequestration.

Cardiac MRI

- Indications:
  - When other diagnostic tests such as echocardiogram do not provide the required information.
- Advantages:
  - No radiation exposure.
  - Larger field of view and multiplanar imaging.
- Disadvantages:
  - Need for sedation.
  - Longer imaging time.
  - Susceptibility to artifact from stents or other hardware limiting its use.
  - Poor evaluation of the lungs when compared with CT imaging.
  - Relatively poor spatial resolution.
- MRI techniques:
  - Spin echo and gradient echo pulse sequences are used for cardiac evaluation.
  - Two types of sequences: black blood imaging and bright blood imaging.
  - ECG triggered steady-state free precision (SSFP) is the most commonly used MRI technique for assessment of cardiac anatomy and for functional evaluation including ventricular function assessment and analysis of regional wall motion.

- Gadolinium-enhanced 3-D MR angiography (MRA) is used for imaging extracardiac vascular anatomy such as imaging of aorta (see Figures 5.47–5.49) and its branches, pulmonary veins, pulmonary arteries, aortopulmonary collaterals, systemic-to-pulmonary artery shunts, conduits, and vascular grafts.
- Quantitative and qualitative assessment of blood flow are used in functional assessment of congenital or acquired pediatric heart diseases.
- Qualitative evaluation includes visual evaluation for abnormal flow patterns that appear as turbulent flow jets related to stenotic or regurgitant valves, or abnormal communication between cardiac chambers or blood vessels.

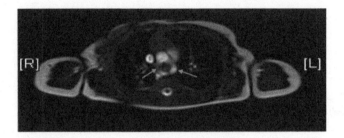

FIGURE 5.47 • **Double Aortic Arch.**

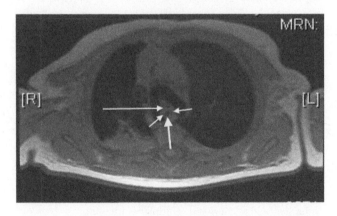

FIGURE 5.48 • **Double Aortic Arch Axial View.**

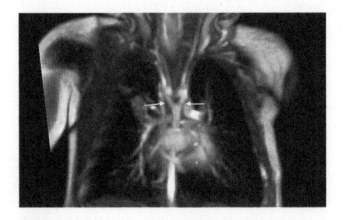

FIGURE 5.49 • **Double Aortic Arch Coronal Projection.**

- Quantitative phase-contrast imaging is used for assessment of direction of flow, flow velocity, flow rate, stroke volume, or minute flow assessment. Clinical examples include measurement of cardiac output, pulmonary to systemic flow ratio in patients with intra- or extracardiac shunts, regurgitation in native or postoperative lesions (e.g., pulmonary regurgitation after repair of Tetralogy of Fallot) in a vessel or at a valve for shunt and regurgitant fraction.
- Provides great tissue characterization and is used for assessment of myocardium, pericardium, vessel walls, and extracardiac tissue for pathologic changes.
- Clinical applications include assessment of ventricular aneurysm, cardiac and pericardial tumors, vessel wall imaging aortitis, dissection, arrhythmogenic right ventricular dysplasia (ARVD), evaluation of pericardium (e.g., constrictive pericarditis), and myocardial iron load.
- Ventricular volume and mass can be calculated using short-axis cine images through the ventricles (see Figure 5.50).
- Additional information that can be obtained includes ejection fraction and stroke volume. Cardiac output (stroke volume × heart rate) and cardiac index (cardiac output/body surface area) can be subsequently calculated from imaging.
- Indications for cardiac MRI; additional consideration for cardiac CT.
  - Tetralogy of Fallot (TOF).
  - Aortic anomalies, including coarctation of aorta.
  - Assessment of ventricular function, valve regurgitation, vascular ring, congenital coronary artery anomalies, ARVD, cardiac tumors, ASD, VSD, among others.
  - More commonly performed in postoperative patients such as postoperative TOF in the second decade of life for assessment of RV volume, or postoperative TGA.
  - Vascular ring.
    - Vascular ring is a form of congenital vascular anomaly in which the trachea and esophagus are surrounded completely by vascular structures. Rings are formed by abnormal embryological development of the aortic arch. Most common are double aortic arch and right arch with left ligamentum arteriosum.

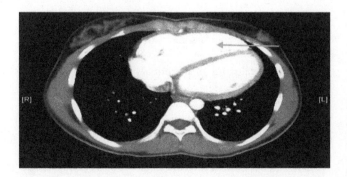

FIGURE 5.50 • **Dilated Right Ventricle**

- Pulmonary sling.
  - Anomalous origin of left PA that arises from proximal right PA and passes leftward between the trachea and esophagus, forming a sling. Associated with severe tracheal compression, displacement of the distal trachea and carina to the left, and complete tracheal rings giving a round rather than oval appearance to the trachea.
- Both CT and MR can demonstrate the course of an aberrant vessel, tracheal compression, and hyperinflation of the right lung (see Figures 5.47–5.49).
- MR provides good visualization of the airways and vasculature with ability of multiplanar imaging without radiation exposure; an important consideration in children.
- Evaluation is usually done by a combination of Gad-enhanced 3-D MRA and spin echo imaging. Double inversion recovery spin echo sequence provides excellent visualization of airway and vasculature.
- Coarctation of aorta.
  - Coarctation is a congenital aortic narrowing in the region of the isthmus.
  - Associated abnormalities include bicuspid aortic valve and cystic medial degeneration that may lead to dilatation of ascending aorta and increased risk of dissection.
  - Angiography has been traditionally used to evaluate coarctation.
  - MR provides the advantage of being noninvasive.
  - Anatomic information can be obtained from Gad-MRA, including anatomy of aorta, cross-sectional measurement of aorta in various locations, and imaging of the collaterals. Cine phase contrast can be used to assess pressure gradient across the coarctation and quantifying collateral flow in descending thoracic aorta.
- Aortic aneurysm and/or dissection can be seen in association with CHD such as bicuspid aortic valve, Tetralogy of Fallot, and in connective tissue disorders such as Marfan's syndrome, and can be assessed with CT or MR.
- Tetralogy of Fallot (TOF).
  - Anatomic features of TOF include VSD involving the outlet portion of the septum, RVOT obstruction, overriding aorta, and right ventricular hypertrophy. MR has an important role in both preoperative and postoperative assessment of TOF.
  - In preoperative cardiac surgery patients, MRA or CTA can be used to assess all sources of pulmonary blood flow to the pulmonary arteries, aortopulmonary collaterals, and ductus arteriosus. Gadolinium-enhanced 3-D MRA is used for assessment of PA anatomy and aortopulmonary collaterals. CTA and MRA are more sensitive than echocardiography for assessment of branch PA stenosis.
  - Short-axis SSFP cine MRI is used for calculation of right and LV volume, function, ejection fraction, RVOT size, and pulmonary valve function.
  - Assessment of the course of coronary arteries to exclude major coronary artery crossing the RVOT (common

associated abnormality includes left anterior descending [LAD] artery arising from right coronary artery).
  - In postoperative patients, MR is used in all ages, particularly in adolescents and adults, in which acoustic echo window is limited.
  - Postoperative TOF patients develop pulmonary regurgitation with progressive RV dilatation and dysfunction.
  - MR is used for quantitative assessment of LV and RV volumes, stroke volume, and ejection fraction; anatomy of RVOT (aneurysm and wide annulus correlated with need for pulmonary valve replacement), pulmonary arteries, aorta, and aortopulmonary collaterals; quantification of pulmonary regurgitation. The anatomy of great vessels may be altered due to prior surgery and resultant fibrosis. CT helps in planning repeat surgery in postoperative patients such as for measurement of distance of PA from sternum.
- TGA:
  - TGA is an abnormal relationship between great arteries and ventricles (ventriculoarterial discordance), where aorta arises from anatomical RV and PA arises from anatomical left ventricle.
  - Normally, pulmonary artery is located anteriorly and to the left of aorta.
  - In TGA, aorta is located anterior and to the right (dextro or D-TGA) or anterior and to the left (levo or L-TGA) of pulmonary artery.
  - Cross-sectional imaging including CT and MR are excellent for depicting anatomy, however are used in preoperative period to answer specific questions raised by echocardiography.
  - MRI is used mainly in postoperative patients.
  - Postoperative atrial switch: quantitative evaluation of size and function of systemic RV, evaluation of RVOT and LVOT for obstruction, imaging of systemic and pulmonary venous pathways or baffles for leak and obstruction.
  - Postoperative arterial switch: Arterial switch patients are prone to PA and branch PA stenosis, which is best evaluated using gadolinium-enhanced MRA. Gadolinium-enhanced respiratory gated MRA to study origin of transposed coronary arteries.
  - Also for assessment of RV and LV size and function, RVOT and LVOT for obstruction.
- Takayasu's arteritis/aortitis.
  - Takayasu's arteritis (TA) is a primary arteritis of unknown cause that commonly affects the aorta and its major branches and the PA.
  - Histologically, TA is characterized by granulomatous inflammation of the arterial wall with intimal proliferation and fibrosis of the media and adventitia, which eventually leads to stenosis, occlusion, and, occasionally, poststenotic dilatations and aneurysm formation.
  - Findings in the acute phase of TA include wall thickening of the aorta and PA, which enhances on

gadolinium-enhanced images. Sometimes, occlusion of the aortic branches or PA or pseudoaneurysm formation is seen in the acute phase.

- Findings in late phase include diffuse narrowing of the descending thoracic and abdominal aorta, stenosis, occlusion, and dilatation.
- Stenotic lesions most commonly involve the proximal portions of aortic branches such as common carotid and subclavian arteries and PA.
- Abrupt occlusion and abrupt transition to collateral vessels are characteristic findings.
- Dilatation commonly involves ascending aorta. Aortic regurgitation caused by dilatation of the ascending aorta is well shown by cine MR.

Echocardiography (ECHO)

Brian F. Joy

- Pediatric echocardiography.
  - An ultrasound beam is transmitted into the chest, and the signal is reflected off interfaces (tissue planes, blood/tissue borders).
  - Ultrasound transducer sends out pulses of ultrasound and listens for returning signal.
  - More dense regions reflect more and transmit less.
- Indications for transthoracic echocardiogram.
  - Suspected CHD.
    - Symptoms of cyanosis, FTT, exercise-induced CP or syncope, respiratory distress, murmurs, CHF, abnormal arterial pulses, cardiomegaly.
    - Certain congenital syndromes, family history of inherited heart disease, extracardiac abnormalities known to be associated with CHD.
    - Abnormal chest radiograph, fetal echocardiogram, ECG, or chromosome analysis.
  - Acquired heart disease and noncardiac diseases.
    - Kawasaki disease, infective endocarditis, rheumatic fever and carditis, myocarditis, pericarditis, HIV infection.
    - Cardiomyopathies.
    - Exposure to cardiotoxic drugs (e.g., chemotherapeutic agents).
    - Systemic hypertension.
    - Pulmonary hypertension.
    - Thromboembolic events.
  - Arrhythmias.
    - Evaluation for underlying structural heart disease.
    - Evaluation for depressed cardiac function.
- Two-dimensional imaging.
  - Multiple pulses sent out along adjacent scan lines.
  - Sector formed by multiple scan lines.
  - Process repeated multiple times for "live" imaging.
- Standard ECHO views.
  - Parasternal long axis (Figure 5.51).

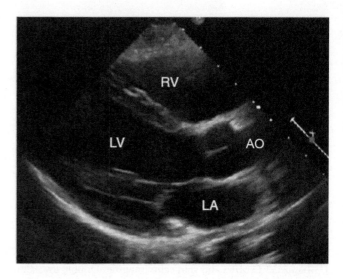

FIGURE 5.51 • **Parasternal Long Axis.** Parasternal long axis. Left atrium (LA), left ventricle (LV), right ventricle (RV), aorta (AO)

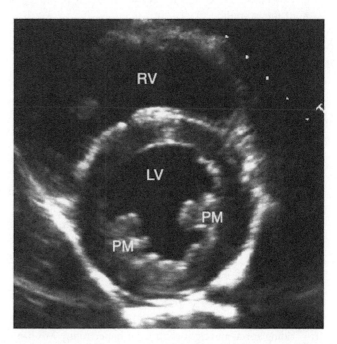

FIGURE 5.52 • **Parasternal Short Axis.** Left ventricle (LV), right ventricle (RV), aorta (AO), Papillary muscle (PM)

  - Parasternal short axis (Figure 5.52).
  - Apical four chambers (Figure 5.53).
  - Suprasternal notch (Figure 5.54).
  - Subcostal.
- M-mode.
  - Multiple pulses sent out along a single line.
  - High temporal resolution—more precise measurement with respect to time.
  - Standard for measuring chamber sizes.
- Doppler—a sound wave reflected from a moving object changes its frequency proportional to the velocity of the object.

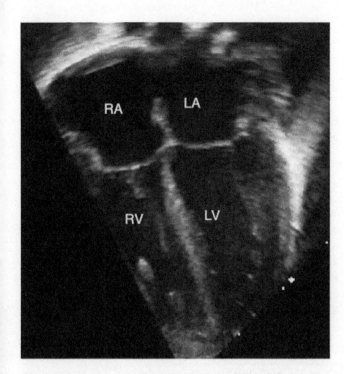

FIGURE 5.53 • **Apical Four Chambers.** Right atrium
(RA), right ventricle (RV), left atrium (LA), left ventricle (LV)

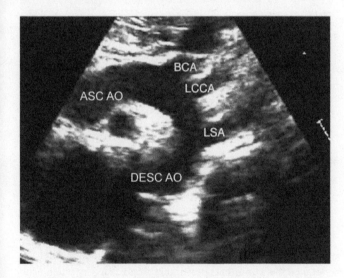

FIGURE 5.54 • **Suprasternal Notch Arch View.**
Ascending aorta (ASC AO), descending aorta (DESC AO),
brachiocephalic artery (BCA), left common carotid artery
(LCCA), left subclavian artery (LSA)

- Color Doppler—use of turbulence map demonstrates velocity, direction, and turbulence.
- Pulse wave Doppler.
  - Determines direction and velocity of blood flow at a specific point.
  - Unable to accurately measure high blood velocities.
- Continuous wave Doppler.
  - Able to measure high blood velocities.

- Unable to measure blood velocity at a specific point along the ultrasound beam.
- Echocardiography provides a basic assessment of the LV.
  - Ventricular chamber size.
    - Chamber dimensions.
    - Chamber volume.
  - Ventricular mass.
    - LV wall thickness.
    - Ventricular hypertrophy.
    - Ventricular geometry.
  - Ventricular systolic function.
  - Ventricular diastolic function.
- Cardiac function.
  - LV shortening fraction.
    - Measurement of systolic function.
    - Calculated from M-mode measurements based on the LV internal dimension at diastole and systole.
      - Normal ≥25%.
      - Inherently limited because it is attempting to assess 3D function in a one-dimensional measurement.
  - LV ejection fraction.
    - Calculated by 2D imaging based on the LV end diastolic and end systolic volumes.
    - Normal ejection fraction ≥55%.
    - Preload and afterload dependent.
    - Does not reflect intrinsic inotropic state.
  - Doppler ultrasound.
    - Assesses ventricular diastolic function.
      - Provides indirect estimates of myocardial relaxation, LV stiffness, and filling pressures.
    - Can be used to calculate cardiac output.
      - Blood velocity in the aorta is calculated using the Doppler principle.
      - Using measured aorta dimensions, velocity time integral is measured, ultimately making it able to calculate the stroke volume.
- Pulmonary hypertension.
  - Echocardiographic signs of pulmonary hypertension.
    - RVH.
    - RV dilation.
    - Reduced right ventricular systolic function.
    - Flattened interventricular septum indicates increased RV pressure.
  - Right ventricular systolic pressure (RVSP) can be estimated by echocardiogram.
  - Systolic PA pressure is considered equal to RVSP (assuming no pulmonary valve stenosis or outflow tract obstruction).
    - RVSP estimated by addition of right atrial pressure (RAP) to the pressure gradient between the right chambers.
    - Pressure gradient calculated by modified Bernoulli equation.
      - $RVSP = 4 * (tricuspid\ regurgitation\ velocity)^2 + RAP$
    - Normal RVSP = 18 to 25 mmHg
    - Precision is debatable—cardiac catheterization is gold standard for measuring the systolic PA pressure.

- Echocardiography is a useful screening method for suspected pulmonary hypertension, but not to determine treatment course or to monitor therapeutic efficacy.
- Transesophageal echocardiogram provides clearer images than transthoracic echocardiogram; especially of structures that are difficult to view from transthoracic windows.
  - Transesophageal ECHO provides better views of aorta, PA, valves of heart, both atria, atrial septum, LA appendage, coronary arteries, and pulmonary veins.
  - Indications for transesophageal echocardiogram.
    - Infective endocarditis.
      - Better delineation of shape and size of vegetations.
    - Evaluation of prosthetic valves—high resolution of valves.
    - Cardioembolic stroke.
      - Assess for atrial communication with or without bubble study.
    - Atrial fibrillation.
      - Assess for atrial thrombus prior to cardioversion.
    - Aortic diseases—aortic dissection, intramural trauma, aortic trauma.
    - Cardiac masses.
    - CHDs and intracardiac shunts with nondiagnostic transthoracic echocardiogram.
    - Perioperative period and during procedures.
    - Critically ill patients with limited acoustic windows.

Endomyocardial Biopsy

Jennifer L. Joiner

Background

- EMB is the gold standard in diagnostic management of cardiac cellular rejection posttransplant and for the determination of myocarditis.

Definition/Rationale:

- Percutaneous intravascular biopsy of the myocardium that remains the gold standard to evaluate for myocardial infection or cardiac transplant rejection.
- Completed at frequent intervals post–cardiac transplant to evaluate for signs of rejection and adequacy of immunosuppressive therapy or in cases when myocarditis is suspected.
  - Rejection may be associated with unexplained fever, tachycardia, fatigue, shortness of breath, joint pain, and personality changes.
  - Cellular rejection categorized from grade 0 to 3. Grade 0 does not detect any signs of rejection.

Laboratory Evaluation

- Qualitative and quantitative polymerase chain reaction (PCR) used to detect viral genomes in myocarditis.
- In suspected rejection, tissue is obtained with biotome forceps, and lymphocyte infiltration with myocardial necrosis is noted.

Management

- Scheduled diagnostic procedure in cardiac catheterization laboratory, where patients will most likely require some sedation or anesthesia.
- Most common site of cannulation to obtain biopsy is right internal jugular vein.
- Most commonly performed with fluoroscopy guidance.
- Management of rejection is based on standardized grading system based on severity of rejection found on EMB from 0 (no rejection) to 4 (severe rejection).
- Steroids are the mainstay of treatment.

Complications

- Thrombosis.
- Bleeding.
- Arrhythmias.
- Infection.
- Vessel injury.
- Cardiac perforation (rare).

Cardiac Catheterization

Jennifer L. Joiner

Background

- Cardiac catheterizations are performed when precise cardiac physiologic measurements are needed.
- Completed in patients when anatomic features are poorly visualized by echocardiography, when electrophysiologic studies are needed, or when therapeutic catheterization studies are needed.

Definition

- Direct catheterization of vessels performed to delineate cardiac anatomy and assess hemodynamics and blood flow patterns, which is done when precise physiologic measurements are needed for management.

Indications

- Patients with congenital cardiac defects who require finely detailed measurements presurgery or postsurgery when echocardiogram or MRI evaluation is not sufficient.
- Evaluation of pulmonary vasculature and reversibility of pulmonary vascular disease.
- Used therapeutically to treat conditions including patent ductus arteriosus (PDA), ASDs, VSDs, collateral vessels.
- Used to perform radiofrequency ablation in malignant or difficult-to-control arrhythmias.

Procedure

- Frequently, sedation and analgesia administration are required; performed by a provider other than the proceduralist. Expertise in airway management and intubation is essential.
- Evaluation for procedure-associated arrhythmias.

Postprocedure

- Evaluation of emergence from sedation/analgesia.
- Monitor catheterization site for evidence of bleeding, hematoma.
- Monitor distal extremity for pulses, perfusion, signs of ischemia/vessel spasm.
- Limit mobility/movement in immediate postcatheterization period per institution protocol.

Near-Infrared Spectroscopy (NIRS) Monitoring

Jennifer L. Joiner

Background

- NIRS is a noninvasive method used to continuously evaluate regional tissue oxygenation.
- Commonly used in pediatric operating rooms and intensive care units to augment other monitoring therapies.

Technology

- Measures regional tissue oxygen saturation by using optical spectrophotometry that elicits real-time information in attempts to determine regional hemoglobin oxygen saturation in a patient's brain.
- Uses a noninvasive skin probe sensor placed on the child's skin (e.g., on the forehead for brain monitoring; over extremity for skeletal muscle tissue evaluation).

Indications

- Infants and children at risk for reduced-flow or no-flow ischemic states/conditions. Commonly used in cardiac surgery patients; applications for use have been expanding.
- Trending the hemoglobin oxygenation saturation of blood in the brain or skeletal muscle below the sensor.
- Should not be used as the sole mechanism for diagnosis, intervention, or therapy. Used as an adjuvant monitoring device.
- Early warning indicator of changes in patient status; deterioration in tissue oxygenation.
- Originally used to measure cerebral oxygen saturation; expanding to measure oxygenation in tissue beyond the brain.

Monitoring

- Cerebral: high flow and high oxygen extraction organ. If cerebral autoregulation is intact, cerebral desaturations are a late indicator of shock.
- Somatic: variable blood flow with lower oxygen extraction rate than cerebral. Somatic desaturations may represent an early indicator of a shock state.
- Regional oxygen saturation is depicted as rSO_2.
- Normal ranges (each patient serves as own control, so trends are most important).
  - Cerebral: typical range: 60 to 80; ≤50% or 20% change from rSO_2 is often a trigger for further evaluation/intervention.
  - Somatic: typical range: 5 to 20 points higher than cerebral rSO_2; changes in this range often trigger further evaluation/intervention.

Considerations

- Infants with NIRS should have it placed high on the frontal eminences above the orbital ridge in cerebral monitoring.
- Readings are trended for rise and fall during surgery and in the intensive care unit.
- Accurate readings may be impacted by skin pigmentation.
- Probes for NIRS monitoring are relatively expensive; recommended replacement every 24 hours.
- Probes should not be placed over nevi, broken skin, hair, or bony prominences.

Complications

- Inability to affix the probe.
- Skin breakdown from probe.
- Inaccurate measurements due to inappropriate placement/securement of probe.

Exercise Stress Testing (EST)

Jennifer L. Joiner

Background

- Cardiac stress testing is based on protocols done on a bicycle or treadmill, where the body is challenged with exercise and its responses to increasing demands are monitored and measured.
- Patients are monitored for responses in heart rate, oxygen saturations, End Tidal pCO_2, BP, and also for symptoms including CP, syncope, arrhythmias, or ischemic changes.
- Exercise stress testing is important when objectively evaluating a patient's cardiovascular function and capabilities.

Definition

- Testing is done to ascertain the maximum aerobic power of the body during exercise when a suspected or documented cardiac problem exists.
- Objective information is gained that reliably informs clinicians on a child's true physical capacity to perform, as measured by the responses of the cardiopulmonary system.

Types

- Treadmill.
- Bicycle.

Indications

- Evaluation of signs/symptoms aggravated by exercise/activity.
- Identification of abnormal responses to exercise in children with underlying cardiopulmonary or other organ system disease.
- Evaluation of prognosis using baseline and serial testing measures.

- Evaluation of efficacy of medical or surgical interventions.
- Determination of baseline data for initiation of cardiopulmonary or musculoskeletal rehabilitation.

Pretesting Considerations

- Patients do not need to be NPO prior to the procedure.
- Recommend caffeine avoidance on the day of the study.
- Recommend avoidance of a large meal prior to the study.
- Loose, comfortable clothes and athletic shoes are appropriate.

Testing

- 10 electrodes are placed on patient's skin.
- Continuous 12-lead ECG and pulse oximetry monitoring.
- Placement of appropriate-sized BP cuff for intermittent monitoring during the study.
- Breathing apparatus is placed prior to the initiation of exercise.
- Exercise typically lasts 10 to 15 minutes.

Findings

- Determines exercise effort, presence of arrhythmias, conduction disturbances, ST segment or T wave changes indicating myocardial ischemia, and QT interval.
- BP changes are reflective of cardiac output and peripheral vascular resistance during exercise. Normally, BP rises with increased intensity; sometimes only modestly. A lack of change in BP may indicate cardiac dysfunction. A fall in BP during exercise may indicate cardiac failure or left-sided obstructive cardiac lesion (e.g., AS).
- Patient-reported symptoms (fatigue, CP, dizziness) also important in the complete cardiac evaluation.

Management

- Most testing centers have protocols for treadmill exercise testing using the Bruce protocol, and less commonly used are bicycle ergometers.
- In the Bruce protocol, the level of exercise is increased in 3-minute stages by elevating both speed and incline.
- Children are monitored for CP and syncope, and are also on continuous ECG monitoring to include BP, ETCO$_2$, and oxygen (O$_2$) saturations.

Support of Cardiovascular Function

Michelle Dokas

Medications to Support Cardiovascular Function

Background/Definition

- Classes of medications used short-term to support cardiac output.
- Have a direct effect on the heart, vascular smooth muscle, central nervous system, and autonomic nervous system.

- β_1-adrenergic stimulation results in increased myocardial contractility and increased heart rate.
- β_2-adrenergic stimulation results in vasodilation.
- α-adrenergic stimulation results in increased systemic vascular resistance through smooth muscle contraction.
- Dopaminergic receptor stimulation results in dilation of the renal and mesenteric vasculature (dose-dependent).
  - Indications for use:
    - Hypotension.
    - Acute heart failure.
    - Impaired vascular tone.

Adrenoreceptor Agents

- Dopamine—central neurotransmitter that stimulates dopamine receptors in the brain and renal vascular beds as well as α-receptors and β-receptors. Results in positive inotropic effects and increases systemic vascular resistance at higher doses.
  - Uses: hypotension after adequate fluid resuscitation, increase cardiac output via positive inotropy.
  - Dose: continuous infusion of 1 to 20 mcg/kg/minute. Effects are dose-dependent.
  - The use of low-dose dopamine (e.g., "renal-dose"dopamine) at 1 to 5 mcg/kg/minute to improve renal function has been discredited as no evidence has been found in adults or children that renal function markers were improved with this therapy.
- Dobutamine—structurally similar to dopamine, but has greater selectivity for β_1-receptors than β_2; provides greater inotropic support and less vasopressor effect.
  - Uses: patients with short-term cardiac decompensation.
  - Dose: continuous infusion of 2 to 20 mcg/kg/minute.
  - Can produce tachycardia in modest doses and is a proarrhythmic agent.
- Epinephrine—endogenous catecholamine with strong affinity for β_1, β_2, and α-receptors in cardiac and smooth muscle. β-effects are more pronounced at lower doses, and α-effects predominate at higher doses.
  - Uses—treatment of shock with myocardial dysfunction and hypotension. Also used in cardiac arrest and treatment of severe allergic reactions. Inhaled forms are used to treat respiratory stridor and bronchospasm.
  - Dose—Continuous infusion of 0.1 to 1 mcg/kg/minute. May titrate up to 5 mcg/kg/minute.
- Alternate dosing is recommended for treatment of allergic reactions and bronchospasm/stridor.
- Epinephrine causes increased myocardial oxygen demand and tachycardia.
- High doses may inhibit end-organ perfusion due to severe vasoconstrictor effects and must be considered with treatment.
- Norepinephrine—endogenous neurotransmitter that has primarily α effects with some β_1 stimulation. This causes powerful vasoconstriction with less potent inotropic effects.
  - Uses: profound hypotension with vasodilation.
  - Dose: continuous infusion of 0.05 to 0.1 mcg/kg/minute. Maximum 1 to 2 mcg/kg/minute.

- Used primarily in patients who are peripherally vasodilated with hypotension due to potent vasoconstrictor effects.
- Isoproterenol—potent β-stimulant with little α-effects, causing increased chronotropy and inotropy with some vasodilatory effects.
  - Uses: bradyarrhythmias or temporary treatment of 3rd degree heart block until pacemaker can be inserted. Also can be used in low cardiac output states.
  - Dose: children—continuous infusions of 0.05 to 2 mcg/kg/minute.
  - Greatly increases myocardial oxygen demand and decreases supply by decreasing coronary filling.
  - Patients should be intravascularly fluid resuscitated before considering this medication.

Vasopressor Agents

- Vasopressin—also known as antidiuretic hormone.
  - Stored in the pituitary gland and released in response to increased osmolality in the plasma, or hypotension.
  - It causes constriction of vascular smooth muscle and increases water reabsorption in the renal collecting duct.
  - An endogenous chemical also available as an exogenous medication.
  - Uses: diabetes insipidus, gastrointestinal hemorrhage, cardiac arrest, and vasodilatory shock unresponsive to exogenous catecholamines and fluid resuscitation.
  - Dose: alternate doses are used for diabetes insipidus and gastrointestinal hemorrhage. Dosing for shock is as follows: Children—continuous infusion of 0.17 to 8 **milliunits**/kg/minute.
  - Urine output and sodium levels should be monitored closely while on this medication due to impact on renal collecting duct.

Phosphodiesterase Inhibitor

- Milrinone: positive inotropic and vasodilatory effects.
  - Use—commonly used to support cardiac output in neonates, infants, and children after heart surgery and in other etiologies resulting in decreased cardiac output (e.g., septic shock). Milrinone increases cardiac output through increasing contractility, reducing systemic and PVR, and decreasing preload.
  - Dose—loading dose of 50 mcg/kg followed by continuous infusion of 0.25 to 0.75 mcg/kg/minute. Loading dose should be administered over at least 15 minutes. A loading dose is not used at all centers.
  - Patients with renal failure have decreased clearance of milrinone; dose adjustment is required based on creatinine clearance.
  - May increase risk of arrhythmias.
  - Milrinone has a long half-life.

Vasodilators

- Sodium Nitroprusside—potent vasodilator via direct action on venous and arterial smooth muscle. Decreases afterload.
  - Use: hypertensive crisis (variety of etiologies). Commonly used after open heart surgery for BP control.

- Dose: continuous infusion of 0.5 to 10 mcg/kg/minute. Start at low dose and titrate to effect.
- Doses above 1.8 mcg/kg/minute have been associated with elevated cyanide levels in children. Monitor cyanide levels to evaluate risk of toxicity.
- Nicardipine—calcium channel antagonist causing vasodilation with minimal negative inotropic effects.
  - Use: short-term treatment of hypertension when oral medications are not tolerated.
  - Dose: continuous infusion of 0.5 to 5 mcg/kg/minute. Titrate to effect.
  - Limited data are available for the use of nicardipine in children.
  - Nicardipine has been found to be as effective as Nitroprusside in adults.
- Esmolol—β-receptor antagonist that is cardioselective, titratable, and has a short duration of action.
  - Use: hypertension, supraventricular tachycardia, and sinus tachycardia.
  - Dose: starting dose continuous infusion of 50 to 75 mcg/kg/minute.
    - In neonates <1 month of age, titrating by 25 to 50 mcg/kg/minute every 20 minutes to desired BP. Starting dose of 100 to 150 mcg/kg/minute in children >1 month of age to 12 years of age, titrating 50 to 100 mcg/kg/minute every 10 minutes to desired BP. Maximum dose 1,000 mcg/kg/minute.
    - Contraindicated in patients with bradycardia; esmolol will decrease heart rate.
    - Use with caution in patients with asthma; risk of bronchospasm.
- Fenoldopam—selective dopamine agonist resulting in vasodilation induces diuresis and natriuresis in the kidneys.
  - Use: treatment of hypertension, increasing creatinine clearance in renal impairment. Also used to prevent and treat acute kidney injury and decreased urine output.
  - Dose: initial dose: continuous infusion of 0.2 mcg/kg/minute. May be increased to 0.3 to 0.5 mcg/kg/minute to a maximum of 0.8 mcg/kg/minute.
  - Use with caution in patients with increased intracranial pressure.

Pacemakers
Elizabeth R. Prentice

Definition

- Cardiac pacing: temporary or permanent pacing leads to sense intrinsic cardiac activity and provide an electrical stimulus to the heart (atrium, ventricle, or both) if no intrinsic cardiac activity is detected.
  - Most commonly used for patients with sinus node dysfunction or atrioventricular block.

- Temporary Pacing: the use of esophageal, epicardial, transvenous, or transcutaneous pacing in patients with unstable arrhythmias.
  - All types of temporary pacing require leads to be connected to an external pacing device.
- Esophageal pacing: A pacing catheter is passed through the nose and into the esophagus, posterior to the LA. Used mainly for atrial overdrive pacing to terminate supraventricular tachycardia.
- Epicardial pacing: used primarily after cardiac surgery. Pacing leads are secured to the epicardial surface of the heart with sutures and directed out through the skin. By convention, atrial wires should always arise from the right side of the chest, and ventricular wires from the left side of the chest.
- Transcutaneous pacing: temporary pacing pads are placed on the chest and back. These pads can also be used for cardioversion or defibrillation.
- Transvenous pacing: requires central venous access through the femoral, internal jugular, or subclavian vein. Pacing catheters are then directed to the endocardial surface of the RV.
- Permanent pacemaker: battery-powered device that is implanted in the chest or abdomen.
  - Pacing leads are generally connected to the epicardial surface of the heart.
  - Transvenous leads can also be used if scarring from cardiac surgery prevents use of epicardial leads.
- Pacemakers can be single or dual-chamber devices.
  - Nomenclature.
    - Standard for all pacemakers to describe type and function.
      - First letter: chamber paced.
        - V = Ventricle.
        - A = Atrium.
        - D = Dual (Both A and V).
        - O = None.
      - Second letter: chamber sensed (V, A, D, O).
      - Third letter: response to sensed event.
        - D = Dual (trigger and inhibit pacing).
        - I = Inhibit pacing.
        - O = None (no response by pacemaker).
      - Example: AAI Pacing.
        - Pacemaker paces the atrium, senses the atrium, and inhibits pacing when an intrinsic atrial contraction is sensed.
- Pacemaker Settings.
  - Mode (DDD, AAI, etc.).
    - The mode selected is dependent on the patient's intrinsic rhythm and whether conduction through the AV node is intact.
      - Example: If complete heart block is present, both the atrium and ventricle will need to be paced in order to provide AV (atrial ventricular) synchrony and improve cardiac output. Therefore, DDD mode would be selected.
  - Rate: dependent on patient age and underlying rhythm. Typically, set at 10 to 20 beats per minute above the intrinsic heart rate to avoid competition.
  - A-output (atrial output): Value selected is dependent on pacing threshold (i.e., the lowest output that consistently causes depolarization of the atrium). Output is usually set at twice the pacing threshold.
- V-output (ventricular output): determined based on the pacing threshold and set at twice the pacing threshold.
- A-V (atrial ventricular) interval: The time from atrial depolarization to ventricular depolarization (i.e., the time from atrial sensing/pacing until ventricular pacing). Actual time is dependent on heart rate.
- A-sensitivity (atrial sensitivity): The degree to which the pacemaker will sense the patient's intrinsic atrial rhythm. A lower sensitivity means the pacemaker is MORE sensitive. Actual setting depends on sensing threshold that is set during pacemaker setup.
- V-sensitivity (ventricular sensitivity): The degree to which the pacemaker will sense the patient's intrinsic ventricular rhythm.
- Upper rate: automatically set at 30 beats per minute. above the set rate. Prevents pacemaker from pacing at very high atrial rates.
- Pacemaker capture.
  - Depolarization of a cardiac chamber (atrium or ventricle) following delivery of a pacing spike.
  - Must be adequate electrical output in order to overcome the depolarization threshold.
  - Pacemaker spike can be visualized on ECG as a thin deflection that occurs prior to the P wave in atrial pacing or prior to the QRS complex in ventricular pacing. DDD pacing will result in 2 pacing spikes if no intrinsic cardiac activity is sensed.
- Pacemaker troubleshooting.
  - Failure to capture: Either complete absence of pacing spikes or spikes that are not followed by cardiac depolarization. Common causes:
    - Lead displacement or disconnection from pacing unit.
    - Pacemaker battery failure.
    - Inappropriately set pacing outputs.
    - Increase in pacing threshold: fibrosis, myocardial ischemia, metabolic abnormalities (e.g., hyperkalemia, acidosis, hypoxemia, hypercarbia), drugs (beta-blockers, class Ia antiarrhythmics, verapamil, flecainide).
  - Failure to sense (undersensing): Pacemaker generates an electrical stimulus with no relation to the patient's intrinsic heart rhythm.
    - Pacing spikes may be seen during the atrial or ventricular refractory period on ECG.
    - Causes: lead displacement or fracture, poor contact with the endocardium, inappropriately set sensitivity, electrolyte imbalances.
  - Failure to pace: A pacemaker spike is not seen even after the set lower heart rate limit has been reached.
  - Oversensing: Pacemaker detects electrical activity that is not originating from the heart and therefore does not generate an output.
    - Can occur due to electrocautery, MRI, myopotentials from skeletal muscle, inappropriately set sensitivity.
    - Other causes: lead displacement or fracture, battery depletion, pulse generator failure.

Implantable Cardioverter Defibrillators (ICD)

Elizabeth R. Prentice

Definition

- An implantable device composed of a pulse generator and one or two leads that is used in patients who are at risk for sudden death due to ventricular tachycardia or ventricular fibrillation.
- All ICDs have a single ventricular lead; an atrial lead can be placed if dual-chamber pacing is needed.
- RV lead is used for sensing ventricular arrhythmias. Shock is delivered between a metal coil in the RV lead and the pulse generator.
- Cardioversion and defibrillation thresholds are set at the time of insertion.

Complications

- Acute: pain, bleeding, pneumothorax, hemothorax, cardiac perforation with or without cardiac tamponade.
- Subacute/long-term: pain, infection, pocket hematoma, wound dehiscence, lead dislodgement/fracture (may lead to inappropriate ICD deactivation), inappropriate shocks (shocking in absence of life-threatening arrhythmia).

Additional Considerations

- If the patient sustains cardiac arrest, chest compressions should be initiated immediately while ICD attempts to shock.
- If ICD is unsuccessful at delivering the shock or the rhythm is refractory to the ICD shocking, proceed with defibrillation with an external device, as needed.
- If rescuers are uncomfortable with the ICD discharge during resuscitation efforts, the device may be deactivated with a magnet (external defibrillator must be immediately available).

Extracorporeal Membrane Oxygenation (ECMO)

Michelle Dokas

Background

- Short-term mechanical support system for severe respiratory and cardiac failure due to a reversible cause that has been refractory to maximal medical support.
- Developed in the early 1970s, progressing from cardiopulmonary bypass in the operating room.

Definition

- System consisting of draining deoxygenated blood from a venous access cannula to a venous drainage reservoir, pumping through a roller or centrifugal pump to a membrane oxygenator where gas exchange occurs, then returning oxygenated blood to the patient.

Types

- Venoarterial (V-A) ECMO—provides biventricular and pulmonary support. Venous access is accomplished either through direct cannulation of the RA through a median sternotomy or through cannulation of the right internal jugular vein. In older children and adults, the femoral vessels may be used. Arterial access is achieved through cannulation of the aorta during surgery or through cannulation of the carotid or femoral artery. Transthoracic cannulation is the method used for patients who are unable to wean off cardiopulmonary bypass in the operating room.
- Venovenous (V-V) ECMO—provides respiratory support but no direct cardiac support. Blood is drained from a large central vein such as the internal jugular or femoral veins, and returned to the venous circulation after passing through the ECMO circuit. This requires the patient to have adequate cardiac function to perfuse the body with oxygenated blood.

Indications

- Respiratory failure without desired response to conventional support.
- Reversible cardiac failure with expected recovery in 5 to 14 days due to surgical or medical etiology (cardiomyopathy, myocarditis, refractory arrhythmias).
- Cardiopulmonary arrest.
- Bridge to cardiac transplantation.

Contraindications (Some are Institution-Specific)

- Gestational age ≤34 weeks.
- Weight <2 kg.
- Irreversible cardiac failure.
- Severe neurologic dysfunction.
- Severe coagulopathy.
- Multisystem organ failure.
- Sepsis (some cases); although ECMO has been used to treat severe sepsis.
- Lethal congenital anomalies.

Management

- Requires extensive knowledge and understanding of the ECMO circuit, the patient's underlying cardiac anatomy, surgical correction (if applicable), and goals for recovery of the patient's cardiac function.
- The team approach should be used, including medical, surgical, nursing, and ECMO pump technicians' expertise when managing these patients.
- LA decompression: Patients with poor LV function on ECMO can develop over distension of the LA causing pulmonary edema or hemorrhage, mitral regurgitation, and poor coronary perfusion. When this occurs, the left side of the heart must be decompressed. This can be accomplished either through direct cannulation of the LA, with a connection to the venous cannula, or through atrial septostomy in the cardiac catheterization lab.
- Hemodynamic support: ECMO flows must be adjusted to obtain adequate cardiac output and systemic BP. Fluid balance must be monitored to maintain adequate preload. Multiple blood products are usually required in the form of packed red blood

cells and platelets. Inotropic support is usually required in low doses. Arrhythmias should be treated aggressively.

- ECMO circuit requires anticoagulation due to the extracorporeal circuit. Heparin is most often used. Activated clotting times (ACT) are followed closely with a goal of maintaining the ACT between 180 and 200. Platelets can be sequestered in the oxygenator of the circuit; therefore, the patient's platelet level must be followed closely and treated if $<100,000/mm^3$. Clotting factors should also be followed and treated appropriately. The patient must be closely monitored for bleeding.

- Ventilator management: Strategies should be used that adequately ventilate the lungs and avoid barotrauma and atelectasis. Lung rest strategies are controversial.

- Fluid balance and nutrition: These patients have high insensible losses due to the extracorporeal circuit and exposure. They also require adequate nutrition, especially if they have undergone a cardiac surgical repair. Most patients require total parental nutrition to meet metabolic demands. Trophic feeding can be utilized and advanced to caloric goals in some patients.

- Infection: These patients are at high risk for hospital-acquired infections from the number of invasive devices for cardiopulmonary support. ECMO cannulas, open chest, central lines, endotracheal tube, foley catheters are all potential sources of infection. Broad-spectrum antibiotics should be used, daily blood cultures should be sent, and any positive culture should be treated aggressively.

- Analgesia and sedation: It is essential to adequately sedate these patients to avoid dislodgement of cannulas. Usually, this is done with narcotic analgesia and sedative infusions such as morphine, fentanyl, and versed. Neuromuscular blockade can be used, although the clinician must be able to assess the patient's neurologic status. Daily head ultrasounds are recommended for infants with an open fontanel to monitor for intracranial hemorrhage.

PEARLS
Extracorporeal cardiac arrest is an expanding area of mechanical circulatory support. This intervention consists of mobilizing the ECMO team after 10 minutes of unsuccessful standard cardiopulmonary resuscitation with the primary goal of establishing cardiac output. This necessitates the rapid deployment of an ECMO team and a pump primed with a crystalloid solution. Some institutions have modified ECMO circuits with small tubing and prime volumes for this purpose. Patients require transition to a traditional circuit if resuscitation efforts are successful.

Ventricular Assist Devices (VAD)

Michelle Dokas

Background

- Circulatory pump devices are of several different types: rotary/centrifugal devices similar to pumps used on ECMO,

axial devices consisting of a magnetically suspended rotating impeller driven by an electric motor, or a pneumatic pulsatile system. VAD systems are preferred for patients who do not require pulmonary support, both short- and long-term.

- Do not require immobilization and promote rehabilitation as patients can ambulate after the initial postoperative recovery period.

- Pediatric VAD support is a developing field and is variable from institution to institution.

Definition

- Mechanical device providing long- or short-term circulatory support without pulmonary support. Most devices require a sternotomy approach for cannulation, although a few percutaneous systems are available for older adolescents. Type of support is determined by origin of heart failure.

Types

- Left ventricular assist device (LVAD): indicated for support of left side of the heart. Cannulation is accomplished via the LA for venous drainage, and the aorta for arterial return, thus "bypassing" the left side of the heart.

- Right ventricular assist device (RVAD): indicated for support of the right side of the heart. Cannulation is accomplished through the RA for venous drainage, and the PA for arterial return, thus "bypassing" the right side of the heart.

- Biventricular assist device (BiVAD): indicated for support of both ventricles. Cannulation is accomplished through the RA for venous drainage and the aorta for arterial return.

Indications

- Bridge to cardiac transplantation.

- Patients with end-stage cardiomyopathy related to congenital or acquired heart failure often require mechanical support until a heart becomes available.

- Bridge to recovery—patients with acute fulminant myocarditis may require mechanical support until heart function recovers.

- Bridge to decision—VAD allows time for patients with severe cardiovascular compromise to determine potential for recovery or cardiac transplantation status.

- Clear goals and end points should be determined before the initiation of VAD support.

Contraindications

- Very low birth weight <1.5 kg, although size of the pump must be considered. Currently, the smallest pump available is a 10 mL pump from Berlin Heart EXCOR⁻.

- Extreme prematurity.

- Chromosomal abnormalities.

- Severe neurologic injury.

- Other considerations: multisystem organ failure, sepsis, severe lung disease.

Management

- Surgical procedure for insertion on most pediatric patients requires cardiopulmonary bypass and hypothermia.

- Anticoagulation: All patients with a VAD require anticoagulation to prevent thrombus formation in the VAD system. Each institution has its own protocol that usually involves a combination of anticoagulant medications.

- General considerations: Adequate nutrition must be provided for growth and healing, usually of the enteral route. Physical and Occupational therapy should be instituted early; patients will not have limited mobility after the initial postoperative period.

Complications

- Postoperative bleeding.
- Neurologic events.
- Infection.
- Thromboembolism.

Cardiac Transplantation

Jennifer L. Joiner

Definition

- Donor heart is transplanted into similar aged recipient in end-stage heart failure when all medical therapy and other surgical options have failed.

Etiology/Types

- Orthotopic
  - Biatrial: Anastomosis of the donor and recipient aorta, pulmonary arteries and atrial cuffs. This technique has higher incidence of thrombus, arrhythmias, conduction problems, and valve regurgitation.
  - Bicaval.
    - Donor RA is preserved with separate caval anastomoses allowing a normal atrial shape, while the LA is separated with small cuffs around the pulmonary veins.
    - This technique has less SA node dysfunction, tachyarrhythmias, tricuspid regurgitation, less need for pacemaker assistance, and better hemodynamics.
  - Heterotopic.
    - Not widely used in pediatrics.
    - This technique preserves the recipient's RV and can be useful in patients who are used to having high RV pressure (pulmonary hypertension).
    - The donor has the systemic veins closed with connection to the PA.

Clinical Presentation

- One-third of all transplants are done on infants <1 year of age due to congenital heart defects.
- In older children, over half of transplants occur secondary to cardiomyopathy.

- As children age, this cause steadily increases over congenital heart defects.
- Symptoms of heart failure that are unresponsive to therapy.
  - Growth failure.
  - Need for inotropic or pulmonary support.
  - Malignant arrhythmias and complete deterioration of ventricular function may also be present.

Diagnostic Evaluation

- Extensive evaluations exist for cardiac transplant recipients prior to transplant.
- Cardiac catheterization is done to assess hemodynamics, anatomy, and PVR.
- Additional cardiac evaluation may include:
  - Echocardiogram.
  - ECG.
  - Cardiac MRI/MRA.
  - Exercise testing.
- End-organ function evaluated with laboratory evaluation of:
  - Complete blood count (CBC).
  - Coagulation panel.
  - Renal function panel.
  - Hepatic function/Liver function tests.
  - Lipid profile.
  - Pulmonary function testing.
  - Immunologic and Infectious testing for:
    - Cytomegalovirus (CMV).
    - Epstein Barr Virus (EBV).
    - Herpes Simplex Virus (HSV).
    - Human Immunodeficiency Virus (HIV).
    - Varicella.
    - Toxoplasmosis.
    - Hepatitis.
    - Tuberculosis.
    - Viral serologies.
    - HLA typing.
    - Panel Reactive Antibody (PRA).
      - Measure of the percentage of human antibodies in the transplant candidate's blood.
    - Isohemagglutinin titers.
  - Psychosocial and financial evaluation.

Management

- The first 72 hours post–transplant remain the most critical.
- Primary management goals are to:
  - Maintain coronary perfusion.
  - Maintain systemic BP.
  - Ensure appropriate cardiac output.
  - Initiate immunosuppression.
  - Reasons for early transplant failure are primary graft failure and right heart failure that is associated with elevated PVR.

1. Inotropes should be avoided in patients with which of the following diagnoses:
   a. Dilated cardiomyopathy.
   b. Septic shock.
   c. Hypoplastic left heart syndrome following Stage I surgical repair.
   d. Hypertrophic cardiomyopathy.

Answer: **D**

Inotropes should be avoided in patients with hypertrophic cardiomyopathy. Enhancing systolic function with inotropes can lead to worsening LV outflow tract obstruction and impaired filling in hypertrophic cardiomyopathy.

2. A 4-year-old who was recently diagnosed with asthma presents to the emergency department (ED) with shortness of breath and difficulty breathing. On examination, inspiratory wheezes and a gallop rhythm are noted. The liver is palpated 4 cm below the right costal margin. The most appropriate intervention is:
   a. Place patient on continuous pulse oximeter and nonrebreather mask, and order an albuterol inhaler.
   b. Place patient on continuous cardiorespiratory monitoring, order an ECG and echocardiogram, and request a cardiology consult.
   c. Order a furosemide 1 mg/kg intravenous and reevaluate in 1 hour.
   d. Order a chest radiograph and request a pulmonology consult.

Answer: **B**

"Cardiac wheezing" is often misdiagnosed as asthma. A gallop rhythm and hepatosplenomegaly are all common presentations of restrictive cardiomyopathy. Initial plan of care for the diagnosis of a cardiomyopathy includes ECG, echocardiogram, continuous cardiorespiratory monitoring, and cardiology consult.

3. Which of the following genetic/metabolic diagnoses raises the most concern for development of a cardiomyopathy, requiring close follow-up by cardiology?
   a. Pompe disease.
   b. Maple syrup urine disease.
   c. Galactosemia.
   d. Turner syndrome.

Answer: **A**

Infiltration of the myocardium occurs in a variety of cardiomyopathies. Pompe disease (a glycogen storage disorder) causes severe hypertrophic cardiomyopathy and is usually fatal in infancy.

4. A 15-year-old presents to the ED with sharp chest pain that is worse on inspiration. Cardiac examination reveals a friction rub on auscultation and a temperature of 38.6°C orally. What is the most likely diagnosis?
   a. Myocarditis.
   b. Pericarditis.
   c. Endocarditis.
   d. Dilated cardiomyopathy.

Answer: **B**

Precordial chest pain exacerbated by respiration is the most commonly reported symptom of pericarditis. Fever is also a common presenting sign of acute pericarditis. The presence of a friction rub strongly suggests a pericardial effusion.

5. Which of the following patients is at highest risk for developing infectious endocarditis:
   a. 7-year-old with asthma.
   b. 5-year-old with history of a repaired ventricular septal defect.
   c. 3-year-old with a prosthetic mitral valve.
   d. 17-year-old with a history of meningitis.

Answer: **C**

The following factors are associated with the highest risk of developing infectious endocarditis: prosthetic valves, previous episode of endocarditis, complex cyanotic CHD, surgically placed systemic-to-pulmonary shunts, injection drug use, and indwelling central catheters.

6. Intravenous immunoglobulin (IVIG) is recommended for the treatment of which of the following diagnoses:
   a. Myocarditis.
   b. Endocarditis.
   c. Dilated cardiomyopathy.
   d. Anomalous origin of the left coronary artery.

Answer: **A**

Administration of intravenous immunoglobulin (IVIG) may be beneficial if administered in the initial phases of myocarditis. IVIG administration is not recommended in endocarditis, dilated cardiomyopathy, or anomalous origin of the left coronary artery.

CASE (REFERS TO NEXT THREE QUESTIONS):

A 6-year-old female is brought to the ED. She has had flulike symptoms for the past 3 days with fever and vomiting. On examination, she is lethargic with the following vital signs: Temperature 37.9°C, HR 165, RR 58, and BP 74/31 mmHg. Her extremities are cold with poor pulses and prolonged capillary refill. Jugular vein distension is noted. Lung sounds include rales and wheezing bilaterally with intercostal retractions. Liver is palpable 4 cm below the right costal margin.

7. What are the best initial steps in managing this child?
   a. Albuterol inhalation treatment, 20 mL/kg fluid bolus, observe in ED
   b. Intubation, 20 mL/kg/fluid bolus, vasopressin infusion at 0.3 mu/kg/minute, and transfer to pediatric intensive care unit.
   c. 100% oxygen by nonrebreather mask, 5 mL/kg fluid bolus repeated if needed, dobutamine infusion at 3 mcg/kg/minute, milrinone at 0.5 mcg/kg/minute, and transfer to the pediatric intensive care unit.
   d. Blow-by 100% oxygen, 20 mL/kg fluid bolus, and observe in the ED.

Answer: **C**

This patient has classic history, signs, and symptoms of acute viral myocarditis causing right and left-sided heart failure. Fluids must be administered judiciously as the child has a history of vomiting and is intravascularly depleted. Fluid boluses of 20 mL/kg would increase the work on the failing heart. Inotropy is needed when hypotension is present. Afterload reduction is the cornerstone of therapy for myocarditis, achieved in this case with milrinone. This child requires monitoring and management in the Pediatric Intensive Care Unit.

8. The patient discussed in the question above has the following arterial blood gas: pH 7.26, pCO_2 32 mmHg, pO_2 85 mmHg, O_2 saturation 95%, HCO_3 20 mEq/L with a base deficit of 6 mmol/L, and a lactate of 5 mg/dL. She is intubated and has a central line placed. Fluid resuscitation has been accomplished, and dobutamine at 8 mcg/kg/minute, milrinone at 0.5 mcg/kg/minute, epinephrine at 0.2 mcg/kg/minute, and norepinephrine at 0.1 mcg/kg/minute are infusing. Her pulse is 158 beats per minute, and her BP is 75/29 mmHg. Her CVP is 19 cm H_2O. She has not had urine output. The next step in her care is:
   a. Consult the ECMO (Extracorporeal Membrane Oxygenation) team for Venoarterial ECMO.
   b. Consult the ECMO team for Venovenous ECMO.
   c. Consult Pediatric Cardiovascular Surgery for VAD placement.
   d. Give another 20 cc/kg fluid bolus, increase the norepinephrine, and increase the rate on the ventilator for the acidosis.

Answer: A

This child is now in potentially reversible, severe, acute heart failure. Her cardiac output is compromised despite maximal inotropic support, now requiring mechanical cardiac support through Venoarterial (VA) ECMO. Venovenous (VV) ECMO is not indicated since she requires circulatory support that VV ECMO cannot provide. VAD placement requires more planning time and is optimally done when the patient is stable enough to go to the operating room. VA ECMO can be done percutaneously at the bedside. The patient is in metabolic acidosis, and, therefore, increasing the rate on the ventilator is contraindicated, as is giving more fluid to this failing heart.

Ongoing case from Question 7
This child has now been on VenoArterial ECMO for 5 days, yet has not been able to be weaned. She is neurologically intact and is on low ventilator settings. She has been hemodynamically stable, has capillary refill <3 seconds, and has adequate urine output. She is on dobutamine at 3 mcg/kg/minute and milrinone of 0.5 mcg/kg/minute.

9. What is the next course of action?
   a. Initiate a family meeting to discuss withdrawing care.
   b. Consult pediatric cardiovascular surgery for VAD placement.
   c. Maximize inotropic support and discontinue ECMO.
   d. Consult the pediatric heart transplant team.

Answer: **B**

Up to 1/3 of children with viral myocarditis will make a full recovery. Withdrawing support is not indicated at this time. Discontinuing ECMO without tolerating a weaning of support would be fatal. This child remains in the acute phase of her illness, so transplantation is not appropriate at this time. Transition to a VAD would allow her to bridge to recovery or bridge to transplantation. She may be awake and extubated after the surgery, allowing her to be mobile and to interact with her therapies as her condition allows.

(The next two questions refer to the following scenario)
A 6-year-old with a history of mitral stenosis that was repaired in infancy presents to the emergency department (ED) with a 2-week history of upper respiratory symptoms, lethargy, and poor oral intake. Physical examination findings reveal a very thin, pale male with circumoral cyanosis, a gallop rhythm, a normal S_1, but narrowly split S_2, holosystolic murmur at the left lower sternal border (LLSB), moderate intercostal retractions with coarse rhonchi bilaterally, and a liver edge 4 cm below the right costal margin. Vital signs are: HR of 140, RR of 36, BP of 82/56 mmHg, and an oxygen saturation of 92%. Chest radiograph reveals cardiomegaly, dilated PA silhouette, and bilateral pulmonary congestion. An echocardiogram reveals a 4 mmHg gradient across the mitral valve, right and left atrial dilation, RVH, moderate tricuspid regurgitation, and a RV pressure estimate of 80/15 mmHg.

10. What is the most likely diagnosis?
    a. Pulmonary hypertension.
    b. Viral myocarditis.
    c. Interstitial lung disease.
    d. Cardiomyopathy.

Answer: **A**

Although the clinical presentation may present as any one of the above diagnoses, the additional information suggests that the patient is displaying signs and symptoms of pulmonary

(continues on page 170)

hypertension. Residual mitral stenosis causes backup of blood in the LA, resulting in LA hypertension and pulmonary congestion. Long-standing pulmonary congestion can result in changes in the pulmonary vasculature and elevated PA pressures. The echocardiogram results indicate the presence of pulmonary hypertension with tricuspid regurgitation, RA dilation, RV hypertrophy, and a RV pressure estimate that is equivalent to systemic.

11. Which of the following diagnostic tests would best determine the diagnosis for the child in the scenario above?
    a. Viral PCR serology.
    b. Chest magnetic resonance imaging.
    c. Right heart catheterization.
    d. Cardiac biopsy.

Answer: **C**

This child has pulmonary hypertension, and a cardiac catheterization is the best choice to confirm the diagnosis. It allows for the pressure and oxygen saturation measurements of the pulmonary arteries and calculation of PVR and cardiac index.

12. A newborn weighing 3.2 kg returns to the ICU following repair of truncus arteriosus and is intubated, sedated, on milrinone of 0.5 mcg/kg/minute, dopamine at 3 mcg/kg/minute, and inhaled nitric oxide at 40 ppm. Ventilator settings: tidal volume = 30 mL; rate = 30, PEEP = 5 cm H_2O, pressure support = 8 cm H_2O, FiO_2 1.0. VS are: HR of 160, BP of 72/38 mmHg, RV pressure of 6 mmHg, and oxygen saturation of 100%. Chest tube output is 2 mL/kg/hour. 4 hours later, the patient is gray, cool, and mottled after being turned and suctioned. Heart rate is 100 beats per minute; BP is 45/25 mmHg, RA pressure is 14 mmHg, and pulse oximetry reading is 50%, although the waveform is dampened. Chest tube output is 1 mL/kg/hour. In addition to bagging the patient with 100% oxygen and giving 10 mL/kg of normal saline, what should be the next intervention?
    a. Administer additional sedation, and give a muscle relaxant.
    b. Increase the dopamine drip, and administer an isuprel bolus.
    c. Obtain a chest radiograph to evaluate endotracheal tube placement.
    d. Obtain an echocardiogram to evaluate pericardial effusion.

Answer: **B**

The patient in this scenario is exhibiting signs of a pulmonary hypertensive crisis. This patient was already at risk for RV dysfunction and elevated PVR due to the type of surgical repair, and need for cardiopulmonary bypass. Based on the changes in hemodynamic parameters and oxygen saturation, the patient's PVR is critically high, resulting in poor forward flow of blood from the RV to the lungs. The patient is in immediate danger of suffering cardiopulmonary collapse. Isuprel is a potent pulmonary vasodilator that can be used to decrease PVR, and dopamine will support RV function.

13. A 6-year-old who has idiopathic pulmonary hypertension is admitted to the ICU for increased work of breathing, lethargy, increased cyanosis, nausea, vomiting, and anorexia. Laboratory results reveal: BUN = 42 mg/dL, creatinine = 1 mg/dL, basic natriuretic peptide = 890 pg/mL, ALT = 1,550 IU/L, AST = 2,100 IU/L. Vital signs reveal: HR of 80 beats per minute, RR of 36 breaths per minute, BP of 85/54 mmHg, and oxygen saturation of 95% on 2 liters nasal cannula. The patient is currently on Sildenafil 10 mg twice a day, Bosentan 62.5 mg twice a day, and Epoprostenol at 45 ng/kg/minute. The dose of Epoprostenol has been gradually decreased from 60 ng/kg/minute due to intolerance. An echocardiogram obtained upon admission revealed worsening LA dilation and RV dysfunction, RVH, moderate tricuspid regurgitation, and a suprasystemic RV pressure estimate, and a cardiac catheterization is scheduled for the next day. Which of the following management strategies would be the best option?
    a. Start a milrinone infusion.
    b. Decrease the Epoprostenol drip rate.
    c. Switch prostacyclin agent to Iloprost.
    d. Start a Dopamine infusion.

Answer: **D**

The patient in this scenario is exhibiting signs of worsening failure and side effects of the current medical therapy. The best option is to start a dopamine infusion for right heart failure. A milrinone infusion could further exacerbate the patient's renal dysfunction.

14. A 10-year-old with new-onset heart failure will have a diagnostic endomyocardial biopsy (EMB). What is the most common complication from this procedure?
    a. Perforation.
    b. Arrhythmia.
    c. Tricuspid damage.
    d. Emboli.

Answer: **A**

In children with thin ventricular walls, as seen in heart failure, there is a greater risk of ventricular wall perforation. During EMB, providers need to obtain a minimum of a 1 mm diameter tissue sample that may lead to perforation in patients with thin myocardial walls. Arrhythmias, tricuspid damage, and emboli may occur, but are very rarely associated with EMB.

15. A cardiac transplant patient has grade 3A rejection found on endomyocardial biopsy (EMB). What initial antirejection medication will be started?
    a. Methylprednisolone.
    b. ATG (Antithymocyte antibody).
    c. Intravenous immunoglobulin (IVIG).
    d. Azathioprine.

Answer: **A**

Methylprednisolone is the initial antirejection medication. Rejection treatment is based on the grade of rejection found in EMB. In grade 1, no acute treatment is started, but nearly 25% of patients will progress to a higher grade. With grade 3 or higher rejection, antirejection therapy is started with methylprednisolone or prednisone with a 2-week taper. If rejection does not respond to steroids, then more aggressive treatments will be initiated to include ATG or monoclonal antibody treatment with Orthoclone OKT3. Azathioprine management not indicated in transplant rejection.

16. A critically ill child in heart failure has suspected myocarditis. What type of sample obtained at the bedside can show strong correlation to support this diagnosis?
   a. Tracheal aspirate.
   b. Endomyocardial biopsy (EMB).
   c. Blood culture.
   d. Cardiac enzymes.

Answer: **A**

PCR detection of viral genomes in tracheal aspirates has shown a strong correlation with the diagnosis of myocarditis. EMB remains the diagnostic study of choice, but is not without risk in the critically ill child, and is not done at the bedside. Blood culture does not support the diagnosis of myocarditis. Cardiac enzymes are elevated in myocarditis, but are not specific and are only trended to monitor for myocardial inflammation.

17. A neonate is being prepared for a cardiac catheterization and is receiving a prostaglandin infusion. What is the most troublesome side effect of this medication?
   a. Apnea.
   b. Hypertension.
   c. Hives.
   d. Vomiting.

Answer: **A**

Apnea is a known and concerning side effect of prostaglandin infusion and may occur at any time during its use. It can cause wide respiratory fluctuations that are not well tolerated by infants and may progress to respiratory failure. Prostaglandins can also cause flushing and hypotension; however, hypertension, hives, and vomiting are not typically associated with prostaglandin infusion.

18. A newborn with suspected CHD has signs of ischemia on ECG and a nondiagnostic echocardiogram. Cardiac catheterization is most sensitive in which congenital heart defect?
   a. Anomalous left coronary artery from the pulmonary artery (ALCAPA).
   b. Total anomalous pulmonary venous return (TAPVR).
   c. Coronary sinus defect.
   d. Coronary artery vasculopathy.

Answer: **A**

ALCAPA is a congenital malformation where coronary artery insufficiency may occur and cause cardiogenic shock in the neonatal period. There are few indications when a cardiac catheterization is essential except in the case of the anomalous left coronary from the pulmonary artery (ALPACA). Other modalities may suggest the diagnosis; however, catheterization with direct root angiography is the most sensitive.

19. An infant on near-infrared spectroscopy (NIRS) monitoring has impedance to readings. What is the most likely cause?
   a. Hair.
   b. Skin.
   c. Bone.
   d. Bilirubin.

Answer: **A**

Melanin pigmentation found in hair attenuates light transmission and impedes NIRS measurements. Melanin found in the skin is confined to the epidermal layer and therefore does not appear to alter NIRS readings. Bilirubin may dampen NIRS readings but does not cause impedance to readings. Optimal placement of the NIRS is high on the frontal eminences above the orbital ridge bone away from the sinuses.

20. A child who has undergone successful Fontan repair is complaining of dyspnea with exercise. What abnormality is the most likely cause of this problem?
   a. Stroke volume.
   b. ST segment changes.
   c. Hypoxemia.
   d. Minute ventilation.

Answer: **A**

In children who have had successful Fontan repair, exercise capacity improves, but remains less than normal. The main reasons for these abnormalities are subnormal heart rate with exercise due to sinus node dysfunction, abnormal stroke volume due to reduced systemic ventricular function, and cardiac arrythmias. In cyanotic congenital heart lesions, hypoxemia and impaired minute ventilation can limit exercise capacity but is not the most likely cause.

21. During exercise stress testing, what other measurement correlates the most when the maximum heart rate in boys and girls is reached?
   a. Oxygen consumption.
   b. Blood pressure.
   c. O₂ saturations.
   d. Respiratory rate.

Answer: **A**

A heart rate of 180 to 200 beats per minute in both boys and girls correlates with maximum oxygen consumption, and all efforts during stress testing should be made to get children to that heart rate. The goal heart rate is calculated with the equation: Peak HR= 220—age in years. Inadequate heart rate increments are seen in sinus node dysfunction (e.g., after Fontan, TOF repair, or Senning procedure). Impairment in chronotropic function is important information to providers as it significantly decreases aerobic capacity and limits exercise ability. BP and respiratory rate fluctuations do not always correlate with maximum heart rate, and oxygen saturations can fall near the normal 90% range at full exercise or go lower in patients with hypoxia during exercise.

(continues on page 172)

22. An infant is postoperative from a transposition of the great arteries (TGA) repair and has done well after extubation 2 days ago, but remains tachypneic with diminished breath sounds on the left side. What study will confirm the diagnosis of pleural effusion?
    a. Right lateral decubitus.
    b. Left lateral decubitus.
    c. Supine CXR.
    d. Prone CXR.

Answer: **B**

To diagnose pleural effusion a lateral chest radiograph will show the dependent layering of fluid. The lateral film is named according to the side that is dependent (down), so in this case, it would be a left lateral decubitus. On a supine film, free fluid appears as an opacification of the lung fields and can look like pulmonary congestion or may be demonstrated as blunted costophrenic angles. On an upright film, even small fluid collections can obscure the costophrenic angle, and larger effusions will cause the diaphragm to appear elevated. In these cases, upright or lateral films should be obtained to elucidate the pleural effusion.

23. When initiating oral feedings on an infant with a chylothorax, a formula that contains which of the following types of fat is recommended?
    a. Medium chain.
    b. Very long chain.
    c. Long chain.
    d. Omega-3 fatty acid.

Answer: **A**

Not all fats require the lymph system for absorption. Medium chain triglycerides (MCT) travel along the GI tract into the portal system and the liver bypassing the lymph system. MCT do not produce chyle and can be consumed by infants with impaired chylus drainage. In most instances, infants are placed on total parenteral nutrition (TPN) and a formula that has MCT only or on TPN with intralipis (IL) as their fat source.

24. An infant with persistent chylothorax is scheduled for pleurodesis. What is the goal of this procedure?
    a. Adhere visceral and parietal pleura.
    b. Minimize chylus output.
    c. Evacuate loculated chylus effusions.
    d. Removal of thoracic duct.

Answer: **A**

Chemical or mechanical pleurodesis is completed when chylothorax is resistant to conservative management. During pleurodesis the visceral and parietal pleura are adhered together so the space between them cannot be occupied with chyle. This obliteration of space sends the fluid on the normal path and promotes its natural drainage. Minimizing chyle output is done before surgery to promote a better outcome. The thoracic duct may be ligated during surgery and evacuation of loculated collections may be done, but it is not the goal during pleurodesis.

25. What is the most likely infectious agent in a postop cardiac transplant patient?
    a. Cytomegalovirus (CMV).
    b. Herpes Simplex Virus (HSV).
    c. Epstein Barr Virus (EBV).
    d. Pneumocystis pneumonia PCP.

Answer: **A**

CMV is a major cause of morbidity and mortality in all patients who have solid organ transplant, and remains the most common infectious agent in pediatric cardiac transplant patients. CMV can lead to the development of acute rejection, posttransplant lymphoproliferative disorder (PTLD), and cardiac allograft vasculopathy (CAV). The highest risk recipients are those who were seronegative and received a heart from a seropositive donor, and those recipients who were sero-positive and received antilymphocytic therapy.

26. A patient who is postop from a cardiac transplant has posttransplant lymphoproliferative disease (PTLD). What is the first-line treatment for this patient?
    a. Reduced immunosuppression.
    b. Chemotherapy.
    c. Monoclonal antibodies.
    d. Antivirals.

Answer: **A**

Diagnosing PTLD is based on rising EBV, tissue sampling histology with staging based on CT scans, bone marrow aspirate, and lumbar puncture. Management is always in conjunction with a pediatric oncologist, and their first-line treatment will be to reduce immunosuppression medications and monitor for rejection. More aggressive treatment will be considered and may include chemotherapy, radiation therapy, tumor debulking, antiviral agents, and monoclonal antibody administration.

27. An infant is eligible to receive an ABO-incompatible heart transplant. What is the benefit of this?
    a. Shorter wait.
    b. Decreased incidence of rejection.
    c. Less ischemia.
    d. Longer survival.

Answer: **A**

Organ donors of appropriate size and blood type for infants are limited in number. Since newborns do not produce isohemagglutinins and their complement system is not fully functional, it allows ABO-incompatible transplants to be performed up to 1 year of age (some even up to 15 months of age). The greatest advantage is that smaller, sicker recipients will have a shorter time to transplant since they can receive any ABO type. Ischemia time for donor hearts is kept to <6 hours and has nothing to do with ABO typing. Data for rejection and long-term survival does not show a difference in infants receiving ABO-compatible or incompatible transplants.

The following stem relates to the following two questions:
A 6-month-old infant undergoes ventricular septal defect
(VSD) surgical repair. 6 hours after surgery, he becomes pro-
gressively tachycardic, hypotensive, with an elevated CVP.
He had a modest response to a total of 20 mL/kg of volume
resuscitation. Mediastinal tube output has been zero in the
last 2 hours. His peripheries are cooler than previous, and
urine output tapered off.

28. The most likely cause of this deterioration is:
    a. Inadequate sedation and analgesia.
    b. Cardiac tamponade secondary to blood clot obstructing
       mediastinal tube drainage.
    c. High ventilator pressure impeding venous blood return.
    d. Tachyarrhythmia causing low cardiac output syndrome.

Answer: **B**

It is very important to ensure that the mediastinal and pleural tubes
are under continuous low suction and intermittently stripped, so
encourage drainage in postoperative cardiac surgery patients. The
drainage should be closely monitored. Excessive drainage as well
as sudden cessation of drainage is cause for alarm. In this case, the
most likely etiology of the child's deterioration in status is cardiac
tamponade as a result of a blocked/clotted mediastinal tube.

29. In the above patient, the care team suspects a cardiac tampon-
    ade. Of the following, which would be the best immediate
    action in the management of this patient:
    a. Perform needle pericardiocentesis.
    b. Strip the mediastinal tube, and watch drainage and
       changes in vitals (e.g., heart rate, BP, CVP).
    c. Order packed red blood cells 50 mL/kg, and reassess after
       administration.
    d. Order furosemide 1 mg/kg intravenously (IV), and reas-
       sess after administration.

Answer: **B**

Clogging of chest tubes is common. Frequent stripping is important in the immediate postoperative period. If drainage did not resume and symptoms resolve, immediate surgical revision will be
indicated. Patient had modest response to fluids; more fluids might
not be the answer to his problem. Low urine output is secondary to
low cardiac output and is unlikely to respond to furosemide.

30. A 13-year-old girl presented to the ED with severe shortness of
    breath and left-sided chest pain. She was kicked in the left side
    of her chest during a soccer game approximately one hour prior
    to presentation. In the ED, she was tachypneic, tachycardic, and
    hypotensive with distended neck veins, muffled heart sounds,
    and diminished breath sounds over the left chest. She appeared
    confused and agitated.
    What is the most urgent action needed for this patient?
    a. Needle pericardiocentesis.
    b. Needle thoracotomy.
    c. Urgent ECHO and Cardiology consult.
    d. Urgent chest radiograph, intubation, and transfer to PICU.

Answer: **B**

The child has suffered a tension pneumothorax; perhaps a broken
rib punctured the left lung. Tension pneumothorax and cardiac
tamponade share most of the same clinical features except that
in cardiac tamponade, breath sounds are normal, while they are
absent or severely diminished in the affected side of the chest in
pneumothorax.

31. A 16-year-old girl presents to the ED with severe shortness of
    breath, chest pain, and hemoptysis. More history is obtained
    after initiating facemask oxygen, IV fluids, and IV pain medica-
    tion. She dropped out of school last year because of bullying
    regarding her weight, she smokes cigarettes and marijuana, and
    has been taking oral contraceptive pills for the last 10 months.
    On examination, she is tachypneic, tachycardic, and hypoten-
    sive with distended neck veins. Breath sounds are clear with a
    loud second heart sound.
    What is the most likely diagnosis?
    a. Conversion disorder.
    b. Cardiac tamponade.
    c. Massive pulmonary embolism.
    d. Tension pneumothorax.

Answer: C

This patient has multiple risk factors for deep vein thrombosis and
pulmonary embolism (PE) and presented with classic signs and
symptoms of PE. In cardiogenic shock and cardiac tamponade,
heart sounds are faint or muffled. In tension pneumothorax, the
breath sounds are severely reduced or absent in the affected side.
Physical signs like hypotension and distended neck veins point toward a somatic disease rather than conversion disorder.

32. Which of the following patients meets diagnostic criteria for
    Acute Rheumatic Fever?
    a. 6-year-old with fever, sore throat, anemia, elevated ESR &
       CRP.
    b. 12-year-old with polyarthritis, fever, elevated C-reactive
       protein and + ASO titer.
    c. 11-year-old with + GAS infection on throat culture and
       fever of 102°F.
    d. 7-year-old with +ASO titer, arthralgia, fever of 104°F.

Answer: **B**

This patient meets Jones criteria: 1 major manifestation (polyarthritis), two minor manifestations (fever, elevated CRP) in the setting of a Streptococcal infection. The 6-year-old does not have
evidence of a *Streptococcal* infection. Options C & D are incorrect,
evidence of a streptococcal infection, fever, and arthralgia alone
does not meet criteria for diagnosis of ARF.

33. A 5-year-old presents to the ED with fever and polyarthritis.
    Her mother reports a history of sore throat approximately
    1 week ago and a positive Group A *Streptococcus* culture at the
    primary care provider's office.
    ED laboratory results are as follows:
    C-reactive protein 18 mg/L.

(continues on page 174)

WBC $20 \times 10^3/\mu$L.

Hemoglobin 8.9 g/dL.

Platelets 225×10^9/L.

What is the initial treatment?

a. Ceftriaxone.

b. Amoxicillin.

c. Vancomycin.

d. Gentamicin.

Answer: **B**

Suspected acute rheumatic fever includes one major manifestation (polyarthritis) and two minor manifestations (fever, elevated CRP). In order to diagnose Rheumatic fever, the patient must exhibit signs of two major or one major and two minor manifestations according to the Jones criteria. Treatment for rheumatic fever includes a macrolide, macrolide, amoxicillin, first generation cephalosporin, clindamycin, or penicillin VK.

34. A 6-month-old has increased work of breathing and stridor with decreased PO intake. History includes three previous diagnoses of viral illness. The infant appears healthy, but is in mild to moderate respiratory distress with clear nasal drainage and a barking cough. The lung fields are clear bilaterally. The mother of the infant reports that "everyone at home has a cold." Chest radiograph is suspicious for a right aortic arch. Which of the imaging studies should be obtained first to evaluate the etiology of the infant's symptoms?

a. Barium swallow.

b. Bronchoscopy.

c. Echocardiography.

d. Magnetic resonance imaging.

Answer: **A**

Classic symptoms of a vascular ring include barking cough, upper airway congestion, and respiratory distress. The radiography is suspicious for a right aortic arch, which supports the diagnosis of a vascular ring, either a right aortic arch with left ligamentum arteriosum or double aortic arch. In most cases, a barium swallow can assist with the diagnosis of a vascular ring. A deep extrinsic indentation of the posterior aspect of the trachea on barium swallow is consistent with a double aortic arch or right aortic arch with left ligamentum arteriosum.

35. A 4-month-old, term male infant is brought to the ED with increased work of breathing. He has not been feeding well for the last few days. Vital signs include temperature 37.5°C, HR 170 beats per minute, RR 62 breaths per minute, and BP 75/45 mmHg. He is noted to be pale with mild respiratory distress including subcostal retractions. He has cool extremities with a capillary refill of 4 seconds. His liver is palpable 4 cm below the right costal margin.

What is the most likely diagnosis in this patient?

a. Septic shock.

b. Viral gastroenteritis.

c. Cardiogenic shock.

d. Pneumonia.

Answer: **C**

Cardiogenic shock presents with not only poor perfusion but also signs of cardiac failure such as hepatomegaly, a gallop heart rhythm, respiratory distress due to pulmonary edema, and peripheral edema. In advanced stages of shock caused by any etiology, depressed cardiac function and excessive fluid administration can result in edema. Anytime an intervention is performed on a patient in shock, the patient should be reassessed for improvement in clinical status. In this patient, the presence of hepatomegaly in the setting of a normal BP leads to the diagnosis of cardiogenic shock rather than other types of shock. Viral gastroenteritis can lead to hypovolemic shock, but these patients generally do not have hepatomegaly. Pneumonia can lead to septic shock in extreme cases; however, these patients generally do not have hepatomegaly. Most patients with septic shock do not have hepatomegaly.

36. The major difference between administering fluid in a patient with septic shock and cardiogenic shock is which of the following?

a. Patients with cardiogenic shock should receive fluid in increments of 5 to 10 mL/kg, and after each fluid bolus, they should be reassessed for signs of fluid overload.

b. There is no difference. The management is the same in both forms of shock.

c. Patients in cardiogenic shock should never be given a fluid bolus.

d. Patients in cardiogenic shock should only receive vasoactive medications.

Answer: **A**

Giving a patient with poor heart function a large volume of fluid quickly can lead to worsening heart failure. The heart is unable to handle the large increase in preload, and the patient can develop peripheral edema, pulmonary edema, and hepatomegaly. In advanced stages of shock caused by any etiology, depressed cardiac function and excessive fluid administration can result in edema. Anytime an intervention is performed on a patient in shock, the patient should be reassessed for improvement in clinical status.

37. An 8-month-old female with a history of unrepaired CHD presents with poor perfusion, tachycardia to 190 beats per minute, a markedly enlarged liver with significant abdominal distension, and poor urine output. A chest radiograph shows clear lung fields and decreased pulmonary vascular markings. What is the most likely lesion?

a. Aortic stenosis.

b. Mitral insufficiency.

c. Pulmonary stenosis.

d. Large VSD.

Answer: **C**

Hepatomegaly, abdominal distension (related to ascites), and clear lung fields all indicate a right-sided cardiac lesion and decompensated right heart failure. This excludes aortic stenosis and mitral insufficiency, which would show signs of pulmonary congestion as more fluid backed up into the lungs. A large VSD could present with right-sided failure, but there would also be increased vascular markings in the lungs as they are seeing increased flow. She is poorly perfused and showing signs of shock secondary to the lack of blood flow going to the left side of the heart, from the right side of the heart (decreased LV preload). Pulmonary stenosis will cause increased afterload on the RV, leading to fluid overload before the lungs with enlarged liver, dependent edema, and ascites. The lung fields would remain clear.

38. A 2-month-old male with history of a large perimembranous VSD is admitted to the pediatric intensive care unit following patch closure of his VSD. The surgery was uneventful; however, when coming off bypass, the patient was noted to be in complete heart block. Temporary pacing was started using epicardial leads placed during surgery. The surgeon tells you the patient is being paced in DDD mode at a rate of 140 beats per minute. Using standard pacemaker nomenclature, how would you describe the current function of the pacemaker?
    a. Both the atrium and the ventricle are being paced, the atrium is being sensed, and pacing is being inhibited when an intrinsic atrial or ventricular contraction is sensed.
    b. The atrium is being paced, the atrium and ventricle are being sensed, pacing is being inhibited when an intrinsic atrial or ventricular contraction is sensed.
    c. The atrium is being paced, the atrium is being sensed, and pacing is being inhibited when an atrial contraction is sensed.
    d. Both the atrium and the ventricle are being paced, both the atrium and the ventricle are being sensed, and pacing is being triggered or inhibited depending on intrinsic cardiac activity.

Answer: **D**

Both the atrium and the ventricle are being paced, both the atrium and the ventricle are being sensed, and pacing is being triggered or inhibited depending on intrinsic cardiac activity. Using standard pacemaker nomenclature, the first letter refers to the chamber being paced, the second letter refers to the chamber being sensed, and the third letter refers to the pacemaker response to a sensed event. The letter D or "dual" mode means that both the atrium and the ventricle are being paced and sensed, and the pacemaker can either trigger or inhibit, depending on the intrinsic cardiac activity sensed.

> *The next two questions relate to this stem.*
> *A 6-year-old female with a history of a Fontan procedure for hypoplastic left heart syndrome on chlorothiazide, metoprolol, and furosemide for chronic heart failure presents to the Emergency Department (ED) with a 3-day history of vomiting and diarrhea. Vital signs include heart rate of 148 beats per minute, respiratory rate of 28 breaths per minute, BP 90/51 mmHg, and oxygen saturation of 94% on room air. On examination, she is lethargic with clear lungs and 4-second capillary refill time.*

39. What is the most important next step in the management of this patient?

    a. Order a dose of intravenous (IV) furosemide to replace oral medications.
    b. Start epinephrine and milrinone infusions.
    c. Intubate the child because of altered mental status.
    d. Give a fluid bolus of 20 mL/kg to maximize the preload.

Answer: **D**

This child's history and presentation are consistent with hypovolemic shock from dehydration. Children on diuretic therapy who develop increased water loss from illness are at risk for dehydration. While at baseline this child may be volume overloaded from her heart failure, she now presents in a hypovolemic state. She does not have enough preload to provide adequate cardiac output, and the first-line therapy would be to give a fluid bolus. She does not show signs of volume overload, so giving extra diuretics would be deleterious in this situation. Epinephrine and milrinone will increase the heart's ability to pump, but without enough preload to pump it will not improve her cardiac output. While the child may need to be intubated, her oxygen saturation is adequate at this time, and her hypovolemia needs to be addressed first. The metoprolol should be discontinued in the acute phase of her illness, but it is an oral drug, and its effects are long lasting. Stopping it now will improve her cardiac output immediately.

40. The 6-year-old female above was subsequently admitted to the PICU for further management. 2 days after resuscitation and stabilization, it is noted on rounds that she has become tachypneic and oxygen saturations are now 90% on 2 L of nasal cannula. A chest radiograph is performed that shows diffuse bilateral pulmonary infiltrates. What is the next step in management?
    a. Start antibiotics as the patient has signs and symptoms of pneumonia.
    b. Add an extra dose of furosemide as the patient is volume overloaded.
    c. Start inotropic support with epinephrine to help cardiac output.
    d. Give the patient a fluid bolus of 20 ml/kg to maximize cardiac output through improving preload.

Answer: **B**

Aggressive resuscitation with IV fluids can result in volume overload. Fluid is an appropriate is appropriate treatment initially, but once her preload has been maximized, any extra fluid is likely to worsen her heart failure. After 2 days, she will have begun to mobilize the fluid that was initially given to her. She is now showing signs of volume overload with pulmonary congestion, tachypnea, and an increased oxygen requirement. She needs to be diuresed until she is euvolemic. New infiltrates are demonstrated on chest radiograph; however, there is no history of fever, making pneumonia less likely. Inotropic support will help with the cardiac output, leading to better urine production, but more acutely, she needs to diurese. She is already showing signs of volume overload, so giving her more fluid at this time will make her worse. She does not have signs of a pleural effusion.

(continues on page 176)

41. Based on standard pacemaker nomenclature, what does each letter in the three-letter sequence represent?
    a. Chamber sensed, chamber paced, response to sensed event.
    b. Chamber sensed, response to sensed event, chamber paced.
    c. Chamber paced, chamber sensed, response to sensed event.
    d. Chamber paced, response to sensed event, chamber sensed.
    e. Response to sensed event, chamber paced, chamber sensed.

Answer: **C**

Standard pacemaker nomenclature is used to signify the function and action of the pacemaker. Three-letter sequences are used, with the first letter indicating the chamber paced, the second letter being the chamber sensed, and the third letter representing the response of the pacemaker to a sensed event.

42. Which of the following would be the most important medication in an infant with a BTS (Blalock–Taussig shunt)?
    a. Coumadin.
    b. Lasix.
    c. ASA.
    d. Digoxin.

Answer: **C**

The most important medication for an infant with a Blalock–Taussig shunt is aspirin (ASA).

43. A teenage girl presents to the ED with a history of syncope in school while walking to class. She is otherwise healthy, with no family history of arrhythmias.
    What is the most likely cause of syncope in this age group?
    a. Seizure.
    b. Migraine.
    c. Structural heart defect.
    d. Dehydration.

Answer: **D**

The incidence of syncope is higher in teenage females. Approximately 75% of children with syncope have vasovagal syncope caused by peripheral venous pooling in the lower extremities, leading to decreased ventricular filling volume. Causes of vasovagal syncope include inadequate fluid intake, caffeine, or inadequate salt intake.

44. An echocardiogram was ordered on a 3-month-old infant who was admitted with respiratory distress and cyanosis. The cardiac sonographer reports that the echocardiogram was limited due to "poor acoustic windows." What is the most likely reason for the poor quality of the echocardiogram?
    a. Pericardial effusion.
    b. Pneumothorax.
    c. Pleural effusion.
    d. Abdominal ascites.

Answer: **B**

"Poor acoustic windows" are any number of factors (e.g., air, edema, adipose tissue, surgical dressings) that impair the ability to obtain echocardiographic images. Ultrasound waves travel extremely poorly through air. Therefore, echocardiograms are difficult to perform on patients with a pneumothorax, pneumo-mediastinum, subcutaneous emphysema, or hyperinflated lungs.

45. A 15-year-old female presents to the ED with an episode of syncope in gym class. Which of the following is the most valuable initial evaluation?
    a. A thorough history and physical.
    b. ECHO.
    c. EEG.
    d. ECG.

Answer: **A**

A thorough history and physical is the most valuable part of an initial evaluation in a child with syncope. A concentrated family history, looking for red flags such as sudden death, arrhythmias, heart disease, structural heart defects, seizures, can aid in directing your focus to the cause of the syncopal episode.

46. What would be the most significant physical finding in a child with suspected coarctation of the aorta?
    a. Hypertension.
    b. Hypotension.
    c. Increased pulse pressure.
    d. Decreased pulse pressure.

Answer: **A**

Hypertension is the most significant physical finding in a child with suspected coarctation of the aorta. Hypotension, increased pulse pressure, and decreased pulse pressure are not associated with coarctation of the aorta.

47. What is the genetic syndrome most commonly associated in a patient with an endocardial cushion defect?
    a. Trisomy 18.
    b. Trisomy 21.
    c. Noonan syndrome.
    d. Di George syndrome.

Answer: **B**

Trisomy 21 is most commonly associated with endocardial cushion defects.

48. A 13-year-old female has lethargy and difficulty breathing. She is difficult to arouse, cold to touch, with weak distal pulses. Her heart rate on the monitor is 30 beats per minute, and BP is 60/30 mmHg. ECG confirms complete heart block. After IV access is established, the patient is given 0.02 mg/kg of atropine. There is no improvement in her heart rate. What is the next most appropriate step in management?
    a. Place an esophageal pacing probe, and begin temporary pacing.
    b. Place transcutaneous pacing pads, and begin temporary pacing.
    c. Place transvenous pacing leads, and begin temporary pacing.
    d. Place a permanent pacemaker.

Answer: **B**

The most appropriate management for this child is to place transcutaneous pacing pads and begin temporary pacing. This patient has presented to the emergency department with bradycardia secondary to complete heart block. Due to her altered mental state, hypotension, and poor perfusion, this would be considered unstable bradycardia. After a dose of atropine is attempted, the next most appropriate step would be to start emergent temporary pacing. The quickest and most readily available means of temporary pacing is transcutaneous pacing. Once the patient is stabilized, she would likely have placement of transvenous pacing leads as this is a more effective and more comfortable way to provide temporary pacing. Esophageal pacing is used primarily for overdrive pacing in the setting of supraventricular tachycardia. Epicardial pacing leads are usually placed only after open heart surgery. Ultimately, if she remains in complete heart block, she would need permanent pacemaker placement; however, this is not the right choice in an unstable patient.

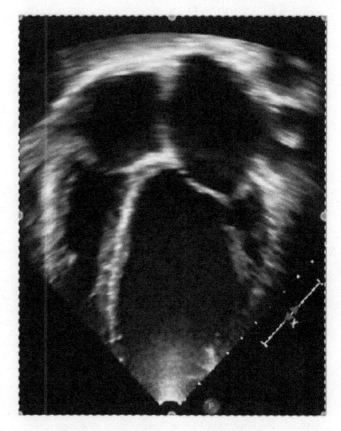

FIGURE 5.55

49. A previously healthy 14-year-old girl presents with shortness of breath. She reports a history of fevers and flulike symptoms 2 weeks ago. On examination, she has a gallop, her liver is down 5 cm below the costal margin, and there are crackles at the bases of her lungs. Echocardiogram shows an ejection fraction of 25%, and a shortening fraction of 8%. What else does the echocardiogram show?
a. Restrictive cardiomyopathy.
b. Hypertrophic cardiomyopathy.
c. Normal echocardiogram.
d. Dilated cardiomyopathy.

Answer: **D**

The history is consistent with a dilated cardiomyopathy, possibly from acute myocarditis (history of recent viral infection). Echocardiographic findings include an extremely dilated LV with poor systolic function. Ventricular systolic function is usually preserved in restrictive and hypertrophic cardiomyopathies. Restrictive cardiomyopathy is characterized with normal ventricular size but severe biatrial dilatation and severe diastolic function. Hypertrophic cardiomyopathy is characterized by thickened myocardium and diastolic dysfunction (Figure 5.55).

50. A 10-year-old develops the following rhythm on postoperative day 4 after repair of aortic stenosis. He is unresponsive and has no palpable femoral pulses (Figure 5.56).
What is the MOST important therapy to initiate:
a. Intubation and mechanical ventilation.
b. Cardiac compressions.
c. Amiodarone.
d. Defibrillation with 2 Joules/kg.

Answer: **D**

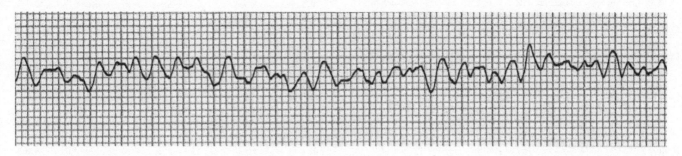

FIGURE 5.56

(continues on page 178)

The patient is in ventricular fibrillation tachycardia without pulses. Until proven otherwise, this is assumed to be pulseless ventricular fibrillation (VF).

Successful treatment of pulseless VT/VF requires immediate defibrillation—survival decreases by 7% to 10% for every minute that defibrillation is delayed. Supportive measures are certainly important, but should not delay defibrillation. From a respiratory perspective, most patients can be supported by bag-valve-mask ventilation adequately until they are hemodynamically stable for intubation. Intubation in this patient would result in pauses in cardiac compressions and delay in defibrillation. Cardiac compressions are only a temporizing measure in this patient—they will not restore a perfusing rhythm. Amiodarone and lidocaine are adjuncts to defibrillation—they are indicated in those patients refractory to initial defibrillation.

Recommended Readings

Abd-Allah, S., & Checcia, P. A. (2007). Heart transplantation. In D. S. Wheeler, H. R. Wong, & T. P. Shanley (Eds.), *Pediatric critical care medicine* (pp. 841–864). London, England: Springer Publishing.

Abman, S. H. (2010). Pulmonary hypertension in children: A historical overview. *Pediatric Critical Care Medicine, 11*(2), S4–S9.

Adatia, I., & Shekerdemian, L. (2010). The role of calcium channel blockers, steroids, anticoagulation, antiplatelets, and endothelian receptor antagonists. *Pediatric Critical Care Medicine, 11*(2), S46–S52.

Ayres, N. A., Miller-Hance, W., Fyfe, D. A., Stevenson, J. G., Sahn, D. J., Young, L. T., . . . Rychik, J. (2005). Indications and guidelines for performance of transesophageal echocardiography in the patient with pediatric acquired or congenital disease. *Journal of the American Society of Echocardiography, 18*, 91–98.

Backer, C. L., & Mavroudis, C. (2003). Vascular rings and pulmonary slings. In C. Mavroudis & C. L. Backer (Eds.), *Pediatric cardiac surgery* (3rd ed., pp. 234–250). Philadelphia, PA: Mosby.

Backer, C. L., Mavroudis, C., Rigsby, C. K., & Holinger, L. D. (2005). Trends in vascular ring surgery. *Journal of the Thoracic Cardiovascular Surgery, 129*, 1339–1347.

Barr, F. E., & Macrae, D. (2010). Inhaled nitric oxide and related therapies. *Pediatric Critical Care Medicine, 11*(2), S30–S36.

Blanco, C. C., & Parekh, J. B. (2010). Pericarditis. *Pediatrics in Review, 31*(2), 83–84.

Border, W. L., Michelfelder, E. C., Hor, K., & Meredith, D. S. (2007). Echocardiography in the pediatric critical care setting. In D. S. Wheeler, H. R. Wong, & T. P. Shanley (Eds.), *Pediatric critical care medicine* (pp. 644–651). London, England: Springer Publishing.

Bronicki, R. A. (2010). Pathophysiology of right ventricular failure in pulmonary hypertension. *Pediatric Critical Care Medicine, 11*(2), S15–S22.

Burch, M., & Prasad, S. (2002). The cardiomyopathies. *Current Paediatrics, 12*, 206–211.

Chan, T. C., Brady, W. J., & Pollack, M. (1999). Electrocardiographic manifestations: acute myopericarditis. *Journal of Emergency Medicine, 17*(5), 865–872.

Chang, A. & McKenzie, E. D. (2006). Myocardial dysfunction, extracorporeal membrane oxygenation, and ventricular assist devices. In B. P. Fuhrman & J. Zimmerman (Eds.), *Pediatric Critical Care* (3rd ed., pp. 346–365). Philadelphia, PA: Mosby.

Charpie, J. R., & Kulik, T. J. (2006). Assessement of cardiovascular function. In B. P. Fuhrman & J. Zimmerman (Eds.), (3rd ed., pp. 265–272). Philadelphia, PA: Mosby.

Colan, S. D. (2011). Treatment of hypertrophic cardiomyopathy in childhood. *Progress in Pediatric Cardiology, 31*, 13–19.

Connolly, D. M., & Eichler, V. (2012). Congestive heart failure. In K. Reuter-Rice & B. Bolick (Eds.), *Pediatric acute care: A guide for interprofessional practice* (pp. 296–304). Burlington, MA: Jones & Bartlett Learning.

Corlett, K. (2012). Chylothorax. In K. Reuter-Rice & B. Bolick (Eds.), *Pediatric acute care: A guide for interprofessional practice* (pp. 260–262). Burlington, MA: Jones & Bartlett Learning.

Corlett, K. (2012). Postpericardiotomy syndrome. In K. Reuter-Rice & B. Bolick (Eds.), *Pediatric acute care: A guide for interprofessional practice* (pp. 308–310). Burlington, MA: Jones & Bartlett Learning.

Curran, M. P., Robinson, D. M., & Keating, G. M. (2006). Intravenous nicardipine: Its use in the short-term treatment of hypertension and various other indications. *Drugs, 66*(13), 1755–1782.

Da Costa, D. (2002). ABC of clinical electrocardiography: Bradycardias and atrioventricular conduction block. *British Medical Journal, 324*(7336), 535–538.

Dalton, H. J., & Duncan, B. W. (2007). Mechanical support of the cardiovascular' system: Extracorporeal life support/extracorporeal membrane oxygenation and ventricular assist devices. In D. S. Wheeler, H. R. Wong, & T. P. Shanley (Eds.), *Pediatric critical care medicine* (pp. 765–777). London, England: Springer Publishing.

Davignon, A., Rautaharju, P., Boisselle, E., Soumis, F., Mégélas, M., & Choquette, A. (1979). Normal ECG standards for infants and children. *Pediatric Cardiology, 1*, 123–131.

Davis, D. (2001). *Quick and accurate 12-lead ECG interpretation* (3rd ed.). Philadelphia, PA: Lippincott Williams & Wilkins.

Deal, B., Wolff, G., & Gelband, H. (1998). *Current concepts in diagnosis and management of arrhythmias in infants and children.* Armonk, NY: Wiley-Blackwell.

Delacretaz, E. Supraventricular tachycardia. (2006). *The New England Journal of Medicine, 354*(10), 1039–1051.

Dickinson, D. F. (2005). The normal ECG in childhood and adolescence. *Heart, 91*(12), 1626–1630.

Doniger, S. J., & Sharieff, G. Q. (2006). Pediatric Dysrhythmias. *Pediatric Clinics of North America, 53*(1), 85–105.

Durani, Y., Giordano, K., & Goudie, B. W. (2010). Myocarditis and pericarditis in children. *Pediatric Clinics of North America, 57*(6), 1281–1303.

Esteban, M. T. T., & Kaski, J. P. (2007). Hypertrophic cadiomyopathy in children. *Pediatrics & Child Health, 17*(1), 19–24.

Extracorporeal Life Support Organization. (2009). *ELSO guidelines for cardiopulmonary extracorporeal life support.* Retrieved from http://www.elso.med.umich.edu/Guidelines.html

Fish, F. A., Kannankeril, P. J., & Johns, J. A. (2006). Assessment of cardiovascular function. In B. P. Fuhrman & J. Zimmerman (Eds.), *Pediatric Critical Care* (3rd ed., pp. 365–394). Philadelphia, PA: Mosby.

Flynn, J. T., & Daniels, S. R. (2006). Pharmacologic treatment of hypertesion in children and adolescents. *The Journal of Pediatrics, 746*–754.

Fraisse, A., & Wessel, D. L. (2010). Acute pulmonary hypertension in infants and children: cGMP-related drugs. *Pediatric Critical Care Medicine, 11*(2), S37–S40.

Fricker, E. J. (2006). Cardiac transplantation. In B. P. Fuhrman & J. Zimmerman (Eds.), *Pediatric Critical Care* (3rd ed., pp. 465–474). Philadelphia, PA: Mosby.

Fuhrman, B. P., & Zimmerman, J. (Eds.). (2011). *Pediatric critical care* (4th ed.). Philadelphia, PA: Elsevier Saunders.

Fuller, J. L., & Hamrick, J. T. (2012). Cardiovascular agents. In K. Reuter-Rice & B. Bolick (Eds.), *Pediatric acute care: A guide for interprofessional practice* (pp. 241–252). Burlington, MA: Jones & Bartlett Learning.

Gambetta, K. (2012). Cardiac transplantation. In K. Reuter-Rice & B. Bolick (Eds.), *Pediatric acute care: A guide for interprofessional practice* (pp. 217–234). Burlington, MA: Jones & Bartlett Learning.

Gandi, S. K. (2009). Ventricular assist devices in children. *Progress in Pediatric Cardiology, 26*, 11–19.

Gesuete, V., Ragni, L., Prandstraller, D., Oppido, G., Formigari, R., Gargiulo, G. D., & Picchio, F. M. (2010). Dilated cardiomyopathy presenting in childhood: Aetiology, diagnostic approach, and clinical course. *Cardiology in the Young, 20*, 680–685.

Gewitz, M. H., & Satou, G. M. (2007). Inflammatory diseases of the heart and pericardium: Dilated cardiomyopathy and myocarditis. In D. S. Wheeler, H. R. Wong, & T. P. Shanley (Eds.), *Pediatric critical care medicine* (pp. 808–821). London, England: Springer Publishing.

Goodacre, S. (2002). ABC of clinical electrocardiography: Atrial arrhythmias. *British Medical Journal, 324*(7337), 594–597.

Grebenik, C. E., & Sinclair, M. E. (2003). Which inotrope? *Current Pediatrics, 13*, 6–11.

Greeley, W. J., Lappe, D. G., Ungerleider, R. M., & Wetzel, R. C. (2006). In D. E. Cameron (Ed.), *Critical heart disease in infants and children* (2nd ed.). Philadelphia, PA: Mosby.

Hanna, B. D. (2012). Physiology and diagnostics. In K. Reuter-Rice & B. Bolick (Eds.), *Pediatric acute care: A guide for interprofessional practice* (pp.189–196). Burlington, MA: Jones & Bartlett Learning.

Hernanz-Schulman, M. (2005). Vascular rings: A practical approach to imaging diagnosis. *Pediatric Radiology, 35*, 961–979.

Hirsch, J. C., Charpie, J. R., Ohye, R. G., & Gurney, J. G. (2009). Near-infrared spectroscopy what we know and what we need to know: a systematic review of the congenital heart disease literature. *Journal of Thoracic and Cardiovascular Surgery, 137*(1), 154–159.

Hirsch, R., & Beekman, R. H. (2007). Cardiac catheterization in the pediatric critical care settting. In D. S. Wheeler, H. R. Wong, & T. P. Shanley (Eds.), *Pediatric critical care medicine* (pp. 651–665). London, England: Springer Publishing.

Hoffman, T. M., Wernovsky, G., Atz, A., Kulik, T. J., Nelson, D. P., Chang, A. C., . . . Wessel, D. L. (2003). Efficacy and safety of milrinone in preventing low cardiac output syndrome in infants and children after corrective surgery for congenital heart disease. *Circulation, 107*, 996–1002.

Hoyer, A., & Silberbach, M. (2005). Infective endocarditis. *Pediatrics in Review, 26*(11), 394–400.

Hurta, J. C. (2006). Echocardiograph and noninvasive diagnosis. In B. P. Fuhrman & J. Zimmerman (Eds.), (3rd ed., pp. 2273–2285). Philadelphia, PA: Mosby.

Jefferies, J. L., Price, J. F., & Morales, D. L. (2010). Mechanical support of childhood heart failure. *Heart Failure Clinics, 6*, 559–573.

Johnson, R. J., Feig, D. I., Nakagawa, T., Sanchez-Lozada, L. G., & Rodriguez-Iturbe, B. (2008). Pathogenesis of essential hypertension: Historical paradigms and modern insights. *Journal of Hypertension, 26*(3), 381–391.

Khan, I. A. (2002). Long QT syndrome: Diagnosis and management. *American Heart Journal, 143*(1), 7–14.

Kleinman, M. E., Chameides, L., Schexnayder, S. M., Samson, R. A., Hazinski, M. F., Atkins, D. L., . . . Zaritsky, A. L. (2010). Pediatric advanced life support: 2010 American Heart Association guidelines for cardiopulmonary resuscitation and emergency cardiovascular care. *Pediatrics, 126*(5), e1361–e1399.

Knilans, T. K. (2007). Arrhythmias. In D. S. Wheeler, H. R. Wong, & T. P. Shanley (Eds.), *Pediatric critical care medicine* (pp. 785–798). London, England: Springer Publishing.

Kuzin, J. (2012). Carditis. In K. Reuter-Rice & B. Bolick (Eds.), *Pediatric acute care: A guide for interprofessional practice* (pp. 252–260). Burlington, MA: Jones & Bartlett Learning.

Kuzin, J. (2012). Rheumatic fever. In K. Reuter-Rice & B. Bolick (Eds.), *Pediatric acute care: A guide for interprofessional practice* (pp. 316–321). Burlington, MA: Jones & Bartlett Learning.

Lai, W. W., Geva, T., Shirali, G. S., Frommelt, P. C., Humes, R. A., Brook, M. M., . . . & Writing Committee. (2006). Guidelines and standards for performance of pediatric echocardiogram: A report from the task force of the pediatric council of the American society of echocardiography. *Journal of the American Society of Echocardiography, 19*, 1413–1430.

Lande, M. B., & Flynn, J. T. (2009). Treatment of hypertension in children and adolescents. *Pediatric Nephrology, 24*(10), 1939–1949.

Lawrence, P. R. (2012). Arrythmias and pacemakers. In K. Reuter-Rice & B. Bolick (Eds.), *Pediatric acute care: A guide for interprofessional practice* (pp. 202–217). Burlington, MA: Jones & Bartlett Learning.

Lexi-Comp, Inc. (2013). *Pediatric & Neonatal Lexi-Drugs Online*™. Hudson, OH: Author.

Magnani, J. W., & Dec, G. W. (2006). Myocarditis: Current trends in diagnosis and treatment. *Circulation, 113*, 876–890.

McCulley, M. E. (2012). Syncope. In K. Reuter-Rice & B. Bolick (Eds.), *Pediatric acute care: A guide for interprofessional practice* (pp. 321–325). Burlington, MA: Jones & Bartlett Learnng.

McDonald, S. (2012). Extracorporeal life support. In K. Reuter-Rice & B. Bolick (Eds.), *Pediatric acute care: A guide for interprofessional practice* (pp. 304–308). Burlington, MA: Jones & Bartlett Learning.

Moffett, B. S., & Price, J. F. (2008). Evaluation of sodium nitroprusside toxicity in pediatric cardiac surgical patients. *The Annals of Pharmacotherapy, 42*, 1600–1604.

Morris, F., & Brady, W. J. (2002). ABC of clinical electrocardiography: Acute myocardial infarction-Part I. *British Medical Journal, 324*(7341), 831–834.

Mourani, P. M., Sontag, M. K., Younoszai, A., Ivy, D. D., & Abman, S. H. (2008). Clinical utility of echocardiography for the diagnosis and management of pulmonary vascular disease in young children with chronic lung disease. *Pediatrics, 121*, 317–325.

Mullen, M. P. (2010). Diagnostic strategies for acute presentation of pulmonary hypertension in children: Particular focus on use of echocardiography, cardiac catheterization, magnetic resonance imaging, chest computed tomography, and lung biopsy. *Pediatric Critical Care Medicine, 11*(2), S23–S29.

Murkin, J. M. & Arango, M. (2009). Near-infared Spectroscopy as an Index of Brain and Tissue Oxygenation. *British Journal of Anesthesia, 103*(suppl 1), i3–i13.

Nally, J. V. (2001). Essential hypertension. In A. Greenberg (Ed.), *Primer on kidney disease* (pp. 475–480). San Diego, CA: Acedemic Press.

National High Blood Pressure Educations Program on High Blood Pressure in Children and Adolescents. (2004). The fourth report on the diagnosis, evaluation, and treatment of high blood pressure in children and adolescents. *Pediatrics, 114* (2 Suppl 4th Report), 555–576.

Nichols, D. G. (Ed.). (2008). *Rogers' textbook of pediatric intensive care.* Philadelphia, PA: Lippincott Williams & Wilkins.

Nieves, J. A., & Kohr, L. (2010). Nursing considerations in the care of patients with pulmonary hypertension. *Pediatric Critical Care Medicine, 11*(2), S74–S78.

O'Connor, M., McDaniel, N., & Brady, W. J. (2008). The pediatric electrocardiogram part II: Dysrhythmias. *The American Journal of Emergency Medicine, 26*(3), 348–358.

Overgaard, C. B., & Dzavik, V. (2008). Inotropes and vasopressors: Review of physiology and clinical use in cardiovascular disease. *Circulation, 118*, 1047–1056.

Park, M. K. (2007). *Pediatric cardiology for practitioners* (5th ed.). St. Louis, MO: Mosby.

Park, M. K., & Guntheroth, W. G. (1992). *How to read pediatric ECGs* (3rd ed.). St. Louis, MO: Mosby.

Pophal, S. G. (2012). Cardiomyopathy. In K. Reuter-Rice & B. Bolick (Eds.), *Pediatric acutecare: A guide for interprofessional practice* (pp. 234–236). Burlington, MA: Jones & Bartlett Learning.

Rijnbeek, P. R., Witsenburg, M., Schrama, E., Hess, J., & Kors, J. A. (2001). New normal limits for the paediatric electrocardiogram. *European Heart Journal, 22*(8), 702–711

Roy, C. L., Minor, M. A., Brookhart, A., & Choudhary, N. K. (2007). Does this patient with a pericardial effusion have cardiac tamponade? *The Journal of the American Association, 297*(16), 1810–1818.

Rosenzweig, E., Feinstein, J., Humpl, T., & Ivy, D. (2009). Pulmonary hypertension in children: Diagnostic work up and challenges. *Progress in Pediatric Cardiology, 27*, 7–11.

Schneider, D. S. (2011). The cardiovascular System. In R. M. Kliegman, K. J. Marcdante, H. B. Jenson, & R. E. Behrman (Eds.), *Nelson's essentials of pediatrics* (5th ed.). Philadelphia, PA: Saunders Elsevier.

Schultz, J. C., Hilliard, A. A., Cooper, L. T., & Rihal, C. S. (2009). Diagnosis and treatment of viral myocarditis. *Mayo Clinic Proceedings, 84*(11), 1001–1009.

Sharieff, G. Q., & Rao, S. O. (2006). The pediatric ECG. *Emergency Medicine Clinics of North America, 24*(1), 195–208, vii–viii.

Simonneau, G., Robbins, I. M., Beghetti, M., & Souza, R. (2009). Updated classification of pulmonary hypertension. *Journal of the American College of Cardiology, 54*(1 suppl), S43–S54.

Smith, L., & Herman, L. (2006). Shock states. In B. P. Fuhrman & J. Zimmerman (Eds.), (3rd ed., pp. 394–411). Philadelphia, PA: Mosby.

Stockwell, J. A., & Preissig, C. M. (Eds.). (2012). *Comprehensive critical care: Pediatric.* Mount Prospect, IL: Society of Critical Care Medicine.

Tibby, S. M., & Murdoch, I. A. (2003). Monitoring cardiac function in intensive care. *Archives of Disease in Childhood, 88*, 46–52.

Towbin, J. A. (2004). Molecular genetic basis of sudden cardiac death. *Pediatric Clinics of North America, 51*(5), 1229–1255.

Troughton, R. W., Asher, C. R., & Klein, A. L. (2004). Pericarditis. *The Lancet, 363*, 717–727.

Tsang, T. S., Oh, J. K., & Seward, J. B. (1999). Diagnosis and management of cardiac tamponade in the era of echocardiography. *Clinical Cardiology, 22*(7),446–452.

Tschudy, M. M., & Arcara, K. M. (2012). *The Harriet Lane handbook* (19th ed.). Philadelphia, PA: Mosby.

Tucker, D., Sullivan, K., Eichler, V., Williams, B., & Amato, J. (2012). Congenital heart disease. In K. Reuter Rice & B. Bolick (Eds.), *Pediatric acute care* (pp. 262–296). Burlington, MA: Jones & Bartlett Learning.

U.S. Department of Health and Human Services National Institutes of Health National Heart, Lung, and Blood Institute. (2005). *The fourth report on the diagnosis, evaluation, and treatment of high blood pressure in children and adolescents.* Retrieved from National Heart Blood and Lung Institute: http://www.nhlbi.nih.gov/health/prof/heart/hbp/hbp_ped.pdf

Van Mieghem, C., Sabbe, M., & Knockaert, D. (2004). The clinical value of the ECG in noncardiac conditions. *Chest, 125*(4), 1561–1576.

Walter, D. (2012). Pulmonary hypertension. In K. Reuter-Rice & B. Bolick (Eds.), *Pediatric acute care: A guide to interprofessional practice* (pp. 310–316). Burlington, MA: Jones & Bartlett Learning.

Webber, S. A. (2008). Primary restrictive cardiomyopathy in childhood. *Progress in Pediatric Cardiology, 25*, 85–90.

Wiest, D. B., Garner, S. S., Uber, W. E., & Sade, R. M. (1998). Esmolol for the management of pediatric hypertension after cardiac operations. *Journal of Thoracic and Cardiovascular Surgery, 115,* 890–897.

Worthen, M. (2012). Cardiogenic shock. In K. Reuter-Rice & B. Bolick (Eds.), *Pediatric acutecare: A guide for interprofessional practice* (pp. 236–241). Burlington, MA: Jones & Bartlett Learning.

Neurologic Disorders

Cranial Nerves

Michele Grimason

- See Table 6.1 and Figure 6.1.

Arteriovenous Malformation

Valarie D. Eichler

Background

- Congenital abnormality in the connection between arteries and veins without a developed capillary; resembling a "bag of worms."
- Most common cause of hemorrhagic strokes in infants and nontraumatic intracranial hemorrhage (ICH) in children.

Definition

- A congenital intracranial malformation distinguished by a persistently abnormal connection between arteries and veins within the brain without an interposed or developed capillary bed.

Etiology/Epidemiology

- Uncommon; etiology is largely unknown.
- Present at birth; formed during the 3rd week of gestation.
- Capillary network fails to develop between the arteries and veins.
- Occurs in approximately 1% of the pediatric population.
- 1:100,000 children have arteriovenous malformations (AVMs); most are asymptomatic.
- Majority of AVMs are supratentorial and within the parenchyma of the brain.
- Less often, located within the brainstem, thalamus, basal ganglia, and cerebellum.
- Infrequently, familial.

- Can be associated with several inherited disorders such as Sturge–Weber syndrome, neurofibromatosis, and von Hippel–Lindau syndrome.

Pathophysiology

- Occurs during fetal development; failed capillary bed development between the cerebral arteries and veins.
- Abnormally high-blood-flow state shunts blood, producing enlarged and engorged vessels.
- Normally the capillary bed dampens the high-velocity flow of blood from the artery to the vein.
- The cluster of veins and arteries is referred to as the nidus or core.
- Because of the high flow state, the AVM steals blood from the surrounding healthy brain tissue, leading to mild hypoxia, progressive neurologic deficits, and more angiogenesis. This is referred as "the steal phenomenon."
- Size can range from 1 mm to >10 cm.
- Smaller defects, usually <2 cm, bleed more often than larger ones and are usually located in the basal ganglia or thalamus.
- Vein of Galen.
  - A distinctive AVM in the infant population that is responsible for more than 30% of AVMs in the general pediatric population.
- Spinal AVMs.
  - Rare.
  - Often associated with cutaneous angiomas such as port-wine stains and hereditary hemorrhagic telangiectasia as seen in Osler–Weber–Rendu syndrome.
- Suspect intracranial AVM when a port-wine stain spans the cutaneous distribution of the trigeminal cranial nerve (CN V).

Clinical Presentation

- Commonly presents between the second and fourth decades of life.
- Usually in healthy children or adolescents.

TABLE 6.1 Cranial Nerves

Cranial Nerve		Function
I	Olfactory	Conveys impulses related to smell.
II	Optic	Conveys impulses related to sight. Visual acuity.
III	Oculomotor	Supplies four extraocular muscles: the medial rectus, superior rectus, inferior rectus, and inferior oblique, which adduct, depress, and elevate the eye. Supplies the levator palpebrae superioris muscle, which controls eye-lid opening. Pupil constriction.
IV	Trochlear	Controls movement of the superior oblique muscle which intorts the eye.
V	Trigeminal	Three branches: maxillary, mandibular, and ophthalmic. Controls chewing movements. Delivers impulses related to touch, pain, and temperature in the facial area. Corneal reflex (with CN VII).
VI	Abducens	Supplies the lateral rectus muscle that abducts the eye.
VII	Facial	Controls the muscles of facial expression including eye-lid closure. Sensation and taste of the anterior two third of the tongue. Controls the tear and salivary glands. Corneal reflex (with CN V).
VIII	Vestibulocochlear	Transmits impulses related to equilibrium and hearing.
IX	Glossopharyngeal	Sensation and taste in the posterior one third of the tongue. Controls swallowing. Controls the salivary glands. Controls viscera in the thorax and abdomen.
X	Vagus	Controls the skeletal muscle movements in the pharynx, larynx, and palate.
XI	Accessory	Controls swallowing. Controls movement of the head.
XII	Hypoglossal	Controls muscles involved in speech and swallowing.

- Often associated with a high morbidity and mortality.
- Associated with ICH ~80% of the time.
- Signs and symptoms of increased intracranial pressure (ICP) due to associated mass effect.
  - Headache (acute or intermittent).
  - Nausea/vomiting.
  - Seizures.
  - Focal neurologic deficits, depending on location of AVM.
  - Infant presentation is usually with vein of Galen.
    - With or without hydrocephalus.
    - With or without macrocephaly.
  - High output cardiac failure.
  - Audible intracranial bruit.
  - Cardiomegaly.

Diagnostic Evaluation

- Computed tomography (CT) is the initial diagnostic tool.
  - Presence of hyperdense tubular structures with calcifications surrounding the AVM.
  - If a hemorrhage is present, the primary AVM may be obliterated or compressed by the hematoma.
  - Evaluates for associated hydrocephalus, cerebral edema (with or without mass effect), and signs of herniation.
- CT angiography.
  - Provides more vascular detail of the AVM.
- Magnetic resonance imaging (MRI)/magnetic resonance angiography (MRA) (once clinically stable).
  - Identifies the structure of the feeding vessels, nidus, draining veins, hemorrhage, hematomas, and presence of vasospasm.

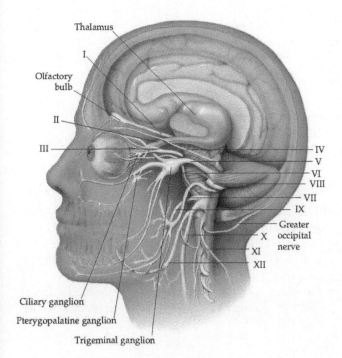

Cranial Nerves

I. Olfactory n.
II. Optic n.
III. Oculomotor n.
IV. Trochlear n.
V. Trigeminal n.
VI. Abducens n.
VII. Facial n.
VIII. Vestibulocochlear n.
IX. Glossopharyngeal n.
X. Vagus n.
XI. Accessory n.
XII. Hypoglossal n.

FIGURE 6.1 • **Cranial Nerves Labeled.**

- Cerebral angiography.
  - Radiologic study of choice or "gold standard."
  - Identifies the dilated feeding arteries, the nidus, and large draining veins.
  - Definitively reveals the origin or morphology of the AVM.
  - When evaluating a ruptured AVM, the child should be clinically stable and ideally in "cooling off" period to allow for resorption of the hematoma.
  - If performed too early, the hematoma and surrounding edema may block or hide the vasculature (Figure 6.2).

Management

- Overall goal is complete elimination of the AVM.
- Presentation with a ruptured AVM is a medical emergency secondary to the likelihood of cerebral edema and increased ICP.
- Goal is prevention of secondary injury.
- Emergent treatment is the same as any patient presenting with signs and symptoms of increased ICP.
- ABCs and controlling increased ICP by positioning, hyperosmolar therapy, mild hyperventilation ($Paco_2$ ~33–35 mmHg), temperature control, seizure control, sedation/analgesia, and pharmacologic paralysis as needed.

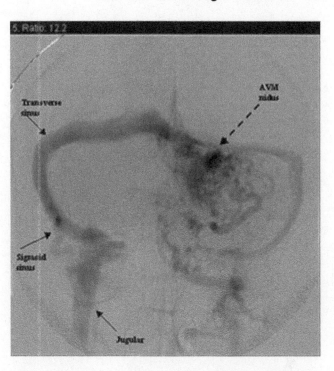

FIGURE 6.2 • **AVM on Cerebral Angiogram.**
Angiogram demonstrates anteroposterior view of left cerebellar arteriovenous malformation (AVM). Dashed arrow points to AVM nidus.

- Further tiered therapy includes placement of an external ventricular drain for cerebrospinal fluid (CSF) removal and barbiturate coma.
- In some cases, a decompressive craniectomy may be performed to allow more room for the brain to swell during the acute phase.
- Surgical excision.
  - Approach depends on the location of the AVM, and usually involves microsurgery and complete obliteration of the AVM.
  - In emergent cases, may be performed to evacuate the hematoma.
  - An angiography or MRA is often performed immediately postoperatively to confirm removal of the AVM.
- Endovascular embolization (with cerebral angiography).
  - Usually a multistage approach and is an adjunct to surgery.
  - Embolization with beads, coils, and glue to reduce the size of the nidus and overall flow to the AVM.
  - Goal is to decrease the morbidity associated with both the AVM and the surgical procedure.
- Stereotactic radiosurgery (Gamma Knife).
  - Used for lesions located deep in the brain parenchyma or when near critical areas such as the basal ganglia, brainstem, or thalamus.
  - A high-dose focused beam of radiation targets the precise area of the AVM while reducing the risk of injury to adjacent tissue.

Botulism
Cathy Haut

Background/Definition

• A progressive descending neurologic disorder caused by the *Clostridium botulinum* bacteria, which causes general muscle weakness that can result in respiratory failure.

Etiology

• The botulinum toxin is a protein that is naturally produced by certain strains of spore-forming *Clostridium* bacteria.
• Clostridia are soil-dwelling organisms that occasionally make their way into food products, especially unpasteurized honey.
• Infants <6 months of age are most often affected.

Pathophysiology

• Botulinum spores are ingested or inhaled from soil, vacuum cleaner dust, honey, or other foods.
• Bacteria multiply, colonize the intestines, and produce toxin, which affects the neuromuscular junction, blocking the release of acetylcholine from nerve endings, resulting in paralysis.

Clinical Presentation

• Symptoms include constipation, poor feeding, lethargy, and increasing weakness.
• Physical examination reveals hypotonia and symmetrical CN palsies.
• Infants have weak cry, expressionless face, ptosis, and sluggish pupillary responses. Gag, suck, and swallow reflexes are diminished or may be absent.

Diagnostic Evaluation

• Presence of botulinum toxin in stool sample.

Management

• Supportive care, monitoring, possibility of intubation, and ventilation.
• Administration of human botulism immune globulin intravenous (BIG-IV).
  • Obtained only through the California Health Department.

Brain Abscess
Cathy Haut

Background/Definition

• A rare, life-threatening condition in children that has decreased in incidence over time.
• Can occur through spread of septic emboli, by direct extension of oropharyngeal infection, or as a result of head trauma.
• Classification of abscess is determined by the mechanism of infection, anatomic area affected and organism causing the infection.

Etiology

• Majority of brain abscesses occur as a result of a suppurative infection in a local area such as sinusitis, mastoiditis, and, occasionally, otitis media.
• Small percentage (10%) associated with trauma.
• Associated with spread from a distant source (e.g., congenital heart disease, AVM, pulmonary infection, skin infections, endocarditis, abdominal and pelvic infections).
• Anaerobic and microaerophilic cocci and gram-negative and gram-positive anaerobic bacilli are the most common isolates, including *Staphylococcus aureus*, *Enterobacter*, and *Streptococcus* species.

Pathophysiology

• Infectious lesion in the intracranial space occurring as a result of a local or distant infection from circulating vascular or cerebrospinal fluid or trauma.

Clinical Presentation

• Presentation can vary, but may include (in order of occurrence) headache, mental status changes, focal neurologic deficits, fever, seizures, nausea and vomiting, nuchal rigidity, and papilledema.
• Localized neurologic signs are related to the area of the lesion (e.g., brainstem lesion will present with facial weakness, headache, fever, vomiting, dysphagia, and hemiparesis).

Diagnostic Evaluation

• Imaging, primarily MRI or CT, of head (Figure 6.3).
• Laboratory evaluation: complete blood count (CBC) with differential, blood culture, erythrocyte sedimentation rate, C-reactive protein (CRP), specific serology.
• In some cases, evaluation of CSF is warranted.
• Culture of involved area via surgical aspiration or stereotactic CT.

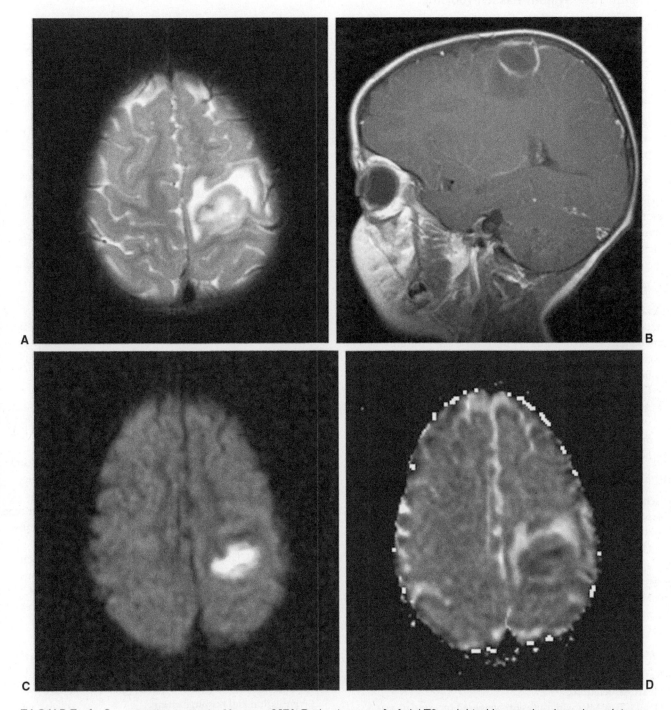

FIGURE 6.3 • **Pediatric Brain Abscess MRI.** Brain abscess. **A:** Axial T2-weighted image showing a hyperintense lesion with hypointense rim and surrounding vasogenic edema in the posterior left frontal lobe. **B:** Sagittal postcontrast T1-weighted image demonstrating hypointense central portion and rim enhancement of the mass. **C:** The lesion is very bright on the axial diffusion-weighted image. **D:** Corresponding apparent diffusion coefficient map revealing the low signal intensity of the mass, consistent with restricted diffusion of water molecules. Surrounding vasogenic edema is hyperintense due to increased diffusion.

Management

- Antimicrobial therapy with good penetration of the intracranial spaces.
- Control of increased ICP, if present.
- Surgical resection, aspiration, or drainage, especially if more than one area is involved.

- Consultation with a neurosurgeon and infectious disease specialist.

PEARL

- *Clinical manifestations are typically nonspecific; so intracranial lesions can go undiagnosed.*

Cerebrovascular Accidents

Michele Grimason

Definition

- A cerebrovascular accident, also known as stroke, is the result of a sudden interruption of arterial or venous blood flow to a focal region of the brain.

Types

- Ischemic: A decrease or disruption of blood flow, leading to dysfunction of brain tissue, caused by systemic hypoperfusion, embolism, thrombus, and sinus venous thrombosis.
- Hemorrhagic: A vessel or aneurysm ruptures and leaks into the surrounding tissue and cells.

Etiology

- About 20% of neonatal and approximately 50% of nonneonatal pediatric strokes are arterial ischemic and the remainder are hemorrhagic or secondary to cerebral sinus thrombosis.
- Most common risk factors for arterial ischemic stroke in children are:
  - Congenital and acquired heart disease.
  - Arteriopathies (e.g., arterial dissection, Moyamoya disease, vasculitis).
  - Sickle cell disease.
  - Hypercoagulable conditions.

Clinical Presentation

- Ischemic.
  - Neonates: seizures, decreased responsiveness, focal weakness.
  - Children: focal neurologic deficits such as hemiparesis, aphasia, visual disturbances, and headache.
- Hemorrhagic.
  - May present with signs of increased ICP such as headache and vomiting.
  - Other signs: irritability, seizures, and hemiparesis.

Diagnostic Evaluation

- National stroke guidelines are available from the American Heart Association.
- Head CT or MRI with diffusion-weighted imaging to assess for ischemic and hemorrhagic infarct.
- Initial CT (hours after infarct) could be negative; thus, serial imaging may be necessary.
- Consider CT angiography or MRA if concern for dissection; consider CT venography or magnetic resonance venography if concerned for venous thrombosis (Figure 6.4).

Management

- Supportive care.
  - Prevention of fever.
  - Maintenance of normoglycemia.
  - Normovolemia to maintenance of adequate substrate delivery.

- Ischemic strokes.
  - Heparin (unfractionated or low molecular weight) may be administered for as long as 1 week.
  - Acetylsalicylic acid (aspirin) 3 to 5 mg/kg has been used for ischemic stroke prophylaxis.
- Hemorrhagic stroke.
  - Neurosurgical evaluation for ICP monitoring.

PEARLS

- *Average time from initial symptoms to diagnosis of stroke is 35 hours; consequently, the patient may have experienced significant ischemia and cell death at the time of diagnosis.*
- *Should be high on the differential when a patient presents with symptoms of headache, seizure, or focal weakness.*

Delirium

Keshava Gowda & Tageldin M. Ahmed

Definition/Background

- A state of acute brain dysfunction.
- Studies have indicated that children who have prolonged ICU stays are more vulnerable to developing delirium.
- Other associated factors include neurologic disorders, including acute brain injury, medications, infection, autoimmune disorders, and multiorgan system failure.
- Postanesthetic emergence delirium is considered another type of delirium, often associated with anxiety in the preoperative period.
- Iatrogenic risk factors include sleep deprivation, restraint use, tubes, catheters, pain, and use of psychoactive medications.
- May occur in as many as 30% of critically ill infants and children.

Etiology/Types

- Hyperactive delirium, often referred as ICU psychosis, manifests as agitated behavior, restlessness, or inattention.
  - Risk increases with duration of length of mechanical ventilation and hospitalization.
- Hypoactive delirium manifests as withdrawal, flat affect, apathy, and lethargy.
- Mixed delirium is a combination of above types.
- Long-term outcomes remain uncertain.

Pathophysiology

- A number of environmental, pharmacologic, and biochemical mechanisms can lead to the final common pathway of delirium.
- There are also patient factors and iatrogenic factors.
- Disruption in the balance of stimulatory and inhibitory neurotransmitters (e.g., dopamine, acetylcholine, gamma-aminobutyric acid).

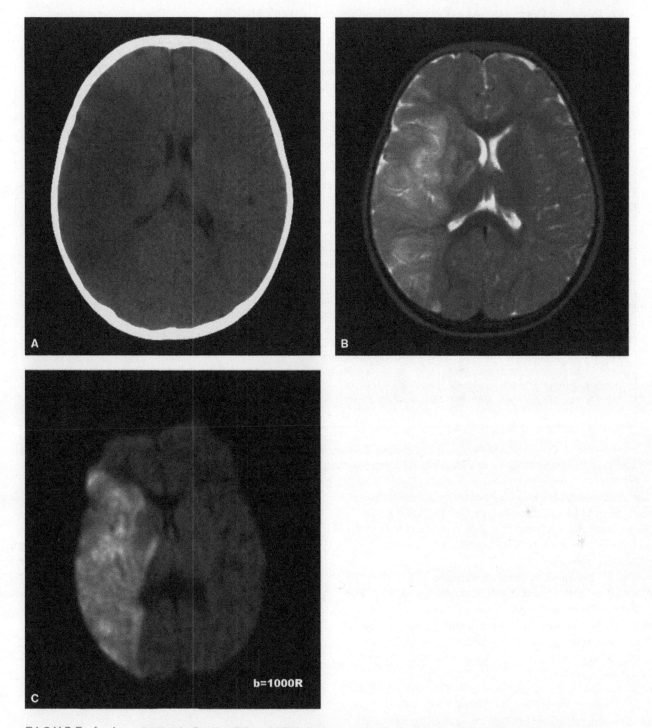

FIGURE 6.4 • **Pediatric Stroke CT and MRI.** A 2-year-old girl who awoke with left hemiparesis and right-gaze preference. **A:** A wedge-shaped area of hypodensity is seen on axial CT. MRI shows **B:** T2 hyperintensity and **C:** corresponding diffusion restriction, indicative of an ischemic stroke in the distribution of the right middle cerebral artery.

Presentation

- Sleep–wake disturbances, disorientation, inattention, purpose-less actions, labile mood or affect, inconsolability, autonomic dysregulation.
- Variation between pediatric and adult presentation emphasizes the benefit to employing a pediatric screening tool.

Diagnostic Evaluation

- Requires complete physical examination including a neuro-logic evaluation and mental status assessment.
- Evaluate for other causes of brain dysfunction (e.g., hypox-emia, new infection, deliriogenic medications, metabolic derangements, pain).

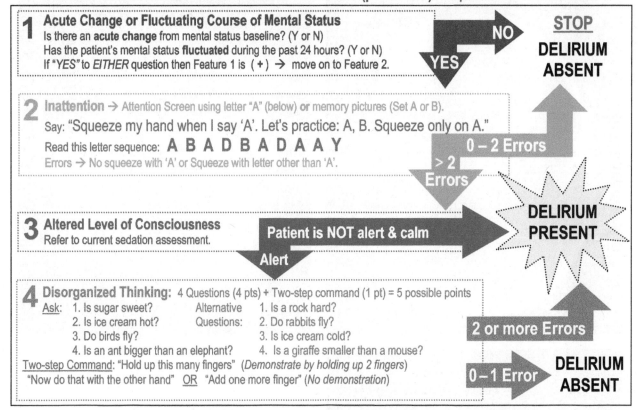

Pediatric Confusion Assessment Method for the ICU (pCAM-ICU): Step 2 Content Assessment

1 Acute Change or Fluctuating Course of Mental Status
Is there an **acute change** from mental status baseline? (Y or N)
Has the patient's mental status **fluctuated** during the past 24 hours? (Y or N)
If "*YES*" to *EITHER* question then Feature 1 is (+) → move on to Feature 2.

NO → STOP **DELIRIUM ABSENT**

YES

2 Inattention → Attention Screen using letter "A" (below) or memory pictures (Set A or B).
Say: "Squeeze my hand when I say 'A'. Let's practice: A, B. Squeeze only on A."
Read this letter sequence: **A B A D B A D A A Y**
Errors → No squeeze with 'A' or Squeeze with letter other than 'A'.

0 – 2 Errors

> 2 Errors

3 Altered Level of Consciousness
Refer to current sedation assessment.

Patient is NOT alert & calm

Alert

DELIRIUM PRESENT

4 Disorganized Thinking: 4 Questions (4 pts) + Two-step command (1 pt) = 5 possible points
Ask: 1. Is sugar sweet?   Alternative   1. Is a rock hard?
          2. Is ice cream hot?   Questions: 2. Do rabbits fly?
          3. Do birds fly?   3. Is ice cream cold?
          4. Is an ant bigger than an elephant?   4. Is a giraffe smaller than a mouse?
Two-step Command: "Hold up this many fingers" (*Demonstrate by holding up 2 fingers*)
   "Now do that with the other hand" OR "Add one more finger" (*No demonstration*)

2 or more Errors

0 – 1 Error → **DELIRIUM ABSENT**

FIGURE 6.5 • **pCAM Pediatric Confusion Assessment.** (Copyright © 2008 Heidi A.B. Smith M.D. and Monroe Carell Jr. Children's Hospital at Vanderbilt. All rights reserved.)

- Use of screening tools including pediatric Confusion Assessment Method for the Intensive Care Unit (pCAM-ICU) or Richmond Agitation Sedation Scale will assist in identifying patients with delirium in PICU (Figure 6.5).
- pCAM-ICU screening tool.
  - Rapid; <2 minutes to complete screening.
  - Specificity 99%; sensitivity 83% in diagnosing delirium in children >5 years of age.
  - Screens for the most fundamental signs of delirium first.
  - Delirium is not present if the child does not display any acute change or fluctuation in mental status or inattention.
- Richmond Agitation Sedation Scale screening tool.
  - Tool to assist in the evaluation of level of consciousness (LOC).
  - Scale from unarousable (−5) to combative (+4).
- Electroencephalogram (EEG) can be utilized for assistance with diagnosis indicating slowing or disorganization.
  - Limitations in evaluation include developmental and cognitive changes in childhood.

Management

- Recognition of the importance of routine delirium evaluation by the interprofessional team.
- Implementation of screening tool (e.g., pCAM-ICU).
- Very little research is available to support therapy.
- Combination of psychosocial and pharmacologic therapies, along with removing or minimizing causative factors, is the best management.

- Minimize known risk factors such as sleep disruption, noise, and environmental disturbances.
- Maintain continuity of care.
- Provide calm, soothing, reassuring environment (e.g., limit extraneous sounds, encourage familiar music/pictures/personal items in child's room).
- Establish day/night routine (as allowed by clinical status) and periods for uninterrupted sleep.
- Encourage family to be present with the child.
- Avoid trigger medications including benzodiazepines.
- Pharmacologic management with haloperidol, droperidol, and risperidone.
- Involve child life therapists/hospital teachers.

Encephalopathy

Michele Grimason

Background

- The brain requires adequate perfusion, acid–base balance, normothermia, as well as a delicate balance of substrates, neurotransmitters, water, and electrolytes, to function correctly.
- Derangement in this milieu can cause disruption of neurotransmitter signals, disturbances of electrical impulses within the brain, and injury to brain cells.

Definition

- Encephalopathy is defined as global brain dysfunction leading to an altered mental state.

Types

- Acute toxic/metabolic encephalopathy.
  - Global cerebral dysfunction resulting in altered consciousness, behavior changes, and/or seizures.
  - Excludes primary structural brain disease, infection, and traumatic brain injury.
  - Etiologies include electrolyte imbalance, medication, environment, organ dysfunction, and inborn errors of metabolism.
- Hypoxic–ischemic encephalopathy.
  - Occurs after an event such as cardiac arrest.
  - Deprives the brain of adequate perfusion or oxygenation, resulting in cerebral ischemia, hypoxia, and cell death.
- Other acute encephalopathies.
  - Infectious.
  - Postinfectious.
  - Vascular disorders.
- Static encephalopathy.
  - Cerebral dysfunction that is permanent and nonprogressive.
  - Etiologies include prematurity, infection, and ischemia.
- Progressive encephalopathies.
  - Most commonly associated with neurodegenerative disorders.
  - May also be associated with autoimmune disorders (e.g., Hashimoto thyroiditis, NMDA receptor antibody encephalitis).
  - These disorders present with progressive deterioration of neurologic dysfunction, sometimes in a previously healthy child, and are the result of specific biochemical or genetic abnormalities, infections, or other unknown causes.

Clinical Presentation

- Mental status changes.
  - Infant: irritability, lethargy, poor feeding.
  - Child: personality or behavioral changes, cognitive decline, concentration problems.
- Other symptoms: seizures, nystagmus, tremor, myoclonus, abnormal movements.

Diagnostic Evaluation

- Since multiple mechanisms (toxins, infection, electrolyte abnormality, cerebral ischemia, or medications) may produce encephalopathy, the diagnostic approach may be broad and is adjusted according to each patient's specific risk factors.
- Laboratory.
  - General: CBC with differential, comprehensive metabolic panel, liver function test, ammonia, coagulation panel, blood gas analysis.
  - Infectious: blood, urine, and CSF cultures.
  - Metabolic: serum amino acids, urine organic acids, lactate, thyroid function tests.
  - Toxic: toxicology screen, medication drug levels, lead level.
  - Inflammatory: CSF for oligoclonal bands; serum for antibodies (thyroid, NMDA).
- CT or MRI.
- EEG to identify seizures and background organization.

- Medications should be reviewed to assess if they are contributing to encephalopathy.

Management

- Electrolyte imbalances should be corrected.
- Antimicrobial, antifungal, and antiviral agents, if indicated, should be initiated promptly.
- Antiepileptics should be administered to treat seizures.
- Steroids should be considered with a postinfectious or autoimmune encephalopathy.

Guillain-Barré Syndrome/Acute Inflammatory Demyelinating Polyradiculoneuropathy

Kelly K. Marcoux

Background

- Both axonal and demyelinating forms have been described.

Definition

- Acute inflammatory peripheral neuropathy.

Etiology/Types

- Specific cause unknown.
- Autoimmune disease triggered by infectious process (particularly viral) as well as immunizations; often preceded by a viral illness or upper respiratory tract infection (URI).

Clinical Presentation

- Progressive extremity weakness, may progress to paralysis, usually ascending; begins distally and progresses to proximal muscles (respiratory, trunk, cranial muscles), maximum weakness usually occurs 1 to 2 weeks after onset of symptoms.
- Areflexia.
- Numbness.
- CN palsies.
- Hypoventilation due to weak respiratory muscles.
- With or without altered LOC.
- With or without ataxia.
- Autonomic instability can occur, including wide fluctuations in blood pressure (BP), diaphoresis, vasoconstriction, pupil dilation and constriction, and cardiac arrhythmias.

Diagnostic Evaluation

- Lumbar puncture (diagnostic): CSF demonstrates elevated protein (>45 mg/dL) and absence of pleocytosis.
- Electromyogram (EMG): diffuse demyelination and delayed motor conduction consistent with lower motor neuron disease.

Management

- Intravenous immunoglobulin (IVIG).
  - IVIG may work via several mechanisms, including blocking macrophage receptors, inhibiting antibody production, inhibiting complement binding, and neutralizing pathologic antibodies.

- Plasmapheresis.
  - Removal of circulating humoral factors (e.g., immunoglobulins and antibodies) responsible for demyelination.
- Supportive care (e.g., airway protection, skin care, physical therapy).
  - Assess functional vital capacity, negative inspiratory force serially (assists in determining trajectory and need for mechanical ventilation).
  - Evaluate BP for autonomic dysfunction.

Hypoxic-Ischemic Encephalopathy

Kelly K. Marcoux

Background

- There are many types of encephalopathy which encompass disorders with acute global brain dysfunction resulting in altered mental status.
- Primary processes leading to hypoxic–ischemic encephalopathy are brain hypoxia and ischemia due to hypoxemia, reduced cerebral blood flow, or both.

Definition

- Type of toxic/metabolic encephalopathy occurring before, during, or after birth due to lack of oxygen or inadequate perfusion, resulting in cerebral ischemia and hypoxia.

Etiology/Types

- Associated with trauma, asphyxiation, congenital abnormality, stroke, medications, and prematurity.
- In older children, can also result from submersion injury, chronic hypoxia from pulmonary disease, respiratory or circulatory arrest, systemic hemorrhage, or carbon monoxide poisoning.

Clinical Presentation

- History:
  - Infants: irritability, poor feeding, change in mental status.
  - Older children: change in mental status, personality or cognitive changes, such as inability to concentrate.
- Examination:
  - Abnormal reflexes.
  - Disorientation.
  - Depressed mental status.
  - Abnormal pupillary response.
  - Abnormal motor response (e.g., tremors, asymmetry, hypotonia, hemiparesis, posturing).
  - Abnormal heart rhythm or perfusion.
  - May have apnea.

Diagnostic Evaluation

- Laboratory evaluation:
  - CBC with differential; comprehensive chemistry, liver function tests with bilirubin, ammonia; coagulation studies; blood gas analysis; toxicology screen; blood, urine, and CSF cultures with viral polymerase chain reaction (PCR).
  - Consider serum amino acids and urine organic acid panels if inborn error of metabolism suspected.

- If endocrine disorder suspected, consider thyroid function tests and cortisol levels.
- Radiologic evaluation.
  - CT brain: initial diagnostic study to evaluate acute hemorrhage, calcifications, mass lesion, cerebral edema.
  - MRI/MRA brain: to identify vascular or hemorrhagic disease.
  - EEG: to evaluate seizure activity, particularly subclinical seizures.

Management

- Supportive care aimed at restoration of adequate oxygenation and ventilation; prevention of secondary injury and increased ICP.
- ABCs; consider endotracheal intubation for airway protection.
- Monitor for increased ICP.
- Correct glucose and electrolyte imbalances; avoid hypo- and hyperosmolar states.
- Hypothermia therapy (e.g., cool cap in neonates).
- Appropriate antibiotic, antiviral, and/or antifungal agents; if indicated, prompt administration.
- Antiepileptic agents to control seizure activity.
- Specialty consultation: neurology, critical care, neurosurgery, cardiology, nephrology, endocrinology, rheumatology, pulmonology, genetics, and rehabilitation medicine.

Intracranial Hypertension

Cathy Haut

Definition/Background

- Three main components inside the skull: brain (80%), CSF (10%), and blood (10%).
  - After birth, the skull becomes relatively inflexible, leaving a fixed space in the skull.
- An increase in any of the three components in the skull requires a decrease in another component (e.g., Monro–Kellie doctrine).
- ICP limits due to fixed space.
- The normal range for ICP varies with age, and the values for children are not well established.
- Typically, accepted normal values are <20–25 cm H_2O in older children and <15–20 mmHg in children <1 year of age.
- ICP can be subatmospheric in newborns, especially in the presence of open fontanels.
- ICP generally peaks 24 to 72 hours after a traumatic injury.
- Cerebral perfusion pressure (CPP) = Mean arterial pressure (MAP) – ICP.
  - Goals: infant >40 mmHg, children >50 mmHg, and adolescents >60 mmHg.
  - Net pressure gradient supplying blood flow to the brain depends on MAP and ICP.
  - MAP is equal to one third systolic BP and two third diastolic BP. Therefore, CPP can be decreased from an increase in ICP, decrease in systemic BP, or a combination of both.

TABLE 6.2	**Causes of Increased Intracranial Pressure**	
Intracranial (Primary)	**Extracranial (Secondary)**	**Postoperative**
• Brain tumor. • Trauma (epidural and subdural hematoma, cerebral contusions). • Nontraumatic intracerebral hemorrhage. • Ischemic stroke. • Hydrocephalus. • Idiopathic or benign intracranial hypertension (pseudotumor cerebri). • Other (e.g., pseudotumor cerebri, pneumoencephalus, abscesses, cysts).	• Airway obstruction or hypoventilation (hypoxia and hypercarbia). • Hypertension or hypotension. • Posture (head rotation). • Hyperpyrexia. • Seizures. • Drug and metabolic (e.g., tetracycline, lead intoxication). • Others (e.g., high-altitude cerebral edema, hepatic failure).	• Mass lesion (hematoma). • Edema. • Increased cerebral blood volume (vasodilation). • Disturbances of CSF.

- Low CPP has been associated with poor outcomes in trauma literature.
- ICP can change easily based on many factors, including intracranial, extracranial, and postoperative situations.
- Idiopathic intracranial hypertension, also known as pseudotumor cerebri, causes increased ICP without evidence of space-occupying lesion or vascular abnormality.

Etiology

- See Table 6.2.

Pathophysiology

- Intracranial hypertension occurs when there is an increase in the volume of any of the intracranial compartments which necessitates a decrease in another, or an increase in ICP will occur (known as Monro–Kellie doctrine).
- The body has various mechanisms by which it keeps the ICP stable, with CSF pressures varying by approximately 1 mmHg in healthy patients through shifts in production and absorption of CSF.
- ICP changes based on normal body functions such as coughing and hyperthermia, but severe changes resulting from trauma or cerebral edema can cause ICP which may be difficult to control, thus contributing to intracranial hypertension and secondary brain injury.
- Persistent increase in ICP can lead to brain herniation and death.
- Cerebral edema may be the result of intracellular swelling (cytotoxic edema), capillary endothelial cell dysfunction, or interstitial edema.

Clinical Presentation

- Traumatic brain injury is the most common problem leading to increased ICP.
- Symptoms of increased ICP include loss of consciousness or altered LOC, vomiting, increased head circumference (especially infant) and tense fontanel, seizures or status epilepticus, coma.
- Cushing triad is an indication of increased ICP with irregular respirations, widening pulse pressure, and bradycardia, indicating impending herniation. *These signs indicate a medical emergency.*

Diagnosis

- Head CT is the initial diagnostic study; rapid with definitive results of cerebral edema and other underlying pathology.
- Increased ICP or intracranial hypertension can be diagnosed and monitored via a ventriculostomy or ICP monitor.
- For more information on ICP monitoring, see Diagnostic Testing later in this section (Figure 6.6).

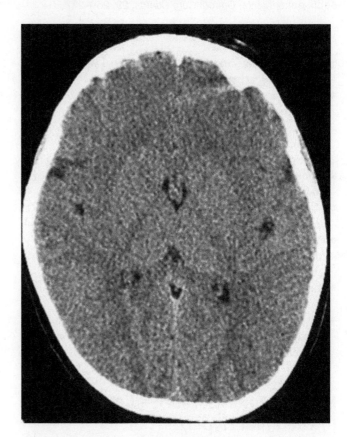

FIGURE 6.6 • **Cerebral Edema Noncontrast CT.** Axial noncontrast CT scan shows diffuse edema manifested as sulcal effacement and low attenuation of the cerebral cortex, resulting in loss of cortical-white matter contrast.

TABLE 1	Empiric Management of Suspected or Documented intracranial hypertension Used at the Children's Hospital of Pittsburgh
Therapy/Intervention	**Comments**
Mannitol 250 mg/kg every 6 h	Place Foley catheter Avoid hypovolemia Monitor serum osmolality and hold dose if >320 mOsm
Hypertonic saline	Desired range serum Na^+ >135 and <150 mEq/L Deliver centrally
Arterial and central venous lines for continuous monitoring of blood pressure and CVP, respectively	Prevent and aggressively treat hypotension
Mechanical ventilation	Maintain $Paco_2$ 35–40 mmHg Maintain Pao_2 >90 mmHg
Temperature control	Prevent and treat hyperthermia Consider hypothermia for refractory status epilepticus
Seizure prophylaxis (refer to text for management of documented seizures)	Consider fosphenytoin or levetiracetam
Glucose management	Prevent and/or aggressively treat hypoglycemia

FIGURE 6.7 • **Management of Increased ICP.** From Simon, D. W., Da Silva, Y. S., Zuccoli, G., & Clark, R. S. B. (2013). Acute encephalitis. *Critical Care Clinics, 29,* 259–277.

Management

- Insert ICP monitoring device, either external ventriculostomy device or parenchymal catheter.
- Maintain adequate CPP.
  - Infants >40 mmHg.
  - Children >50 mmHg.
  - Adolescents >60 mmHg.
  - Elevations in ICP typically peak 24 to 72 hours following injury.
- Monitor ICP; if increased, control extrinsic factors, and/or drain CSF (if ventriculostomy drain present).
- Medical management should include sedation, drainage of CSF, and osmotic diuresis with either mannitol or hypertonic saline.
- Position with head of bed elevated and midline.
- Mild hyperventilation is helpful in decreasing ICP, with goal CO_2 30 to 35 mmHg.
- If evidence of cerebral ischemia and no contraindications, consider hypothermia.
- For intracranial hypertension refractory to initial medical management, barbiturate coma, hypothermia, or decompressive craniectomy should be considered (Figure 6.7).

Pseudotumor Cerebri: Idiopathic Intracranial Hypertension

Cathy Haut

Clinical Presentation

- Often presents in obese or overweight adolescent females with persistent headache and visual loss or diplopia.

- These patients are often referred from primary care providers who have evaluated papilledema as an accompanying physical feature.

Diagnosis

- Opening-pressure evaluation with lumbar puncture.
- Imaging, usually MRI, which is completed to document normal results.
- Ophthalmology examination with visual fields.
- Associated conditions or risk factors: obesity, hypernatremia, medications such as tetracyclines, fluoroquinolones, oral contraceptives, vitamin A, isotretinoin, sulfamethoxazole, growth hormone, lithium.

Management

- Medications for the management of headache symptoms and acetazolamide (Diamox).
- Draining CSF with repeated lumbar punctures, surgery.
- Identify/Address any secondary cause.
- Main goal of treatment is to prevent or reverse visual loss.

Bacterial Meningitis

Denise C. Schiel

Definition/Background

- Inflammation of the membranes lining the brain and spinal cord.
- Infectious etiologies include acute bacterial, viral, fungal, parasitic.

- Usually purulent and involves the fluid in the subarachnoid space.
- Most common acute central nervous system (CNS) infection.
- More than two third of cases involve children <15 years of age.
- Peak incidence in 3 to 12 months of age, with decreasing incidence after age 2 years.
- Peak season is late fall and early winter.

Risk Factors

- Males > females.
- Urban areas, crowded living conditions, poverty.
- Underlying chronic illness/immunosuppression, asplenia.

Routes of CNS Invasion

- Causative agent varies with age and route of infection.
- Hematogenous dissemination.
- Sinuses, middle ear, mastoid, other pericranial structures.
- Congenital or acquired defects in the skull or spinal cord (Table 6.3).

Pathophysiology

- Colonization and penetration of the nasopharyngeal epithelium or direct extension from a distant site of infection.
- Hematogenous dissemination.
- Bacteria enter the CNS and circulate to CSF/subarachnoid space.
- Bacterial-/endotoxin-induced local inflammation of the meninges, CSF, and ventricles.
- Polymorphonuclear infiltration of the subarachnoid space.

Mechanism of CNS Injury

- Alterations in CBF.
- Initial hyperemia followed by a reduction of CBF with progressive infection/inflammation.
- Impaired delivery of metabolic substrate (e.g., oxygen and glucose) to the brain tissue with resultant ischemia and infarction.

Infection-Mediated Loss of Capillary Integrity

- Altered cerebral metabolism.
- Impairment of CSF flow and drainage.
- Inflammation may block the reuptake of CSF by arachnoid villi, causing communicating hydrocephalus.
- Infection within the ventricles (ventriculitis) or at the base of the brain may cause obstructive hydrocephalus.
- Cortical ischemia.
- Increased ICP.
  - Due to cerebral edema, hydrocephalus, venous congestion (Table 6.4).

Clinical Presentation

- Sudden or insidious onset.
- Systemic symptoms:
  - Fever/chills.
  - Anorexia/poor feeding.
  - Myalgias/arthralgias.
  - URI symptoms.
  - Tachycardia/hypotension.
  - Cutaneous signs: petechiae, purpura, erythematous macular rash.
- Meningeal signs:
  - Severe throbbing headache, photophobia.
  - Nuchal rigidity.
  - Kernig sign:
    - Passive extension of the knee in supine position, resulting in back pain and resistance.
  - Brudzinski sign:
    - Passive flexion of the neck, resulting in involuntary flexion of the knees and hips.
- Neurologic signs:
  - Increased ICP: Cushing triad (i.e., bradycardia, hypertension, abnormal respirations), emesis, bulging fontanel, widening of the cranial sutures.
  - Posturing, seizures, alterations in LOC, irritability, stupor, coma.
  - CN palsies.
  - Focal neurologic deficits.

TABLE 6.3	Age-Associated Pathogens for Meningitis
Age	**Common Organisms**
<1 mo	Group B streptococcus. *E. coli.* *Listeria monocytogenes.* *Klebsiella* species.
1–2 mo	*Strep. pneumoniae.* *H. influenzae* type B. *N. meningitidis.* Group B streptococcus. *E. coli.*
2 mo to 5 y	*Strep. pneumoniae.* *H. influenzae* type B. *N. meningitidis.*
5 y	*N. meningitidis.* *Strep. pneumoniae.*

TABLE 6.4	CSF Changes Associated with Bacterial Meningitis
Diagnostic Finding	**Explanation**
↑ WBC	Usually polymorphonuclear leukocytes.
↑ Protein	Transudation across injured capillaries.
↓ Glucose	Decreased transport and increased utilization.
↑ Pressure	Cerebral edema and hydrocephalus.
↑ Lactate	Altered cerebral metabolism, if >25 mg/dL, indicative of bacterial meningitis.

Diagnosis

- Clinical signs and symptoms.
- Head CT to evaluate for abscess or space-occupying lesion.
- Lumbar puncture for CSF analysis.
- Blood culture (~80% will have a positive blood culture).
- CSF information.
  - Traumatic tap.
    - In the context of a traumatic or "bloody" spinal tap, the predicted WBC count can be calculated as follows:
      - Predicted CSF WBC = CSF RBC × (serum WBC/serum RBC).
  - WBC: RBC ratio of CSF should be similar to that of the serum (i.e., ~1:700).
  - Some guidelines suggest allowing 1 WBC for every 500 to 700 RBCs and 0.01 g/L protein for every 1,000 RBCs.
  - Rules based on a "predicted" WBC count in the CSF are not reliable.
  - Guidelines on decisions about whom not to treat for possible meningitis should be conservative.
  - The safest interpretation of a traumatic tap is to count the total number of WBCs, and disregard the RBC count; if there are more WBCs than the normal range for age, then the safest option is treatment.

Management

- Prompt definitive treatment.
- Immediate administration of antibiotics; if child is too unstable to undergo a lumbar puncture, do not wait to obtain cultures prior to initiating antibiotic therapy.
- Antibiotic therapy based on most likely organism according to history, age, and presentation.
  - Recent neurosurgery or ventricular shunt: coagulase-negative staphylococci (*Staphylococcus epidermidis*), methicillin-susceptible and methicillin-resistant *Staph. aureus* (i.e., MSSA, MRSA), aerobic gram-negative bacilli (*Pseudomonas aeruginosa*), *Propionibacterium acnes*.
    - Management: vancomycin + cefepime; vancomycin + ceftazidime; or vancomycin + meropenem.
  - Basilar skull fracture: *Streptococcus pneumoniae*, *Neisseria meningitidis*, *Strep. pyogenes*.
    - Management: vancomycin + 3rd-generation cephalosporin.
- Supportive treatment of systemic and metabolic consequences of infection.
  - Sepsis/shock/respiratory failure/disseminated intravascular coagulation.
  - Hypothalamic/pituitary dysfunction.
- Treatment of neurologic sequelae.
  - Increased ICP/cerebral edema/hydrocephalus/seizures/vasospasm.
- Evacuation of loculated infection.
  - Abscess or empyema.
- Adjunctive therapy.
  - Dexamethasone.
    - Proven benefit is only in patients with known *Haemophilus influenzae* type B infection.
    - Decreased risk of neurosensory hearing loss.

TABLE 6.5	Normal CSF Findings		
	Protein (mg/dL)	Glucose (mg/dL)	WBC (mm³)
Newborn	20–170	34–119	0–22
Child >1 mo	5–40	40–80	0–7

- Dose: 0.15 mg/kg every 6 hours for 2 to 4 days if given 10 to 20 minutes prior to or at least concomitantly with the first dose of antibiotics.
- No proven benefit for children who have already received antibiotics.
- Use in children with pneumococcal meningitis is controversial.

Prognosis

- Mortality is 5% to 15%.
- 20% to 30% develop severe long-term neurodevelopmental sequelae.
- Hearing loss, neurologic impairment, seizures, visual impairment, delay in language acquisition, chronic residual hydrocephalus.
- 50% develop neurobehavioral morbidities: behavior problems, attention deficit, hyperactivity, and others (Table 6.5).

Viral Meningitis

Denise C. Schiel

Definition/Etiology

- Most common cause of meningitis in children.
- Specific agent usually not identified.
  - Enteroviruses account for >80% of cases.
  - Echovirus, coxsackievirus.
  - Arboviruses, mumps, Epstein–Barr virus, cytomegalovirus, varicella, adenovirus, and herpes simplex virus are other causes.
- Peak incidence in late summer/early fall.

Pathophysiology

- Viral replication in the initial organ system, with access to the bloodstream and then CSF.
- Primary viremia introduces the virus to the reticuloendothelial organs, specifically liver, spleen, and lymph nodes, and replication occurs.
  - If the replication persists despite immunologic defenses, secondary viremia occurs, which is thought to be responsible for seeding of the CNS.
  - The rapidity of viral replication probably plays a major role in overcoming the host defenses.
  - The mechanism of viral penetration into the CNS is not well understood. The virus may cross the blood–brain barrier directly at the capillary endothelial level.

- Hematogenous spread is the most common route for viral penetration of most known pathogens.
- Neural penetration along the nerve roots: usually limited to herpes viruses (HSV-1, HSV-2, and varicella zoster virus), and possibly some enteroviruses.
- Typically, local and systemic immune responses, skin and mucosal barriers, and the blood–brain barrier prevent the viral inoculum from being effective in causing clinically significant infection.
- Inflammatory response is noted as pleocytosis; polymorphonuclear leukocytes predominate the differential cell count in the first 24 to 48 hours, followed later by increasing numbers of monocytes and lymphocytes.

Diagnosis

- Associated CSF changes
  - Glucose normal to slightly decreased.
  - Protein slightly increased.
  - WBC: mildly increased with neutrophil predominance early, followed by lymphocyte predominance.
- CSF PCR for HSV is the "gold standard" for diagnosis of HSV meningitis.

Clinical Presentation

- Signs and symptoms similar to bacterial meningitis (although may not appear as "toxic").
- Acute-onset fever/lethargy/irritability.
- Increased ICP, autoregulation.
- Anorexia/vomiting.
- Hyper/hyporeflexia.
- Bulging fontanel, increased ICP.
- Seizures.
- Skin rash (varicella, enteroviruses).
- Diarrhea (enteroviruses).
- URI (enteroviruses).
- Older children:
  - Headache.
  - Meningeal signs.
  - Photophobia.
- Characteristics of HSV meningitis:
  - EEG: sharp waves superimposed on a slow background in the temporal region.
  - CSF may contain RBCs/xanthochromia.
  - CT or MRI: temporal hypodensity or edema.

Management

- Usually self-limited and resolves in 7 to 10 days, largely supportive care and support of vital functions.
- Control of seizures.
- Specific antiviral therapy if HSV suspected.
  - Herpes meningitis (meningoencephalitis).
  - Presentation similar to viral meningitis.
- May have associated changes in cortical function: ataxia, focal neurologic signs, acute encephalopathy (high suspicion).
- Decreased morbidity and mortality with prompt antiviral therapy.
- If HSV meningitis is suspected, most important treatment is prompt initiation of antiviral agent: acyclovir IV.

Encephalitis
Cathy Haut

Background/Definition

- An inflammatory process of the brain parenchyma which is usually caused by an infectious process or can be a hyperimmune reaction.
- Indicates brain parenchymal involvement and is most often associated with meningitis.
- Viral etiologies are most common; however, many cases do not have an identifiable cause.
- Pathologic diagnosis involving neuroinflammation, brain tissue damage, pathogen.
- High morbidity and mortality for survivors.

Etiology

- Can occur with bacterial meningitis and with organisms such as *Borrelia burgdorferi* (Lyme disease), *Bartonella* (cat scratch disease), and *Treponema pallidum* (syphilis).
- Fungal encephalitis includes cryptococcus, and is concerning for immunocompromised children.
- Acute viral encephalitis can be caused by rabies virus, herpes simplex virus, and other etiologies.
- Immune-mediated encephalitis can also occur in children, but poses more difficulty with diagnosis.

Pathophysiology

- An inflammatory process of the brain parenchyma which results in altered neurologic status/function.

Clinical Presentation

- Fever.
- Altered consciousness.
- Seizures.
- Focal neurologic signs.
- Neonates/infants may present with shock, lethargy, irritability, poor feeding, seizures, and apnea.
- Distinguish from bacterial meningitis and other causes of encephalopathy.
- Diagnosis made on the constellation of symptoms.
- Clinical features vary based on the causal agent.

Etiology

- In many cases, it is not identified despite an extensive evaluation.

Diagnostic Evaluation

- EEG: nonspecific, sensitive for brain dysfunction; abnormal in approximately 90% of cases.
- MRI brain.
  - MRI preferred over CT imaging, though CT with IV contrast may be sufficient when MRI is contraindicated.
  - MRI with diffusion-weighted imaging can detect early lesions and depict lesion borders.
- Neuroimaging is abnormal in approximately 50% of cases.

- Lumbar puncture.
  - Consider delaying in patients with altered mental status (may be a sign of increased ICP).
  - Neuroimaging is often insensitive to the presence of cerebral edema in cases of meningoencephalitis.
  - When safe to perform:
    - CSF is usually clear and colorless.
    - Opening pressure may be normal or elevated.
    - Typically, mononuclear pleocytosis (>5 WBC/μL).
    - Polymorphonuclear cells may be noted if sampled early in the course of illness.
    - Protein and glucose usually normal.
    - Bacterial culture; negative result excludes bacterial meningitis.
    - Viral culture; low yield, though helpful if positive.

Management

- ABCs.
- Intubation for Glasgow Coma Scale ≤8.
- Antibiotic and antiviral therapy; prompt administration.
  - Until infectious etiology and bacterial meningitis are excluded.
  - Acyclovir until herpes simplex virus can be excluded.
  - Tailor therapy if causative pathogen identified.
- If seizures, anticonvulsant therapy.
  - Lorazepam or diazepam for immediate management.
- Intracranial hypertension; management as outlined in ICP section.
- Avoid/prevent secondary brain injury.
- Physical and occupational therapy evaluations when stable.
- Long-term sequelae may include irreversible brain damage.
- Consultation with a pediatric infectious disease specialist.

PEARL

- *The etiology of encephalitis remains elusive in many cases.*

Myasthenia Gravis

Denise C. Schiel

Definition/Background

- Literal meaning "grave muscle weakness."
- Chronic neuromuscular disease characterized by varying degrees of weakness and fatigability of the skeletal muscles.
- Due to autoimmune destruction of the acetylcholine receptors at the neuromuscular junction.
- Adult and juvenile forms are clinically identical, occurs in all ethnic groups.
- Onset of juvenile myasthenia gravis (MG) is 3 months to 16 years.

Types

- Transient neonatal:
  - Occurs in approximately 10% to 12% of mothers with autoimmune MG.
  - Due to transplacental transfer of maternal antibodies.
  - Typically presents shortly after birth and can last for 1 week to 2 months.
  - Symptoms include hypotonia, ptosis, weak suck and cry, and respiratory insufficiency or failure.
  - Diagnosis is based on serum antibody titers and maternal history.
  - Treatment is anticholinesterase and symptomatic support.
- Congenital:
  - Usually presents in childhood.
  - Symptoms are similar to juvenile MG.
  - Autosomal dominant, recessive or sporadic.
  - Acetylcholine receptor (AChR) antibody negative (therefore not autoimmune).
  - Due to congenital abnormalities resulting in presynaptic, synaptic, or postsynaptic defects of the neuromuscular junction.
  - No role for immunosuppressants.
  - Variable response to anticholinesterase medications.
- Juvenile:
  - Although uncommon, it is the most common form in pediatrics, clinically identical to the adult form.
  - Onset of juvenile MG is 3 months to 16 years.
  - Subtypes:
    - Ocular: localized form limited to the muscles of the eye; weakness is asymmetric.
      - Symptoms include ptosis and diplopia.
      - Does not progress to generalized weakness.
      - Pupillary response is unaffected.
    - Generalized: may begin with ocular symptoms and progress to generalized weakness, or initial presentation may be generalized weakness.
    - Presentation:
      - Hallmark is muscle weakness that worsens during periods of exercise or activity and improves after periods of rest.
      - May present with ocular symptoms alone or in combination with facial muscle weakness, difficulty chewing, talking, or swallowing, weakness of the extremities and neck, and shortness of breath.

Diagnosis

- Based on clinical presentation, history, and physical examination, including a detailed neurologic assessment.
- If MG is suspected, a confirmatory test should be sought.
- Approximately 80% of patients will have AChR antibodies.
  - 30% to 40% of those without AChR antibodies will have antibodies to muscle-specific kinase (anti-MuSK antibodies).
  - Neither antibody may be present in some individuals, particularly those with ocular MG.
- The classic bedside test is the edrophonium or Tensilon test. Edrophonium is a rapid-onset (30–90 seconds), short-acting (5 minutes) anticholinesterase that temporarily blocks the degradation of acetylcholine.
- Some patients may not show a response to edrophonium or it may not be widely available, in which case neostigmine or

pyridostigmine may be substituted, which has a short onset but its effect may last for hours.

- Patients should be on a cardiac monitor and atropine available to treat any muscarinic adverse effects such as bradycardia, increased bronchial secretions, and bronchospasm.
- Repetitive nerve stimulation test: tests for gradual muscle fatigue due to repetitive nerve stimulation and impaired nerve-to-muscle transmission.
- Diagnostic imaging of the chest to evaluate for thymoma.
  - Some individuals with MG develop tumors of the thymus gland.
  - The relationship between MG and the presence of thymomas is not clear; some researchers believe they play a role in auto-immunity and the formation of AChR antibodies.

Treatment

- Consult neurology specialist.
- Pharmacologic treatment: anticholinesterase medications such as pyridostigmine or neostigmine.
- Immunosuppressants such as corticosteroids, azathioprine, cyclophosphamide, cyclosporine, methotrexate, mycopheno-late, and tacrolimus.
- IVIG.

Other Therapies

- Plasmapheresis.
- Thymectomy: recommended for those with thymoma, but may also alleviate symptoms in some patients without thymoma.

Myasthenic Crisis

- Life-threatening emergency.
- Triggered by infection, or sometimes an adverse reaction to a medication.
- An exacerbation of MG that results in severe weakness of the respiratory muscles, the diaphragm, and the upper airway muscles, leading to respiratory failure.
- Admission to the pediatric intensive care unit is indicated for advanced airway management.

PEARL

- *Most children with MG will lead normal lives with treatment, with temporary or permanent remission.*

Neurocutaneous Disorders

Denise C. Schiel

Definition

- A group of inherited disorders, mostly autosomal dominant, that are characterized by tumors in the brain, spine, skin, and eye.
- Neurofibromatosis: common form with development of mul-tiple soft tumors, called neurofibromas, of the skin and CNS.

- Two types:
  - Neurofibromatosis 1 (NF1): accounting for approximately 90% of cases, affecting approximately 1 in every 2,500 to 3,000 individuals.
    - Mutation of neurofibromin, responsible for regulating cell growth of neurocutaneous tissues.
    - 30% to 50% of new cases arise spontaneously through genetic mutation.
  - Neurofibromatosis 2 (NF2): much less common, accounting for approximately 10% of cases, affecting approximately 1 in 40,000 individuals.
    - Mutation in the NF2 gene that encodes merlin, a protein believed to play a role in controlling cell growth, motility, and remodeling.

Presentation

- NF1
  - Typically present at birth or in the first few years of life, usually by age 10 years.
  - Café au lait spots are present in greater than 90% of all patients and are often the first clinical manifestation in infants and young children.
  - Lisch nodules (hamartomas of the iris) are pathognomonic for NF1.
  - Tumors of the peripheral nerves, known as neurofibromas, are the most common nerve-associated tumor.
    - Usually benign, but 3% to 5% may become malignant.
  - Scoliosis is the most common osseous disorder, affecting 10% to 30% of individuals, with other abnormalities includ-ing short stature, tibial dysplasia, and abnormalities of the sphenoid bone.
  - Optic gliomas are present in about 15% of patients, usually as-ymptomatic, and typically occur within the first decade of life.
  - Cardiac manifestations include hypertension, congenital anomalies, and vasculopathies, with renal artery stenosis being the most common in pediatric patients with NF1, and the most common cause for hypertension.
- NF2
  - Typically present in early adulthood.
  - Develop hearing loss or ringing in the ears due to the hallmark finding of slow-growing tumors on the 8th CN, known as vestibular schwannomas.
  - May have cutaneous schwannomas (small flesh-colored skin flaps), but rarely have café au lait spots.

Diagnosis

- See Table 6.6.

Management

- No specific therapeutic management; treatment tailored to the individual.
- Surgery is recommended for tumors that become symptom-atic or malignant or for cosmetic reasons.
- Biannual physical examinations during childhood and annually thereafter, including neurologic and ophthalmologic evaluation.
- Formal neurodevelopmental and behavioral evaluation is warranted.

TABLE 6.6   NIH Diagnostic Criteria: NF1 and NF2

NF1	NF2
Present with two or more of the following: Six or more café au lait macules measuring more than 5 mm in diameter in children and more than 15 mm in adolescents and adults. Two or more neurofibromas, or one plexiform neurofibroma. Freckling in the axilla or inguinal region. Tumor on the optic nerve (optic glioma). Two or more Lisch nodules (iris hamartomas). Abnormal development of the spine, tibia, or sphenoid bone. A first-degree relative with NF1.	Bilateral CN VIII mass detectable on MRI or CT (vestibular schwannomas). A first-degree relative with NF2 plus a unilateral vestibular schwannoma before the age of 30 or any two of the following: Glioma. Meningioma. Schwannoma. Juvenile posterior subcapsular/lenticular opacity (cataract).

- Patients with NF2 should undergo annual neurologic and ophthalmologic evaluation in addition to audiometry and brain MRI.

PEARLS

- *Patients with NF1 are at increased risk for neurocognitive and behavioral deficits, including attention deficit hyperactivity disorder, autism spectrum disorders, and language and motor deficits, and for malignancies such as pheochromocytomas and chronic myeloid leukemia.*
- *Patients with NF2 are at risk for developing other nervous system tumors such as gliomas, meningiomas, schwannomas, and neurofibromas.*
- *Early onset of symptoms and the presence of meningiomas are associated with a poor prognosis in patients with NF2.*

Tuberous Sclerosis Complex

Denise C. Schiel

Definition/Background

- Autosomal dominant neurocutaneous disorder characterized by the development of benign tumors (hamartomas) that grow most commonly in the brain, skin, and kidneys, but can be present in any organ system.
- Incidence is approximately 1 in 6,000 to 7,000 individuals.
- Can be inherited from one affected parent, although most cases are sporadic owing to new spontaneous genetic mutations.

Clinical Presentation

- Average age of diagnosis is 5 years.
- Symptoms range from mild to severe, and the clinical course varies between individuals, making definitive diagnosis prior to age 2 years challenging.
- Infants typically present with seizures or infantile spasms, hypomelanotic skin lesions (ash leaf spots), or cardiac rhabdomyomas.

- Tumors can form in any organ, but are most common in the brain, heart, lungs, kidneys, and skin, and are rarely malignant.
- Seizures are common, which are often refractory to multiple antiepileptic drugs.

Diagnosis

- There are no pathognomonic clinical signs of tuberous sclerosis complex (TSC).
- Diagnosis is based on detailed physical examination and diagnostic imaging.
- Diagnostic criteria:
  - Definite TSC: presence of two major features or one major feature plus two minor features.
  - Probable TSC: one major plus one minor feature.
  - Possible TSC: either one major feature or two or more minor features (Table 6.7).

Management

- No cure for TSC; an interprofessional approach to care should be directed at symptom management, including antiepileptic drugs to control seizures.
- Prognosis is variable and dependent on the severity of symptoms.
- The immunosuppressant rapamycin has been shown to be an effective nonsurgical option in the treatment of brain astrocytomas; however, its use in patients with TSC is not yet approved by the United States Food and Drug Administration.

Neuropathy

Denise C. Schiel

Background/Definition

- General term which refers to disease or malfunction of the nerves.
- Categorized according to the type or location of the nerves affected: disorders of the nerve, the neuromuscular junction, or the muscle.

TABLE 6.7   Major and Minor Features of Tuberous Sclerosis Complex

Major Features	Minor Features
Facial angiofibromas or forehead plaque.	Multiple, randomly distributed pits in dental enamel.
Ungual or periungual fibroma.	Hamartomatous rectal polyps.
Hypomelanotic macules (>3).	Bone cysts.
Shagreen patch.	Cerebral white matter radial migration lines.
Multiple retinal nodular hamartoma.	Gingival fibromas.
Cortical tuber.	Nonrenal hamartoma.
Subependymal giant cell astrocytoma.	Retinal achromic patch.
Subependymal nodule.	Confetti-like skin lesions.
Cardiac rhabdomyoma, single or multiple.	Multiple renal cysts.
Lymphangioleiomyomatosis, renal angiomyolipoma, or both.	

- Characterized by dysfunction of the nerve signal, destruction or inflammation of the neuron, or destruction of the myelin sheath.
- Neuropathy is not a disease but rather a symptom of a disease with various potential causes.
- Distribution of weakness and any sensory abnormalities will help to distinguish the etiology.

Categories

- Motor: weakness or paralysis.
- Sensory: numbness, dysesthesia, ataxia.
- Autonomic: arrhythmia, hypotension, bowel and bladder problems, abnormal sweating.
- Mixed: a combination of the aforementioned.

Types

- Congenital: spinal muscle atrophy, Friedreich ataxia, mitochondrial disorders, congenital muscular dystrophy, Charcot–Marie–Tooth disease, and others.
- Autoimmune: MG, Guillain–Barré syndrome.
- Acquired: postinfectious, such as transverse myelitis, vitamin deficiencies (usually B vitamins), toxicities, trauma, critical illness polyneuropathy.

Presentation

- Cardinal sign of neuropathy is a reduction or absence of reflexes on physical examination.
- Varying degrees of weakness or paralysis.
- Severity of symptoms varies depending on the etiology and the disease process (e.g., respiratory insufficiency or failure due to respiratory muscle weakness, chronic

aspiration due to bulbar dysfunction, pain, or sensory abnormalities).
- Weakness in patients with prolonged ICU admission, sepsis, systemic inflammatory response syndrome, the use of chronic steroids, neuromuscular blocking medications, or aminoglycoside antibiotics are at risk for critical illness polyneuropathy.

Diagnosis

- Diagnostic evaluation is based on comprehensive history and physical examination, including a detailed neurologic examination and may include the following:
  - Radiographic imaging of the brain and spinal cord.
  - Evaluation of CSF (protein and WBC count).
  - Serum creatine kinase (CK) (reflects skeletal or cardiac muscle injury).
  - Antibody testing (AChR, ganglioside antibodies).
  - Electrolytes (sodium, potassium, calcium, magnesium, phosphorus).
  - Nerve conduction studies and single-fiber EMG (can localize the pathology to the nerve, neuromuscular junction, or muscle and distinguish between an axonal or demyelinating process).
  - Metabolic workup, toxicology screen, heavy metals.
  - Nerve or muscle biopsy.

Management

- Acute treatment is directed at symptom management with careful attention to the potential for weakness, especially respiratory muscle weakness.
- Treatment of acute or chronic neuropathic pain (e.g., opioids, nonsteroidal anti-inflammatory drugs, and gabapentin).

- Neuropathies may present as acute or chronic and, therefore, the course may be protracted, and an interprofessional approach is necessary with specialties including neurology, pulmonology, physical, occupational, and speech therapies, rehabilitation medicine, and others as indicated.

Seizures and Status Epilepticus
Michele Grimason

Background/Definition

- A seizure is a disturbance of brain function caused by paroxysmal discharges within the neuronal system.
- The surge of electrical activity can affect motor control, sensory perception, or autonomic functions.
- Many children (~25%) with a first-time unprovoked seizure will demonstrate a normal neurologic examination and have few or no recurrent seizures.
- Status epilepticus is defined as a single seizure lasting longer than 30 minutes or two or more consecutive seizures without return to baseline LOC.
- One third of children with febrile seizure will experience another episode in future.
- Refractory status epilepticus is considered in patients with ongoing seizure activity after the administration of two appropriately dosed anticonvulsant medications.

Etiology

- Genetic or abnormal cortical development.
- Metabolic (e.g., hyponatremia, hypoglycemia).
- Infection (e.g., meningitis).
- Fever.
- Stroke.
- Traumatic brain injury.
- Toxic ingestion/exposure.
- Subtherapeutic anticonvulsant medication levels, in cases of epilepsy.
- Unknown.

Pathophysiology

- Hypersynchronous discharges within the cortex combine with high-frequency bursts of the action potentials to generate a seizure.

Clinical Presentation

- Generalized: Seizure originates and engages bilateral hemispheres.
- Absence: brief, usually 15- to 20-second periods of impaired consciousness or confusion.
- Myoclonic seizures: brief muscle movements usually lasting <1 second.
- Clonic seizures: rhythmic, repetitive movements of head, trunk, and extremities.
- Tonic seizures: sustained extension or flexion of head, trunk, and extremities.

- Tonic–clonic seizures: consist of the combination of tonic and clonic movements.
- Atonic seizures: sudden loss of muscle tone.
- Focal: Seizure originates within in one hemisphere.
- Unknown/unclassified epileptic seizures.

Potential Complications of Status Epilepticus

- Rhabdomyolysis.
- Hyperthermia.
- Cerebral edema.
- Respiratory failure.

Evaluation

- First-time seizure
  - CBC, serum electrolytes, glucose, calcium, magnesium.
    - Order based on individual circumstances (e.g., vomiting, diarrhea, dehydration, failure to return to baseline promptly).
    - In the majority of febrile and nonfebrile seizures, laboratory study results are often unremarkable.
  - Lumbar puncture in seizure associated with fever.
    - Evaluates for CNS infection.
  - If toxic exposure possibility, toxicology screen warranted.
  - EEG.
    - Ordered selectively.
    - May be useful for future comparison.
  - Imaging.
    - If postictal focal deficit noted (e.g., Todd paralysis), prolonged seizure, or in patients who have not returned to baseline within several hours of seizure.
    - MRI is the preferred imaging study.
  - Anticonvulsant therapy.
    - Only after thoughtful analysis of variables; potential benefits must outweigh risks.
    - Significant risk of adverse side effects with approximately 30% of anticonvulsant therapy (e.g., hepatotoxicity, aplastic anemia, brain development).
- Recurrent seizure(s).
  - Require prompt diagnostic evaluation.

Management

- Stabilize ABCs.
- Obtain IV access.
- Lorazepam is the first-line therapy outside of neonatal period.
  - Rapid onset.
  - Ceases seizure activity in most patients in 2 to 5 minutes.
  - May repeat dose.
- Fosphenytoin or phenobarbital for persistent seizures.
- Identify and treat underlying etiology, when possible (e.g., hypoglycemia, hyponatremia).
- Refractory seizures may require drug-induced coma (e.g., pentobarbital, high-dose benzodiazepine infusion) (Figure 6.8).
  - Goal of therapy is burst suppression or electrocerebral silence.
  - Continuous EEG monitoring and cardiopulmonary monitoring are needed for patients.
- Refractory seizures may require surgical resection (e.g., hemispherectomy) or vagal nerve stimulator for long-term therapy.

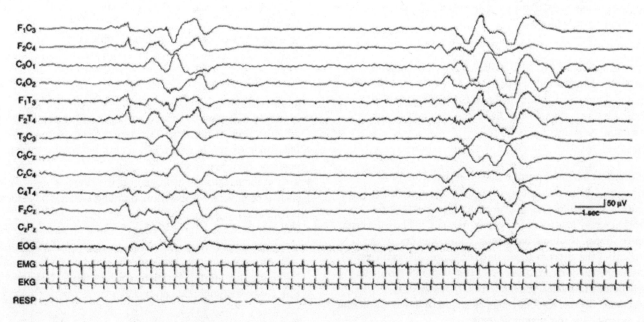

F₁C₃
F₂C₄
C₃O₁
C₄O₂
F₁T₃
F₂T₄
T₃C₃
C₃Cᵤ
CᵤC₄
CᵤT₄
FᵤCᵤ
CᵤPᵤ
EOG
EMG
EKG
RESP

50 µV
1 sec

FIGURE 6.8 • **EEG Burst Suppression.** Burst suppression pattern in a 37-week infant with hypoxic–ischemic encephalopathy.

Family Education

- Administration of rectal diazepam.
- Seizure recognition.
- Maintaining anticonvulsant therapy medication, when indicated.
- Seek medication attention.
  - First-time seizure.
  - Seizure lasting more than 5 minutes.
  - High fever.
  - Risk for head injury.
  - Compromised respiratory or cardiac function.

Shunt Malfunction and Infection

Katherine Worst

Background/Definition

- Hydrocephalus is defined as a condition in which the formation, flow, or absorption of CSF is disturbed.
- Untreated hydrocephalus has a mortality rate of 50% to 60%, while surgically treated hydrocephalus in children with minimal or no irreversible brain damage has a mortality rate of 10%.
- CSF shunts are essential to maintain normal ICP in children with hydrocephalus.
- As a mechanical device, a shunt can be expected to fail at a rate of approximately 10% each year and have an infection rate of 8% to 12%.
- Young age and a principal diagnosis of obstructive hydrocephalus are associated with high risk for shunt failure.
- Highest incidence of shunt infection is in children less than 6 months of age.

- Shunt survival rates decrease once a patient requires a revision.

Pathophysiology

- CSF is an ultrafiltrate of the blood, produced primarily in the choroid plexus and deposited within the ventricular system.
- CSF flows through the ventricular system and central spinal canal to be ultimately absorbed into the bloodstream and arachnoid granuloma.
- CSF serves multiple functions that aid in normal brain activity, including the provision of nutrients, proteins, and a protective cushion for the brain and spinal cord, and assists in the removal of metabolic wastes and creates a proper environment for neurotransmission.
- When CSF is overproduced, obstructed, or improperly absorbed, the CSF volume can increase in the rather fixed spaces of the skull, leading to an increased ICP.

Types and Description

- Valve-regulated shunt systems have become the mainstay of treatment for hydrocephalus, with over 30,000 shunt procedures performed each year in the United States.
- Ventricular and lumbar shunts are the most commonly used devices to redirect CSF.
- Ventricular catheters are placed within the lateral ventricles of the brain and drain to an absorptive surface in the peritoneum, pleural cavity, right atrium, or liver.
- Lumbar catheters are proximally placed in the lumbar subarachnoid space, with a distal site matching those of a ventricular device.
- Ventriculoperitoneal shunt devices use either differential pressure valves or programmable valves to assure adequate CSF drainage. The differential pressure valves open when the intraventricular pressure exceeds a predetermined threshold.

Programmable valves have the ability to externally adjust their opening-pressure limits.

Epidemiology

- Approximately 30% to 40% of shunts placed in pediatric patients fail within the first year.
- Median lifespan of a shunt before it must be replaced or revised is 2 years in a child <2 years of age and 8 to 10 years in a child >2 years of age.

Etiology

- CSF shunts may malfunction due to obstruction (most common), disconnection, migration, fracture, ascites, abdominal pseudocysts, infections, and/or constipation.
- Blockage may be caused by ependymal cells, glial tissue, brain debris, fibrin, or blood, but is most commonly due to the growth of the choroid plexus into the ventricular catheter.
- Distal obstructions are often associated with infection, but may be due to ascites, pseudocysts, or constipation.
- Disconnection is rare following placement of a new shunt, but is generally due to a technical error.
- Fractures in a shunt system are often due to chronic mechanical stress related to patient growth and movement.

Pathophysiology

- Shunt infection is the cause of malfunction in 3% to 8% of patients and typically occurs when pathologic organisms enter the surgical wound from the patient's adjacent skin or via surgical gloves or instruments contaminated with the patient's flora during an operation.
- Over half of ventriculoperitoneal shunt infections are caused by coagulase-negative staphylococci, with methicillin-resistant *Staph. epidermidis* being the most commonly isolated organism. Other organisms include streptococci, gram-negative bacteria, anaerobes, mycobacteria, and fungi depending on the acute illness and location of the shunt.

Clinical Presentation

- Fever, headache, nausea, vomiting, upgaze paralysis, and papilledema.
- Drowsiness was found to be the best predictive symptom for shunt malfunction in children.
- Depressed LOC, irritability, abdominal pain, and bulging fontanels with accelerated head growth in infants.
- With a concurrent infection, fever and vomiting are the most common symptoms of malfunction, but fever may or may not be present.
- Infections may also present with purulent leakage around the insertion site and/or redness and swelling along the shunt tract.

Diagnosis

- Diagnostic imaging studies may include an ultrasound for infants with open fontanels, a CT, or an MRI. Anterior and lateral radiographs are also often obtained to assess for continuity of the shunt (evaluates for shunt fracture).
- CBC with differential, erythrocyte sedimentation rate, and CRP values.
- Respiratory, stool, urine, and blood cultures.
- CSF for WBCs, glucose, protein, Gram staining, and culture.

Management

- Shunt malfunction can be a *medical emergency*.
- Increased ICP must be treated promptly with osmotic agents, diuretics, and/or steroids.
- Placement of an external ventricular drain may be needed and possibly shunt placement or revision.
- Treatment is focused on eliminating the cause of shunt failure, such as removal of obstruction, draining ascites, and resolving constipation.
- Infection: administration of empiric antibiotics including vancomycin and gram-negative coverage, removal of the shunt with external drainage, antibiotic therapy, and replacement of the shunt once sterile. Antibiotic therapy should be guided by CSF Gram stainings and cultures.

PEARLS

- *Symptoms of shunt malfunction can mimic other childhood infections and diseases, so caution in making diagnosis is necessary.*
- *Neuroimaging has a low sensitivity for identifying shunt malfunction independently; so shunt series radiographies or CT should be considered carefully.*

Spinal Muscle Atrophy

Denise C. Schiel

Definition/Background

- Autosomal recessive disorder of the anterior horn cells in the brainstem and spinal cord.
- Degenerative disease characterized by progressive denervation of the muscle, leading to progressive hypotonia and muscle weakness.
- Most common cause of degenerative neurologic disease in children, with an incidence in the United States of 1 in 6,000 to 27,500 live births.
- Males are more commonly affected than females.
- Three types that are genetically similar but differ in their clinical presentation and age of onset.

Etiology

- Due to a mutation in the survival motor neuron gene on chromosome 5 which is responsible for arresting programmed cell death, or apoptosis.

Pathophysiology

- See Table 6.8.

TABLE 6.8	**Clinical Presentation of Spinal Muscle Atrophy Types 1, 2, and 3**	
SMA Type 1	**SMA Type 2**	**SMA Type 3**
Presentation by 6 months of age in most cases Floppy infant. Unable to achieve milestones of rolling or sitting independently. Weakness is greater in proximal muscle groups vs. distal and lower extremities are more severely affected. Infants have poor head control. Demonstrate a weak cry or cough and have difficulty with feeding, swallowing, or handling oral secretions due to bulbar dysfunction. Paradoxical breathing due to intercostal muscle weakness with sparing of the diaphragm. Often have characteristic bell-shaped trunk and abdominal protrusion. When supine, assume the frog-legged position Areflexia, fine tremor (most notably in the hands), tongue fasciculations, facial weakness, and normal sensation are reported.	Characterized by fairly normal development for the first 6 mo. May sit independently and demonstrate head control, but are never able to stand or walk independently. Fine motor tremor of the hands and tongue fasciculations are present. May also demonstrate diaphragmatic breathing and have difficulty with swallowing or handling secretions. Prone to scoliosis and contractures. Life expectancy is variable and with aggressive pulmonary management; may survive beyond adolescence.	Weakness is greater in the proximal muscle groups vs. distal. Lower extremities more severely affected than the upper extremities. Patients typically achieve the ability to walk independently, but many are wheelchair-bound by the fourth decade of life. With aggressive symptomatic treatment, they may have a normal life expectancy.

Diagnostic Evaluation

- Based on age of onset of clinical symptoms.
- Electromyography (EMG) testing: demonstrates acute denervation due to malfunction of the motor neurons, but motor and sensory conduction velocities are normal.
- Serum CK: may be normal or slightly elevated (opposed to muscular dystrophy, in which CK is classically very elevated).
- Muscle biopsy (may not be necessary if confirmatory genetic testing is done).
- Genetic testing: survival motor neuron gene testing.
- Prenatal DNA testing is also available.

Management

- There is no cure, no specific therapy, or pharmacologic treatment for spinal muscle atrophy.
- Management is directed at aggressive treatment of symptoms and associated complications (e.g., respiratory insufficiency or failure, feeding difficulties, orthopedic issues).
  - Oxygen.
  - Noninvasive or conventional mechanical ventilation (tracheostomy).
  - Feeding tubes (nasogastric or gastrostomy).
  - Bracing or surgical spinal fusion.
- Consultation with a interprofessional team including neurology, pulmonology, orthopedics, and physical and occupational therapy is warranted.
- Genetic counseling.

Common Diagnostic Testing

Michele Grimason

Laboratory Studies

- Background: Many different laboratory studies are indicated in neurologic illnesses and neurologic demise. Chemistry studies can provide information about metabolic disease, electrolyte imbalances, liver and kidney functions, as well as drug levels.
- Antiepileptic medications can contribute to poor liver or kidney function, requiring monitoring of liver and renal functions. Other laboratory studies to consider in neurologic disease include the following:
  - Lactate: may identify resulting acidosis after prolonged seizures or the presence of septic shock in meningitis.
  - Ammonia: Ammonia levels assist in determining the presence of metabolic disease with seizures.
  - CBC with differential: infectious process or identification of anemia while managing increased ICP, among other indications.
  - Newborn screening test: identifies inborn errors of metabolism which can result in neurologic presentations such as seizures.
  - Infectious disease titers or levels: can be obtained via serum or CSF or both.
  - Lyme, CMV, herpes, rubella, EBV, toxoplasmosis, and other viral origins.

Drug Levels

Definition/Background

- Important when monitoring antiepileptic therapy; levels are used to help guide therapy with specific medications.
- For patients with well-controlled epilepsy and no adverse effects, drug levels are not routinely used as therapy is titrated to clinical efficacy, not to the drug level.
- Drugs typically requiring drug-level monitoring:
  - Fosphenytoin.
  - Phenobarbital.
  - Valproic acid.
  - Carbamazepine.
- Indications:
  - Initiation of drug to establish therapeutic level or range.
  - Breakthrough seizures in a previously stable patient.
  - Monitor adherence to medication.
  - Measure changes in levels with addition of second medication with known interactions.
- Timing.
  - Antiepileptic medication levels should be drawn as trough levels 30 minutes prior to dose administration.
- Goal levels.
  - Phenytoin.
    - Total (protein and non–protein-bound phenytoin): 10 to 20 μg/mL.
    - Free (non–protein-bound phenytoin): 1 to 2.5 μg/mL.
    - Fosphenytoin is protein-bound; therefore, an albumin level should be collected when institutions do not have access to phenytoin free levels.
    - Calculation for correction of phenytoin level with low albumin:

$$\text{Corrected level} = \text{Measured phenytoin level}/[(\text{albumin} \times 0.1) + 0.1]$$

  - Phenobarbital: 15 to 40 μg/mL.
  - Valproic acid: 50 to 100 μg/mL.
  - Carbamazepine: 4 to 12 μg/mL.

Electroencephalography

Background/Definition

- Noninvasive diagnostic procedure that provides a continuous recording of the brain's electrical activity using multiple reference electrodes placed on the scalp.
- Neuronal electrical signals from the cerebral cortex are displayed on a graphic grid to be interpreted by the neurologist.
- The tracing records the frequency, amplitude, and characteristics of the brain waves.

Indications

- Evaluation of events suspected to be seizures.
- Seizure localization.
- Assessment of subclinical seizures.
- Evaluation of altered LOC.
- Adjunct diagnostic test in the determination of brain death.

Contraindications

- Scalp infection.
- Scalp skin breakdown.

Complications

- Scalp burn from glue, typically with prolonged studies.

Classification of Brain Waves

- Brain waves are classified by the number of cycles per second (frequency) and are recorded in hertz (Hz).
- There are four frequency bands that are used when interpreting brain waves.
  - Delta: 1 to 3 Hz.
  - Theta: 4 to 7 Hz.
  - Alpha: 8 to 12 Hz.
  - Beta: 13 to 20 Hz.
- Frequency increases from birth to adulthood.

EEG Abnormalities

- Spikes: waves that are paroxysmal, sharp, and of high voltage.
- Epileptiform activity: single or repetitive spikes that can be focal, multifocal, or generalized.
- Slow waves: waves in the 1- to 7-Hz range.
  - Focal: can be secondary to a specific lesion such as an infarction, hematoma, localized infection, or tumor.
  - Generalized: often noted in toxic or metabolic encephalopathy, degenerative conditions, inflammatory processes, widespread infection, and postictal states.
- Silence: absence of all brain electrical activity, seen with brain death.

Imaging Modalities

Background

- CT and MRI are imaging techniques used for diagnostic evaluation of abnormalities in the intracranial and intraspinal structures.
- Both are noninvasive studies that have independent advantages and disadvantages.

CT

- Background:
  - A CT generates an image with the use of X-ray beams that pass through the anatomic structure in multiple directions.
  - These beams differentiate tissues based on physical density and generate profiles which a computer then integrates to create a dimensional image.
- Brain or head CT images are used in the clinical evaluation of:
  - Bony abnormalities.
  - Hydrocephalus.
  - ICH.
  - Cerebral edema.
  - Space-occupying lesions.
  - Intracranial calcifications.

MRI

- Background:
  - MRI uses a magnetic field to align hydrogen atoms.
  - Radio waves are then released, which excite the atoms and cause them to spin into their normal position.
  - The movement of the atoms is detected by the computer to create an image.
  - By varying the timing of the excitation, the magnetic resonance signal can be manipulated to obtain the best image of the type of tissue under study.
- Brain MRI is used in the clinical evaluation of:
  - Ischemia or infarct.
  - Degenerative diseases.
  - Congenital anomalies.
  - Arteriovenous malformations.
  - Lesions in the posterior fossa and spinal cord (Table 6.9).

Brain Magnetic Resonance Angiogram

- Background:
  - MRA is a type of MRI that uses pulses of radio wave energy to provide images of blood vessels inside the body.
- MRA images are useful in the clinical evaluation of:
  - Reduced blood flow.
  - Aneurysm.
  - Arteriovenous malformations.

Cerebral Perfusion Scan

- Background:
  - Cerebral perfusion scan uses xenon-133, a radioactive dye, which is injected prior to the scan.

- Adequately perfused brain tissue will have uptake of the dye.
- Cerebral perfusion scan may be considered in the clinical evaluation of:
  - Brain death.
  - Acute stroke.

Lumbar Puncture

Background

- A lumbar puncture is performed to obtain CSF as a therapeutic measure or to support a diagnosis of CNS infection, malignancy, autoimmune disease, or inflammatory process.

Indications

- Suspected infectious, immunologic, or inflammatory process involving the CNS.
- Measurement of opening pressure.
- Administration of intrathecal medications (e.g., anesthesia or chemotherapy).
- Therapeutic CSF removal to relieve increased ICP due to pseudotumor cerebri.

Contraindications

- Increased ICP—as evidenced by clinical manifestations or on radiographic images.
- Platelet dysfunction, bleeding disorder.
- Respiratory or hemodynamic instability.
- Skin infection near the site of entry.
- Spinal cord trauma or compression.
- Posterior spinal cord fusion in lumbar region.
- Focal neurologic deficit.

Potential Complications

- Bleeding.
- Infection.
- Back pain.
- Headache.
- CSF leak.
- Epidural or subdural spinal hematoma.
- Herniation, rarely.

Laboratory Studies

- CSF is obtained for the presence of white and red blood cell counts, culture, Gram staining and sensitivities, PCR and certain titers, and other neurologic studies.
- Normal results are found in the discussion of meningitis in this section.

PEARLS

- *Perform a head CT on any patient with suspected increased ICP or suspected space-occupying lesion prior to performing an lumbar puncture.*
- *A negative head CT does not completely exclude the possibility of increased ICP.*

TABLE 6.9	Comparison of CT and MRI
Advantages of CT	More sensitive in detecting blood, making it ideal for trauma evaluation. Scan is quick, making it an option to perform on a conscious patient.
Advantages of MRI	Does not use ionizing radiation and eliminates exposure risk. Higher level or gray/white differentiation. Provides higher-resolution detail at skull bases and orbits.
Disadvantages to CT	Uses ionizing radiation expose to generate images.
Disadvantages to MRI	Patients with metallic devices are unable to enter the scanner at risk of device dislodgement. Longer imaging time, usually sedation required.

Intracranial Monitoring with Ventriculostomy

Background/Definition

- A ventriculostomy catheter is the preferred device for monitoring ICP and can also be used for draining CSF.
- It is connected to an external pressure transducer and monitor and can be easily calibrated.
- A waveform indicates respiratory variations and pulse pressure, as well as ICP.
- There are other monitoring devices available, which include a microsensor transducer and a fiber-optic transducer that work without a fluid-filled system, but cannot usually be calibrated once in place.

Indications

- Children with traumatic brain injury, especially those with an elevated ICP or potential for elevated ICP.
- Cardiopulmonary resuscitation, along with an abnormal head CT scan on admission, and/or a Glasgow Coma Scale of less than 8 after resuscitation, in some cases.
- Children with low-density or high-density lesions, including contusions; epidural, subdural, or intraparenchymal hematomas; compression of basal cisterns; and edema.

Goals of ICP Monitoring

- Maintain ICP <20 to 25 mmHg in older children and <15 to 20 mmHg in children <1 year of age.
- Maintain CPP by maintaining adequate MAP; goal CPP >60 mmHg in adolescents, >50 mmHg in children, >40 mmHg in infants.
- Avoid factors that aggravate or precipitate elevated ICP.
  - Agitation and pain.
  - Obstruction of venous return (e.g., keep head in neutral position).
  - Respiratory insufficiency such as airway obstruction, hypoxia, or hypercapnia.
  - Fever (increases metabolic rate and is vasodilator).
  - Hypertension.
  - Hyponatremia.
  - Anemia.
  - Seizures (increased cerebral metabolic demand).

1. A 4-year-old with repaired congenital heart disease presents with new-onset right-sided hemiparesis. His speech is difficult to understand, even for his mother. Which one of the following imaging modalities would be the most appropriate for the initial evaluation of this patient?
 a. CT of head.
 b. MRI of head.
 c. Head ultrasound.
 d. Skull X-ray.

Answer: **A**

Obtaining a head CT would be the most appropriate diagnostic study to evaluate symptoms of stroke. Prior to anticoagulation or antiplatelet therapy for ischemic stroke, it must be confirmed that the child does not have an ICH. Due to time sensitivity, a CT is a more appropriate scan compared to an MRI. At 4 years of age, the fontanel has closed, thus making a head ultrasound an unattainable option. A skull X-ray provides information only on bone, not brain parenchyma.

2. A 3-week-old infant with a congenital heart defect returns to the cardiac intensive care unit on extracorporeal membrane oxygenation (ECMO) postoperatively. The bedside nurse notes anisocoria on initial evaluation of the baby. Which one of the following would be the most appropriate initial imaging study?
 a. CT.
 b. MRI.
 c. Head ultrasound.
 d. MRA.

Answer: **C**

Head ultrasound is the most appropriate imaging modality for an unstable neonate with an open fontanel. Ultrasound is a bedside procedure and can identify hemorrhage as a cause for anisocoria. The ECMO circuit contains metal, and therefore, MRI would not be an appropriate imaging choice at this point in the infant's hospital course.

3. A 3-month-old is brought into the emergency department (ED) with decreased PO intake for the past 12 hours. He has been sleepier than usual and just "hasn't been acting right." On examination, the infant is lethargic, but opens his eyes to painful stimulation. Which one of the following imaging studies would be the first choice for this patient?
 a. CT.
 b. MRI.
 c. Head ultrasound.
 d. Skull X-ray.

Answer: **A**

If there is concern for cerebral trauma, a head CT should be the first imaging choice. A head ultrasound would be possible to evaluate the possibility of a brain hemorrhage, but a head CT will offer other information, including findings of hydrocephalus, hemorrhage, or skull fracture.

4. A 6-year-old with no medical history arrives at the ED with generalized tonic–clonic seizures. What is the initial management?
 a. Administer lorazepam.
 b. Load with fosphenytoin.
 c. Obtain a STAT head CT.
 d. Obtain an EEG.

Answer: **A**

Administering lorazepam to control the seizure activity is the initial treatment of choice due to the rapid onset of action. If seizures continue despite giving the benzodiazepine, then loading with fosphenytoin or phenobarbital would be appropriate. A CT is indicated; however, it requires cessation of seizure for the patient to be still during the procedure to obtain the necessary images.

5. Which one of the following descriptions indicates a diagnosis of status epilepticus?
 a. A 4-year-old with a history of cerebral palsy, who presents to the hospital after 5 minutes of tonic–clonic activity.
 b. A febrile 9-month-old with a history of febrile seizures, who presents after a 3-minute seizure.
 c. A 7-year-old with known seizure disorder, who presents after a 25-minute seizure at home which has resolved.
 d. A 3-year-old who presents after having three seizures at home and does not follow commands and is very drowsy on presentation.

Answer: **D**

A history of three consecutive seizures with continuing altered neurologic status could indicate status epilepticus which is defined as one seizure lasting greater than 30 minutes or two or more consecutive seizures without return to baseline mental status.

6. A previously healthy 3-year-old presents to the ED with acute onset of nausea/emesis, headache, generalized tonic–clonic seizure, and is now obtunded. Vital signs are: heart rate, 58 beats per minute; BP, 158/98 mmHg; respiratory rate, 6 breaths per minute; right pupil, 6 mm nonreactive ; and left pupil, 4 mm sluggish. What is the most important initial intervention?
 a. ABCs with securing of the airway.
 b. Administer Ativan 2 mg IV.
 c. Order hypertonic 3% saline 5 mL/kg bolus.
 d. Order a STAT MRI/MRA.

Answer: **A**

(continues on page 208)

In any situation when a child has an altered neurologic status and is presumed unresponsive, stabilizing and protecting the airway is always the first priority. Following ABCs and treatment for increased ICP and seizures would be appropriate while preparing to determine diagnostic studies. If intubating the child, mild hyperventilation (Paco$_2$ ~32–35 mmHg) also assists in decreasing the blood flow to the brain, therefore decreasing blood volume in the cranial vault, in turn lowering the ICP. Often, these interventions are happening simultaneously.

7. In a *symptomatic,* unstable, pediatric patient what is the best diagnostic study to obtain to best identify the presence of an AVM?
   a. Transcranial Doppler.
   b. CT.
   c. MRI/MRA.
   d. Cerebral angiography.

Answer: **B**

Although the cerebral angiography is the most important technique to show an exact depiction of the AVM, its feeder vessels, nidus, and draining veins, it is a study that should be done once the patient is stabilized. In the symptomatic patient, a CT will allow for immediate viewing of the general location of the AVM, if there is a rupture resulting in hemorrhage, and the presence of edema with mass effect. It is quick, available in any hospital, and does not require a specialized team of interventional radiologists to obtain.

8. A 6-month-old with congenital heart disease presents to the ED with fever, first-time seizure, and right leg weakness. What condition should be first on the differential list, and what studies should be obtained?
   a. Febrile seizure; obtain a blood culture.
   b. Ischemic or hemorrhagic stroke; order CT and MRI.
   c. Meningitis; obtain a head CT and lumbar puncture.
   d. Seizure with a Todd paralysis; order CT and EEG.

Answer: **B**

The presence of congenital heart disease is one of the most common risk factors for stroke in the pediatric population. When a pediatric patient presents with focal weakness and seizure, stroke should be high on the differential list. CT should be obtained immediately to evaluate for an ICH and an MRI with diffusion to establish the diagnosis of a stroke.

9. A 16-year-old boy with a history of pulmonary valvular stenosis presents with headache and vomiting. His initial head CT demonstrates a large subarachnoid hemorrhage with midline shift. What should be done first?
   a. Obtain a CTA to assess for aneurysm.
   b. Order a blood transfusion.
   c. Consult neurosurgery.
   d. Administer steroids for cerebral edema.

Answer: **C**

Consult a neurosurgeon if there is a concern for increased ICP. The neurosurgeon should be contacted for possible hematoma evacuation or pressure monitoring placement.

10. A previously healthy 13-year-old girl required surgery with general anesthesia, for repair of multiple pelvic fractures after a motor vehicle accident. Immediately after awakening, she is found to be agitated, restless, and confused. Which one of the following should be highest on the differential list?
    a. Behavioral response.
    b. Emergence delirium.
    c. Meningitis.
    d. Hypoglycemia.

Answer: **B**

Emergence delirium is a well-described phenomenon observed in children within the first 30 minutes after emerging from anesthesia and is diagnosed by symptoms or behavior.

11. What is the first step in managing a child who is thought to have emergence delirium in an intensive care unit?
    a. Call parents for help.
    b. Protect child from bodily injury.
    c. Administer benzodiazepines.
    d. Administer haloperidol.

Answer: **B**

The most important task of managing a child with delirium is protection from bodily injury. Emergence delirium is a self-limited condition with variable duration. If injury to the patient or caregivers is a possibility, pharmacologic management (e.g., benzodiazepine) can be considered.

12. A 4-month-old infant presents with a 3-day history of constipation and poor feeding. There is no fever or other signs of illness. Which one of the following should be highest on the differential diagnosis list?
    a. Guillian–Barré syndrome.
    b. Infant botulism.
    c. Sepsis.
    d. Seizures.

Answer: **B**

Infant botulism is a progressive, neuromuscular disease which typically presents with poor feeding, weakness, constipation, weak cry, and other neurologic symptoms. If it is not recognized early, progression of further neurologic symptoms, including respiratory failure, can occur.

13. Which one of the following practices is most important to minimize the infection rate in a child with a ventriculoperitoneal (VP) shunt in place?
    a. Routine infection surveillance with CSF analysis every 6 months.
    b. Antibiotic prophylaxis for dental procedures.
    c. Antibiotic prophylaxis with individually tailored specifications following shunt placement.
    d. Avoidance of gastrostomy tube (GT) placement.

Answer: **C**

Following VP shunt placement, all patients should be placed on antibiotic prophylaxis in the immediate preoperative period and postoperatively to reduce infection rates. Alternatively, routine surveillance for CSF infection is not recommended because it is a poor predictor of infection and may actually increase a patient's probability of contracting an iatrogenic infection. Patients who have a VP shunt are also not required to have prophylaxis for dental procedures. Most VP shunt infections result from microorganisms not of oral origin, but associated with surgical implantation and other acute infections. Finally, placing a GT in a patient with a VP shunt is considered to be safe practice, with evidence supporting that GT placement does not have any effect on the shunt's infection rate and/or survival.

14. Which one of the following is the most common cause of CSF shunt malfunction?
a. Disconnection.
b. Obstruction.
c. Infection.
d. Migration.

Answer: **B**

Obstruction is the most common cause of shunt failure in pediatrics, most commonly at the proximal end of the catheter. Disconnection of a shunt is rare and usually due to a technical error at the time of placement. Infection occurs in only 3% to 8% of patients with shunt malfunction, and while migration can also occur, it is far less common.

15. Which one of the following is indicative of a bacterial infection in CSF?
a. WBC 450 cells/µL and protein 35 mg/dL.
b. RBC 5 cells/µL and glucose 69 mg/dL.
c. WBC 1,200 cells/µL and protein 150 mg/dL.
d. RBC 35 cells/µL and glucose 85 mg/dL.

Answer: **C**

A bacterial infection in CSF can be identified by an elevated WBC count (>1,000), increased protein (>100 mg/dL), and decreased glucose (<60% of the serum glucose). Normal values include a WBC count of 0 to 5 cells/µL, a protein level of 15 to 60 mg/dL, and a glucose level of 50 to 80 mg/dL. RBCs found in CSF can indicate bleeding during the tap or a viral infection.

16. A 6-year-old with a normal developmental history presents with behavioral changes (irritability, confusion), headache, and vision changes. He is not febrile and has no focal neurologic findings on examination. Which one of the following history questions is most pertinent?
a. Is there a family history of substance use?
b. Is there a family history of stroke?
c. Is there a family history of malignancy/cancer?
d. Has your son recently been sick?

Answer: **D**

Acute disseminated encephalomyelitis is a type of parainfectious encephalopathy which can cause behavioral changes, altered mental status, fatigue, fever, headache, nausea, vomiting, and seizures. Disseminated encephalomyelitis often occurs following a viral illness, so a history question should be included that addresses recent past illnesses.

17. A 3-month-old infant presents with seizures, lethargy, and emesis. Laboratory results indicate a serum sodium of 116 mEq/L, and the caregiver reports giving the baby only water since she has been sick. With slow correction of the infant's sodium level, the seizures subsided and the infant is more responsive. Which one of the following is highest on the differential list?
a. Syndrome of inappropriate antidiuretic hormone.
b. Metabolic encephalopathy secondary to water intoxication.
c. Cerebral salt wasting.
d. Diabetes insipidus.

Answer: **B**

Metabolic/toxic encephalopathy results from water intoxication which can lead to hyponatremia and secondary seizures with altered mental status. Slow sodium correction will improve neurologic status, stop seizure activity, and it will be anticipated that mental status should improve to baseline.

18. A 12-year-old boy with seizures, cerebral palsy, and static encephalopathy presents with altered mental status. Parents report no fever, recent illness, or clinical seizures. At baseline he takes Keppra for seizure prophylaxis. Which one of the following diagnostic tests should be ordered first?
a. Keppra level.
b. Head CT.
c. Toxicology screen.
d. CSF cell count and culture.

Answer: **A**

With onset of seizure activity or altered mental status in a previously healthy child with an underlying seizure disorder, attention to medication levels should be the first priority. Encephalopathy can occur with toxic drug levels, and seizures can occur when levels are low. It is important to review all of the patient's medications to assess if they could be contributing to the encephalopathic state.

19. A 3-year-old who has had an ischemic stroke located in the pons diagnosed with imaging has an asymmetric smile on examination. Which one of the following CNs is affected?
a. Trigeminal nerve (V).
b. Facial nerve (VII).
c. Glossopharyngeal nerve (IX).
d. Vagus nerve (X).

Answer: **B**

The facial nerve (VII) controls the muscles of facial expression.

20. A full-term infant suffered severe anoxia during delivery. He currently has sluggish pupils and minimal response to stimuli. Which one of the following is the most likely diagnosis?
a. Duchenne muscular dystrophy.
b. Encephalitis.
c. Intraventricular hemorrhage.
d. Hypoxic–ischemic encephalopathy (HIE).

Answer: **D**

(continues on page 210)

HIE results when the brain suffers a hypoxic event and is not sufficiently oxygenated. This can occur in many situations, including birth injuries. The outcome of a child with HIE can include severe developmental delays as well as physical disabilities.

21. A 14-year-old gymnast presents to the ED with lower extremity weakness and areflexia. She reports having a flu-like illness 2 weeks earlier. The initial diagnostic test that should be considered is:
    a. Lower extremity radiographies.
    b. Lumbar puncture.
    c. EMG.
    d. EEG.

Answer: **B**

The presentation of a patient who recently experienced a viral illness and has new-onset weakness and areflexia is highly suspicious for Guillain–Barré syndrome. A lumbar puncture will provide the definitive diagnosis. The other diagnostic tests are supportive, not diagnostic.

22. A 17-year-old is being admitted with a diagnosis of Guillain–Barré syndrome. What serial evaluation is most important in assessing her respiratory status?
    a. EMG.
    b. Negative inspiratory force (NIF).
    c. Peak flow monitoring.
    d. Head CT.

Answer: **B**

Guillain–Barré syndrome is a demyelinating disease of peripheral nerves, causing acute and progressive weakness. A major life-threatening complication is ascending paralysis which impairs respiration and results in hypoventilation requiring endotracheal intubation. Obtaining pulmonary function testing using NIF evaluation assists in determining worsening of respiratory drive.

23. In which patient would an EEG be indicated?
    a. A 5-year-old who presented with clinical seizures and is now unresponsive.
    b. A 3-year-old with a brain tumor who is interactive and playing with toys.
    c. A 15-year-old patient with seizures that began 2 years following a diagnosis of meningitis.
    d. A 7-year-old newly diagnosed with spinal muscular atrophy.

Answer: **A**

There are many indications for EEG monitoring, with the most frequent including evaluation of events that are suspected to be seizures, seizure localization, assessment for subclinical seizures, evaluation of altered LOC, adjunct diagnostic test in the determination of brain death.

24. A 3-year-old presents with seizures and is started on fosphenytoin therapy. At what time should the phenytoin level be obtained?
    a. 30 minutes after dose administration.
    b. 30 minutes prior to dose administration.
    c. 4 hours after dose administration.
    d. 4 hours before dose administration.

Answer: **B**

Phenytoin levels should be trough levels, drawn 30 minutes prior to dose administration. Phenytoin levels are also helpful in determining whether the bolus or loading dose has created a therapeutic level. In this case, the level can be drawn 1 hour following the load.

25. A febrile 8-week-old arrives at the PICU with a diagnosis of suspected meningitis. Blood and urine cultures were sent to the ED, but this patient is in need of a LP to complete the evaluation. Which one of the following is a contraindication to performing an LP on this infant?
    a. Full fontanel.
    b. Current temperature 38°C.
    c. Platelet count of $60,000/mm^3$.
    d. BP of 124/60 mmHg.

Answer: **A**

An infant with a full or tense anterior fontanel, especially in the scenario of other neurologic symptoms or diagnoses, may be exhibiting signs of increased ICP and an LP should be withheld until a head CT is completed. Performing an LP on a patient with increased ICP can result in transtentorial herniation or herniation of the cerebellar tonsils.

26. A 7-year-old who had been previously diagnosed with attention deficit hyperactivity disorder is brought to the ED because he was "staring into space" and was unable to be aroused. This has also happened several times in the past, both at home and in school. The most likely diagnosis and needed evaluation include:
    a. Encephalopathy and lumbar puncture.
    b. Absence seizures and EEG.
    c. Meningitis and lumbar puncture.
    d. Atonic seizures and EEG.

Answer: **B**

Absence seizures are brief, usually 15- to 20-second periods of impaired consciousness or confusion, and can be followed by a postictal period. Children who have been diagnosed with other behavioral or attention-related disorders could potentially be having seizures as the underlying cause of their inattention. An EEG or video EEG can be helpful in diagnosing the presence of absence or subclinical seizures.

27. Which one of the following is the "gold standard" study for a child with a suspected arteriovenous malformation?
a. MRI of brain.
b. Cerebral angiography.
c. Lumbar puncture with opening pressure.
d. Head CT.

Answer: **B**

When considering the presence of an arteriovenous malformation, a head CT can be the initial study for a child. The cerebral angiography is the gold standard of diagnosis and identifies the dilated feeding arteries, the nidus, and large draining veins.

28. An infant was considered "floppy" in the first few weeks of life and is now 5 months old. He currently does not roll over and will not maintain a sitting position when propped in the corner of the couch. She was born weighing 7 lb, and is now 9 lb and 3 oz. Which one of the following is the most likely diagnosis?
a. Human botulism.
b. Infantile spasms.
c. Spinal muscular atrophy.
d. Muscular dystrophy.

Answer: **C**

Spinal muscle atrophy, type 1, usually is present at birth and diagnosed within the first 6 months of life. Typical findings include "floppy" muscle tone, inability to meet milestones, not rolling over by 6 months of life, poor head control, feeding and swallowing problems, and other neurologic symptoms.

29. Which one of the following is the most effective method to monitor increased ICP in a child?
a. Continuous assessment of neurologic examination.
b. Ventriculostomy and monitoring.
c. Ophthalmologic examination.
d. Serial head CTs.

Answer: **B**

Children who experience traumatic brain injury or have space-occupying brain lesions have a high incidence of increased ICP and potentially intracranial hypertension. If a child presents with a Glasgow Coma Scale of less than 8, requires resuscitation following traumatic brain injury or has other significant neurologic symptoms, placement of a ventriculostomy tube is warranted with monitoring to maintain specific intracranial parameters.

30. An 18-year-old complains of high fever for the past 2 days, has a severe headache, and is unable to put his chin to his chest. The diagnostic study of choice for this child is:
a. Lumbar puncture.
b. CBC with differential.
c. Brain MRI.
d. Lateral neck X-ray.

Answer: **A**

Symptoms of fever, severe headache, and nuchal rigidity are classic signs of meningitis. A lumbar puncture to evaluate for the presence of bacteria and cell count is the most important diagnostic test with these presenting symptoms.

Recommended Readings

Aoun, S. G., Bendok, B. R., & Batjer, H. H. (2012). Acute management of ruptured arteriovenous malformations and dural arteriovenous fistulas. *Neurosurgery Clinics of North America, 23,* 87–103.

Berg, A., & Scheffer, I. (2011). New concepts in classification of the epilepsies: Entering the 21st century. *Epilepsia, 52*(6), 1058–1062.

Craig, V. L. (2012). Botulism and guillian-barre syndrome. In K. Reuter-Rice & B. Bolick (Eds.), *Pediatric acute care: A guide for interprofessional pratice* (pp. 1026–1029). Burlington, MA: Jones & Bartlett Learning.

Felisher, G., & Ludwig, S. (2012). *Pediatric emergency medicine* (6th ed., pp. 1502). Philadelphia, PA: Lippincott Williams & Wilkins.

Ghotme, K., Drake, J., Shunts, J. A., & Duhaime, A. C. (2013). *Pediatric handbook.* Schaumburg, IL: Congress of Neurological Surgeons, University of Neurosurgery. Retrieved from http://w3.cns.org/university/pediatrics/index2.asp

Gillis, J., & Ryan, M. M. (2009). Chronic neuromuscular disease. In M. A. Helfaer & D. G. Nichols (Eds.), *Rogers' handbook of pediatric intensive care* (4th ed., pp. 229–237). Philadelphia, PA: Lippincott Williams & Wilkins.

Grimason, M., Wainwright, M. S., & Eichler, V. (2012). Neuropathy. In K. Reuter-Rice & B. Bolick (Eds.), *Pediatric acute care: A guide for interprofessional practice* (pp. 951–954). Burlington, MA: Jones & Bartlett Learning.

Lam, A. (2012). Meningitis and encephalitis. In K. Reuter-Rice & B. Bolick (Eds.), *Pediatric acute care: A guide for interprofessional practice* (pp. 943–945). Burlington, MA: Jones & Bartlett Learning.

Lang, S. S., Beslow, L. A., Bailey, R. L., Vossough, A., Ekstrom, J., Heuer, G. G., & Storm, P. B. (2012). Follow-up imaging to detect recurrence of surgically treated pediatric arteriovenous malformations. *Journal of Pediatric Neurosurgery, 9*(5), 497–504.

Marcoux, K. (2012). Arteriovenous malformation. In: Reuter-Rice K & Bolick, B (Eds.) *Pediatric acute care: A guide for interprofessional practice.* Burlington, MA: Jones & Bartlett Learning.

Marlin, A., & Gaskil, S. (2011). Neurosurgical shunts and their compliations. *Neurology Medlink.* Retrieved from www.medlink.com/medlinkcontent.asp

Milonovich, L. (2012). Neurocutaneous disorders. In K. Reuter-Rice & B. Bolick (Eds.), *Pediatric acute care: A guide for interprofessional practice* (pp. 948–951). Burlington, MA: Jones & Bartlett Learning.

Milonovich, L., & Eichler, V. (2013). Neurological disorders. In M. F. Hazinski (Ed.), *Nursing care of the critically ill child* (3rd ed., pp. 587–677). St. Louis, MO: Elsevier.

National Institutes of Health, National Institute of neurological Disorders and Stroke. (2012). Neurofibromatosis. Retrieved from www.ninds.nih.gov/disorders/myasthenia_gravis/detail_myasthenia_gravis.htm

National Institutes of Health, National Institute of neurological Disorders and Stroke.(2012). Neuropathy. Retrieved from www.ninds.nih.gov/disorders/peripheralneuropathy/peripheralneuropathy.htm

Niazi, T. N., Klimo, P., Anderson, R. C., & Raffel, C. (2010). Diagnosis and management of arteriovenous malformations in children. *Neurosurgery Clinics of North America, 21,* 443–456.

Recinos, P. F., Rahmathulla, G., Pearl, M., Recinos, V. R., Jallo, G. I., Gailloud, P., & Ahn, E. S. (2012). Vein of Galen malformations: Epidemiology, clinical presentations, management. *Neurosurgery Clinics of North America, 23*(1), 165–177.

Rowin, M. E., Reade, E. P., & Christenson, J. C. (2011). Central nervous system infections presenting to the pediatric intensive care unit. In B. Fuhrman &

J. Zimmerman (Eds.), *Pediatric critical care* (4th ed., pp. 918–932). Philadelphia, PA: Elsevier Saunders.

Sanchez, G. M. (2012). Encephalopathy. In K. Reuter-Rice & B. Bolick (Eds.), *Pediatric acute care: A guide for interprofessional practice* (pp. 280–284). Burlington, MA: Jones & Bartlett Learning.

Simon, D. W., Da Silva, Y. S., Zuccoli, G., & Clark, R. S. B. (2013). Acute encephalitis. *Critical Care Clinics, 29,* 259–277.

Singhi, P. D., Singhi, S. C., Newton, R. J. C., & Simon, J. (2009). Central nervous system infections. In M. A. Helfaer & D. G. Nichols (Eds.), *Rogers' handbook of pediatric intensive care* (4th ed., pp. 500–511). Philadelphia, PA: Lippincott Williams & Wilkins.

Smith, A. B., Berutti, T., Brink, E., Strohler, B., Fuchs, D. C., Ely, E. W., & Pandharipande, P. P. (2013). Pediatric critical care perceptions on analgesia, sedation, and delirium. *Seminars in Respiratory and Critical Care Medicine, 34*(2), 244–261.

Smith, A. B., Brink, E., Fuchs, D. C., Ely, E. W., & Pandharipande, P. P. (2013). Pediatric delirium: Monitoring and management in the pediatric intensive care unit. *Pediatric Clinics of North America, 60*(3), 740–761.

Tamargo, R. J., & Huang, J. (2012). Cranial arteriovenous malformations and cranial dural arteriovenous fistulas. *Neurosurgery Clinics of North America, 23*(1), 1–198.

Tristram, D. A. (2008). Encephalitis. In R. M. Perkin, J. D Swift, D. A. Newton, & N. G. Anas (Eds.), *Pediatric hospital medicine: Textbook of inpatient management* (2nd ed., pp. 430–432). Philadelphia, PA: Lippincott Williams & Wilkins.

Weil, A. G., Li, S. & Zhao, J. Z. (2011). Recurrence of a cerebral arteriovenous malformation following surgical resection: A case report and review of literature. *Surgical Neurology International, 2*(1), 175–179.

Weimer, M. B., Reese, Jr. J.J., & Tilton, A.H. (2011). Acute neuromuscular diseases and disorders. In B. Fuhrman & J. Zimmerman (Eds.), *Pediatric critical care* (4th ed., pp. 914–915). Philadelphia, PA: Elsevier Saunders.

Yilmaz, A., Dalgia, N., Musluman, M., Sancer, M., Colak, I., & Aydin, Y. (2010). Linezolid treatment of shunt-related cerebrospinal fluid infections in children. *Journal of Neurosurgery: Pediatrics, 5,* 443–448.

Yogev, R., & Bar-Meir, M. (2004). Management of brain abscesses in children. *Pediatric Infectious Disease Journal, 23*(2), 157–159.

Endocrine Disorders

Adrenal Insufficiency

Mary P. White

Background

- Adrenal glands, located on the kidneys, produce three types of hormones:
  - Glucocorticoid hormones (e.g., cortisol, corticosterone).
    - Maintain glucose control by affecting protein and carbohydrate metabolism.
    - Inhibit glucose uptake in muscle and adipose tissue.
    - Stimulate gluconeogenesis, particularly in the liver.
    - Respond to stress by upregulating the expression of antiinflammatory mediators and downregulating the expression of proinflammatory mediators.
    - If prolonged exposure to glucocorticoids, Cushing syndrome develops.
      - Obesity, muscle wasting/weakness, decreased glucose tolerance/hyperglycemia, buffalo hump.
  - Mineralocorticoid hormones (e.g., aldosterone, dehydroepiandrosterone).
    - Maintain the balance of sodium and potassium in the body.
    - When aldosterone is increased, aldosteronism develops.
      - Hypernatremia and hyperkalemia, resulting in hypertension.
    - If androgens are increased, sex characteristics will be affected.
  - Sex hormones (e.g., androgens, progestins, and estrogens).
- Disorders affecting the adrenal cortex lead to inadequate or absent production of hormone(s).
- Disorders are either congenital or acquired.
- Adrenal insufficiencies can be *acute* (adrenal crisis) or *chronic* (Addison disease).
  - The most common causes of acute adrenal insufficiency are Waterhouse–Friderichsen syndrome, sudden withdrawal of long-term corticosteroid therapy, and stress states in patients with chronic adrenal insufficiency.

Primary Adrenal Insufficiency

Definition

- Impairment in the adrenal glands.
- Glucocorticoid and mineralocorticoid hormones, particularly cortisol, are not produced in sufficient amounts.

Etiology/Types

- Congenital primary adrenal insufficiency.
  - Congenital adrenal hyperplasia (CAH) is the most commonly identified cause of primary adrenal insufficiency in children.
    - Autosomal recessive disorder: defect in an enzyme (largely, 21-hydroxylase deficiency) required in the synthesis of cortisol to cholesterol.
    - Results in dysfunction in the synthesis of adrenal steroids.
    - Incidence: 1 in 10,000 to 18,000 live births.
      - Females have higher incidence; most commonly diagnosed at birth.
      - Males usually present with a life-threatening saltwasting crisis in the first month of life.
    - Newborn screen has incorporated CAH testing in most states in the United States, decreasing the time to diagnosis, particularly for males.
- Acquired primary adrenal insufficiency.
  - Includes autoimmune etiologies (autoimmune destruction of adrenal cortex) and iatrogenic causes such as hemorrhage, trauma, drug effects, pituitary tumor, or infection.

Clinical Presentation

- CAH.
  - Ambiguous genitalia at birth.
  - If not diagnosed at birth, symptoms will present within 1 to 4 weeks of life.
    - Vomiting, dehydration, cardiac arrhythmias, hyponatremia, hyperkalemia, or salt-losing crisis, resulting in circulatory collapse.
- Adrenal insufficiency.
  - Symptoms can be slower to progress.

- Fatigue, loss of weight, hyperpigmentation of the creases of the skin, nausea, vomiting.
- Prolonged recovery from an illness may prompt further investigation of multiple vague symptoms, leading to the diagnosis.
- Adrenal crisis.
  - Acute symptoms: life-threatening disorder.
    - Vomiting, abdominal pain, hypovolemic shock.
    - May occur in individuals with chronic adrenal insufficiency experiencing a stressor such as an intercurrent illness, surgical procedure, or in cases of abrupt cessation of glucocorticoid administration.

Diagnostic Evaluation

- 17-OHP levels; often completed on newborn screening.
- Morning 17-OHP levels may be elevated in a partial enzyme deficiency.
- Testosterone level; females (elevated).
- Androstenedione; males and females.
- Karyotyping important for ambiguous genitalia.
- Adrenocorticotropic hormone (ACTH) stimulation test may be necessary to confirm diagnosis.
  - Significant rise in cortisol level 30 to 60 minutes following ACTH injection.
  - Decreased cortisol response also seen in some cases.

Secondary Adrenal Insufficiency

Definition

- Caused by an impairment in the hypothalamus or pituitary gland.
- Lack of corticotrophin-releasing hormone from the hypothalamus and/or ACTH secretion from the pituitary, resulting in poor function of the adrenal cortex.
- *Mineralocorticoid function is preserved in secondary adrenal insufficiency.*
- Congenital secondary adrenal insufficiency.
  - Congenital causes of secondary adrenal insufficiency include septo-optic dysplasia, corticotropin-releasing hormone deficiency, and maternal hypercortisolemia.
- Acquired secondary adrenal insufficiency.
  - Most common cause is abrupt discontinuation of glucocorticoid therapy.
  - Glucocorticoids, administered in any route, can result in suppression of the hypothalamic–pituitary–adrenal axis.
  - This occurs with glucocorticoid therapy of as short as 2 weeks' duration.
  - Inflammatory disorders, tumors, radiation therapy, or trauma are other causes.

Diagnosis

- Metabolic acidosis, hyponatremia, hypoglycemia, hyperkalemia, low or normal plasma cortisol, elevated ACTH.
- ACTH stimulation test.
  - Measures how well the adrenal glands respond to the administration of ACTH.
  - See Common Diagnostic Testing at the end of this chapter for more information.

Management: Primary and Secondary Adrenal Insufficiency

- Glucocorticoid administration.
  - Goal is to replace physiologic glucocorticoid production.
    - CAH: 10 to 20 mg/m^2/day of oral hydrocortisone daily.
    - Adrenal insufficiency: 6 to 9 mg/m^2/day oral hydrocortisone daily.
  - The dose of glucocorticoid should be adjusted in patients with fever or illness to reflect the normal physiologic response to stress (stressed states result in elevated cortisol levels in a normal host).
  - Stress dosing: hydrocortisone 25 to 50 mg/m^2/day IV/IM.
  - For severe illness or surgical procedures, higher doses may be indicated: hydrocortisone 50 to 123 mg/m^2/day IV.
- Mineral corticoid maintenance.
  - CAH and salt-losing forms of adrenal insufficiency: 0.1 to 0.2 mg oral fludrocortisone acetate daily.
  - Infants require 17 to 34 mEq of sodium supplementation daily.
  - Monitor blood pressure and electrolytes.

PEARL

- *Adrenal insufficiency can be life-threatening and should always be considered in an individual recently receiving steroids.*

Cerebral Salt Wasting

Michele Goodwin & Sharon Y. Irving

Background

- Occurs following an acute central nervous system (CNS) injury.
- Occurs in the setting of *both* hypovolemia and hyponatremia.
- Reports of cerebral salt wasting (CSW) in the pediatric population first appeared in the 1980s.
- Syndrome of inappropriate antidiuretic hormone (SIADH) is more common than CSW in patients with hyponatremia and CNS disease.
- *It is important to distinguish between SIADH and CSW as treatments for the disorders are different.*

Definition

- Characterized by increased renal loss of salt during or following intracranial insult.
- Results in volume depletion and hyponatremia.
- Can be described as a volume-depleted clinical state accompanied by renal salt wasting.
- Typically, the onset occurs within the first few days of an inciting intracranial injury, surgery, or disease process.

Etiology

- Unclear etiology.
- Strong association with elevation in the circulating brain and atrial natriuretic peptides, along with an alteration in the neuronal control of the kidneys.

- May lead to the inhibition of the renin–angiotensin–aldosterone system, causing abnormal renal reabsorption of sodium and triggering the release of antidiuretic hormone (ADH) necessary to maintain intravascular volume.
- May be associated with the following clinical conditions:
  - Traumatic brain injury.
  - Intracranial surgery.
  - Meningitis.
  - Encephalitis.
  - Subarachnoid hemorrhage.

Pathophysiology

- Poorly understood.
- Hypothesized mechanisms are thought to be related to impaired sodium reabsorption likely due to the release of brain natriuretic peptide, increased atrial natriuretic peptide, and/or decreased central sympathetic activity.
- The natriuretic peptides are believed to cause the inhibition of renal salt reabsorption by the kidneys and the restriction of renin and aldosterone release; both affect sodium levels and fluid volume (Figure 7.1).

Clinical Presentation

- Headache.
- Nausea/vomiting.
- Depressed/altered mental status.
- Lethargy.
- Dehydration.
- Agitation.
- Seizures.
- Hypotension.
- Coma.
- *The rate of renal sodium loss, the degree of hyponatremia, and the overall fluid status impact the severity of the presenting symptoms.*

Diagnostic Evaluation

- Laboratory studies:
  - Serum sodium <135 mEq/L.
  - Serum osmolarity <280 mOsm/kg.
  - Urine sodium >80 mEq/L.
  - Urine osmolarity >200 mOsm/kg.
  - Urine specific gravity >1.010.

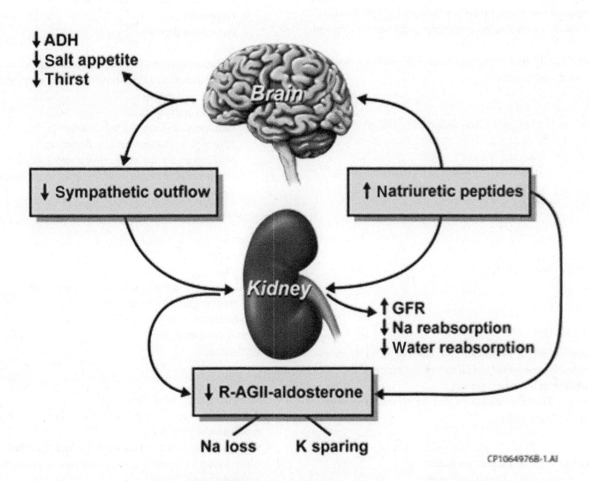

FIGURE 7.1 • **Cerebral Salt-Wasting Pathophysiology.** (From Yee, A. H., Burns, J. D., & Wijdicks, E. F. (2010). Cerebral salt wasting: Pathophysiology, diagnosis, and treatment. *Neurosurgical Clinics of North America, 21*, 339–352 with permission.)

- Urine output 2 to 3 mL/kg/hour.
- Head CT/MRI.
  - Can identify structural abnormalities/pathophysiologic changes (e.g., arteriovenous malformation, tumor or other space-occupying lesion, hemorrhage).
- Lumbar puncture.
  - CNS infection (in cases of CNS-infection-triggered CSW).

Management

- Distinguish between CSW and SIADH.
  - Treatment is different for these conditions.
  - Identify and treat the underlying cause.
  - Frequent monitoring of serum sodium levels and fluid balance.
  - Sodium replacement using a non–dextrose-containing isotonic or hypertonic fluid at an approximate rate of 0.5 to 1 mEq/hour.
  - Limit serum sodium level rise to no more than 10 to 12 mEq/day.
    - The demyelination that occurs with rapid osmotic fluid shifts can result in irreversible neurologic damage.
    - If the patient presented with acute neurologic changes, this may be related to the rate of serum sodium loss.
      - In this instance, it may be more appropriate to provide non–glucose-containing hypertonic fluid until symptoms abate.
- Consultation with appropriate subspecialty services, including neurosurgery and neurology.
- Patient/family education regarding CSW etiology, diagnostic testing, and treatment.

PEARLS

- *CSW should always be considered in early-onset hyponatremia accompanied by hypovolemia that follows an intracranial insult.*
- *Avoiding too rapid a rise in serum sodium levels can reduce the risk of central pontine demyelination of white matter in brain.*

Diabetes Insipidus

Allison Thompson

Background

- A disorder caused by insufficient secretion of ADH by the pituitary gland (neurogenic), *or* failure of the kidneys to respond to circulating ADH (nephrogenic).
- Characterized by increased thirst and the excretion of large amounts of dilute urine.

Etiology

- Neurogenic (central diabetes insipidus [DI]).
  - Genetic: typically X-linked recessive.
    - Examples: Wolfram syndrome.
      - A rare inherited autosomal recessive condition.
      - Affects 1 in 770,000 children.
      - Characterized by central DI, diabetes mellitus, optic atrophy, and deafness.
      - In this disorder, central DI is caused by the loss of ADH-secreting neurons in the supraoptic nucleus and impaired processing within the hypothalamus.
  - Congenital.
    - Often associated with midline craniofacial defects such as holoprosencephaly and septo-optic dysplasia.
  - Acquired.
    - Can result from damage to the pituitary gland or posterior hypothalamus from neurosurgery, trauma, tumors or other brain lesions, meningitis, or encephalitis.
    - *May be either a temporary or a permanent disorder depending on the injury.*
- Nephrogenic DI.
  - Congenital.
    - Typically X-linked recessive involving mutations of VR2 or AQP2.
  - Acquired.
    - Variety of conditions that lead to the inability of the kidneys to respond to ADH.
      - Chronic renal failure.
      - Renal tubulointerstitial diseases.
      - Hypercalcemia.
      - Potassium depletion.
      - Sickle cell disease.
    - Medication-induced from drugs, including alcohol, lithium, diuretics, amphotericin B, demeclocycline.
    - Dietary abnormalities.
      - Primary polydipsia.
      - Decreased sodium chloride intake.
      - Severe protein restriction or depletion.
      - *Nephrogenic DI that results from a metabolic condition may be reversed if the medication is stopped or the metabolic condition is corrected.*

Clinical Presentation

- Polyuria.
- Dilute urine.
- Polydipsia.
- Inappropriately low urine sodium and osmolality.
- Urine specific gravity <1.005.
- Hypernatremia.
- Serum hypo-osmolality.
- Dehydration.

Diagnostic Evaluation

- History and differential diagnoses.
  - The primary causes of polyuria and polydipsia are diabetes mellitus and central DI.
  - Other causes include urinary tract infection, relief of renal obstruction, and psychogenic polydipsia (characterized by excessive water intake).
  - Once hyperglycemia has been excluded, history should include age of initiation and rate of onset of polyuria (will reflect primary vs. secondary cause).

- Serum laboratory studies.
  - Sodium >150 mEq/L.
  - Osmolality ≧295 mOsm/kg.
- Urinary laboratory studies.
  - Sodium <30 mEq/L.
  - Osmolality <200 mOsm/L.
  - Specific gravity <1.005.
- Brain imaging studies.
  - Head CT/MRI.
    - Presence of intracranial mass, abnormal findings of hypothalamic/pituitary stalk.
- Water deprivation testing.
  - Only performed in acute care setting under close medical monitoring and supervision.
  - Fluids are restricted until as much as 5% of body weight has been lost to evaluate urinary response when the serum osmolality exceeds 295 mOsm/kg.
    - Central DI.
      - Concentrated urine and decreased urine output following ADH administration.
    - Nephrogenic DI.
      - Excessive, dilute urine despite hypernatremia and hyperosmolality.

Management

- Restore hemodynamics.
- Replace water deficits and correct electrolyte disturbances.
- Decrease urine output to within normal range (e.g., vasopressin, desmopressin).
- Treat underlying condition, when possible.
- Volume replacement.
  - Maintenance IV fluids, *plus* mL per mL urine output replacement (usually allow 1–2-mL/kg/hour urine output and replace the remainder).
- Monitor serum sodium closely.
- Primary plan for central DI is ADH replacement to control polyuria.
  - ADH preparation depends on acuity of illness and the ability of the patient to tolerate oral intake.
  - Dose varies based on the preparation/formulation and include:
    - Vasopressin.
      - Continuous IV infusion.
      - Used in the critical care or perioperative setting due to its short half-life (10–20 minutes) and easy titration.
      - Initiated at a dose of 0.5 milliunits/kg/hour and titrated until urine output is decreased.
      - Titrated to obtain urine output less than 4 mL/kg/hour.
    - Desmopressin.
      - Used in all other settings.
      - Available in oral and intranasal formulations.
      - Chronic therapy: Dose range is 5 to 30 μg/day, with a peak effect within 1 to 5 hours.
      - *Nephrogenic DI is resistant to vasopressin administration* (Figure 7.2).

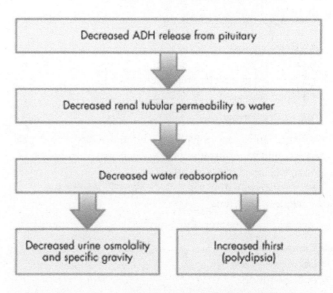

FIGURE 7.2 • **Diabetes Insipidus Flowchart.**

PEARL
- *Pediatric patients with a known history of DI who are acutely ill may quickly develop signs of dehydration or hypovolemic shock.*

Diabetic Ketoacidosis

Keshava Gowda & Tageldin M. Ahmed

Background/Definition

- Potentially life-threatening complication of type 1 diabetes.
- Stimulated by insulin deficiency.
  - Insulin must be present to bind to receptor sites, allowing glucose to enter cells.
  - Without insulin, the body breaks down fat for fuel, resulting in ketosis.
- Diabetic ketoacidosis (DKA) is diagnosed when blood glucose is >200 mg/dL, presence of serum ketones (ketonemia), urine ketones (ketonuria), blood pH <7.3, and serum bicarbonate <15 mmol/L.

Epidemiology/Etiology

- Previous diagnosis of type I diabetes:
  - Insulin dose omission.
  - Intercurrent illness.
    - Stress increases counterregulatory hormone levels, promoting gluconeogenesis and insulin resistance.
  - Unrecognized disruption in insulin pump therapy (if applicable).
- New onset of type diabetes

Pathophysiology

- Insulin deficiency or insulin inefficiency due to counterregulatory hormones is the main stimulus in DKA.

- Hyperglycemia leads to:
  - Osmotic diuresis.
  - Electrolyte loss.
  - Dehydration.
  - Decreased glomerular filtration.
  - Hyperosmolarity.

Clinical Presentation

- Polyuria, polydipsia, polyphagia, abdominal discomfort/pain, nausea and vomiting, nonspecific weakness, fruity breath odor, Kussmaul respirations.
  - Severe presentation can include altered mental status, seizures, and coma.

Physical Examination Findings

- Tachycardia.
- Decreased pulses.
- Poor perfusion.
- Dry mucus membranes.
- Enophthalmos.
- Poor skin turgor.
- Hypotension.
- Deep or labored breathing.

Diagnostic Evaluation

- Blood glucose >200 mg/dL, serum pH <7.3, bicarbonate <15 mmol/L.
- Serum electrolytes, blood urea nitrogen (BUN), creatinine, calcium, magnesium, phosphorus.
- High serum osmolality.
- Positive serum/urine ketones.
- Hemoglobin $A1_C$.
- Complete blood count with differential.
  - Leukocytosis is not a reliable marker of infection.
  - Elevation in stress hormones may mimic infection.
- Autoimmune markers.
  - GAD-65 (glutamic acid decarboxylase), IA-2, IA-2β.
  - Insulin auto-antibodies.
  - May be evaluated for evidence of associated autoimmune conditions.

Management

- Monitoring.
  - Cardiac monitoring.
    - Assess T wave alterations with hyper- or hypokalemia.
  - Cerebral edema.
    - Most serious complication and frequent cause of death.
    - Survivors often experience neurologic sequelae.
    - Occurs in approximately 1% of cases.
    - Has been reported prior to the initiation of therapy, but typically occurs after the start of treatment.
    - Risk factors.
      - Young age.
      - New-onset diabetes.
      - Longer duration of symptoms.
    - Signs and symptoms of cerebral edema (see Section 6: Neurologic Disorders).

- *Requires rapid recognition and treatment.*
  - Elevate head of bed.
  - Administer hyperosmolar therapy.
    - Preferred treatment is hypertonic saline (e.g., 3% saline).
      - 5 to 10 mL/kg.
    - Mannitol.
      - 0.5 to 1 g/kg IV.
      - May be repeated if no response.
  - Intubation and mechanical ventilation if progression of symptoms.
  - Head CT is not routinely completed prior to start of therapy, but can be obtained to evaluate and document presence of cerebral edema.
- Respiratory support.
  - Supplemental oxygen.
    - If respiratory distress, circulatory impairment, or shock.
  - If altered mental status, consider mechanical ventilator support.
- Access.
  - Establish multiple peripheral IV catheters.
  - May require arterial line for frequent laboratory sampling.
- Judicious fluid replacement.
  - Avoid overaggressive fluid replacement with frequent evaluation and repeated boluses, as needed.
  - Moderate to severe DKA with poor perfusion.
    - Start with 0.9 normal saline (NS) 10 to 20 mL/kg bolus.
    - Repeat bolus if poor perfusion/hypotension persists.
    - Obtain repeat blood gas, finger-stick glucose, and basic metabolic panel after initial fluid resuscitation.
    - Remaining fluids are calculated deficits and replaced over 36 to 48 hours using isotonic fluid (e.g., 0.9 NS).
      - Subtract the volume administered in boluses from 24 hours fluid calculation.
  - Withhold potassium from fluids until evidence of adequate kidney function and serum potassium level decreasing.
  - Consider use of two-bag method when ready for introduction of glucose.
    - Allows regulation of glucose from D5W to D10W.
    - Equal electrolyte supplements are added to each bag when using two-bag method.
  - *Add dextrose to IV fluids when blood glucose level is 200 to 250 mg/dL.*
  - *Adjust glucose to prevent rapid drop in blood glucose (e.g., >100 mg/dL/hour).*
- Insulin therapy.
  - Insulin infusion is typically started at 0.1 unit/kg/hour.
  - Follow hourly blood glucose levels.
  - *Adjust the amount of dextrose in the IV fluids rather than decreasing the insulin.*
  - Decrease the insulin infusion only in cases when patient demonstrates extreme sensitivity to insulin (e.g., usually young children).
  - Continue the infusion until the pH is >7.3 and bicarbonate level >18 mmol/L, or ketonemia has resolved.

- Sodium.
  - Replace using 0.9 NS or Ringer lactate for first several hours of DKA therapy.
  - Follow this initial therapy with 0.45 NS.
  - Hyperglycemia results in a lower serum sodium concentration.
    - Results in dilutional hyponatremia, due to the movement of water into the extracellular fluid.
    - Calculation:
      Corrected Sodium $= [Na^+] + [1.6 \times$ (plasma concentration mg/dL $- 100$)]/100
    - As hyperglycemia improves, serum sodium should improve.
    - If sodium level increases or does not begin to fall, there is concern for the development of cerebral edema.
- Potassium.
  - Serum potassium levels may be low, normal, or high in DKA presentation.
  - Potassium loss is an effect of movement of water out of the cells due to the increase in serum osmolarity, resulting in concentrated potassium level.
  - Add potassium to IV fluid when potassium level <6 mEq/L, based on institutional protocol.
  - Correction of hyperglycemia and administration of insulin result in shift of potassium back into the cells, evidenced by a decrease in serum potassium.
- Phosphorus.
  - Depletion of intracellular phosphorus is a result of acidosis, osmotic diuresis, and insulin administration.
- Bicarbonate administration.
  - Only indicated in extreme circumstances.
  - No clinical trial support for its use in DKA.
  - Risks of administration include:
    - CNS acidosis.
    - Hypokalemia.
    - Association with cerebral edema.
- Antibiotics.
  - If identified infection or if highly suspicious of bacterial infection.
- Monitoring.
  - Hourly blood glucose, blood gas, serum electrolytes, serum ketones, osmolarity based on institution protocols.
  - Urine ketones based on institution protocols.
- Transitioning to subcutaneous insulin.
  - Best time to convert is *preceding* a meal.
  - Administer subcutaneous dose of rapid-acting insulin 10 to 15 minutes prior to discontinuing insulin infusion.
  - Most newly diagnosed patients.
    - Multiple doses per day regimen.
      - Basal and bolus insulin.
    - Basal as long-acting insulin is given daily.
    - Bolus doses.
      - Calculated on premeal glucose and carbohydrate content of meal.
      - Example: 1 unit insulin for every 15 g of carbohydrate, plus 1 unit insulin for every 50 g/dL over 150 mg/dL on measured blood glucose.

- Blood glucose monitoring.
  - Prior to meals and 2 hours after meal ends, based on the institution or specialty guidelines.
  - At bedtime.
    - Evaluates the appropriateness of the basal dose.

PEARLS
- *Cerebral edema is the most serious complication of pediatric DKA.*
- *DKA flow sheet is helpful for hourly clinical and laboratory findings.*
- *Prevention of DKA is key through proper education of patient and family which includes an interdisciplinary approach.*
- *Check all home equipment (e.g., pumps, glucometers) for malfunction as precipitating factor in DKA admission.*
- *Remove insulin pump prior to beginning therapy for DKA.*

Hyperglycemic Hyperosmolar State

Laura Crisanti

Background

- Hyperglycemic hyperosmolar state (HHS) is a potentially fatal complication of diabetes, usually type 2, due to an insulin deficiency and an increase in counterregulatory hormones.

Etiology

- Accounts for <1% of primary diabetic admissions.
- Mortality rate is approximately 11% to 15%.

Pathophysiology

- Insulin deficiency and an increase in counterregulatory hormones.
- Enough endogenous insulin to suppress ketosis, although an insufficient amount of insulin to prevent hyperglycemia.
- Accumulation of ketoacids that cause gap metabolic acidosis in DKA patients does *not* occur in HHS.

Clinical Presentation

- Severe dehydration, polyuria, polydipsia, weight loss, altered mental status, hyperglycemia, increased serum osmolality.

Diagnostic Evaluation

- Laboratory studies.
  - BUN, creatinine, calcium, magnesium, phosphate, pH analysis, serum ketones, urine analysis, serum osmolality, hemoglobin $A1_C$.
- Diagnostic criteria.
  - Plasma glucose >600 mg/dL, arterial pH >7.30, serum bicarbonate >15 mmol/L.
  - Small ketonuria.
  - Mild or absent ketonemia.

- Serum osmolality >320 mOsm/kg.
- Altered mental status; stupor, coma.

Management

- ABCs.
  - May require intubation if unable to protect airway.
- Restore circulatory volume and correct fluid deficit.
- Correct hyperglycemia, hyperosmolality, and electrolyte imbalances.
  - Fluid management alone is often sufficient; however, insulin therapy at doses similar to DKA therapy may facilitate the correction of hyperglycemia.
- Frequent laboratory evaluation.
  - Hourly serum glucose in acute phase, electrolytes, and other laboratory studies per institution.
- Treat underlying cause.
  - Infection is the most common precipitating factor.
- Monitor for signs of cerebral edema.
  - Correcting fluids over a longer time period (e.g., 48 hours) may reduce the risk of cerebral edema.

PEARLS

- *Evaluation for infection should be completed as it can be a precipitating factor of hyperglycemic crisis.*
- *Careful titration of fluids and insulin prevents rapid fluid shifts and reduces the risk of cerebral edema and hypotension.*

Thyroid Disorders

Mary P. White

Background

- Thyroid disorders occur as a result of over- or underproduction of thyroid hormone. Dysfunction can be chronic or occur acutely.

Pathophysiology

- The thyroid gland regulates metabolism through the secretion of T_3 and T_4, which are produced in the presence of iodine and based on the secretion of thyroid-stimulating hormone (TSH).
- The hypothalamus releases thyrotropin-releasing hormone, which then stimulates the pituitary gland to secrete TSH.
- An increase in serum levels of T_3 and T_4 will result in lower levels of TSH. A decrease in serum levels of T_3 and T_4 will result in higher levels of TSH.

Etiology/Types

- Hypothyroidism:
  - Congenital hypothyroidism.
    - Abnormal fetal thyroid development or a disturbance in the production of thyroid hormone.
  - Acquired hypothyroidism.
    - Autoimmune and iatrogenic causes.

- Autoimmune hypothyroidism.
  - Immune system response results in damage and altered function of thyroid.
  - Most common autoimmune thyroid disorder is chronic lymphocytic thyroiditis or Hashimoto thyroiditis.
    - Chronic lymphocytic thyroiditis affects females more often than males.
    - Common comorbidities include type 1 diabetes, juvenile rheumatoid arthritis, trisomy 21.
- Iatrogenic hypothyroidism.
  - Can be caused by head or neck radiation therapy, surgery, or induced by drugs that increase thyroxine metabolism.
- Hyperthyroidism:
  - Congenital or neonatal hyperthyroidism.
    - Occurs in infants of mothers with Graves disease, causing a transplacental transfer of the thyroid-stimulating immunoglobulin (TSI) from the mother to the infant.
  - Acquired hyperthyroidism.
    - Autoimmune and iatrogenic causes.
    - Graves disease.
      - Most common cause of acquired hyperthyroidism resulting in an overproduction of the thyroid hormone.
    - Hashimoto thyroiditis.
      - Autoimmune disorder resulting in hyperthyroid state, often associated with other disorders such a type 1 diabetes mellitus or celiac disease.
      - Autoimmune destruction of thyroid tissues, causing an initial surge of thyroid hormone, followed, over time, by a state of hypothyroidism.

Clinical and Diagnostic Presentation

- Congenital hypothyroidism.
  - Symptoms typically develop within the first 2 to 6 weeks of life.
  - *Early diagnosis is critical due to the risk of irreversible neurocognitive deficits if untreated.*
  - Symptoms include lethargy, hoarse cry, bradycardia, large size for gestational age, large fontanels, constipation, hypothermia, jaundice, and dry skin.
  - Diagnostic evaluation: Positive Newborn Screening results, free T_4, TSH elevated.
- Acquired hypothyroidism.
  - Symptoms and clinical findings.
    - Linear growth deceleration.
    - Weight gain, fatigue, dry skin, brittle hair.
    - Muscle cramps, cold intolerance.
    - Delayed tooth eruption.
  - Laboratory studies: elevated TSH, low T_4, and free T_4 levels.
    - If Hashimoto thyroiditis is the cause of the hypothyroidism, increased thyroid peroxidase antibodies, antimicrosomal antibodies, and thyroglobulin antibody titers will be present.
- Congenital hyperthyroidism.
  - Findings usually develop in the initial days after birth, including small fontanels, fever, irritability, tachycardia, vomiting, diarrhea, poor weight gain despite increased feeding.

- Birth history may be positive for intrauterine growth retardation or premature birth.
- Diagnostic evaluation: elevated free T_3 and T_4 levels and decreased TSH level.
  - Antithyroid peroxisomal antibodies may be present.
- Acquired hyperthyroidism.
  - Symptoms and clinical findings.
    - Diffuse enlargement of the thyroid.
    - Anxiety, sweating, weight loss, tachycardia.
    - Eyelid lag or retraction, periorbital edema, and exophthalmus.
    - Diagnostic evaluation: elevated T_3 and T_4 levels and decreased TSH.
      - May or may not have antithyroid peroxisomal antibodies present.
    - *Radiographic testing for any thyroid disorders is not commonly used in screening.*
      - Ultrasound may be used to evaluate the soft tissues of the thyroid.
      - Scintigraphy is used to evaluate the function of the thyroid gland.

Management

- Congenital hypothyroidism.
  - L-Thyroxine administration and monitoring for life.
    - Normalization of T_4.
- Congenital hyperthyroidism.
  - Propylthiouracil or methimazole.
    - Blocks thyroid hormone stimulation.
  - Iodine.
    - Blocks the release of thyroid hormone already synthesized with the administration of iodine.
- Acquired hypothyroidism.
  - L-Thyroxine.
    - Thyroid replacement.
- Acquired hyperthyroidism.
  - Propylthiouracil or methimazole.
  - Radioactive iodine.
  - Surgery (some cases).
- Intermittent monitoring of serum thyroid hormone levels.

PEARL

- *Profound neurologic impairment can occur in cases of delayed diagnosis and therapy in congenital hypothyroidism.*

Parathyroid Disorders

Mary P. White

Background

- Primary function of the parathyroid gland and parathyroid hormone (PTH) is to regulate the amount of calcium present in blood and bones.

Definitions

- Hypoparathyroidism.
  - Decreased function or absence of the parathyroid gland, causing a decrease in PTH.
- Hyperparathyroidism.
  - Excessive secretion of PTH, leads to hypocalcemia, hypocalciuria, hypophosphatemia, and hyperphosphaturia.

Pathophysiology

- Secretion of PTH is triggered by a reduction in the serum calcium level. When released, PTH targets musculoskeletal, renal, and gastrointestinal systems to regulate serum calcium levels.
- PTH triggers increased bone resorption, resulting in an elevation in serum calcium and serum phosphate.
- In the kidney, PTH stimulates the reuptake of calcium and magnesium and increases phosphorus excretion.
- In the intestine, PTH activates the enzyme responsible for vitamin D absorption, which then controls the absorption of intestinal calcium.

Etiology/Types

- Congenital hypoparathyroidism.
  - DiGeorge syndrome (22q11 deletion).
    - The most common congenital cause of hypoparathyroidism.
- Hypoparathyroidism.
  - Autoimmune.
    - Usually associated with Addison disease or other endocrine diseases such as adrenal insufficiency with polyglandular autoimmune syndrome type 1.
  - Acquired.
    - Injury to parathyroid gland.
    - Ingestion of certain medications.
      - Anticonvulsants causing hypocalcemia.
      - Radioactive iodine treatment.
  - Primary hyperparathyroidism.
    - Associated with multiple endocrine neoplasia syndromes or adenomas.
  - Secondary hyperparathyroidism.
    - Largely due to hypocalcemic states associated with chronic renal failure, vitamin D deficiency, rickets.

Clinical Presentation

- Congenital hypoparathyroidism.
  - Neonatal hypocalcemia.
  - Micrognathia.
  - Hypertelorism.
  - Short or hypoplastic philtrum.
  - Congenital heart disease (e.g., tetralogy of Fallot, truncus arteriosus, right aortic arch).
- Hypoparathyroidism.
  - Hypocalcemia.
  - Muscle twitching, cramping, tetany.
  - Seizures.
  - Abdominal pain.
  - Dry hair and skin, brittle nails.

Diagnostic Evaluation

- Hypoparathyroidism.
  - PTH level decreased.
  - Serum and urinary calcium decreased.
  - Hyperphosphatemia.
  - Electrocardiography (EKG) with shortened or prolonged QTc interval.
- Primary hyperparathyroidism.
  - Hypercalcemia.
  - Abdominal pain, vomiting, and constipation.
  - Bone pain and paresthesias.
  - Renal stones.
  - Hypertension.
  - Diagnostic evaluation: PTH elevated, hypercalcemia, hypophosphatemia, alkaline phosphatase normal or elevated.
- Secondary hyperparathyroidism.
  - Hypercalcemia.
  - Abdominal pain, vomiting, constipation.
  - Bone pain.
  - Renal stones.
  - Paresthesias.
  - Hypertension.
  - Diagnostic evaluation: Serum calcium levels are low or normal; EKG with prolonged QTc interval, nephrolithiasis, parathyroid adenoma.

Management

- Hypoparathyroidism.
  - Calcium and vitamin D supplementation.
  - Electrocardiograph monitoring.
  - Long-term monitoring of dietary calcium intake.
  - Close monitoring (e.g., every 3–6 months) of serum calcium and phosphorus, serum magnesium, alkaline phosphate levels, 25-(OH)D$_3$ and 1,25-(OH)$_2$D$_3$.
  - Urine calcium-to-creatinine level monitoring.
- Hyperparathyroidism.
  - Aggressive hydration and diuretics.
  - Restriction of calcium and vitamin D intake.
  - Hydrocortisone.
  - Calcitonin.
  - Surgical removal of parathyroid glands.

Pheochromocytomas
Andrea M. Kline-Tilford

Background

- Neuroendocrine tumor.
  - Arising from the adrenal medulla.
  - Specifically from the catecholamine-producing chromaffin cells.
- May be benign or malignant.
- Often bilateral.

- Often extra-adrenal.
- May be associated with von Hippel–Lindau disease, multiple endocrine neoplasia type 2, familial paraganglioma syndrome, or neurofibromatosis type 1.

Pathophysiology

- Failure of extra-adrenal chromaffin tissue to involute during development.
- Results in secretion of catecholamines.

Presentation

- Hypertension; typically sustained.
  - Result of tumor-associated catecholamine release.
- Triad.
  - Headache, diaphoresis, palpitations.
    - Less common in pediatric presentation when compared with adults.
- Tachycardia.
- Abnormal skin sensation.
- Anxiety.
- Hyperglycemia.

Diagnosis

- Metanephrine or catecholamine levels; plasma or urine.
  - 24 hour urine collection.
- Urinary vanillylmandelic acid.
- Evaluation for other causes of catecholamine release/adrenergic excess.
- CT scan: head, neck, chest, abdomen.
  - Tumor localization.
- Scintigraphy or positron emission tomography may also be used to localize tumor.

Management

- Hypertension control.
  - Typically, α- or β-blockers may be used presurgically.
- Surgical resection.
- Metastatic pheochromocytoma requires antineoplastic therapy.

Prognosis

- Depends on size and extent of tumor, ability to resect the tumor, and presence of metastasis.

Syndrome of Inappropriate Antidiuretic Hormone
Kristin M. Print

Background

- A common cause of hyponatremia.

Definition

- Excessive release of ADH from the pituitary gland.

Etiology/Types

- CNS disorders.
- Pulmonary disorders.
- Surgically induced.
- Medication-induced.

Clinical Presentation

- Hyponatremia.
- Decreased serum osmolarity and increased urine osmolarity.
- Decreased urine output with increased urine concentration.
- Cerebral edema may ensue in severe cases of hyponatremia.

Diagnostic Evaluation

- Serum sodium <135 mEq/L, serum osmolarity <280 mOsm/L, urine osmolarity >200 mOsm/L.
- BUN <10 mg/dL.
- Urine specific gravity >1.020.
- Urine sodium >25 mEq/L.
- Refer to Table 7.1.

Management

- Identify and treat underlying cause.
- Fluid restriction to <75% daily maintenance fluid requirement.
- Avoid hypotonic IV fluids.
- Correct hyponatremia slowly by 0.5 to 1 mEq/hour.
- For severe hyponatremia, correct sodium to 125 mEq/L with 3% hypertonic saline (Figure 7.3).

Na$^+$ deficit = (Body weight in kg) × (0.6 % in extracellular fluid: ECF) × (Desired serum sodium level [125] − Actual serum sodium level) = mEq.

Common Diagnostic Testing

Diabetic Evaluation

- Laboratory testing for diabetes has several purposes, including differentiating between type 1 and type 2 diabetes diagnoses,

determining the presence of ketoacidosis, and identifying other specific patient characteristics.
- Initial evaluation for child newly diagnosed with diabetes:
  - Laboratory testing:
    - Complete blood count with differential.
    - Basic or comprehensive metabolic panel.
      - Hemoglobin A1$_C$.
      - Marker of chronic glycemia.
      - Provides an average measure of glucose level over the course of 2 to 3 months.
      - Also known as glycosylated hemoglobin (i.e., the percentage of hemoglobin that is coated with glucose).
      - Correlates with micro- and macrovascular complications.
      - Level ≥6.5% supports diagnosis of type 2 diabetes.
  - Insulin level.
    - Peptide hormone produced by the β-cells in the pancreas.
    - Decreased in type 1 diabetes.
  - Insulin antibodies.
    - Includes islet cell antibodies and GAD-65.
  - C-peptide.
    - Levels can assist in determining the distinction between types 1 and 2 diabetes.
    - Low in type 1 and high in type 2.
    - *Values should be obtained prior to initiating insulin therapy.*
    - Oral glucose-tolerance testing.
      - Level ≥200 mg/dL diagnostic of diabetes.
      - Fasting plasma glucose: if measures greater than or equal to 126 mg/dL, diagnostic of diabetes.
      - 12-Lead EKG may be indicated to assist in documenting hyperkalemia.
      - Also consider evaluation for other autoimmunities.
        - Celiac disease.
        - Thyroiditis (Table 7.2).

TABLE 7.1	**Comparison of Clinical Findings for Diabetes Insipidus, SIADH, and Cerebral Salt Wasting**					
	Serum Na (mEq/L)	Serum Osmo (mOsm/kg)	Urine Na (mEq/L)	Urine Osmo (mOsm/kg)	Urine Specific Gravity	Urine Output (mL/kg/hr)
Diabetes Insipidus	>150	>295	<30	<200	<1.005	>4
SIADH	<135	<280	>30	>200	>1.020	≤1
Cerebral Salt Wasting	<135	<280	>80	>200	>1.010	2–3

Na, Sodium; Osmo, Osmolarity

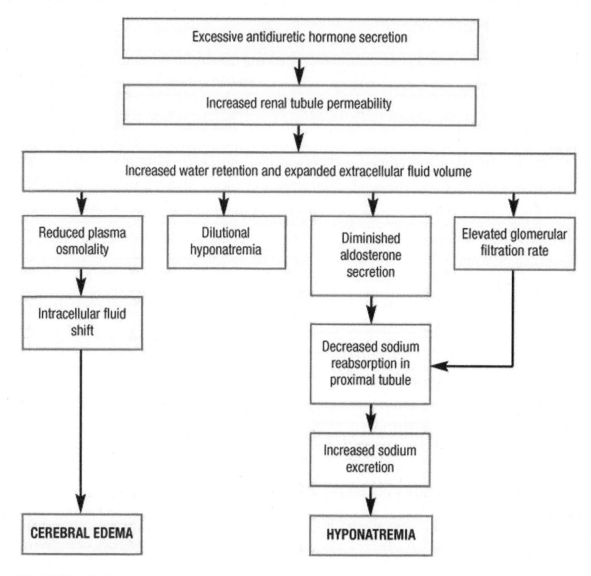

FIGURE 7.3 • **SIADH Flowchart**.

TABLE 7.2 Diagnostic Criteria: Type 1 Diabetes*	
ONE of the following must be present:	
Diagnostic Test	**Additional Information**
Hemoglobin A1$_c$ ≥6.5%.	Testing in a laboratory with a certified method.
Oral glucose-tolerance test: 2 hr plasma glucose ≥200 mg/dL.	Must include a glucose load of 75 g of anhydrous glucose dissolved in water.
Fasting plasma glucose ≥126 mg/dL.	Fasting = No caloric intake for >8 hr.
Random plasma glucose >200 mg/dL in a patient with symptoms of hyperglycemia or hyperglycemia crisis.	

*Tests with unequivocal results should be retested to confirm diagnosis
Adapted from American Diabetes Association. (2013). *Standards of medical care of diabetes 2013*. Retrieved from
http://care.diabetesjournals.org/content/36/Supplement_1/S11/T2.expansion.html

ACTH Stimulation Testing

Mary P. White

- Measures adrenal gland response to administration of ACTH.
- Performing the test.
  - Obtain baseline cortisol level prior to ACTH administration.

- About 30 to 60 minutes following the injection, a second cortisol level is obtained.
- Results: Cortisol levels.
  - <16 µg/dL (440 nmol/L) suggests failing or insufficient response.
  - 18 to 20 µg/dL (500–550 nmol/L) is minimal response.
  - >30 µg/dL (825 nmol/L) is a normal response (Figure 7.4).

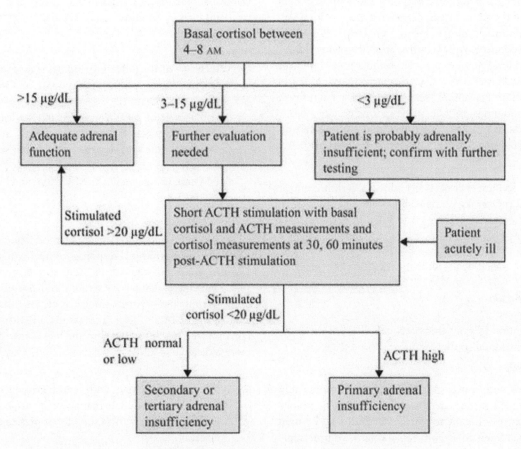

FIGURE 7.4 • **Adrenal Insufficiency Diagnosis Algorithm.** Adrenocorticotropic hormone (ACTH).

1. A 10-year-old, who weighs 30 kg, suffered a subarachnoid hemorrhage as the result of a motor vehicle accident 1 week ago and is now complaining of a headache. Her blood pressure is 75/40 mmHg, and her urine output is 2 to 3 mL/kg/hour. Which one of the laboratory findings is consistent with CSW?
   a. Serum sodium 143 mEq/L, serum osmolarity 285 mOsm/kg, urine sodium 60 mEq/L, urine specific gravity 1.020.
   b. Serum sodium 130 mEq/L, serum osmolarity 275 mOsm/kg, urine sodium 90 mEq/L, urine specific gravity 1.030.
   c. Serum sodium 125 mEq/L, serum osmolarity 350 mOsm/kg, urine sodium 90 mEq/L, urine specific gravity 1.005.
   d. Serum sodium 135 mEq/L, serum osmolarity 200 mOsm/kg, urine sodium 65 mEq/L, urine specific gravity 1.010.

Answer: **B**

In CSW, serum sodium will be <135 mEq/L, serum osmolarity will be <280 mOsm/kg, urine sodium will be >80 mEq/L, and urine specific gravity will be >1.010 due to excess sodium excreted in the urine.

2. Which one of the following is the most appropriate treatment for CSW?
   a. Fluid restriction.
   b. Sodium repletion.
   c. Administration of a mineralocorticoid.
   d. Vasopressin administration.

Answer: **B**

Sodium repletion with a non–glucose-containing isotonic solution is recommended. If the patient is exhibiting acute neurologic signs, a non–dextrose-containing hypertonic fluid may be more appropriate. In addition to sodium replacement, volume repletion is necessary to suppress the release of ADH, permitting excretion of excess water and sodium correction.

3. A 5-year-old boy is on postoperative day 2 from an astrocytoma resection. He is awake, alert, and has been tolerating oral feeds. His morning laboratory values reveal a serum osmolarity of 250 mOsm, serum sodium of 133 mEq/L, and urine sodium of 100 mEq/L.
   Which one of the following is the best intervention to correct his electrolyte imbalances?
   a. Give IV fluid replacement with 0.9% sodium chloride.
   b. Allow him to drink fluids that he likes and can tolerate.
   c. Write an order for him to be NPO.
   d. No intervention needed; the laboratory value will correct over time.

Answer: **B**

The route of sodium and fluid replacement is based on the patient's acuity and ability to tolerate enteral intake. If oral intake

is well tolerated and can be accurately monitored, sodium replacement can occur by replacing measured urinary sodium losses and by providing ongoing maintenance sodium needs. Careful monitoring of fluid intake and output, as well as serum and urinary sodium, is an essential component of patient management.

4. Which one of the following findings is diagnostic of DI?
   a. Oliguria, urine specific gravity 1.001, and serum osmolality of 250 mOsm/L.
   b. Polyuria, urine specific gravity 1.001, and serum osmolality of 300 mOsm/L.
   c. Oliguria, urine specific gravity 1.015, and serum sodium 128 mEq/L.
   d. Polyuria, urine specific gravity 1.015, and blood glucose of 450 mg/dL.

Answer: **B**

DI is associated with a deficiency of production or secretion of ADH or a decreased renal response to ADH with resulting excessive urine output of dilute urine, urine specific gravity of less than 1.005, and increased serum sodium and osmolality. Decreased urine output and serum osmolality of 250 mOsm/L is more indicative of SIADH. DI is not associated with hyperglycemia. Polyuria with low serum sodium and high urine specific gravity is more indicative of CSW.

5. When treating a patient with central DI, which one of the following is the appropriate management strategy?
   a. Fluid replacement, titration of vasopressin continuous infusion.
   b. Fluid restriction to half maintenance rate, diuretics.
   c. Fluid replacement, sodium supplementation.
   d. Fluid restriction, titration of insulin continuous infusion.

Answer: **A**

The primary management strategy in DI is to restore hemodynamics, replace water deficits, correct electrolyte disturbances, and decrease urine output to a normal range. This can be accomplished by administering maintenance IV fluids as well as urine output replacement. Vasopressin therapy is initiated and titrated until urine output is less than 4 mL/kg/hour. Fluid restriction is not appropriate in the management of DI because of the severe dehydration that can occur in this clinical state. Sodium supplementation is not warranted in the management of DI because serum sodium levels are elevated (though, partly due to hemoconcentration). Finally, hyperglycemia is not associated with DI; therefore, insulin administration is not part of DI therapy.

6. Symptoms of congenital hypothyroidism include which of the following?
   a. Hoarse cry, large fontanels, and hypothermia.
   b. Tachycardia, small fontanels, and diarrhea.
   c. Constipation, bradycardia, and irritability.
   d. Lethargy, poor weight gain, and vomiting.

Answer: A

A hoarse cry, large fontanels, and hypothermia are symptoms of congenital hypothyroidism. Tachycardia, small fontanels, and hypothermia are characterized by congenital hyperthyroidism. Irritability is common in congenital hyperthyroidism, while constipation and bradycardia are symptoms of congenital hypothyroidism. Vomiting and poor weight gain are symptoms of congenital hyperthyroidism.

7. A child with Graves disease will typically have which of the following laboratory findings?
   a. Increased T_3 and T_4, increased TSH, and negative TSI.
   b. Decreased T_3 and T_4, increased TSH, and positive TSI.
   c. Increased T_3 and T_4, decreased TSH, and positive .
   d. TSI.
   e. Decreased T_3 and T_4, decreased TSH, and negative TSI.

Answer: C

Graves disease is a form of hyperthyroidism resulting from an autoimmune disorder resulting in a positive TSI. Hyperthyroidism will result in increased T_3 and T_4 and decreased TSH. Hypothyroidism will result in decreased T_3 and T_4 and increased TSH.

8. PTH targets which of the following organs to regulate calcium levels?
   a. Musculoskeletal, cardiovascular, and kidney.
   b. Musculoskeletal, kidney, and gastrointestinal.
   c. Cardiovascular, musculoskeletal, and gastrointestinal.
   d. Cardiovascular, kidney, and musculoskeletal.

Answer: B

When released into the circulation, PTH targets three organ systems to ultimately regulate serum calcium levels. These organ systems include musculoskeletal, kidney, and gastrointestinal. In the bone, PTH triggers increased bone resorption, causing an elevation in serum calcium and serum phosphate. In the kidney, PTH stimulates the reuptake of calcium and magnesium and increases phosphorus excretion. In the intestine, PTH activates the enzyme responsible for vitamin D absorption, which then controls the absorption of intestinal calcium.

9. In determining the presence of adrenal insufficiency, which cortisol level would support the diagnosis?
   a. 16 μg/dL (440 nmol/L).
   b. 18 μg/dL (500 nmol/L).
   c. 25.4 μg/dL (700 nmol/L).
   d. 30 μg/dL (825 nmol/L).

Answer: A

A cortisol level of <16 μg/dL, or 440 nmol/L, is highly suggestive of adrenal insufficiency. The minimum expected response results in a level of 18 to 20 μg/dL (500–550 nmol/L). A cortisol level >30 μg/dL (825 nmol/L) does not support the diagnosis of adrenal insufficiency.

10. A 5-year-old patient with a history of chronic renal failure is admitted to the pediatric intensive care unit for an acute illness and is noted to have polyuria with urine output of 6 mL/kg/hour, serum sodium of 167 mEq/L, urine specific gravity of 1.001, and serum osmolality of 300 mOsm/kg. The ICU team has initiated fluid replacement and a vasopressin infusion. Despite titrating the vasopressin up every 30 minutes, the patient's urine output remains 6 mL/kg/hour. What is the likely cause?
    a. Central DI.
    b. Diabetes mellitus.
    c. CSW.
    d. Nephrogenic DI.

Answer: D

Nephrogenic DI is resistant to the administration of vasopressin. It is caused by conditions in which the kidneys do not respond to circulating ADH. Central DI is responsive to administration of vasopressin because it is characterized by low circulating levels of ADH. Diabetes mellitus and CSW involve different management strategies, which do not include the initiation of vasopressin therapy. Individuals with nephrogenic DI need to consume the same amount of fluid that is produced in the urine. Some patients have demonstrated improvement with the administration of hydrochlorothiazide and amiloride. A low-salt and low-protein diet is recommended in some cases.

11. A 15-year-old boy with a history of type 1 diabetes is admitted to ICU with DKA. Two hours into treatment he becomes agitated, complains of severe headache, begins to vomit, and becomes lethargic.

    Which one of the following diagnoses is highest on the differential list?
    a. Worsening DKA.
    b. Cerebral edema.
    c. Hypoglycemia.
    d. Meningitis.

Answer: B

If there are any acute changes in mental status during the first few hours of DKA treatment, cerebral edema should always be considered as a possibility. It is not always necessary to obtain imaging in this case. Assessment of clinical findings and adjusting therapy are the appropriate management.

12. What is the first step in managing a child who is diagnosed with DKA and is suspected of developing cerebral edema?
    a. Morphine.
    b. CT of brain.
    c. 3% Saline bolus.
    d. Intubation.

Answer: C

(continues on page 228)

All steps should be taken to identify and treat cerebral edema. Reducing elevated intracranial pressure with head position to 30 degree, using an osmotic agent such as mannitol or 3% saline, and avoiding narcotics and sedatives are important. Imaging may or may not be appropriate, depending on the current status of the patient and the risk of radiation exposure.

13. A previously healthy 7-year-old boy, on postoperative day 1 status brain tumor resection, is normotensive, warm, and well perfused with normal pulses and a capillary refill time of 3 seconds. He has been without urine output for 10 hours. Which of the following laboratory results are consistent with SIADH?
    a. Serum sodium 150 mEq/L, serum osmolarity 310 mOsm/kg, urine sodium 10 mEq/L, urine osmolarity 120 mOsm/kg.
    b. Serum sodium 130 mEq/L, serum osmolarity 270 mOsm/kg, urine sodium 95 mEq/L, urine osmolarity 240 mOsm/kg.
    c. Serum sodium 140 mEq/L, serum osmolarity 200 mOsm/kg, urine sodium 30 mEq/L, urine osmolarity 200 mOsm/kg.
    d. Serum sodium 125 mEq/L, serum osmolarity 270 mOsm/kg, urine sodium 40 mEq/L, urine osmolarity 240 mOsm/kg.

Answer: **D**

SIADH can develop from various mechanisms, including brain injury or brain surgery, and is characterized by serum sodium <135 mEq/L, serum osmolarity <280 mOsm/kg, urine sodium >30 mEq/L, and urine osmolarity >200 mOsm/kg.

14. Which one of the following is a potential complication of rapid correction of hyponatremia?
    a. Acute kidney injury.
    b. Cardiac arrhythmias.
    c. Central pontine myelinolysis.
    d. Pulmonary edema.

Answer: **C**

Hyponatremia should be corrected at a rate of 0.5 to 1 mEq/hour to avoid rapid fluid shifts, and serum sodium levels should rise at no more than 10 mEq per 24-hour period to avoid central pontine myelinolysis. Central pontine myelinolysis occurs when free water rapidly moves out of the cells to compensate for the hypertonicity of the extracellular fluid, resulting in shrinking of the brain cells and ultimately demyelination of the axons.

15. What is the recommended goal serum sodium correction level for a child with severe hyponatremia who presents with status epilepticus?
    a. 10 to 12 mEq/L in the first 24 hours.
    b. 14 to 16 mEq/L in the first 24 hours.
    c. 10 to 12 mEq/L in the first 12 hours.
    d. 14 to 16 mEq/L in the first 12 hours.

Answer: **D**

Correct severe hyponatremia with 3% hypertonic saline initially to increase the sodium level in order to prevent further seizure activity. At this point, the goal is to then slowly correct sodium with a goal of 12 to 14 mEq/L/day to normal levels of 135 to 145 mEq/L.

CASE STUDY: QUESTIONS 16–18 FROM FOLLOWING SCENARIO
A 5-year-old boy (weight 20 kg) is on postoperative day 1 from a thoracic rib expansion for congenital restrictive lung disease. Overnight his urine output decreased to <0.5 mL/kg/hour. His morning laboratory values include the following results: Serum sodium 130 mEq/L, Serum osmolarity 270 mOsm/L, BUN 8 mg/dL, urine specific gravity 1.030, urine osmolarity 230 mOsm/L, and urine sodium 35 mEq/L.

16. What is the most likely diagnosis?
    a. CSW.
    b. DI.
    c. DKA.
    d. SIADH.

Answer: **D**

Hyponatremia, decreased serum osmolarity, increased urine osmolarity, increased specific gravity, normal BUN, as well as decreased urine output in the face of a euvolemic fluid status are consistent with SIADH.

17. What is the appropriate management for SIADH?
    a. Bolus with 20 mL/kg NS and increase maintenance fluids to 1.5 times the daily requirement.
    b. Continue D5 0.45 NS at maintenance rate.
    c. Restrict the IV fluid to <75% of total daily maintenance.
    d. Bolus with 3% hypertonic saline (1 mL/kg/hour).

Answer: **C**

Fluid restriction to <75% of total daily maintenance is needed to decrease the free-water reabsorption and excess sodium intake while addressing the underlying cause of SIADH.

18. If the serum sodium level was 120 mEq/L, calculate the amount of 3% hypertonic saline (513 mEq of sodium/L) needed to correct his serum sodium level to 125 mEq/L.
    a. 10 mL.
    b. 15 mL.
    c. 20 mL.
    d. 30 mL.

Answer: **D**

Correct severe hyponatremia with 3% hypertonic saline using the following equation:

Na + deficit = (Body weight in kg) × 0.6 (% in ECF) × (Desired serum sodium level [125] – Actual serum sodium level) = mEq

$$20 \text{ kg} \times 0.6 \times 125 - 120 = 60 \text{ mEq}$$
$$30 \text{ mEq} \times 0.513 \text{mEq/mL (3\% NaCl)} = 30 \text{ mL}$$

19. When ordering an insulin infusion, it is important for the health care team to be aware of which of the following?
    a. IV tubing must be protected from light.
    b. IV tubing must be completely flushed with the insulin.
    c. IV tubing must be changed every 4 hours.
    d. IV insulin is not compatible with any other fluids.

Answer: B

Insulin adheres to IV tubing, requiring that the tubing be completely flushed with the insulin prior to initiating therapy.

20. When discussing the long-term care of nephrogenic DI with a patient and family, the counseling will include instructions for which of the following?
    a. Finger-stick glucose monitoring.
    b. Urine ketone monitoring.
    c. Intake and output monitoring.
    d. Blood pressure monitoring.

Answer: C

Essential to the successful management of nephrogenic DI is ensuring that the child's intake closely matches the output. In nephrogenic DI, the kidneys do not respond to ADH, which is important in body fluid regulation. Blood glucose, urine ketones, and blood pressure monitoring are not required in the child's daily routine.

21. When admitting a child with a history of adrenal insufficiency for a surgical procedure, which one of the following medications needs to be ordered for the perioperative period?
    a. Hydrocortisone.
    b. Dopamine.
    c. Magnesium sulfate.
    d. Fludrocortisone acetate.

Answer: A

A child with adrenal insufficiency will require higher doses of glucocorticoid administration during times of stress. The appropriate medication to order at stress dosing for this child is hydrocortisone. If the adrenal replacement therapy is not adequate, it is possible that fluid resuscitation and/or pressor therapy may be required. Magnesium sulfate is not routinely required in the treatment of adrenal insufficiency. Fludrocortisone acetate is an oral replacement therapy used for long-term management of adrenal insufficiency; however, it is not appropriate for managing adrenal insufficiency during periods of acute stress, as in surgical procedures.

CASE STUDY: QUESTIONS 22 AND 23

A 9-year-old girl diagnosed with diabetes mellitus 2 years ago presents to the emergency room with headache, vomiting, and upper abdominal pain. She was at a family picnic the day before and had a sleepover with her cousins the night before.

22. What is the most likely diagnosis?
    a. Food poisoning.
    b. DKA.
    c. Viral gastroenteritis.
    d. Hypoglycemia.

Answer: B

Presentation with headache, vomiting, and abdominal pain are classic manifestations of DKA, although other differentials may be considered after exclusion of DKA. In addition, other illnesses such as gastroenteritis can predispose a child with diabetes to develop DKA.

23. In this case study scenario, which is the first diagnostic test that should be considered for this patient?
    a. Abdominal X-ray.
    b. Blood glucose test.
    c. Urine drug screen.
    d. Urine specific gravity.

Answer: B

A blood glucose level with a blood gas and electrolytes are essential to confirm a diagnosis of DKA. A low serum pH and bicarbonate level assist in supporting the diagnosis.

CASE STUDY: QUESTIONS 24–26

A 15-year-old underwent a craniotomy secondary to a bleeding arteriovenous malformation. On postsurgery day 2, he presented with a new-onset generalized seizure that was self-limited at 2 minutes. Following the seizure, he was lethargic.

Laboratory findings include the following:
Serum sodium 124 mEq/L, serum osmolarity 200 mOsm/kg, urine sodium 160 mEq/L, urine osmolarity 350 mOsm/kg, and urine specific gravity 1.035.

24. Based on history and the laboratory results for this patient, which diagnosis is most likely?
    a. SIADH.
    b. DI.
    c. CSW.
    d. Water intoxication.

Answer: C

A low serum sodium, low serum osmolarity, and a high urine osmolarity and specific gravity are consistent with CSW.

25. The immediate course of action based on these laboratory results is to:
    a. administer 3% hypertonic saline fluid bolus.
    b. administer oral sodium replacement.
    c. restrict fluid intake.
    d. administer a 0.9% saline fluid bolus.

Answer: D

Correcting the low sodium level is the first objective to prevent continuing seizure activity. A fluid bolus using isotonic 0.9% NS is the appropriate next step to correct CSW.

26. Which one of the following is the best strategy to normalize the serum sodium value?
    a. Rapidly correct serum sodium level to a range of 135 to 145 mEq/L.
    b. No intervention—it will correct on its own over time.
    c. Correct sodium level at a rate of 0.5 to 1 mEq/hour.
    d. Restrict the fluid and sodium intake and the levels will rise.

Answer: C
(continues on page 230)

Slow correction of serum sodium is essential to help prevent acute neurologic changes due to central pontine myelinosis, a symmetric, noninflammatory demyelination of the mid brain, thalamus, basal nuclei, and cerebellum.

27. Which one of the following patients presenting to the emergency department (ED) meets diagnostic criteria for HHS?

   a. A 5-year-old presents to the ED with lethargy, serum glucose of 650 mg/dL, arterial pH 7.12, and serum bicarbonate 11 mmol/L.

   b. A 10-year-old girl presents to the ED difficult to arouse, laboratory values significant for serum glucose of 700 mg/dL, serum bicarbonate of 20 mmol/L, arterial pH 7.35, with a serum osmolality of 324 mOsm/kg.

   c. A 6-year-old boy presents with polydipsia, polyuria, serum pH of 7.16, and serum glucose of 400 mg/dL.

   d. An 8-year-old girl presents unresponsive, with serum glucose of 600 mg/dL, serum bicarbonate of 14 mmol/L, and an arterial pH of 6.9.

Answer: **B**

Diagnostic criteria for HHS include plasma glucose >600 mg/dL, arterial pH >7.30, serum bicarbonate >15 mmol/L, small ketonuria, mild- or absent ketonemia, serum osmolality >320 mOsm/kg. Diagnostic criteria for DKA include blood glucose >250 mg/dL, arterial pH <7.30, serum bicarbonate <15 mEq/L, and moderate ketonemia or ketonuria.

Recommended Readings

American Diabetes Association. (2013). *Standards of medical care of diabetes 2013*. Retrieved from http://care.diabetesjournals.org/content/36/Supplement_1/S11/T2.expansion.html

Bettinelli, A., Longoni, L., Tammaro, F., Faré, P. B., Garzoni, L., & Bianchetti, M. G. (2012). Renal salt wasting syndrome in children with intracranial disorders. *Pediatric Nephrology, 27*(5), 733–739.

Briars, R. (2012). Diabetes ketoacidosis. In K. Reuter-Rice & B. Bolick (Eds.), *Pediatric acute care: A guide for interprofessional practice* (pp. 385–394). Burlington, MA: Jones & Bartlett Learning.

Buzby, M. (2012). Endocrine disorders: Physiology and diagnostics. In K. Reuter-Rice & B. Bolick (Eds.), *Pediatric acute care: A guide for interprofessional practice* (pp. 364–369). Burlington, MA: Jones & Bartlett Learning.

Eichler, V. (2012). Adrenal disorders. In K. Reuter-Rice & B. Bolick (Eds.), *Pediatric acute care: A guide for interprofessional practice* (pp. 369–376). Burlington, MA: Jones & Bartlett Learning.

Gallagher, M. P., & Oberfield, S. E. (2007). Disorders of pituitary function. In L. B. Zaoutis & V. W. Chiang (Eds.), *Comprehensive pediatric hospital medicine* (pp. 590–591). Philadelphia, PA: Mosby Elsevier.

Lynch, R. E., & Wood, E. G. (2011). Fluid and electrolyte issues in pediatric critical illness. In B. Fuhrman & J. Zimmerman (Eds.), *Pediatric critical care* (4th ed., pp. 944–962). Philadelphia, PA: Elsevier Saunders.

Olivieri, L., & Rose, C. (2013). Diabetic ketoacidosis in the pediatric emergency department. *Emergency Medicine Clinics of North America, 31*(3), 755–773.

Ranadive, S. A., & Rosenthal, S. M. (2011). Pediatric disorders of water balance. *Pediatric Clinics of North America, 58*(5), 1271–1280.

Simone, S. (2012). Diabetes insipidus, syndrome of inappropriate antidiuretic hormone, and cerebral salt wasting. In K. Reuter-Rice & B. Bolick (Eds.), *Pediatric acute care: A guide for interprofessional practice* (pp. 383–385). Burlington, MA: Jones & Bartlett Learning.

Von Saint Andre-von Arnim, A., Farris, R., Roberts, J. S., Yanay, O., Brogan, T. V., & Zimmerman, J. J. (2013). Common endocrine issues in the pediatric intensive care unit. *Critical Care Clinics, 29*(2), 335–358.

Waguespack, S. G. (2011). Adrenal tumors. In R. M. Kliegman (Ed.), *Nelson textbook of pediatrics* (19th ed., chap 500.5). Philadelphia, PA: Saunders Elsevier.

Wolfsdorf, J. I., Allgrove, J., Craig, M. E., Edge, J., Glaser, N., Jain, V., . . . Hanas, R. (2014). Diabetic ketoacidosis and hyperglycemic hyperosmolar state. *Pediatric Diabetes, 15*, 154–179.

Yee, A. H., Burns, J. D., & Wijdicks, E. F. (2010). Cerebral salt wasting: Pathophysiology, diagnosis and treatment. *Neurosurgical Clinics of North America, 21*(2), 339–352.

Fluid and Electrolytes

General Principles
Cathy Haut

- Fluid management is an important part of the care of hospitalized children.
- As much as 70% of lean body mass in infants is water.
- Children, in general, have approximately 60% of lean body mass as water and an overall higher concentration of extracellular fluid than adults.
- Daily maintenance fluids for healthy children include fluid for physiologic needs, daily output, and insensible losses.
- Dehydration is a concern for morbidity and mortality in children <5 years of age.
- Gastroenteritis is responsible for 200,000 hospitalizations per year for children with resulting dehydration.
- There is a known, although not thoroughly precise, relationship between caloric expenditure, fluid requirements, and body weight.

Calculating Maintenance Fluid Requirements

- H_2O is generated in the process of metabolism.
  - Heat regulation requires H_2O.
  - Solute excretion requires H_2O.
  - Metabolic rate is related to body surface area (BSA) and to weight.
  - Metabolic rate (kcals/day) approximates fluid requirement (mL/day).

Box 8.1 Holliday-Segar Method

Weight:

2–10 kg: 100 mL/kg.

11–20 kg: 1,000 mL + 50 mL/kg for each kg between 11 and 20 kg.

21–70 kg: 1,500 mL + 20 mL/kg for each kg between 21 and 70 kg.

Calculate the total volume for 24 hours and then divide by 24 to reach the hourly intravenous fluid rate.

- The Holliday-Segar method is commonly used to calculate maintenance fluid requirements for a 24-hour period in children.
- 4-2-1 Method: An additional method of calculating maintenance fluid requirements. This provides the *hourly* calculated rate rather than a volume for a 24-hour period.

Box 8.2 4-2-1 Method

For the first 10 kg of body weight: 4 mL of fluid is administered per kg (e.g., 4-kg patient. 5 kg × 4 mL = 20 mL/hour);

For the second 10 kg (e.g., 11–19 kg), 2 mL/kg is administered; *and*

Each additional kg over 20 kg, 1 mL/hour should be given.

(e.g., 25-kg patient. 40 mL [first 10 kg] + 20 mL [2nd 10 kg] + 5 mL [each kg over 20 kg] = 65 mL/hour).

- BSA calculation.
  - Use a nomogram to find BSA in meters squared (m^2). The patient's height and weight are needed for nomogram.
  - Or, to calculate the BSA using height and weight:

Box 8.3 BSA Calculation

$$BSA = \sqrt{Weight\ (kg) \times Height\ (cm)/3600}$$

Maintenance fluids calculation using BSA = 1,500–2,000 mL/m^2/day.

Evaluation of Hydration
Cathy Haut

Background/Definition

- Hydration refers to the proper balance between water and electrolytes.

Box 8.4 Conditions Resulting in Alterations in Maintenance Fluid Requirement

Fever

Tachypnea, hyperpnea

Postoperative state

Increased physical activity

Diarrheal illness

Altered kidney function (e.g., anuria, polyuria)

Very low-birth-weight infants: decreased skin integrity, increased surface area to weight ratio

Burns

Trauma

Excessive sweating

Endocrine disorders (e.g., syndrome if inappropriate antidiuretic hormone, diabetes insipidus, hyperthyroidism)

- Fluid and electrolyte therapies require careful calculation with careful attention to detail.
- Dehydration can be estimated based on clinical status. In children, usually 3%, 6%, or 9%. In infants, observed as 5%, 10%, or 15%. Other evaluation methods describe dehydration as mild, moderate, or severe based on physical assessment.
- Moderate to severe dehydration can lead to hypovolemic shock. Treating hypovolemia and maintaining euvolemia are critical.

Pathophysiology

- Fluid and electrolytes are involved in the dehydration and rehydration process.
- Shifts from intracellular to extracellular spaces can explain changing laboratory values in many cases.
- Clinical features can assist in determining the level of dehydration or overhydration.
- Aldosterone is released in response to the renin–angiotensin–aldosterone release in cases of extracellular volume depletion.
- Antidiuretic hormone (ADH) is released in response to volume depletion, which results in decreased urine output and increased absorption of water by the kidneys.

Clinical Presentation

- It is most important to evaluate the child's history to determine and treat the etiology of fluid loss as early as possible.
- There are characteristic findings associated with both dehydration and overhydration.
- Dehydration is more common in young children and has classic components on physical examination, which are assessed based on percentage of hydration: mild, moderate, or severe.
  - Assessment of dehydration includes parameters of mental status, heart rate, presence of tears, skin condition, capillary refill, blood pressure, and urine output.
- Hydration can be classified based on serum sodium levels (Table 8.1).

TABLE 8.1 Classification of Dehydration

Determined by Serum Sodium Concentration (mEq/L)	
Isotonic	130–150
Hypotonic/Hyponatremic	<130
Hypertonic/Hypernatremic	>150

Goals of Dehydration Fluid Therapy

- Restore circulating volume to prevent or treat shock using fluid boluses 20 mL/kg of crystalloid fluid until improvement in circulation, urine output, and capillary refill time.
- Some underlying medical conditions (e.g., kidney disease, cardiac disease) require exquisite care and evaluation during fluid resuscitation to prevent fluid overload and subsequent decompensation.
- Restore intracellular and extracellular water and electrolyte deficits within 24 hours in hyponatremic and isonatremic dehydration; restore over 48 hours in hypernatremic dehydration.
- Replace ongoing losses, as appropriate.
- Correct acid–base imbalances; may be achieved solely through treating the underlying cause.

Evaluation of Overhydration

- Children can experience overhydration or water intoxication through processes that correct hyponatremia too quickly or by administering intravenous (IV) fluids including plain D5W or other hypotonic solutions.
- Infants can develop hyponatremia from incorrect mixing of formula with too much water.
- Overhydration can occur as a result of other pathologic problems, including nephrotic syndrome and syndrome of inappropriate antidiuretic hormone (SIADH).
- Children are vulnerable to cerebral edema through correcting hyponatremia too quickly.

Calculating Fluid Deficit

- Methods of calculating fluid deficit.
  - Determine clinical/physical features that represent % dehydration.
  - Current weight × 1,000 × % dehydration = volume of fluid to replace.
  - The most precise method of determining fluid deficit is weight loss, but it is not typical to have recent pre-illness weight results.

Box 8.5 Fluid-Deficit Calculation Example

Fluid deficit = Pre-illness weight − Illness weight.

% Dehydration = (Pre-illness weight − Illness weight)/ Illness weight × 100%.

Once the fluid deficit is calculated, subtract any fluid bolus before determining the hourly rate.

TABLE 8.2   Oral Rehydration Fluids

Type of Fluid	Na (mEq/L)	K (mEq/L)	Glucose (mEq/L)	Base/Bicarbonate (mEq/L)	Osmolarity
World Health Organization ORT	90	20	2	30	310
Pedialyte	45	20	2.5	30	270
Ricelyte	50	25	3	34	290
Gatorade	20	3	4.6	3	330
Ginger Ale	3	1	5–15	4	540
Apple Juice	3	28	10–15	0	700
Tea	0	5	0	0	5

ORT, oral rehydration therapy

Fluid and Electrolyte Replacement

- Maintenance fluid calculation is addressed in the previous section.
- Calculation of fluid deficit can be accomplished in several ways:
  - Calculate percentage of weight loss, if known.
  - Estimate the percentage of fluid loss based on clinical evaluation.
  - Percentage of dehydration × Weight in kg × 10 = mL fluid needs.
- Replacement of fluid deficit can be accomplished either through oral rehydration therapy if shock is not present, or with IV fluids.
- Oral rehydration fluids should have goal of replacing deficit volume over 4 to 6 hours, then to replace ongoing losses (Table 8.2).

Intravenous Fluid Replacement

- See Table 8.3.

Isotonic and Hyponatremic Dehydration

- Replace half of the deficit plus one-third of the maintenance over 8 hours, then the remaining half of the deficit and two-third of the maintenance over the next 16 hours, or replace the whole deficit over 8 hours, then the whole day's maintenance over 16 hours.

Hypernatremic Dehydration

- Combine the total volume deficit plus the maintenance volume for 48 hours; administer this total volume divided over 48 hours. *Prevents osmotic fluid shifts resulting in cerebral edema and seizures.* Ensure serum sodium level is not corrected by >10 mEq/L/day.

TABLE 8.3   Intravenous Fluid Composition

Type of Fluid	Glucose (g/L)	Sodium (g/L)	Chloride (g/L)	Potassium (g/L)
Isotonic solutions:				
Normal saline (0.9)	0	154	154	0
Lactated Ringers	0	130	109	4
Albumin	0	100–160	<120	0
Other fluids:				
D5 ½ NS (D5 0.45 NS)	50	77	77	0
D5 ¼ NS (D5 0.2 NS)	50	38.5	38.5	0
½ NS	0	77	77	0
¼ NS	0	38.5	38.5	0
Hypertonic saline	0	513	513	0

Insensible Fluid Losses

- Fluid losses normally occurring through the skin, respiratory tract, and gastrointestinal (GI) tract.
- Losses through the kidney system are not insensible losses.

- In some conditions (e.g., diabetes insipidus (DI), kidney disease), calculation of insensible fluid losses may be used to determine appropriate fluid administration (e.g., replacing insensible losses and urine output or replacing insensible losses only).

Box 8.6 Insensible Fluid Loss Calculation

300 mL × BSA = approximated insensible losses for 24 hours.

Divide this amount by 24 to obtain the hourly rate of insensible loss replacement.

Box 8.7 Insensible Fluid Loss Calculation Example

A child with a BSA of 0.8 m^2.

300 mL × 0.8 = 240 mL of insensible losses per 24 hours, or a rate of 10 mL/hour.

Electrolyte Replacement

- Prescription for daily electrolytes:
  - Sodium: 2 to 3 mEq/100 mL of fluid.
  - Potassium: 2 mEq/100 mL of fluid.
  - Chloride: 5 to 6 mEq/100 mL of fluid.
- Replacement for electrolyte loss:
  - Sodium replacement: calculating the sodium deficit.
  - *Only correct sodium quickly to avoid compromise such as seizures.*

    Na deficit = (135 − measured Na) mEq/L × 100/L

  - It is difficult to accurately assess potassium deficit, as potassium is mainly intracellular and shifts based on catabolism, cell injury, and acid–base balance.
  - It is estimated that 1 mEq/L potassium loss = 10% to 30% total body potassium loss.

Specific Electrolyte Disorders

Jessica S. Farber

Electrolyte Imbalances: Calcium

Background

- Calcium is a component of multisystem body functions, including neuronal activity, muscular contraction, myocardial contraction, hemocoagulation, and bone formation.
- Calcium is present in three forms in plasma.
  - Bound to albumin (plasma protein).
  - Diffusible (such as calcium citrate or calcium phosphate).
  - Unbound ion.
- Ionized calcium is the form most important for body functions.
- Calcium concentration is regulated by renal, skeletal, and GI systems.

Definitions

- Hypocalcemia: serum calcium <9 mg/dL; ionized calcium <1.1 mmol/L.
- Hypercalcemia: serum calcium >10 mg/dL.

Etiology/Types

- Hypocalcemia.
  - Binding of ionized calcium to citrate after red cell transfusion, ethylene glycol ingestion, malabsorption, hypoparathyroidism, renal failure, rhabdomyolysis, sepsis, tumor lysis syndrome, and pancreatitis.
  - DiGeorge syndrome, malnutrition, certain medications such as furosemide.
  - Electrolyte abnormalities of hyperphosphatemia and hypomagnesemia.
- Hypercalcemia.
  - Williams syndrome.
  - Excessive intake, excessive vitamins A and D intake, hyperparathyroidism, immobility, malignancy, sarcoidosis, and thiazide diuretics.

Pathophysiology

- Calcium regulation.
  - Regulation via GI, renal, and bone.
  - Primary regulation by parathyroid hormone (PTH).
  - PTH promotes calcium absorption from the bone and decreases renal excretion of calcium.
  - PTH mediates the process of conversion of vitamin D to active form, thus increasing intestinal absorption of calcium.
  - Risk of hypocalcemia in neonates is increased due to decreased calcium intake, increased fetal calcium levels leading to transient parathyroid suppression, and PTH resistance.

Clinical Presentation

- Hypocalcemia.
  - Can include neuromuscular irritability, Chvostek sign, confusion, irritability, laryngospasm, muscle cramps, numbness and tingling, paresthesias and weakness, seizures, tetany, and Trousseau sign.
  - ECG changes include sinus tachycardia, long QT interval, and AV blocks.
  - Evidence of myocardial irritability with severe hypocalcemia can include hypotension and bradycardia.
- Hypercalcemia.
  - Can be asymptomatic.
  - Severe hypercalcemia is indicated by GI signs of nausea, anorexia, constipation, neurologic signs such as anxiety, depression, headache, lethargy, hypotonia, seizures, and coma. Cardiac arrhythmias include shortened QT interval, sinus bradycardia, first-degree heart block, and ventricular tachycardia.
  - Hypercalcemia can result in polyuria, renal calculi, and renal tubular dysfunction.

Diagnostic Evaluation

- Hypocalcemia.

- Serum laboratory analysis should include total serum calcium, ionized calcium, and complete metabolic panel, PTH, pH, and 25-hydroxy vitamin D and 1,25–dihydroxy vitamin D.
- Urine calcium, phosphate, and creatinine.
- Radiographs of ankle and wrist for bone density.
- Chest radiograph for evaluation of presence of thymus.
- ECG.
- Hypercalcemia.
  - Serum laboratory analysis should include total serum calcium, ionized calcium, complete metabolic panel, PTH, pH, 25-hydroxy vitamin D and 1,25–dihydroxy vitamin D, and urine electrolytes. PTH-related protein level if suspected malignancy and fluorescence in situ hybridization probe for Williams syndrome.
  - ECG.
  - Abdominal radiography (kidneys, ureters, and bladder [KUB]) or renal ultrasound to evaluate for renal calculi.

Management

- Hypocalcemia.
  - Symptomatic hypocalcemia, acute repletion:
    - Parenteral calcium replacement:
      - Calcium chloride (10–20 mg/kg/dose) given through central venous catheter only.
      - Calcium gluconate (100 mg/kg/dose) given through either peripheral or central venous catheter.
    - Chronic hypocalcemia, subacute or chronic repletion:
      - Enteral supplements such as calcium carbonate, citrate, calcium gluconate, glubionate, lactate, along with vitamin D supplements and 1,25-dihydroxy vitamin D for patients unable to convert vitamin D.
- Hypercalcemia.
  - Identification and treatment of underlying disease.
  - Hydration with normal saline (NS) (often 2–3 times maintenance rate).
    - Hypercalcemia may cause increased urinary output, resulting in dehydration.
    - Increased urinary sodium excretion enhances calcium excretion.
  - Diuresis with loop diuretics, which aids in calcium excretion.
    - Avoid thiazide diuretics that reduce calcium excretion in urine.
  - Glucocorticoids—reduce effects and level of vitamin D.
  - Only calcitonin for rapid correction of calcium or if hypercalcemia is refractory to hydration and diuresis.
  - Bisphosphonates for rapid treatment of severe hyperphosphatemia, in consultation with endocrinologist.
  - If severe or refractory, hemodialysis may be indicated.

PEARLS

- *Ionized calcium should be interpreted in relation to serum pH.*
- *Hypomagnesemia may lead to hypocalcemia.*
- *If hypocalcemia is refractory, replace magnesium.*
- *Correct severe hyperphosphatemia prior to correction of related hypocalcemia to avoid soft tissue calcification.*

Electrolyte Imbalances: Chloride

Background

- The major role of chloride is to maintain electrical neutrality by balancing cations (usually sodium) in the blood.
- Functions as a regulator of acid–base balance in the body due to inverse relationship with bicarbonate.

Definitions

- Hypochloremia: serum chloride <97 mmol/L.
- Hyperchloremia: serum chloride >108 mmol/L.

Etiology/Types

- Hypochloremia is associated with:
  - Bartter syndrome.
  - Cystic fibrosis.
  - Bulimia nervosa.
  - Diuretic usage.
  - Removal of gastric secretions by nasogastric tube.
  - Permissive hypercapnia.
  - Metabolic alkalosis contributes to hypochloremia.
- Hyperchloremia: associated with:
  - Diarrhea.
  - Excessive chloride administration.
  - Metabolic acidosis.
  - Renal tubular acidosis (RTA).
  - Urinary diversion into the colon or ileum.

Pathophysiology

- Chloride regulation is by renal and GI mechanisms.
- Indirectly affected by aldosterone, as it passively follows renal sodium reabsorption.
- Passively follows sodium absorption in GI tract.
- Actively absorbed in the presence of bicarbonate excretion in intestine.
- Hydrochloric acid represents active secretion of chloride by stomach.

Clinical Presentation

- Hypochloremia.
  - Rarely occurs as sole electrolyte abnormality.
  - When associated with metabolic alkalosis, may exhibit arrhythmias, decreased respiratory effort, seizures in severe states.
  - When associated with volume depletion or dehydration, may exhibit thirst, lethargy, tachycardia, tachypnea, and delayed capillary refill.
  - Hypocalcemia, due to increased binding of calcium to albumin.
- Hyperchloremia.
  - Often does not result in any symptoms.
  - May exhibit Kussmaul respirations (especially in diabetes ketoacidosis); possible neurologic symptoms include lethargy, headache, and confusion.
  - Altered cardiac function and response to inotropes.
  - Associated with hypernatremia and hyperkalemia.

Diagnostic Evaluation

- Hypochloremia.
  - Serum electrolyte evaluation and serum pH.
  - Urine chloride and sodium.
- Hyperchloremia.
  - Laboratory studies will be based on determining the cause of hyperchloremia and associated acidosis.

Management

- Hypochloremia: First address known causes, including fluid resuscitation, and add potassium-sparing diuretics or acetazolamide to reduce reabsorption of bicarbonate.
  - Chloride repletion: can be replaced with sodium, potassium, and ammonium chloride compositions. Arginine chloride or hydrochloric acid can be used for severe hypochloremia-related seizures, arrhythmias, or respiratory depression.
- Hyperchloremia: Address underlying cause and treat associated acidosis.
  - Consider sodium bicarbonate IV if severe metabolic acidosis.

PEARLS

- *Chloride has a direct relationship with sodium (e.g., when sodium levels are elevated, chloride levels are elevated).*
- *Chloride has an inverse relationship with bicarbonate.*

Electrolyte Imbalances: Magnesium

Background

- Serum magnesium level is a poor indicator of total body magnesium level.
- About 50% of magnesium stores are contained in bone.
- Majority of remaining magnesium is in intracellular spaces or soft tissue.
- Less than 1% of total magnesium is extracellular.
- Magnesium is important for adenosine triphosphate (ATP) generation, DNA transcription, protein synthesis, membrane stabilization, regulation of potassium excretion, and is a cofactor for ion transport channels.
- Magnesium is absorbed in large part in the upper small intestine and is primarily excreted and regulated in the kidney. Excretion may be altered by diuretics, presence of hypercalcemia, pH, PTH, calcitonin, and vasopressin levels.

Definitions

- Hypomagnesemia: serum magnesium <1.7 mg/dL.
- Hypermagnesemia: serum magnesium >2.2 mg/dL.

Etiology

- Hypomagnesemia.
  - GI losses with diarrhea, vomiting, steatorrhea, refeeding syndrome, pancreatitis.
  - Celiac disease, cystic fibrosis, inflammatory bowel disease, and short gut syndrome.

- Renal: hypercalcemia, chemotherapy, chronic adrenergic stimulants, diuretic use, hypercalciuria, nephrocalcinosis, and RTA.
- Medications: amphotericin, cisplatin, loop and osmotic diuretics.
- Endocrine: diabetes mellitus, diabetic ketoacidosis (DKA), excessive bone uptake after parathyroidectomy, hyperaldosteronism, and PTH disorders.
- Bartter and Gitelman syndromes, autosomal dominant hypoparathyroidism, and mitochondrial hypomagnesemia.
- Hypermagnesemia.
  - Excessive intake, including magnesium-containing laxatives or antacids, total parenteral nutrition, maternal magnesium therapy in neonates.
  - Altered renal function, renal failure, tumor lysis syndrome, milk alkali syndrome, and lithium ingestion.

Pathophysiology

- Hypomagnesemia may result from altered absorption or excretion or from overhydration.
- Decreased sodium reabsorption with volume expansion, results in reduced magnesium reabsorption.
- Decreased magnesium intake with administration of non–magnesium-containing IV fluids.
- Neonates may experience transient hypomagnesemia or develop idiopathic hypomagnesemia, particularly in association with maternal magnesium depletion.

Clinical Presentation

- Hypomagnesemia.
  - GI: anorexia, nausea, and vomiting.
  - Neurologic: depression, malaise, nonspecific psychiatric symptoms, hyperreflexia, seizures, paresthesias, ataxia, tetany, decreased deep tendon reflexes, weakness, paralysis, muscle weakness, delirium, carpopedal spasm, and clonus.
  - Cardiac: ECG changes, atrial or ventricular ectopy, torsades de pointes, and long QT interval.
  - Endocrine: Hyperglycemia can occur if hypomagnesemia is related to insulin resistance.
- Hypermagnesemia.
  - Neurologic: impairment of the neuromuscular junction; hypotonia, decreased deep tendon reflexes, weakness, paralysis, CNS depression, lethargy, and confusion.
  - Cardiac: altered vascular tone, hypotension, flushing, possible ECG changes (prolonged PR, QRS, or QT intervals), heart block.
  - GI: abdominal cramping, nausea, and vomiting.
  - Respiratory failure can occur in severe cases.

Diagnostic Evaluation

- Hypomagnesemia: serum laboratory studies; basic metabolic panel with magnesium and ionized calcium; ECG and arrhythmia monitoring.
- Hypermagnesemia: serum laboratory studies; basic metabolic panel with magnesium and ionized calcium; ECG and arrhythmia monitoring.

Management

- Hypomagnesemia.
  - Severe, acute management.
    - Magnesium sulfate or magnesium chloride.
    - Consider potassium repletion, particularly if refractory.
  - Mild, subacute management.
    - Magnesium gluconate, oxide, or sulfate.
- Hypermagnesemia.
  - Cessation of magnesium intake.
  - Monitoring of renal function and support of cardiovascular and respiratory function.
  - Parenteral calcium supplements (calcium chloride or calcium gluconate) for heart block.
  - Removal of magnesium with volume expansion, forced diuresis, loop diuretics, dialysis if life-threatening or exchange transfusion if life-threatening and unable to perform dialysis.

PEARLS

- *Hypomagnesemia may result in refractory hypokalemia.*
- *A rapid increase in serum magnesium related to rapid bolus may result in increased magnesium excretion. Therefore, unless treating hypomagnesium-related seizures or arrhythmia, a slow infusion rate is preferred.*
- *If torsades de pointes rhythm noted on ECG, administer magnesium.*

Electrolyte Imbalances: Phosphorus

Jessica S. Farber

Background

- Phosphate shifts easily from intracellular to extracellular.
- Important functions in membrane structure, energy storage and transport, most metabolic processes, glycolysis, ATP, 2,3-diphosphoglycerate, creatine phosphokinase.
- Absorbed through jejunum.
- Excreted through kidneys.
- Approximately 12% of phosphorus is protein-bound.
- Levels vary with circadian rhythm and age.

Definitions

- Hypophosphatemia: serum phosphorus <2.5 mg/dL.
- Hyperphosphatemia: serum phosphorus >4.1 mg/dL.

Etiology/Types

- Hypophosphatemia.
  - Malnutrition or starvation situations such as protein energy malnutrition or malabsorption, respiratory or metabolic alkalosis.
  - DKA treatment without adequate repletion.
  - Corticosteroid use.
  - Renal tubular defects or diuretic use.
  - Vitamin D deficiency and vitamin D-resistant rickets.
  - Reduced intake/supplementation in very low-birth-weight infants.
  - Chronic use of aluminum-containing antacids.
  - Tumor-induced osteomalacia resulting in renal phosphorus wasting.
  - Extensive burns.
  - Hyperparathyroidism.
- Hyperphosphatemia.
  - Excessive administration or intake.
  - Tumor lysis syndrome.
  - Hypoparathyroidism.
  - Rhabdomyolysis.
  - Renal failure when decreased glomerular filtration rate <25% or smaller glomerular filtration rate reductions in neonates.

Pathophysiology

- Many of the clinical manifestations of phosphorus imbalances are related to either shifting (intracellular to extracellular) or the role of phosphorus in ATP, 2,3-diphosphoglycerate, and creatine phosphokinase.
- A sudden increase in serum phosphorus may result in precipitation of calcium, thus resulting in symptoms of hypocalcemia such as tetany.
- Chronic hyperphosphatemia may result in calcium precipitation or deposition in soft tissues.

Clinical Presentation

- Hypophosphatemia (level <1 mg/dL).
  - Neurologic signs of confusion, irritability, coma, muscle weakness, paresthesias, seizures, and apnea in very low-birth-weight infants.
  - Hemolytic anemia.
  - Hypoxia.
  - Impaired granulocyte activity.
  - Thrombocytopenia.
  - Rhabdomyolysis.
  - Myocardial depression.
  - Rickets.
- Hyperphosphatemia.
  - Altered mental status, seizures.
  - Tetany, weakness, paresthesias.
  - Fatigue.
  - Cramping.
  - Laryngospasm.
  - Neuromuscular irritability.
  - Cardiac arrhythmias.
  - Chronic hyperphosphatemia may result in calcium deposits in soft tissue.

Diagnostic Evaluation

- Hypophosphatemia.
  - Serum: basic metabolic panel, phosphorous, magnesium and ionized calcium, vitamin D levels, and PTH.
  - Urine: calcium, phosphorous, creatinine, pH.

- Hyperphosphatemia.
  - Serum: basic metabolic panel, ionized calcium, phosphorous and magnesium, PTH, vitamin D, complete blood count, and arterial blood gas.
  - Urine: calcium, phosphorous, creatinine.

Management

- Hypophosphatemia.
  - Acute.
    - Parenteral repletion is indicated with potassium or sodium phosphate.
  - Subacute or gradual onset of symptoms.
    - Replace with potassium or sodium phosphate enteral supplements.
    - Hyperphosphatemia: restrict dietary intake of phosphorus (protein restriction).
    - Phosphate binders which include sevelamer hydrochloride, lanthanum carbonate, calcium carbonate, or aluminum hydroxide.
    - If cell lysis with normal renal function, forced diuresis with NS and osmotic diuretic such as mannitol.
    - Consider dialysis if severe and underlying poor renal function; dialysis may be of limited effectiveness.

PEARL

- *Risk of calcium–phosphorus precipitation, particularly with tumor lysis syndrome or renal failure.*

Electrolyte Imbalances: Potassium

Jessica S. Farber

Background

- Primarily found in intracellular space; excretion and regulation through kidneys.
- Balance between intracellular and extracellular potassium concentration regulated by several mechanisms:
  - Insulin and β-adrenergic catecholamines produce an intracellular shift.
  - α-Adrenergic catecholamines produce extracellular potassium shift.
  - Aldosterone is important in potassium regulation by the kidney.
  - PTH causes a decrease in intracellular potassium; however, exerts a mild effect.
  - Mineralocorticoids result in mild reduction in potassium levels.

Definitions

- Hypokalemia: serum potassium <3.7 mEq/L.
- Hyperkalemia: serum potassium >5.2 mEq/L.

Etiology

- Hypokalemia.
  - Medications: amphotericin B, decongestants, diuretics, dopamine, dobutamine, and bronchodilators.

- Anorexia nervosa.
- Bartter and Cushing syndromes.
- Fanconi, Liddle, and Gitelman syndromes.
- Hematologic: leukemia.
- GI: diarrhea, use of laxatives and enemas, and vomiting.
- Endocrine causes: DKA, hyperaldosteronism, increased insulin levels, and excess mineralocorticoid.
- Renal: increased renin levels, renovascular disease, metabolic alkalosis, and type I RTA.
- Magnesium depletion and malnutrition.
- Hyperkalemia.
  - Acidosis, acute increase in serum osmolarity.
  - Addison disease, aldosterone insensitivity, hypoaldosteronism, pseudohypoaldosteronism, and associated aldosterone resistance.
  - Medications: angiotensin II receptor blockers, ACE inhibitors, theophylline, and nonsteroidal anti-inflammatory drugs.
  - Congenital adrenal hyperplasia.
  - Trauma: crush injury.
  - Excess supplementation.
  - Rhabdomyolysis.
  - Tumor lysis syndrome.
  - Renal impairment or RTA.
  - Spitzer–Weinstein syndrome.
  - Technical problems in obtaining a blood sample can result in hyperkalemia if the blood is hemolyzed, if there is existing thrombocytosis, or leukocytosis at the time of serum sample, or if the child has received blood that has been stored for a long time.

Pathophysiology

- Potassium homeostasis is influenced by pH and osmolarity.
  - Increased osmolarity results in an extracellular shift of potassium and water.
  - Acidosis may result in a significant extracellular shift in potassium; however, the level may vary based on the nature of the acidosis (hyperkalemia).
  - Conversely, alkalosis produces a reduction in extracellular potassium (hypokalemia).

Clinical Presentation

- Hypokalemia.
  - Often, no symptoms.
  - Diastolic dysfunction, hypertension, or ventricular arrhythmias in patients with heart disease, heart failure, or left ventricular hypertrophy.
  - ECG changes can include delayed depolarization, flat or absent T waves, long QT, prolonged QRS, ST changes, and the presence of U waves.
  - Cramping.
  - Decreased perfusion.
  - Fatigue.
  - Ileus.
  - Impaired insulin release.

- Impaired muscle contraction, paralysis.
- Polyuria.
- Hyperkalemia.
  - ECG changes: most commonly peaked T waves, low-voltage P waves, prolonged PR and QRS interval, ST changes, AV block, ventricular tachycardia and fibrillation, loss of PR interval, merging of QRS, and T waves to produce a sine wave pattern, asystole.
  - Neurologic: muscle weakness, paresthesias, and tetany with severe hyperkalemia (≥9 mEq/L).

Diagnostic Evaluation

- Hypokalemia.
  - Serum: basic metabolic panel with magnesium, creatine kinase, renin, pH, and cortisol levels.
  - Urine studies: urinalysis, electrolytes, osmolality, and urine 17-ketosteroids.
  - ECG.
- Hyperkalemia.
  - Serum: basic metabolic panel with magnesium, creatine kinase, renin, pH, and cortisol levels.
  - Urine studies: urinalysis, electrolytes, osmolality, and urine 17-ketosteroids.
  - ECG.

Management

- Hypokalemia.
  - Identification of cause.
  - Potassium repletion.
  - Acute, risk for arrhythmia.
    - Calculate electrolyte deficiency to minimize risk of hyperkalemia with treatment.
    - Potassium chloride 0.5 to 1 mEq/kg/dose IV; maximum 20 mEq/dose; central administration is preferred and cardiac monitoring required.
  - Subacute, chronic repletion.
    - Potassium chloride, phosphate, or bicarbonate enteral supplement, based on etiology.
- Hyperkalemia.
  - Evaluate for accuracy of the laboratory sample (may be falsely elevated with hemolysis, thrombocytosis, or leukocytosis).
  - Remove all exogenous potassium sources.
  - Hyperkalemia with ECG changes.
    - Administer calcium chloride or calcium gluconate IV for membrane stabilization.
    - Administer IV insulin and glucose (e.g., D25 or D50), IV sodium bicarbonate, inhaled β-agonists (e.g., albuterol); all temporarily shifts potassium intracellularly.
    - Diuretics, if normal renal function (results in potassium removal).
    - Cation exchange resin, such as sodium polystyrene sulfonate (exchanges potassium for sodium in the GI tract, resulting in potassium removal).
    - Hemodialysis, if refractory to conventional therapy or with renal failure.

PEARLS
- *Potassium should be interpreted in relation to serum pH as it shifts intracellularly with alkalosis and extracellularly with acidosis.*
- *Severe hyperkalemia (potassium level >7 mEq/L) is a medical emergency.*

Electrolyte Imbalances: Sodium

Jessica S. Farber

Background

- Sodium has significant roles in the maintenance of intravascular and interstitial volumes.
- Sodium is integral to skeletal muscle function, nerve and myocardial action potentials, acid–base balance.
- The regulation of sodium intake is not well developed in children.

Definitions

- Hyponatremia: serum sodium <135 mEq/L.
- Hypernatremia: serum sodium >145 mEq/L.

Etiology/Types

- Hyponatremia: hypervolemic, euvolemic, or hypovolemic.
  - Hypervolemic.
    - Congestive heart failure.
    - Renal failure.
    - Nephrotic syndrome.
    - Water intoxication.
    - Cirrhosis.
  - Hypovolemic.
    - Renal losses through osmotic diuresis or RTA.
    - Extrarenal losses through diarrhea, vomiting, burns, or pancreatitis.
  - Normovolemic: SIADH, adrenal insufficiency.
    - CNS diseases: cerebral salt wasting, meningitis, intracranial tumors.
    - Pulmonary disease: cystic fibrosis.
    - Diuretic use.
- Hyponatremia.
  - May be characterized by a comparison of pre-illness weight to current weight.
  - Decreased weight.
    - Renal losses: sodium-losing enteropathy, diuretics, adrenal insufficiency, and cerebral salt wasting.
    - Extrarenal losses: GI losses, skin losses, tissue third spacing, and cystic fibrosis.
    - Increased weight or normal weight: nephrotic syndrome, congestive heart failure, SIADH, renal failure, water intoxication, cirrhosis, excess salt-poor infusions.
- Hypernatremia.
  - May be hypervolemic, euvolemic, or hypovolemic.

- Excessive sodium intake: inappropriately concentrated formula, use of sodium supplements, sodium bicarbonate administration.
- Excessive free-water loss: breast-feeding failure without supplementation, diarrhea, DI, renal tubular disorders, and postobstructive diuresis.
- May be characterized by a comparison of pre-illness weight to current weight.
  - Decreased weight.
    - Renal losses: nephropathy, use of diuretics, DI, postobstructive diuresis, acute tubular necrosis diuretic phase.
    - Extrarenal losses: GI, skin, or free-water loss from respiratory system.
  - Increased weight.
    - Exogenous sodium administration.
    - Mineralocorticoid excess.
    - Hyperaldosteronism.

Pathophysiology

- Changes in serum sodium, fluid balance, and serum osmolality often occur simultaneously.
- Fluctuations in serum sodium are typically attributed to water reabsorption.
  - Excess water intake and altered urinary diluting capacity produce hyponatremia; inadequate water intake and poor urinary concentration produce hypernatremia.
- Sodium absorption occurs through the GI tract, primarily through the jejunum.
- Sodium- and potassium-activated ATP transport mechanism facilitates sodium absorption.
- ATP-facilitated sodium absorption is influenced by aldosterone or desoxycorticosterone acetate.
- Sodium excretion via sweat, stool, and urine: 99% of sodium is reabsorbed in the renal tubule and 1% excreted in urine.
- Sodium levels are maintained because the percentages of filtered sodium and water reabsorption are proportional based on extracellular fluid volume.
- Renal regulation of sodium: Based on a balance of glomerular and tubular functions in association with osmoreceptors in the hypothalamus that regulates secretion of ADH and vasopressin.

Clinical Presentation

- Hyponatremia.
  - Acute hyponatremia.
    - Rapid decrease in serum sodium level is associated with more severe symptoms.
    - Irritability, poor feeding, nausea, lethargy, seizures, coma, seizures.
    - Can lead to cerebral edema.
- Hypernatremia.
  - Acute hypernatremia.
    - Weakness, lethargy, decreased deep tendon reflexes, fever, high-pitched cry, irritability, muscle cramps, rhabdomyolysis, renal failure, respiratory failure, altered mental status, seizures.

Diagnostic Evaluation

- Hyponatremia.
  - Serum: sodium and osmolality.
  - Urine: sodium, specific gravity, and osmolality.
- Hypernatremia.
  - Serum: sodium and osmolality.
  - Urine: sodium, specific gravity, and osmolality.

Management

- Hyponatremia.
  - Identify and treat cause of hyponatremia.
  - Restore normal intravascular volume.
  - Replete sodium deficit.
    - Serum sodium correction must be done in a slow, controlled manner to avoid central pontine myelinolysis.
      - *Goal rate of sodium rise is 2 to 4 mEq/L every 4 hours or 10 to 20 mEq/L in 24 hours.*
  - If seizures are present, goal is to raise serum sodium acutely to 125 mEq/L for seizure cessation.
    - Hypertonic saline solution; NS bolus 20 mL/kg may be administered if hypertonic saline is not available.
    - Hypertonic saline is calculated based on this formula: mEq sodium to raise sodium to desired level.
      - $0.6 \times$ (Weight in kg) $\times$ (target sodium − measured sodium).
- Hypernatremia.
  - Avoid decreasing serum sodium more than 15 mEq/L in 24 hours to minimize risk for cerebral edema or no faster than 0.5 to 1.0 mEq/L/hour.
  - Therapy is guided by a combination of sodium level and serum osmolarity, and intravascular volume status.
  - Hypernatremic, hypovolemic dehydration.
    - Calculation of free-water deficit, solute fluid deficit, solute sodium deficit, solute potassium deficit, maintenance fluid requirements, and ongoing losses determines composition of IV fluids and rate of administration.
  - Hypernatremic, hypervolemic dehydration.
    - May require natriuretic agent for increased weight.

PEARLS

- *Reported sodium concentration may be low in association with hyperlipidemia, hyperproteinemia, or hyperglycemia.*
- *Thirst is a protective mechanism for hypernatremia and hypovolemic dehydration. Infants, small children, those with developmental delay, altered level of consciousness, or critical illness may not be able to respond to their intrinsic thirst mechanism and thus are at increased risk for hypernatremia and associated hypovolemic dehydration.*
- *A serum sodium level of <125 mEq/L places a child at high risk for seizure activity (Table 8.4).*

TABLE 8.4 **Summary of Key Features of Electrolyte Disturbances**

Critical Electrolyte Disturbance	Critical Results
Hyperkalemia	Peaked T waves on ECG
Hypokalemia	Ventricular arrhythmias, prominent U waves, ST segment depression
Hyponatremia Hypernatremia Hypophosphatemia Hypochloremia Hypocalcemia Hypercalcemia	Seizures
Hypomagnesemia	Ventricular ectopy, torsades de pointes
Hypermagnesemia	Hypotension, AV block
Hypocalcemia	Long QT interval, AV block

Acid-Base/Osmolar Gap Disorders

Please find information on acid–base disorders in Sections 7 (Endocrinology), 13 (Toxicology), and 16 (Kidney and Genitourinary Disorders).

Eating Disorders: Anorexia Nervosa and Bulimia Nervosa

Jessica S. Farber

Background

- Both anorexia nervosa and bulimia nervosa are characterized by a restriction of calories.
- Binge eating in bulimia nervosa is likely a result of hunger.
- May include calorie restriction, purging, and/or excessive exercise; often characterized by an obsession or preoccupation with food.

Definitions

- Anorexia nervosa.
  - Refusal to maintain normal body weight for age and height: generally body weight <85% expected.
  - Fear of weight gain or becoming "fat" despite being underweight.
  - Body image disturbance.
  - Primary or secondary amenorrhea in postmenarchal females.
- Bulimia nervosa.
  - Recurrent episodes of binge eating characterized by inability to control eating during episodes.

- Recurrent behaviors in an effort to avoid weight gain, including induced vomiting, abuse of laxatives, diuretics, fasting, excessive exercise.
- Self-evaluation that is abnormally influenced by body shape and weight.

Pathophysiology

- Weight loss is often associated with a desire to further reduce weight and leads to an inability to modulate emotions.
- Associated electrolyte abnormalities; chloride-responsive metabolic alkalosis and significant hypophosphatemia.
- Intravascular volume depletion or shock.
- Risk for cardiac arrhythmias due to electrolyte abnormalities: depletion of total body potassium, hypomagnesemia, serum hypophosphatemia, and altered acid–base balance.
- Bone marrow failure may develop.

Clinical Presentation

- Patients with anorexia nervosa and bulimia nervosa both can have:
  - Emaciated body habitus, cachectic appearance, decreased body temperature, bradycardia, hypotension, acrocyanosis, edema, dry skin with discoloration, cold extremities, scalp hair loss, increased lanugo, decreased deep tendon reflexes, arrhythmias, evidence of dehydration, and/or shock.
- Patients with bulimia nervosa may be of normal weight and body habitus with enlarged parotid glands or tonsils, erosion of tooth enamel, superficial ulceration, calluses, or scarring on dorsum of fingers, decreased or absent gag reflex, and swelling of hands and feet related to hypoalbuminemia.
- Subjective complaints include fatigue, muscle weakness, cramps, abdominal pain, constipation, headache, chest pain, palpitations, easy bruising, sore throat, sleep disturbances, difficulty concentrating, increased physical activity, dizziness, fainting.

Diagnostic Evaluation

- Evaluation of degree of malnutrition: serum complete metabolic panel, carotene levels, zinc, copper, prealbumin, amylase and lipase, cholesterol, and liver function tests.
- Endocrine evaluation: thyroid function tests, estradiol levels.
- Urinalysis: urine electrolytes.
- ECG.
- Evaluation for possible malignancy, inflammatory bowel disease, malabsorption syndrome such as celiac disease, diabetes mellitus, hyperthyroidism, hypopituitarism, or other chronic disease as appropriate based on history and clinical findings.

Management

- Medical stabilization: correct intravascular volume depletion and normalize electrolytes.
  - Reverse hypotension, tachycardia.
- Referral for psychiatric evaluation and therapy: developmental history, family history, medical history, and history of present illness.
- Elicit history of anxiety, difficulty with separation from parents, peer relationships.

- *Patients with bulimia nervosa may appear of normal or increased weight and may not appear grossly malnourished.*

Review of General Principles: Laboratory Studies in Fluid and Electrolyte Evaluation

- A basic metabolic panel or comprehensive metabolic panel.
  - Serves as the primary chemistry laboratory analysis for fluid and electrolyte evaluation.
  - Results of other laboratory studies can support assessment of fluid status.
- Serum electrolytes (basic metabolic panel).
  - BUN can indicate dehydration but is not predictive alone.
  - Serum bicarbonate levels of <17 mEq/L along with clinical findings of dehydration may identify children with moderate to severe dehydration.
  - Serum bicarbonate levels of <13 mEq/L typically are associated with high risk of failure of oral rehydration therapy.
  - Normal sodium levels range from 135 to 145 mEq/L, chloride levels range from 98 to 108 mEq/L, and potassium from 3.5 to 4.5 mEq/L.

- Comprehensive metabolic panel.
  - Typically consists of electrolytes, including sodium, potassium, chloride, carbon dioxide, BUN, creatinine, magnesium, phosphorous; liver function tests, including AST (aspartate aminotransferase) or SGOT (serum glutamic-oxaloacetic transaminase) and ALT (alanine aminotransferase) or SGPT (serum glutamic–pyruvic transaminase), which are liver enzyme levels; bilirubin level, serum total protein, and alkaline phosphatase.
- Blood gas values: pH of less than 7.35 with normal Pco_2 and normal or low bicarbonate may indicate dehydration.
- Urinalysis: dark color, high specific gravity, and presence of ketones can indicate dehydration.
- Urine electrolytes: If urine sodium is low, kidneys may be conserving sodium due to dehydration.
- Fractional excretion of sodium: A comparison between the amounts of sodium and creatinine in the blood compared to the urine. It assists in differentiating between dehydration and poor kidney function.
- Urine and serum osmolarity: Urine and serum osmolarity are elevated in dehydration.
- Complete blood count: Elevated red blood cell count, white blood cell count, or both, along with clinical findings, can assist in identifying dehydration.

1. A high school football player presents with hyperthermia and dehydration. Which one of the following findings is associated with hypokalemia in this athlete?
   a. Enhanced diastolic function.
   b. Peaked T waves.
   c. Atrial arrhythmias.
   d. Muscle weakness/fatigue.

Answer: **D**

Muscle weakness and fatigue are associated with hypokalemia, which can occur for a variety of reasons and often result from fluid shifts. Ventricular arrhythmias, flattened T waves, and decreased diastolic function are also found in patients with hypokalemia. Peaked T waves typically occur with hyperkalemia.

2. A 30-kg child has had repair of a congenital heart lesion, with poor cardiac function, and currently a potassium level of 2.2 mEq/L. Cardiac monitor indicates intermittent premature ventricular contractions. What is the most appropriate choice for potassium replacement?
   a. Potassium chloride 30 mEq (1 mEq/kg) over 1 hour.
   b. Potassium chloride 20 mEq (0.67 mEq/kg) over 90 minutes.
   c. Potassium phosphate 2.4 mmol (0.08 mmol/kg) over 4 to 6 hours.
   d. Potassium phosphate 2.4 mmol (0.08 mmol/kg) over 1 hour.

Answer: **B**

A potassium level of less than 3 mEq/L in a child with underlying cardiac disorder requires urgent treatment. The recommended dose of potassium chloride is 0.5 to 1 mEq/kg/dose, not to exceed 20 mEq per dose at a rate of 0.5 mEq/kg/hour. Potassium phosphate must be administered over 4 to 6 hours and is used primarily for phosphorus supplementation.

3. Initial treatment of hyperkalemia with ECG changes includes which one of the following?
   a. Magnesium sulfate 25 mg/kg.
   b. Magnesium sulfate 50 mg/kg.
   c. Calcium chloride 10 mg/kg.
   d. Calcium gluconate 25 mg/kg.

Answer: **C**

Hyperkalemia and associated ECG changes should be considered a life-threatening emergency and treated immediately. Calcium chloride 10 mg/kg by central venous catheter or calcium gluconate 100 mg/kg by peripheral IV should be administered to stabilize the myocardium until additional therapy can be administered which will shift potassium intracellular and remove from circulation. Magnesium sulfate is not indicated in the therapy for hypokalemia.

4. Which one of the following is a finding in a child with hypophosphatemia?
   a. Thrombocytosis.
   b. Tetany.
   c. Laryngospasm.
   d. Muscle weakness.

Answer: **D**

Critically low phosphorus levels (<1 mg/dL) can result in symptoms that include muscle weakness including respiratory muscle function. Hypophosphatemia may be associated with thrombocytopenia, not thrombocytosis. Laryngospasm and tetany may be symptoms of hyperphosphatemia.

5. The acute treatment of clinically significant hypophosphatemia includes which one of the following in a patient with normal renal function and a serum potassium level of 2.8 mEq/L and serum sodium level of 140 mEq/L?
   a. IV potassium phosphate infused over 4 to 6 hours.
   b. IV sodium phosphate infused over 1 hour.
   c. IV potassium phosphate infused over 20 to 30 minutes.
   d. Enteral phosphorus supplement.

Answer: **A**

The appropriate type of phosphorous supplement is often based on the child's current potassium level. Potassium phosphate should be administered slowly, as rapid infusion may result in renal failure, hypocalcemic tetany, hyperphosphatemia, and ECG changes. Oral supplements are indicated for mild or chronic hypophosphatemia.

6. A 12-month-old child has had diarrhea for 6 days and has lost 1.5 lb since his last visit 3 weeks prior. He has tears, has had two wet diapers in the past 5 hours, and is taking sips of water and milk. What is the first step in his management?
   a. Determining level of dehydration by clinical assessment.
   b. Obtaining serum electrolytes and urine for specific gravity.
   c. Administering an IV fluid bolus of 20 mL/kg of isotonic solution.
   d. Observing his ability to take oral fluids.

Answer: **A**

The first step in managing a child who may be dehydrated is to determine his clinical level of hydration which includes obtaining vital signs, noting condition of mucous membranes, urine output, and weight among other clinical criteria.

(continues on page 244)

7. Which one of the following situations/conditions can be the rationale for hypermagnesemia in the acutely ill child?
   a. Hepatic failure and associated bleeding.
   b. Renal failure, excessive magnesium intake/supplementation, tumor lysis syndrome.
   c. Decreased calcium and potassium intake.
   d. Hypoalbuminemia, hyponatremia, and hypoglycemia.

Answer: **B**

Renal failure may cause a mild elevation in serum magnesium due to altered renal excretion. Excessive magnesium intake or repletion is also a common cause in the hospitalized child. Tumor lysis syndrome may also be associated with hypermagnesemia.

8. Calculate the hourly rate of IV fluid infusion for a 4-year-old who weighs 44 lb and requires maintenance fluid therapy.
   a. 30 mL/hour.
   b. 44 mL/hour.
   c. 62.5 mL/hour.
   d. 88 mL/hour.

Answer: **C**

When calculating fluid therapy for a child, the weight is noted in kilograms, which for this 44-lb child would be 20 kg. The first 10 kg is calculated at 10 mL/kg or 1,000 mL/day. The second 10 kg is calculated at 5 mL/kg or 500 mL, to equal a total of 1,500 mL over 24 hours. The 1,500 mL divided by 24 hours of therapy equals 62.5 mL/hour of IV fluids.

9. The treatment of DKA may result in hypomagnesemia because:
   a. Osmotic diuresis leads to depletion of total body magnesium stores.
   b. Treatment with insulin suppresses uptake of magnesium by the cells.
   c. Fluids are restricted in DKA, causing increased magnesium excretion.
   d. Acidosis causes shifting of magnesium into the cells and therefore eliminates urinary excretion.

Answer: **A**

Osmotic diuresis leads to depletion of total body magnesium stores. Treatment with insulin actually stimulates cellular uptake of magnesium, which leads to hypomagnesemia. Fluids are not restricted in DKA; rather, patients receive replacement of losses.

10. Which of the following are possible clinical signs of both hyponatremia and hypernatremia?
    a. Seizures, irritability, lethargy.
    b. Decreased deep tendon reflexes, signs of cerebral edema.
    c. Renal failure, hypertension.
    d. Arrhythmia, seizures, diarrhea.

Answer: **A**

Both hyponatremia and hypernatremia result in primary neurologic symptoms, including seizures, irritability, lethargy, and others.

11. An adolescent who is thin admits to purposefully vomiting after eating large meals. Which one of the following findings would be associated with bulimia nervosa?
    a. Clubbing of fingers.
    b. Hyperreactive gag reflex.
    c. Peripheral edema.
    d. Strawberry tongue.

Answer: **C**

Swelling of the hands and feet related to hypoalbuminemia may be noted in patients with bulimia nervosa and other eating disorders in which nutrition is challenged.

12. The management of hyponatremia is based on the etiology and typically includes which of the following?
    a. Volume expansion without fluid restriction.
    b. Volume expansion, fluid restriction, or diuretic use.
    c. Fluid restriction and maintenance IV fluids.
    d. Diuretic use and replacement of sodium with NS.

Answer: **B**

The management of hyponatremia depends on the underlying cause. Volume expansion, fluid restriction, or diuretic use may be indicated based on etiology. Replacement and maintenance fluids should be calculated to determine appropriate electrolyte composition of IV fluids and IV fluid rate, especially if using 3% sodium chloride. Serial serum sodium levels should be measured routinely to closely monitor rate of increase in serum sodium level.

13. An adolescent who weighs 54 kg is admitted with a diagnosis of status asthmaticus and is placed on continuous albuterol therapy. His orders include potassium supplement and IV fluids at two-thirds maintenance. What is the best choice for IV infusion?
    a. D5.45 NS with 20 mEq KCl/L at 45 mL/hour.
    b. 0.9 NS at 85 mL/hour.
    c. D5.45 NS with 20 mEq KCl/L at 60 mL/hour.
    d. 0.9 NS with 30 mEq KCl/L at 65 mL/hour.

Answer: **C**

Albuterol administration can result in decreased serum potassium levels. Two-thirds maintenance fluid would be 65 mL/hour, so the best choice is D5.45 NS with 20 mEq/L KCl, which is considered physiologic.

14. What is the appropriate rate of rise in serum sodium for a patient with asymptomatic hyponatremia?
    a. 2 to 4 mEq/L every 4 hours or 10 to 20 mEq/L in 24 hours.
    b. 4 to 6 mEq/L every 4 hours or 24 to 36 mEq/L in 24 hours.
    c. 1 to 2 mEq/L every 8 hours or 3 to 6 mEq/L in 24 hours.
    d. The goal of therapy is to correct sodium to normal levels in 24 hours regardless of the rate of rise.

Answer: **A**

Serum sodium correction must be done in a slow, controlled manner to avoid central pontine myelinolysis. If patient is asymptomatic, goal rate of sodium rise is 2 to 4 mEq/L every 4 hours or 10 to 20 mEq/L in 24 hours.

15. Which one of the following genetic syndromes is associated with hypochloremia?
    a. Bartter syndrome.
    b. DiGeorge syndrome.
    c. Prader–Willi syndrome.
    d. Fanconi anemia.

Answer: **A**

Bartter syndrome includes a group of autosomal recessive genetic disorders defined by an impairment of salt reabsorption with significant salt wasting, hypokalemic metabolic alkalosis, and hypercalciuria.

16. Which one of the following may contribute to hypernatremia, especially in a young infant?
    a. Inappropriately concentrated infant formula.
    b. SIADH.
    c. Adrenal insufficiency.
    d. Cystic fibrosis with frequent diuretic use.

Answer: **A**

Caregivers who do not understand the rationale behind appropriately concentrated infant formula can contribute to their infants' altered electrolyte status. Inappropriately concentrated infant formula may contribute to significant hypernatremia. Infants and young children are at increased risk for hypernatremia and dehydration due to inability to communicate thirst.

17. An infant presents for care with active seizure activity and a serum sodium level of 121 mEq/L. What is the most appropriate initial treatment?
    a. Hypertonic saline calculated by formula [0.6 × (weight in kg) × (target sodium − measured sodium)] to achieve a target sodium level of 135 mEq/L.
    b. Hypertonic saline calculated by body weight at a dose of 2 mL/kg.
    c. NS bolus in increments of 20 mL/kg to restore intravascular volume. Hypertonic saline is not indicated.
    d. Hypertonic saline calculated by formula [0.6 × (weight in kg) × (target sodium − measured sodium)] to achieve a target sodium level of 125 mEq/L.

Answer: **D**

Hypertonic saline calculated by formula to achieve a target sodium level of 125 mEq/L is indicated for active seizure activity and documented hyponatremia. If hypertonic saline is not available, a NS bolus may be administered in the interim.

18. Which one of the following mechanisms is primarily responsible for calcium regulation?
    a. Cortisol.

b. Thyroid hormone.
c. PTH.
d. Aldosterone.

Answer: **C**

GI, renal, and skeletal mechanisms are components of calcium regulation. However, PTH is primarily responsible for calcium regulation. PTH regulates calcium absorption from bone and renal excretion of calcium.

19. Serum calcium level measurement is affected by which of the following?
    a. Albumin levels.
    b. Hemoglobin.
    c. Creatinine.
    d. Sodium.

Answer: **A**

Serum or plasma calcium is bound to proteins, and the measurement of serum calcium is effected by albumin. In contrast, serum albumin levels do not affect the measurement of ionized calcium, as the ionized form is the unbound/free calcium ion.

20. A genetic disorder associated with significant hypocalcemia and that can present with hypocalcemia is:
    a. DiGeorge syndrome.
    b. Angelman syndrome.
    c. Sturge–Weber syndrome.
    d. Turner syndrome.

Answer: **A**

DiGeorge syndrome is associated with absence or hypoplasia of the parathyroid and therefore is associated with significant hypocalcemia.

21. An adolescent with a metabolic condition has a high chloride level on basic metabolic panel. The treatment of hyperchloremia includes which of the following?
    a. Identification and treatment of the underlying cause.
    b. Administration of sodium bicarbonate as first-line therapy for mild-to-moderate hyperchloremia.
    c. Administration of sodium chloride as first-line therapy for severe hyperchloremia.
    d. Respiratory support for respiratory acidosis.

Answer: **A**

The most critical aspect of treatment for hyperchloremia is the identification and treatment of the underlying cause of metabolic acidosis. The administration of sodium bicarbonate is indicated only for patients with severe acidosis and is not generally considered first-line therapy. Patients with hyperchloremia and associated metabolic acidosis may develop Kussmaul breathing as a compensatory mechanism and do not generally develop a respiratory acidosis.

22. A 14-year-old wrestler is suspected of having an eating disorder. Which of the following should be routinely included in

(continues on page 246)

the initial evaluation to help assist in the diagnosis of intravascular volume depletion?

a. Orthostatic vital signs.
b. Doppler pulses.
c. Cardiac ECHO.
d. Abdominal ultrasound.

Answer: **A**

Assessment of orthostatic vital signs is a component of the evaluation for intravascular volume depletion in adolescents who are suspected of having eating disorders.

23. What is the physiologic reason that young infants with fluid losses will have more severe dehydration over a shorter period of time than their older counterparts?

a. Infants have as much as 70% lean body mass as water.
b. Infants have as much as 50% lean body mass as water.
c. Secretion of aldosterone results in a decrease in production of ADH.
d. Secretion of ADH results in secretion of aldosterone, resulting in excess urine output.

Answer: **A**

Children in general have bodies that are composed of more water per lean body mass than their adult counterparts. Young infants have as much as 70% lean body mass as water, which, with disease processes such as gastroenteritis and fever, will result in dehydration very early in the disease process.

24. A child with a nasogastric tube attached to suction/gastric decompression has hypochloremia. Which type of medication could be considered if the cessation of nasogastric suctioning and removal of gastric secretions is not a treatment option?

a. Magnesium supplement.
b. β-Blocker.
c. Proton-pump inhibitor.
d. Loop diuretic.

Answer: **C**

Proton-pump inhibitors may decrease the loss of gastric acid. Loop diuretics result in chloride loss and should be avoided.

25. A 3-month-old infant with a history of severe diarrhea presents with a 3-minute tonic–clonic seizure. Initial electrolytes include a sodium level of 124 mEq/L, potassium of 3.0 mEq/L, chloride of 86 mmol/L, and sodium bicarbonate of 12 mmol/L. After an initial bolus infusion of NS, what is the most important initial management?

a. Infusion of 3% saline solution.
b. IV fluids containing sodium acetate.
c. Potassium infusion of 10 mEq/L.
d. Maintenance IV solution with ½ NS (0.45 NS).

Answer: **A**

Replacement of sodium will assist in preventing continued seizure activity, as a low sodium level could contribute to seizures. Rapidly increasing the sodium to above the seizure threshold is best accomplished with the use of 3% saline infusion. The low bicarbonate level is indicative of dehydration, and low potassium will not cause seizure activity.

Recommended Readings

Bouquegneau, A., Dubois, B. E., Krzesinski, J. M., & Delanaye, P. (2012). Anorexia and the kidney. *American Journal of Kidney Disease, 60*(2), 299–307.

Friedman, A. (2010). Fluid and electrolyte therapy: A primer. *Pediatric Nephrology, 25,* 843–846.

Fuchs, S., LeRoy, K., Goodman, D., Mead, J., Strokosh, G., Ruppel, R., & Madden, M. (2012). Fluid, electrolytes, and nutrition. In K. Reuter-Rice & B. Bolic (Eds.), *Pediatric acute care: A guide for interprofessional practice* (pp. 403–465). Burlington, MA: Jones & Bartlett Learning.

Herrin, J. T. (2013). Management of fluid and electrolyte abnormalities in children. In D. B. Mount, M. H. Sayegh, & A. K. Singh (Eds.), *Core concepts in the disorders of fluids, electrolytes and acid-base balance* (pp. 147–170). Philadelphia, PA: Springer.

Hines, E. Q. (2012). Fluids and electrolytes. In M. M. Tschudy & K. M. Arcara (Eds.), *The Harriet Lane handbook* (19th ed., pp. 271–292). Philadelphia, PA: Mosby.

LabCorp. (2013, January 15). *Serum chloride.* Retrieved from https://www.Labcorps.com

Lexicomp Online. (2013). *Calcium chloride: Pediatric drug information.* Retrieved from http://online.lexi.com/crlsql/servlet/crlonline

Lexicomp Online. (2013). *Calcium gluconate: Pediatric drug information.* Retrieved from http://online.lexi.com/crlsql/servlet/crlonline

Lexicomp Online. (2013). *Magnesium sulfate: Pediatric drug information.* Retrieved from http://online.lexi.com/crlsql/servlet/crlonline

Lexicomp Online. (2013). *Potassium chloride: Pediatric drug information.* Retrieved from http://online.lexi.com/crlsql/servlet/crlonline

Lexicomp Online. (2013). *Potassium phosphate: Pediatric drug information.* Retrieved from http://online.lexi.com/crlsql/servlet/crlonline

Lexicomp Online. (2013). *Sodium chloride preparations: Pediatric drug information.* Retrieved from http://online.lexi.com/crlsql/servlet/crlonline

Lexicomp Online. (2013). *Sodium phosphate: Pediatric drug information.* Retrieved from http://online.lexi.com/crlsql/servlet/crlonline

Norington, A., Stanley, R., Tremlet, M., & Birrell, G. (2012). Medical management of acute severe anorexia nervosa. *Archives of Disease in Childhood: Education and Practice Edition, 97,* 48–54.

Online Mendelian Inheritance in Man. (2005). *Liddle syndrome.* Retrieved from http://www.Omim.org

Online Mendelian Inheritance in Man. (2011, updated 2 May). *Bartter syndrome.* Retrieved from http://www.Omim.org

Online Mendelian Inheritance in Man. (2011). *Fanconi renotubular syndrome.* Retrieved from http://www.Omim.org

Online Mendelian Inheritance in Man. (2011). *Prader-Willi syndrome.* Retrieved from http://www.Omim.org

Online Mendelian Inheritance in Man. (2012). *DiGeorge syndrome.* Retrieved from http://www.Omim.org

Online Mendelian Inheritance in Man. (2013). *Gitelman syndrome.* Retrieved from http://www.Omim.org

Metabolic Disorders

Inborn Errors of Metabolism

Shari Simone

Background

- Genetic metabolic disorders, also known as inborn errors of metabolism (IEM), are individually rare, but collectively numerous and occur in 1 of 1,500 children.
- Most metabolic disorders are inherited as autosomal recessive traits.

Definition

- Genetic metabolic disorders are a group of disorders that result in abnormalities in the synthesis or catabolism of proteins, carbohydrates, or fats.
- Most disorders result from the absence or abnormality of an enzyme or its cofactor essential for normal function of specific metabolic pathways.
- The disrupted metabolic pathway has various consequences, including a deficiency of a particular end product or excessive, toxic accumulation of a substrate.

General Classification

- Disorders of protein metabolism.
  - Amino acid disorders (e.g., phenylketonuria or PKU).
  - Organic acid disorders (e.g., propionic acidemia).
  - Urea cycle disorders (e.g., ornithine transcarbamylase (OTC) deficiency).
- Disorders of glucose metabolism.
  - Glycogen storage disease (GSD) (e.g., Pompe disease).
  - Other carbohydrate disorders (e.g., galactosemia).
- Disorders of fat metabolism.
  - Fatty acid oxidation disorders (e.g., medium-chain acyl-CoA dehydrogenase (MCAD) deficiency).
- Disorders of organelles.
  - Mitochondrial disorders (e.g., Leigh syndrome).
  - Lysosomal storage disorders (e.g., mucopolysaccharidosis such as Hurler syndrome, sphingolipidoses such as Tay–Sachs disease).
  - Peroxisomal disorders (e.g., Zellweger syndrome).

- Other disorders: purine and pyrimidine disorders, porphyrias, metal disorders (e.g., Wilson disease).
  - These disorders are extremely rare and only Wilson disease will be discussed.

Pathophysiology

- In normal circumstances, the dietary intake of glucose and tissue glycogen stores is sufficient for adenosine triphosphate (ATP) production (Figure 9.1).
- If the supply of glucose cannot be maintained, the body changes to a catabolic state and fat and protein are mobilized to supply substrates to make ATP.
- Protein metabolism (Figure 9.2).
  - Protein is made up of amino acids, composed of an amino and an organic acid group.
  - The amino group is metabolized in the form of ammonia, which is degraded in the urea cycle and forms blood urea nitrogen (BUN).
  - Organic acids are metabolized into intermediates of energy pathways (e.g., pyruvate, acetyl CoA, and ketones) and are converted to ATP through a cascade of reactions when they enter the Krebs cycle.
  - Amino acid metabolism also involves conversion of some amino acids to other amino acids.
  - Failure of, or deficiencies in, any of these pathways can lead to toxic accumulation of proteins or by-products of protein metabolism.
- Carbohydrate metabolism.
  - Glucose is generated by mobilization of glycogen tissue stores or dietary intake of carbohydrates, and through the

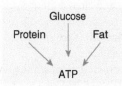

FIGURE 9.1 • **Production of ATP under Normal Condition.**

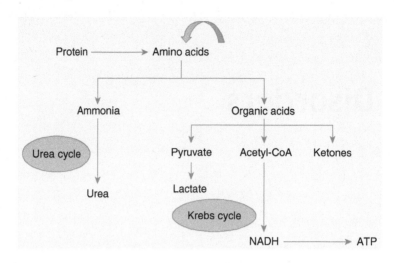

FIGURE 9.2 • **Protein Metabolism.**

process of glycolysis, it is converted to pyruvate and acetyl CoA and then enters the Krebs cycle.

- In the Krebs cycle, acetyl CoA is converted to nicotinamide adenine dinucleotide (NADH).
- NADH is then carried through a cascade of reactions within the mitochondria, known as oxidative phosphorylation, in which the chemical energy locked within NADH is transferred to ATP.
- Fat metabolism (Figure 9.3).
  - Triglycerides are hydrolyzed and broken down into fatty acids and glycerol.
  - Through the process of β-oxidation, 2-carbon units (acetyl CoA) are removed from the fatty acid molecule and enter the Krebs cycle to produce ATP.
  - During fat breakdown, the massive flux of acetyl CoA results in formation of ketone bodies and produces ketosis.
  - Carnitine is a cofactor and helps transport fatty acids into the mitochondria.
- Metal metabolism.
  - A small amount of copper is needed for the body to function properly.
  - Excess copper is toxic.
  - Normally, excess copper is metabolized through the liver and excreted in the bile.
  - In Wilson disease, copper is not excreted in the bile, and builds up in the liver, releasing copper into the bloodstream.
  - Results in damage to brain, kidneys, and eyes.
- General findings of IEM (Table 9.1).
  - Disorders often mimic other diseases or infections.
  - Most common presentations are feeding intolerance, history of vomiting, and altered mental status.
- General urine odors associated with IEM: see Table 9.2.
  - Characteristic urine odors are associated with some amino acid and organic acid disorders.
- General diagnostic evaluation for acute presentation of IEM.
  - Blood and urine laboratory screening tests should be obtained upon suspicion of a metabolic disorder (Table 9.3).
  - Consider head CT or MRI if neurologic symptoms.

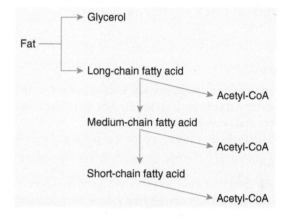

FIGURE 9.3 • **Fat Metabolism.**

TABLE 9.1	General Acute vs. Chronic Findings of IEM	
Acute Findings	**Chronic Findings**
Seizures/lethargy/coma	Hypotonia
Poor feeding/vomiting	Failure to thrive
Hypoglycemia	Recurrent unexplained illnesses
Signs of sepsis	Developmental delay/loss of milestones
Hyperammonemia	Cardiomegaly
Ketosis	Macro/Microcephaly
Metabolic/Lactic acidosis	Eye/Hair/Skin abnormalities
Abnormal urine odor	"Coarse" appearance

TABLE 9.2	Urine Odors Associated with IEM
Disorder	**Urine Odor**
Maple syrup urine disease	Maple syrup
Phenylketonuria	Musty
Isovaleric/Glutaric acidemia	Sweaty feet
Tyrosinemia	Boiled cabbage
Trimethylaminuria	Fishy

TABLE 9.3	Blood and Urine Laboratory Screening Tests for IEM	
First Set of Screening Laboratory: Blood Tests	**First Set of Screening Laboratory: Urine Tests**
Complete blood count (CBC)	Urinalysis
Blood gas (evaluate pH)	Urine pH
Serum glucose (evaluate for hypoglycemia)	Urine color and specific gravity
Serum electrolyte panel (evaluate anion gap)	Odor
Liver function tests Ammonia (evaluate for hyperammonemia)	Urine ketones (evaluate for inappropriateness for state of nutrition)

If abnormality of any of the above tests raises suspicion for IEM, then obtain:

Blood Tests	**Urine Tests**
Plasma amino acids	Urine amino acids
Acylcarnitine profile	Urine organic acids
Lactate	Urine-reducing substances

- Check newborn screen; however, normal results do not exclude IEM.
- General management principles for acute presentation of IEM.
- Maintain a high index of suspicion.
- Suspect diagnosis based on history, physical examination, and diagnostic studies, especially if no improvement seen with standard therapy (e.g., continued metabolic acidosis despite fluid resuscitation).

- Early genetic consultation as treatment is disease-specific.
- NPO to stop intake of suspected toxic substrate (e.g., protein, galactose).
- Stop catabolism by providing high energy with glucose infusion of D10 plus electrolytes at 1.5 times maintenance.
- If hyperammonemia is present, correct to a goal of <100 mmol/L.
- Reduce ammonia serum level by discontinuing protein intake.
- Consider intravenous arginine or sodium benzoate.
- Hemodialysis indicated for severe hyperammonemia and encephalopathy or if refractory to pharmacologic treatment.
- Correct acidosis and dehydration.
- Treat the "trigger" (e.g., infection).
- Treat complications (e.g., increased intracranial pressure).
- Initiate any specific therapies guided by genetics consult (e.g., carnitine, biotin).

Specific Metabolic Disorders

Disorders of Protein Metabolism

- Amino acid disorders.
  - Pathophysiology.
    - A defect in the metabolic pathways of amino acids resulting in abnormal accumulation of amino acids in the plasma.
    - Examples: PKU, nonketotic hyperglycinemia.
  - Clinical presentation.
    - Often presents in newborns who may initially be well and then become acutely symptomatic.
    - May experience metabolic decompensation with poor feeding and lethargy after a period of protein feeding.
    - Symptoms in newborn range from none to metabolic acidosis, hyperammonemia, hypoglycemia, ketosis, and liver dysfunction.
    - May progress to encephalopathy, coma, or death if not recognized.
  - Diagnostic evaluation.
    - Quantitative plasma amino acids and qualitative urine organic acids.
    - Specific enzyme analysis.
  - Management.
    - Complete protein restriction initially, then change to amino acid–restricted diet (i.e., phenylalanine-restricted diet) when specific amino acid disorder identified.
    - Infants and children should be monitored regularly during the developmental period.
    - Strict dietary therapy is recommended to be continued for life for some disorders (i.e., maple syrup urine disease).
- Urea cycle disorders.
  - Pathophysiology.
    - Deficiency of an enzyme or cofactor that transforms nitrogen to urea for excretion and results in the accumulation of ammonia and other precursor metabolites.
    - Severity of disease is based on the position of the defective enzyme in the urea cycle pathway and the severity of the enzyme defect.

- OTC deficiency, an X-linked disorder, is the most common urea cycle disorder.
- Clinical presentation.
  - Classic form presents few days after birth with poor feeding, vomiting, tachypnea, and altered mental status after a period of protein feeding.
  - Patients with partial enzyme activity deficiency present later and with milder symptoms.
  - Laboratory findings include hyperammonemia (>150 mmol/L), respiratory alkalosis, and low BUN.
- Diagnostic evaluation.
  - Main criterion for diagnosis is hyperammonemia with normal anion gap.
  - Amino acid levels and enzyme assay for differentiation.
  - Urine organic acids and urine orotic acid (positive urine orotic acid in OTC deficiency).
- Management.
  - NPO status to remove protein load.
  - Administer intravenous glucose infusion with D10 or higher glucose concentration plus electrolytes at 1.5 times maintenance for high glucose infusion rate to reverse catabolism.
  - Removal of ammonia.
    - Immediate: administer sodium benzoate, dialysis (if severe).
    - Long-term: protein-restricted diet, sodium phenylacetate, arginine supplementation, agents for ammonia excretion.
  - Once a diagnosis is made, treatment is tailored for the specific urea cycle disorder.
  - Certain individuals may benefit from liver transplantation.
- Organic acidemias.
  - Pathophysiology.
    - Enzyme deficiency or abnormal step in pathways of amino acid degradation.
    - Characterized by accumulation of abnormal organic acid metabolites and increased excretion of organic acids in the urine.
    - Some organic acids are excreted bound to carnitine and can lead to carnitine deficiency.
      - Examples: propionic acidemia, maple syrup urine disease.
  - Clinical presentation.
    - Develops during newborn period or early infancy.
    - Initially well, develop a life-threatening episode of metabolic decompensation.
    - Poor feeding, vomiting, lethargy progressing to coma if not treated.
    - Metabolic acidosis with increased anion gap and ketosis (positive urine ketones) is common finding.
    - Mild to moderate hyperammonemia.
    - Hypoglycemia and liver dysfunction.
  - Diagnostic evaluation.
    - Quantitative plasma amino acids and qualitative urine organic acids.

- Acylcarnitine profile, total and free carnitine to diagnose a secondary carnitine deficiency.
- Enzyme analysis.
- Management.
  - NPO and intravenous fluids with D10 plus electrolytes at 1.5 times maintenance to provide a high glucose infusion rate.
  - Dietary protein restriction of the precursor amino acid.
  - Specific formula or foods deficient in particular precursor amino acids but with essential amino acids are the critical part of management.
  - Carnitine supplementation can facilitate excretion of organic acids.
  - May progress to requiring liver transplantation.

Disorders of Carbohydrate Metabolism

- Galactosemia.
  - Pathophysiology.
    - Deficiency of galactose-1-phosphate uridyl transferase, disorders of glycogen breakdown.
  - Clinical presentation.
    - Typically presents in first couple of weeks of life with vomiting, diarrhea, poor weight gain, jaundice, and hepatomegaly.
    - Infants with galactosemia are prone to sepsis from *Escherichia coli*.
    - Untreated infants may develop severe growth failure, mental retardation, cataracts, and liver cirrhosis.
  - Diagnostic evaluation.
    - Laboratory findings of elevated liver transaminases, hypoglycemia, metabolic acidosis, and hyperbilirubinemia.
    - Newborn screening.
    - Positive urine-reducing substances.
    - Diagnosis is confirmed with enzyme assay.
  - Management.
    - Main treatment for infants is initiating lactose-free formula.
    - Dietary restriction of lactose-containing foods later in life.
- GSD.
  - Pathophysiology.
    - Disorder of glycogen breakdown.
    - Subdivided into disorders presenting primarily with liver disease, muscle and liver disease, and disorders primarily affecting muscle.
    - Examples: GSD types 1, 2, 4, Pompe disease (type 2).
  - Clinical presentation.
    - Pompe disease presents classically in first month of life with hypotonia, cardiomegaly, hepatomegaly, feeding difficulties, and failure to thrive.
    - Seizures may occur if hypoglycemia present with GSD.
  - Diagnostic evaluation.
    - Laboratory studies to include glucose, liver enzymes, and creatine phosphokinase (CPK).
      - Hypoglycemia and elevated liver enzymes and CPK seen in classic infantile-onset Pompe disease and in older children with GSD.

- Chest radiography may reveal cardiomegaly.
- Echocardiography may reveal hypertrophic cardiomyopathy.
- Positive urinary oligosaccharides are highly sensitive in Pompe disease.
- Muscle biopsy for definitive diagnosis.
- Management.
  - Begins with treatment of the manifestations of GSD (i.e., cardiac).
  - Cornstarch supplementation for GSD with hypoglycemia.
  - Enzyme replacement therapy with alglucosidase alfa (Myozyme) for Pompe disease.

Disorders of Fat Metabolism

- Fatty acid oxidation disorders.
  - Pathophysiology.
    - Fatty acid oxidation is a major source of energy for peripheral tissues once glycogen stores become depleted during fasting and periods of high energy demands.
    - Fatty acid oxidation disorders involve single-enzyme defects either in one of the β-oxidation steps for fatty acids or in the pathway that transfers electrons from flavin adenine dinucleotide to the electron transport chain.
    - Examples: MCAD deficiency, very long-chain acyl-CoA dehydrogenase deficiency.
    - MCAD deficiency is the most common fatty acid oxidation disorder.
    - Triggers in infancy include prolonged fasting or common illness or infections.
  - Clinical presentation.
    - Previously normal child presents with vomiting, altered mental status/lethargy/coma, occasionally seizures, with or without hepatomegaly.
  - Diagnostic evaluation.
    - Low urinary and plasma hypoglycemia with inappropriately low ketones (hypoketotic hypoglycemia) is classic finding.
    - Other common findings include mild acidosis, hyperammonemia, elevated liver enzymes and CPK.
    - Elevated acylcarnitines.
    - Positive organic acids in urine also suggestive of disorder.
    - Skin biopsy may be needed for enzyme analysis.
  - Management.
    - Acute.
      - Intravenous glucose infusion with D10 and electrolytes at 1.5 times maintenance.
      - Carnitine supplementation.
      - Treat the precipitating illness.
    - Chronic.
      - Avoid fasting (frequent feeding and bedtime feeding).
      - Diet moderately light in fat for some of these disorders.

Disorders of Organelles

- Mitochondrial diseases.
  - Pathophysiology.

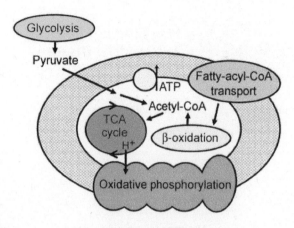

FIGURE 9.4 • **Mitochondrial Functions.**

- Group of disorders that occur as a result of dysfunction of the mitochondrial respiratory chain or oxidative phosphorylation (Figure 9.4).
- The respiratory chain is the essential final common pathway for aerobic metabolism.
- Mitochondria also have a role in fatty acid oxidation and in the urea cycle.
- Mitochondrial disorders may affect only a single organ, but usually involve multiple organ systems with prominent neurologic and myopathic features.
- Consider in differential diagnosis of any progressive multisystem disorder and in children with complex neurologic symptoms.
- Clinical presentation.
  - Wide range of symptoms if multisystem organ involvement.
  - May present at any age.
  - Red flag findings (Table 9.4).
- Diagnostic evaluation.
  - Based on findings.
  - Neuroimaging is indicated in children with suspected CNS disease.
  - Supportive findings of mitochondrial disease include:
    - Head CT revealing basal ganglia calcification and/or diffuse atrophy.
    - Brain MRI revealing atrophy of the cortex or cerebellum or generalized leukoencephalopathy.
    - Electroencephalography showing generalized slow wave activity or generalized or focal spikes with seizures.
    - Electromyography is indicated in children with limb weakness, sensory symptoms, or areflexia, but often findings are normal.
    - Electrocardiography and echocardiography may reveal cardiac involvement such as cardiomyopathy.
    - Serum lactate and pyruvate indicated in children with features of myopathy or CNS disease and markedly

TABLE 9.4	Red Flag Findings Suggestive of Mitochondrial Disease	
System	**Clinical or Diagnostic Findings**	
Neurologic	Encephalopathy	
	Ataxia	
	Myoclonus	
	Seizures	
	Neurodegenerative findings	
Cardiovascular	Cardiomyopathy	
	Unexplained heart block	
Ophthalmologic	Visual disturbances	
	Ptosis/dysconjugate eye movements	
Gastrointestinal	Unexplained liver failure	
	Severe dysmotility	
MELAS	Mitochondrial encephalomyopathy with lactic acidosis and stroke-like episodes	
Other	Unexplained hypotonia	
	Weakness	
	Failure to thrive	
	Metabolic acidosis	

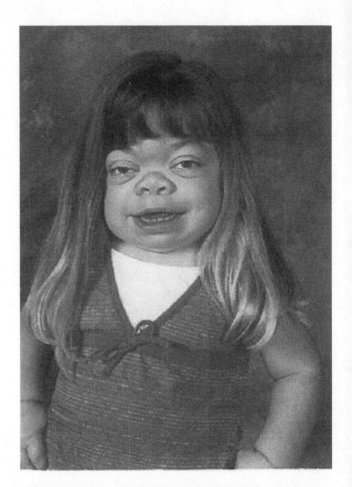

FIGURE 9.5 • **Lysosomal Storage Disorders: Hurler Syndrome.** Young woman with characteristic prominent forehead and depressed nasal bridge, commonly noted in Hurler syndrome.

elevated lactate (properly obtained and no evidence of dehydration or seizure activity) should raise suspicion for mitochondrial disease.
- Lumbar puncture is also important to evaluate for raised CSF lactate and a mild protein elevation consistent with mitochondrial disease.
- Definitive diagnosis is made with a skeletal muscle biopsy.
- Management.
  - Primarily supportive of complications of disease process.
  - Variety of vitamins and cofactors have been used, but evidence supporting their use is lacking.
  - Supplements are generally well tolerated and may include coenzyme Q10, carnitine, creatine, biotin, thiamine, riboflavin, and others.
- Lysosomal storage diseases.
  - Pathophysiology.

- Deficiency of lysosomal enzymes leading to excessive tissue storage of lipid material or incomplete degradation and storage of mucopolysaccharides.
- More than 50 different lysosomal storage disorders.
- Type 1 Gaucher disease is the most common lysosomal storage disorder and typically presents with hepatosplenomegaly, pancytopenia, and destructive bone disease.
- Other examples: Hurler syndrome, Tay–Sachs disease, Hunter syndrome.
- Clinical presentation.
  - Developmental delay/cognitive impairment or only somatic.
  - Symptoms: hepatomegaly, splenomegaly, neurologic regression, short stature, coarse facial features, limitation of small and large joints, and cardiac disease (Figure 9.5).
- Diagnostic evaluation.
  - Urinary measurement of glycosaminoglycans (polysaccharides) and oligosaccharides (simpler polysaccharides) are suggestive of lysosomal storage disorder.
  - Diagnosis is confirmed by enzyme assay.

- Management.
  - Supportive care for complications of disorder.
  - Enzyme replacement if available, but has had limited success.
  - Hematopoietic stem cell transplantation or bone marrow transplantation is used to treat some disorders.
  - Gene therapy is under development, but the goal is to provide therapeutic levels of the deficient enzyme to all involved organs.
- Peroxisomal disorders.
  - Pathophysiology.
    - Cellular organelles involved in β-oxidation of very long-chain fatty acids.
      - Examples: infantile Refsum disease and Zellweger syndrome (most severe of peroxisomal disorders).
  - Clinical presentation/findings.
    - Zellweger syndrome has classic dysmorphic features: high forehead, flat occiput, large anterior fontanelle, hypoplastic superior orbital ridges, epicanthal folds, broad nasal bridge, anteverted nostrils, camptodactyly, and micrognathia (Figure 9.6).
    - Seizures, brain defects (i.e., neuronal migration defect), severe intellectual disability.
    - Liver disease (dysfunction and cirrhosis) and adrenal insufficiency.
  - Diagnostic evaluation.
    - Diagnosis confirmed with enzyme assay.
  - Management.
    - Supportive.

Metal Metabolism Disorders

- Pathophysiology.
  - Abnormal gene on long arm of chromosome 13 (13q14.3).
  - Results in reduced copper excretion, inability of copper incorporation into ceruloplasmin, and accumulation of copper in hepatocytes.
  - Over time, copper overload is distributed to brain and kidneys; inhibits enzymatic processes.
  - Example: Wilson disease.
- Presentation.
  - Liver dysfunction; hepatomegaly, cirrhosis, portal hypertension; variceal bleeding, hepatitis, ascites, edema, delayed puberty, amenorrhea, coagulation disorders.
  - May present with acute hepatic failure; more common in females.
  - Neurologic: intention tremor, dysarthria, dystonia, choreiform movements, decreased coordination, changes in school performance, behavioral changes.
  - Psychiatric: depression, personality changes, anxiety, psychosis.
  - Fanconi syndrome.
  - Bone/muscle disease.

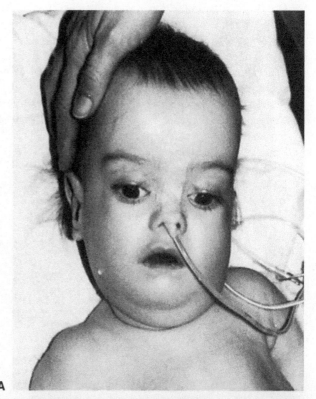
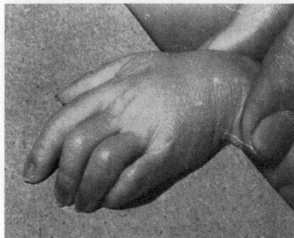

FIGURE 9.6 • **Zellweger Syndrome and Characteristic Dysmorphic Features. A:** Typical facies with high forehead and flat facies. Redundant skin of the neck is seen. (Courtesy of the late Dr. H. Zellweger, University of Iowa, Iowa City, IA.) **B:** Hand, demonstrating camptodactyly of the third, fourth, and fifth fingers.

- Presentations are variable; tendency toward familial patterns.
- Diagnostic evaluation.
  - Ceruloplasmin level <20 mg/dL.
  - Increased serum copper level; increased urinary copper excretion (>100 μg/day).

- Ophthalmologic evaluation: Kayser–Fleischer ring; slit lamp examination demonstrates brown discoloration at outer rim of cornea as a result of copper deposition.
- Liver biopsy: determines extent and severity of disease; determines elevated hepatic copper content ($>250\,\mu g/g$ dry weight).
- Management.
  - Restrict dietary copper (e.g., shellfish, liver, nuts, chocolate).
  - Copper-chelating agents (e.g., d-penicillamine, triethylene tetramine dihydrochloride).
  - Zinc.
  - Liver transplantation is curative.
  - Early initiation of chelation or zinc therapy of asymptomatic siblings can prevent expression of the disease.
  - Untreated disease can be fatal.

PEARLS

- *Suspect IEM in an infant or child who presents with acute illness and metabolic acidosis but without evidence of shock, seizures, or documented asphyxia.*
- *Proof of another diagnosis does not exclude IEM; make certain the diagnosis explains all of the patient's presentation (e.g., sepsis may be the precipitating event that unmasks IEM disorder).*
- *There are few clinical clues to the presence of hyperammonemia; however, this symptom is a respiratory stimulant, so should suspect hyperammonemia in an infant or child with unexplained tachypnea (e.g. no signs of respiratory illness, congestive heart failure, etc.).*

1. A 6-day-old term infant with poor feeding, nonbilious, non-bloody emesis, and increased lethargy presents to the emergency room. On examination, respirations are deep and labored. Initial laboratory evaluation reveals serum sodium of 135 mEq/L, potassium 4.9 mEq/L, chloride 103 mEq/L, BUN 5 mg/dL, creatinine 0.3 mg/dL, bicarbonate 28 mEq/L, glucose 85 mg/dL, and arterial pH 7.47. Which one of the following laboratory tests would be *most* helpful in determining diagnosis?
   a. Plasma amino acids.
   b. Urine organic acids.
   c. Arterial lactate and pyruvate levels.
   d. Serum ammonia level.

Answer: D

Laboratory data reveals metabolic alkalosis and low BUN despite a presentation of dehydration. A typical presentation for an infant with urea cycle disorder includes normal birth and initially well but develops severe emesis and altered mental status after a period of protein feeding. The inability to break down ammonia leads to toxic accumulation and a low serum BUN. Elevated ammonia is a potent respiratory stimulant and causes metabolic alkalosis. Obtaining an ammonia level is important for urea cycle disorder diagnosis.

2. A previously healthy 16-month-old is admitted with vomiting and diarrhea secondary to gastroenteritis. Twenty-four hours after admission, the infant develops generalized seizures and decreased level of consciousness. Laboratory analysis reveals normal electrolytes but serum glucose is 25 mg/dL. Urinalysis reveals no ketones. Among the following, the *most* likely diagnosis is:
   a. GSD type 1.
   b. MCAD deficiency.
   c. OTC deficiency.
   d. Pompe disease.

Answer: B

Classic feature of a fatty acid disorder is hypoketotic hypoglycemia. During periods of fasting when glucose and glycogen stores are depleted, fat and protein are mobilized for energy. During fat breakdown, there is a massive flux of acyl-CoA that results in the formation of ketones. In fatty acid disorders, such as MCAD deficiency, there is a deficiency in acyl-CoA dehydrogenase, which prevents fatty acids from crossing the mitochondrial membrane to be used for energy, and therefore, ketone bodies are not generated.

3. A 2-month-old infant with a history of poor feeding and lethargy is admitted with initial working diagnosis of sepsis and concern for IEM. Which one of the following is a critical initial management strategy for the treatment of suspected IEM?
   a. Normal saline bolus.
   b. NPO and intravenous fluids with D10 .45 NS.
   c. NPO and intravenous fluids with D5 0.45 NS.
   d. Initiate carnitine supplementation.

Answer: B

Critical initial management is stopping the suspected toxic substrate (e.g., protein, galactose) which includes all oral intake and stopping catabolism by providing high-energy glucose infusion.

4. PKU is an illness that is considered:
   a. Carbohydrate disorder of metabolism.
   b. Amino acid disorder.
   c. Glycogen storage defect.
   d. Zellweger syndrome.

Answer: B

PKU is an autosomal recessive metabolic genetic disorder characterized by a mutation in the gene for the hepatic enzyme phenylalanine hydroxylase. PKU is an illness in which children can develop seizures or neurologic sequelae if phenylalanine is ingested by the child. Early testing for PKU is indicated and done through the newborn metabolic screen.

5. A metabolic disorder that presents with hepatosplenomegaly, pancytopenia, and destructive bone disease is known as:
   a. Zellweger syndrome.
   b. PKU.
   c. Gaucher disease.
   d. Hurler syndrome.

Answer: C

Gaucher disease is caused by a hereditary enzyme deficiency of the enzyme glucocerebrosidase which results in manifestations including an enlarged liver and spleen, fatty skin deposits, and painful bone lesions. Liver dysfunction can result in pancytopenia.

6. A full-term infant who is now 24 hours old develops tachypnea at rest while being observed by his mother in her postpartum room. He was small for gestational age, but has no other maternal or neonatal history. Which diagnostic test is *most* important to be included in his workup today?
   a. Echocardiography.
   b. Ammonia level.
   c. Metabolic screening.
   d. Liver function tests.

Answer: B

(continues on page 256)

Any infant who presents with unexplained tachypnea should have a workup for a metabolic disorder which always includes an ammonia level. Hyperammonemia is a respiratory stimulant, thus contributing to tachypnea.

7. After presenting with a serious illness, a 2-week-old infant is diagnosed with galactosemia. Which one of the following is the most appropriate infant formula for this baby?
   a. Nutramigen.
   b. Similac sensitive.
   c. Enfamil Prosobee.
   d. Pregestimil.

Answer: **C**

Galactosemia is a carbohydrate disorder that typically presents in the first couple of weeks of life with vomiting, diarrhea, poor weight gain, jaundice, and hepatomegaly. The management of an infant with galactosemia is nutrition with a lactose-free formula which would include Enfamil Prosobee and Similac Isomil.

8. Appropriate laboratory evaluation for a child with a suspected fatty acid oxidation disorder should include:
   a. Complete blood count with differential, blood cultures, and complete metabolic panel.
   b. Glucose, ketones, ammonia level, liver function tests, and CPK.
   c. Glucose, complete blood count with differential, CPK, and thyroid function tests.
   d. Thyroid function tests, ammonia level, and complete metabolic panel.

Answer: **B**

Fatty acid oxidation is a major source of energy for peripheral tissues once glycogen stores become depleted during fasting and periods of high energy demands. Fatty acid oxidation disorders involve single-enzyme defects either in one of the β-oxidation steps for fatty acids or in the pathway that transfers electrons from flavin adenine dinucleotide to the electron transport chain. Infants will present with hypoglycemia and inappropriately low ketones as well as hyperammonemia, altered liver function tests, and high CPK.

9. The acute treatment of fatty acid oxidation disorder includes administration of which of the following?
   a. Intravenous fluids with D10W and electrolytes.
   b. Fluid bolus of normal saline at 10 mL/kg.
   c. Sodium bicarbonate in electrolyte solution.
   d. Intravenous fluids with D5 ½ NS and potassium.

Answer: **A**

Typically fatty acid oxidation disorder includes presentation of hypoglycemia. The acute management involves administration of an intravenous solution containing D10W and electrolytes at 1.5 times maintenance rates.

10. Which isolated symptom/finding in a newborn would warrant a full metabolic evaluation?
    a. Hypoglycemia.
    b. Small for gestational age.
    c. Hyperbilirubinemia.
    d. Seizure activity.

Answer: **D**

An infant who has seizures in the newborn period should have a full evaluation for sepsis, hypoxic injuries, genetic neurologic disorders, and metabolic disease. Seizures can indicate an electrolyte abnormality that could correspond to a metabolic diagnosis or a diagnosis such as mitochondrial disorder.

Recommended Reading

Balistreri, W. F., & Carey, R. G. (2011). Wilson disease. In R. M. Kliegman, B. F. Stanton, J. W. St Gemelll, N. F. Schor, & R. E. Behrman (Eds.), *Kliegman: Nelson textbook of pediatrics* (19th ed., pp. 1391–1392). Philadelphia, PA: Saunders Elsevier.

Edmond, J. C. (2009). Mitochondrial disorders. *International Ophthalmology Clinics, 49*(3), 27–33.

Hansen, K., & Waibel, E. M. (2012). Inborn errors of metabolism. In K. Reuter-Rice & B. Bolick (Eds.), *Pediatric acute care: A guide for interprofessional practice* (pp. 586–588). Burlington, MA: Jones & Bartlett Learning.

Kwon, K., & Tsai, V. (2007). Metabolic emergencies. *Emergency Clinics of North America, 25*(4), 1041–1060.

Levy, P. A. (2009). Inborn errors of metabolism. Part 1: Overview. *Pediatrics in Review, 30*(4), 131–138.

Levy, P. A. (2009). Inborn errors of metabolism. Part 2: Specific disorders. *Pediatrics in Review, 30*(4), e22–e28.

Paprocka, J., & Jamroz, E. (2012). Hyperammonemia in children on the crossroad of different disorders. *The Neurologist, 18*(5), 261–265.

Hematology and Oncology Disorders

Anemia: Acute

Christine A. Schindler

Background/Definition

- Anemia is a reduction in red blood cell (RBC) mass or blood hemoglobin concentration that is more than two standard deviations below the mean for the reference population. Most commonly defined by reduction in either hematocrit or hemoglobin.

Etiology/Types

- Increased red cell destruction (hemolysis) caused by hemoglobinopathies, membrane and enzyme defects, autoimmune hemolytic anemia, drug-associated hemolytic anemias, disseminated intravascular coagulation (DIC), and hemolytic uremic syndrome (HUS).
- Excessive blood loss (hemorrhage).
- Deficient red cell production (ineffective hematopoiesis).
  - Disorders of heme and globin production such as non-nutritional disorders of hemoglobin synthesis, thalassemia syndromes, lead poisoning, iron deficiency, chronic inflammatory diseases, chronic infections, chronic renal disease, and hyper/hypothyroidism.

Pathophysiology

- RBCs develop in the bone marrow and circulate for approximately 100 to 120 days in the body before their components are recycled by macrophages.
- Rate of RBC destruction exceeds the rate of production, resulting in hemolysis.
- Rate of blood loss exceeds rate of production from hemorrhage.
- Ineffective hematopoiesis: Rate of RBC production is slower than the rate of destruction.

- Transient Erythroblastopenia of childhood: transient or temporary red cell aplasia; typically presents following viral illness, with anemia in the range of 6 to 8 mg/dL (although can be lower) and reticulocytopenia.

Clinical Presentation

- Weakness, fatigue, confusion, and palpitations.
- Pallor, tachycardia, flow murmur, diminished peripheral pulses, and sometimes jaundice.

Diagnostic Evaluation

- Marked decrease in hematocrit and hemoglobin.
- RBC indices and morphology.
  - Increased reticulocyte count and low mean corpuscular volume (MCV) includes hemoglobinopathies (e.g., thalassemia syndromes).
  - Increased reticulocyte count and normal MCV indicates Membrane, Enzyme, or Immune disorders, Microangiopathic anemias, DIC, infection-induced hemolysis or chronic blood loss.
  - Low, normal, or slightly elevated reticulocytes and low MCV: iron deficiency anemia, lead toxicity, Thalassemia trait, Sideroblastic anemia, or anemia of chronic disease.
  - Low, normal, or slightly elevated reticulocytes, and high MCV: congenital hypoplastic or aplastic anemia, acquired hypoplastic or aplastic anemia (malignancies), aplastic crisis with underlying hemolytic anemia (HbSS), megoblastic anemia (Folate or B_{12} deficiency), immune disorders, Hypersplenism, anemia of chronic disease.

Management

- Treat underlying cause, maintain oxygenation.
- If hypovolemic shock present, volume expansion with packed RBC (PRBC) transfusion is indicated.
- Dietary counseling; in iron deficiency anemia and iron supplement.

Aplastic Anemia

Christine A. Schindler

Background/Definition

- Aplastic anemia is a life-threatening disease of bone marrow failure resulting in decreased production of hematopoietic stem cells that results in peripheral pancytopenia and bone marrow aplasia. Rare condition; 0.6 to 6.1 cases per 1 million population.

Etiology/Types

- Congenital aplastic anemia occurs in approximately 20% of cases.
- Acquired aplastic anemia occurs in approximately 80% of cases. Acquired aplastic anemia may be a result of exposure to drugs, chemicals, ionizing radiation, or viruses.

Pathophysiology

- The causative injury in aplastic anemia is thought to be a direct injury to the pluripotent stem cells.

Clinical Presentation

- History: mucosal/gingival bleeding, headaches, fatigue, easy bruising, rash, fever, mucosal ulcerations, or recurrent viral infections.
- Symptoms: pallor, tachycardia, petechial rash, purpura, ecchymoses, or jaundice.
- Symptom severity depends on the level of pancytopenia.

Diagnostic Evaluation

- Decrease in hemoglobin, white blood cell (WBC) count, and platelet count.
- Reduction in or absence of the absolute number of reticulocytes.
- Peripheral blood smear; no abnormal cells.
- Reduction or absence of hematopoietic elements from bone marrow aspirate.

Management

- Transfusions of RBCs and platelets.
- Antibiotic therapy.
- Bone marrow transplantation (BMT).
- Immunosuppressive therapy if unable to receive a BMT.

Diamond-Blackfan Anemia (Diamond-Blackfan Anemia)

Christine A. Schindler

Background/Definition

- A rare congenital hypoplastic anemia resulting in constitutional bone marrow failure.

Etiology/Types

- Mutation for Diamond–Blackfan is on chromosome 19, which encodes for a ribosomal protein known as RPS19.

Pathophysiology

- The definitive cause is unknown; hypothesized that it is an autosomal dominant disorder of faulty ribosome biogenesis that results in proapoptotic erythropoiesis, leading to marrow failure.

Clinical Presentation

- Symptoms: pallor, fatigue, irritability, syncope, and dyspnea during feeding.
- Physical examination: irregular heartbeat, hypotonia, short stature, and evidence of failure to thrive.
- Associated with physical defects including craniofacial, hands, upper limbs, cardiac, or genitourinary.

Diagnostic Evaluation

- Profound macrocytic anemia; WBCs and platelet count generally normal.
- Reticulocytopenia.
- Increased percentage of hemoglobin F for age.
- Elevated erythrocyte adenosine deaminase activity.
- Decreased or absent erythroid precursors in bone marrow aspirate.
- Genetic screening; Diamond–Blackfan anemia—mutation in RPS19.

Management

- Corticosteroids, frequent blood transfusion, BMT in some cases.
- Hematology, BMT, and endocrinology team involvement.

Coagulation Disorders

Disseminated Intravascular Coagulation (DIC)

Sheree H. Allen

Background/Definition

- DIC, also referred to as defibrination syndrome or consumptive coagulopathy, is a life-threatening complication of systemic or localized tissue injury causing a disturbance of the normal coagulation cascade that results in uncontrolled intravascular coagulation coupled with the consumption of coagulation factors and platelets, which triggers concurrent thrombosis and hemorrhage.

Etiology

- Acquired condition resulting from single or multiple underlying conditions or disease processes.
- Associated with significant mortality and may *not* resolve with treatment of the underlying cause.
- Infection—most common cause (approximately 35% of all cases).
  - Gram-negative (most commonly associated with DIC) or gram-positive sepsis.
  - Viral processes.

- Fungal infection.
- Severe pancreatitis.
- Trauma; penetrating brain injury, burns, or multiple trauma.
- Hematologic malignancies; hemolytic processes.
- Acute respiratory distress syndrome.
- Obstetrical complication.
- Necrotizing enterocolitis.
- Extra Corporeal Membrane Oxygenation.
- Graft-versus-host disease (GVHD).

Pathophysiology

- Acute or chronic process in which there is concurrent acceleration of the clotting cascade and the fibrinolytic system causing simultaneous hemorrhage and microvascular clotting.
- Uncontrolled, intravascular coagulation secondary to:
  - Excessive fibrin and platelets deposited into microvascular system causing microfibrin threads and thrombi.
  - Consumption of platelets—thrombocytopenia.
  - Intravascular thrombosis, purpura, petechiae, end organ ischemia, and infarction.
- Hemorrhage secondary to:
  - Depletion of coagulation factors and platelets.
  - Prolonged protime (PT).
  - Prolonged activated partial thromboblastin time (PTT).
  - Activation of fibrinolytic system—increased plasmin production and release of fibrin degradation products.
- Hemorrhage causes a rapid release of procoagulant into circulation, causing further depletion of coagulation factors, and ultimately results in increased bleeding.
- Multiple organ system failure secondary to microinfarction, tissue ischemia and necrosis, end organ failure, and shock.

Clinical Presentation

- No predictable pattern. DIC is not a primary disorder, but is always a complication preceded by a significant illness or injury.
- Symptoms: headache, altered level of consciousness, bleeding, disproportionate bruising.
- Findings: diffuse bleeding; often initial symptom, petechiae, ecchymosis, purpura, and hematoma, gingival bleeding and epistaxis, hematuria, hematemesis and melena, intrahepatic hemorrhage, signs and symptoms of shock, thrombosis can be present, cool mottled skin, pallor, poor perfusion, tissue necrosis, and gangrene.
- Multiorgan system failure can occur related to ischemia and/or necrosis, resulting in respiratory insufficiency or failure, renal failure, and altered level of consciousness.

Diagnostic Evaluation

- Laboratory testing—may change depending on the length of illness; there is not one confirmatory laboratory study to diagnose DIC. The following findings are consistent with DIC:
  - Prolonged PT.
  - Prolonged activated partial thromboblastin time.
  - Increased international normalized ratio (INR).
  - Decreased fibrinogen and platelet count.
  - Schistocytes (fragmented RBCs) on complete blood count (CBC) smear.
  - Elevated fibrin split product (FSP).
  - Positive/elevated D-dimer (marker is sensitive to endogenous generation of thrombin and plasmin).

Management

- Supportive therapy should target specific organ symptoms affected while maintaining perfusion of vital organs until DIC is controlled.
- Monitor vital signs, central venous pressure, and oxygen saturation.
- Administer oxygen as needed; additional respiratory strategies as needed.
- Antibiotics—organism specific for presumed or identified infectious etiology.
- Fluid and electrolyte balance; correct acidosis and shock.
- Administer vitamin K as indicated.
- Frequent evaluation of laboratory studies—coagulopathy profile, CBC, chemistry, and acid–base balance (arterial or venous blood gases).
- Blood product administration and replacement.
- Cryoprecipitate—provides fibrinogen, factor VIII, and vonWillebrand factor.
- Consider anticoagulation (e.g., heparin); controversial and not widely recommended; inhibits thrombin generation; efficacy has not been demonstrated in clinical trials.
- Antithrombin III (ATIII)—An α2-globulin that inhibits coagulation.
- Consider Aprotinin—slows fibrinolysis, but not routinely used.

PEARLS
- *Thrombocytopenia is the most common laboratory finding in DIC.*
- *Differential diagnosis includes liver disease, which produces similar coagulopathies. However, in liver disease, factor VII is significantly decreased, and factor VIII may be normal or increased.*
- *Early detection and prompt management of DIC may prevent complications and death.*

Hemolytic Uremic Syndrome
Sheree H. Allen

Background/Definition

- HUS, a disease of the microcirculation, is characterized by hemolytic anemia, thrombocytopenia, and acute renal failure (ARF). Occurs most frequently in children <4 years of age and is the most common cause of ARF.

Etiology

- Contamination of water, meat, fruits, and vegetables with infectious bacteria; peak incidence during summer.
- *E. coli* 0157:H7 is the most common etiology of postdiarrheal (D$^+$) HUS.

Types

- D$^+$ HUS—Postdiarrheal or typical HUS; occurs in previously healthy children who have had recent gastroenteritis. Mortality rate is 3% to 5%; associated with renal failure in 50% to 70% of patients affected. Bacterial verotoxins, absorbed through intestinal mucosa, are produced by *E. coli* O157:H7 infection (Shiga toxin; most common cause), *Shigella dysenteriae*, *Citrobacter freundii*, and other subtypes of *E. coli* (also Shiga toxin).
- D$^-$HUS—Atypical or sporadic HUS is less common and more severe than D$^+$HUS with an approximately 25% mortality rate. It is associated with end-stage renal disease in approximately 50% of cases. More common in adulthood, atypical D$^-$HUS infection may have a familial link and may also begin in the neonatal period; occurs year round with no gastrointestinal (GI) prodrome. Causative factors include Inherited factor H deficiency (10%–20%); inhibits complement activation, Membrane cofactor protein mutations, *Streptococcus pneumoniae* infection, medications including Cyclosporine and Tacrolimus.

Pathophysiology

- D$^+$HUS occurs as a result of verotoxins, especially Shiga toxin, absorbed by the intestinal mucosa, which damage endothelial cells and erythrocytes, producing a prodrome of hemorrhagic enterocolitis.
- Endothelial swelling of the glomerular arterioles in the kidneys results in a decrease in glomerular filtration rate, proteinuria, and hematuria.
- This characteristic microangiopathy precipitates the release of clotting factors, platelet aggregation, and fibrin deposition in the small vessels of the kidney, gut, and central nervous system (CNS), resulting in hemolytic anemia; shearing of RBC's as they pass through narrowed vessels, renal cortical injury and ARF, and thrombocytopenia.

Clinical Presentation (Typical D$^+$HUS)

- Previously healthy child with exposure to contaminated source, incubation period 3 to 5 days.
- Symptoms: abdominal pain; watery, nonbloody diarrhea, fever, weakness, lethargy, irritability.
- Progression to hemorrhagic colitis occurs 5 to 7 days after onset of diarrhea.
- Findings: pallor, petechiae, ecchymoses, hematuria, oliguria, azotemia, hypertension; may progress to anuria, hepatomegaly, splenomegaly, hematemesis, edema.
- Tremor and seizures (approximately 20% of cases).

Diagnostic Evaluation

- HUS diagnosis is supported by patient history and the presence of microangiopathic hemolytic anemia, thrombocytopenia, and ARF.
- Reticulocytosis and abnormal RBC morphology.
- Schistocytes, burr, and helmet cells on smear; fragmented erythrocytes.
- Anemia; decreased plasma haptoglobin.
- Thrombocytopenia.

- Leukocytosis is common.
- Coagulation profile is often normal.
- Stool cultures are often positive for *E. coli* O157:H7, or other toxin-producing bacteria; however, not always detected.
- Serum ELISA testing—should be done at diagnosis and repeated 2 weeks later (determines presence of antibodies to Shiga toxin *E. coli* serotypes).
- Elevated BUN, serum creatinine, bilirubin, and potassium.
- Coombs negative.
- Microscopic hematuria, proteinuria, and casts on urinalysis.

Management

- Typical D$^+$HUS.
  - Supportive therapy—90% of patients survive the acute phase.
    - Greater than 50% recover full renal function.
    - Antibiotics are not indicated (may stimulate the bacteria to release more toxins that can damage platelets, blood vessels, and kidneys).
    - Dialysis—(approximately 50% of patients).
    - Correct electrolyte imbalances, azotemia, manage fluid overload.
    - Maintain adequate nutrition and caloric intake while observing renal protective diet.
    - Correct anemia—75% of patients require PRBC transfusion.
    - Control hypertension.
    - Oral calcium channel blocker (e.g., nifedipine).
    - Intravenous (IV) calcium channel blocker (e.g., nicardipine) or nitroprusside.
  - Long-term follow-up:
    - Monitor blood pressure (BP) and urinalysis.
    - Complications are uncommon; however, proteinuria, decreased glomerular filtration rate, and hypertension may recur up to 1 year later.
- Atypical D$^-$HUS.
  - Plasmapheresis—consider for patients with factor H deficiency; may limit renal involvement temporarily, but does NOT prevent progression to end-stage renal disease and has not been shown to prevent recurrence of D$^-$HUS.
  - Kidney transplantation—8% to 30% if recurrence persists.
  - Long-term follow-up with monitoring of BP and urinalysis.
    - Proteinuria, decreased glomerular filtration rate, and hypertension may recur up to 1 year later.

Hemophagocytic Lymphohistiocytosis
Daniel K. Choi

Background/Definition

- Syndrome of immune overactivation leading to systemic inflammation and resulting damage to any organ(s) in the body.
- Overall rare condition; estimated at 1 in 3,000 inpatient admissions.

- One condition in the spectrum of histiocytic disorders that occurs in adults and children.

Etiology/Types

- Primary hemophagocytic lymphohistiocytosis (HLH): primarily in newborns and young children.
  - Often associated with a family history of HLH and/or in patients with genetic mutations associated with specific immune cell defects that lead to HLH.
  - Gene defects associated with increased risk of HLH: Perforin (PRF), MUNC (UNC13D), Syntaxin 11 (STX11), and SAP (SH2-D1A).
- Secondary HLH: Older children, usually secondary to an underlying medical condition with an underlying immune system defect that acts as a "trigger."
  - Conditions associated with malignancy, autoimmune disease, immune deficiency, and specific infections (e.g., Ebstein–Barr virus, cytomegalovirus [CMV]).

Pathophysiology

- Complex immune dysregulation; molecular mechanism not completely understood.
- When the immune system is activated, critical immune cells (e.g., T-cells, macrophages) are not downregulated appropriately.
- Overactivated critical immune cells (e.g., T-cells/macrophages) stimulate other immune cells to release additional inflammatory cytokines, leading to a self-perpetuating "cytokine storm."
- End organ damage occurs from immune cell damage and inflammation.

Clinical Presentation

- Variable presentation; often appear quite ill.
- Most "common" presentation is prolonged high fever (≥38.5°C), hepatosplenomegaly, hepatitis, and cytopenias (at least two cell lines).
- Can affect any organ system; notable systems include the skin, pulmonary, and CNS.
- A high index of suspicion is needed; the diagnosis can often be confused with malignancy, Kawasaki Disease, and severe infection.

Diagnostic Evaluation

- Criteria first proposed in 1994, and updated in 2004, and are often referred to as the HLH-2004 Criteria:
  - A molecular diagnosis consistent with HLH: pathologic mutations of PRF1, UNC13D, Munc18-2, Rab27a, STX11, SH2D1A, or BIRC4; or
  - Five out of the eight criteria listed below are fulfilled:
    - Fever ≥38.5°C.
    - Splenomegaly.
    - Cytopenias (affecting at least two of three lineages in the peripheral blood):
      - Hemoglobin <9 g/dL (in infants <4 weeks: hemoglobin <10 g/dL).
      - Platelets <100×10^3 cells/mL.
      - Neutrophils <1×10^3 cells/mL.

- Hypertriglyceridemia (fasting >265 mg/dL) and/or hypofibrinogenemia (<150 mg/dL).
- Hemophagocytosis in bone marrow or spleen or lymph nodes or liver.
- Low or absent NK-cell activity.
- Ferritin >500 ng/mL (usually much higher in HLH).
- Elevated Soluble CD25 (alpha chain of soluble IL-2 receptor).
- *Important to note that these are suggested criteria, and that a high clinical suspicion and consultation with a pediatric hematologist/oncologist is warranted.*

Management

- Children are often acutely ill, and usually require close pediatric intensive care unit support and monitoring.
- Therapy is generally initiated even if there are coinciding infections.
- Human leukocyte antigen (HLA) typing is usually sent early in the treatment course for possible stem cell transplantation.
- Induction therapy is generally with dexamethasone, etoposide +/− cyclosporine, with treatment weaning over 8 weeks.
- In patients with genetic/familial predisposition or recurrent/refractory disease, an allogeneic stem cell transplant with a HLA-matched donor is indicated.
  - Risk of recurrence is much higher in this patient population.
  - Caution must be used with a HLA-matched sibling, as they may also have the genetic/familial predisposition to HLH.

Hemophilia

Sheree H. Allen

Background/Definition

- Hemophilia is an X-linked, recessive coagulation disorder that occurs most commonly in males and is caused by specific clotting factor deficiencies. Females may rarely be affected, as in the case of a carrier mother and affected father. There is no racial or ethnic predilection for hemophilia. The majority of cases are diagnosed at birth due to a positive family history. Approximately one-third of hemophilia patients have no family history of hemophilia and develop the disease as a result of a new gene mutation.

Etiology

- Hemophilia A—"Classic hemophilia"— is a deficiency of Factor VIII, occurring 1 in 5,000 male births.
  - The most common and severe form; 80% to 85% of all hemophilia.
- Hemophilia B—"Christmas disease" is a deficiency of Factor IX deficiency.
  - 1 in 30,000 male births.

Pathophysiology

- When injury occurs, both intrinsic and extrinsic pathways of the clotting cascade are activated to form a stable fibrin clot and achieve secondary hemostasis. The severity of bleeding is dependent upon the degree of factor deficiency.

- Severe disease—persons with <1% of normal factor activity; may experience spontaneous or excessive bleeding following minimal trauma. Risk for trauma-induced hemorrhage.
- Moderate disease—persons with 2% to 5% of normal factor activity; typically bleed with trauma or surgery.
- Mild disease—persons with greater than 5% of normal factor activity; generally, experience only delayed clotting/bleeding associated with significant hemostatic challenges.

Clinical Presentation

- Symptoms: slow, persistent bleeding after minor injury, hematemesis or melena, epistaxis, hematuria, joint pain, swelling, and decreased range of motion due to bleeding into the joints (especially knees, ankles, and elbows), causing hemarthroses, ecchymosis, and subcutaneous hematoma.
  - Uncontrollable bleeding after injury.
    - 30% to 50% of patients experience earliest symptom during and after circumcision.
- Neonatal considerations include cephalohematoma, subdural, and periosteal bleeding during delivery, and intracranial hemorrhage (up to 2% of infants).

Diagnostic Evaluation

- Factor assay to determine deficiency.
  - Hemophilia A: factor VIII assay decreased, prolonged PTT, normal platelets.
  - Hemophilia B: factor IX assay decreased, prolonged PTT.
- Hematocrit may be decreased in presence of excessive bleeding, normal platelet count.
- PT will be normal, and PTT prolonged >60 seconds.

Management

- Blood Product Administration: fresh frozen plasma (FFP), Cryoprecipitate, PRBC.
- Factor Administration.
  - Prompt factor replacement minimizes the morbidity from hemorrhage.
    - Major bleeding—100% factor replacement.
    - Minor bleeding into muscles and joints—50% to 60% factor replacement.
    1. Mucocutaneous bleeding—30% to 50% replacement.
  - Factor VIII—(half-life 8–12 hours).
  - Factor IX—(half-life 12–24 hours).
  - 1-deamino-8-D-arginine vasopressin (DDAVP) for mild to moderate hemophilia A.
    - Parenteral DDAVP or Intranasal DDAVP.
  - Patients should be *pretreated* with 100% recombinant clotting factor concentrate prior to any surgical or invasive procedure.

Patient and Family Education

- Genetic counseling.
- *Avoid* medications that inhibit platelets or coagulation factors including NSAIDS, aspirin, anticoagulants, and certain antibiotics.
- Contact sports are not recommended.

- Vaccination for hepatitis A and hepatitis B is recommended.
- Maintain a healthy weight, exercise to increase muscle strength and protect joints.
- Annual evaluation at a Hemophilia Treatment Center.

Immune Thrombocytopenic Purpura

Sheree H. Allen

Background/Definition

- ITP is an acquired autoimmune disorder that results in destruction of platelets, which presents in healthy children. Peak age for presentation is from 2 to 6 years of age, with equal distribution between males and females until adolescence, when there is an increase in females with ITP.

Etiology

- Cause is unknown; may be acute or chronic.
- Frequently precipitated by a viral illness.
- Estimated incidence is 4 to 8 cases per 100,000 population per year (United States).
- Acute ITP is self-limiting in children <12 years of age; resolves within 6 months.
- Approximately 10% of children will develop chronic ITP.

Pathophysiology

- Antibodies develop.
- IgG, IgA, or IgM autoantibodies coat the platelets.
- Platelets are destroyed in the spleen with resulting splenic sequestration.
- Antibodies contribute to immature platelet production by the bone marrow.
- New platelets are destroyed within hours.
- Bleeding may occur as platelet count falls.

Clinical Presentation

- Bruising and petechiae, epistaxis, GI bleeding, hematuria, menorrhagia, spontaneous bleeding from mucous membranes and gingiva.
- Intracranial bleeding and splenomegaly are possible.

Diagnostic Evaluation

- Platelet count <100,000; large platelets on smear.
- PT and PTT (normal), Fibrinogen (normal), Fibrin degradation products (normal).
- Diagnosis may be confirmed by bone marrow aspiration; normocellular result with elevated megakaryocytes.

Management

- Acute ITP—goal is to restore the platelet count.
  - Oral corticosteroids; course may be weeks to months.
  - IV gamma globulin (IVIG) OR Anti D immunoglobulin (WinRho-D).
  - Recurrent monitoring of platelet count guides therapy.
  - Avoid NSAIDS and aspirin.

- Chronic ITP—(ITP lasting longer than 6 months).
  - Regular administration of IVIG or WinRho-D.
  - Splenectomy.

Henoch-Schönlein Purpura

Sheree H. Allen

Background/Definition

- An acute, systematic, immune complex mediated, small-vessel vasculitis, which is self-limiting and resolves within about 4 weeks, considered the most common vasculitis of childhood. Incidence of 10 to 20 cases per 100,000 children. Peak age at presentation is between 2 and 8, affecting more males than females and occurring primarily in fall, winter, and spring months. Renal impairment is the most serious complication.

Etiology

- Usually precipitated by an upper respiratory tract infection, medication, or other environmental trigger.
- Associated with many infectious agents, with most prevalent organism group A streptococcus; approximately 50% of patients with Henoch–Schönlein purpura have antistreptolysin O antibodies.

Pathophysiology

- Pathogenesis is not completely understood.
- IgA complexes are deposited in the small vessels of the renal glomeruli, skin, and GI tract, causing petechiae, purpura, GI bleeding, and glomerulonephritis.

Clinical Presentation

- Recent upper respiratory tract infection and prodrome of fever and fatigue.
- Commonly presents with tetrad of symptoms:
  - Rash: nonpruritic, erythematous papules or wheals that progress to petechiae, and nonblanching, palpable, purpuric lesions >10 mm diameter; found in dependent areas of body that are subject to pressure and extensor surfaces of the extremities. Trunk is usually spared, and lesions fade over 10 to 12 days.
  - Polyarthralgias: pain, swelling, decreased range of motion; Lower extremity joints most frequently involved.
  - "Bowel angina" - diffuse, colicky abdominal pain with melena and vomiting; approximately 70% of patients.
  - Renal symptoms with hematuria, proteinuria, and hypertension; approximately 20–60 % of patients weeks to months after initial presentation
    - Mild renal impairment may progress to nephrotic syndrome and ARF.
    - Renal biopsy consistent with focal and proliferative glomerulonephritis.

Diagnostic Evaluation

- Based on clinical features and presenting symptoms; renal function should be evaluated at baseline.
- Platelets normal or elevated.
- BUN and creatinine may be elevated.
- Normal coagulation studies.
- Immune antibody panel—Presence of IgA antibodies in the blood, skin, or glomeruli may help to confirm diagnosis.
- Urinalysis for evaluation of blood and protein.

Management

- Rest and activity limitations, with symptomatic management of systemic complications, NSAIDS.
- Oral prednisone; indicated for patients with kidney involvement.
- Henoch-Schönlein purpura resulting in severe kidney disease may require plasma exchange, high-dose IV immunoglobulin (IVIG), or immunosuppressant agents.
- Long-term management of hypertension may be required.

PEARL

- *Differential diagnosis should include IgA nephritis; evaluation for autoimmune conditions including systemic lupus erythematosus, acute hemorrhagic edema of infancy, septicemia, and other forms of vasculitis.*

Heparin-Induced Thrombocytopenia

Melanie Muller

Background

- Heparin-induced thrombosis (HIT) occurs in approximately 2% to 3% of pediatric patients who receive heparin.

Definition

- An immune mediated drug reaction that places the patient at a higher risk of thrombosis development.

Pathophysiology

- Presence of heparin in the body causes the formation of IgG antibodies that recognize platelet factor 4 (PF4), a protein on the surface of the platelet that is bound to the heparin.
- The IgG antibodies attach to the PF4–heparin complex, resulting in platelet activation and subsequent thrombin generation and formation of thrombosis.
- Thrombocytopenia results from increased platelet aggregation and consumption.

Etiology

- Exposure to heparin.
  - Duration and extent of exposure.

Clinical Presentation

- Thrombocytopenia; platelets decrease by >50% within the first 4 to 14 days after initiation of heparin.
- Occasionally, development of thrombosis is the first sign of HIT, more commonly venous thrombosis.
- In some patients, rapid onset of thrombocytopenia, occurring within minutes to hours after heparin exposure. This usually occurs as a result of heparin exposure in the previous 100 days.

Diagnostic Evaluation

- Diagnosis is made based on clinical presentation.
- Serotonin release assay, heparin-induces platelet activation test, and flow cytometric tests to detect platelet microparticle release may be used
- Evaluating for other etiologies of thrombocytopenia, including cardiopulmonary bypass within the last 48 hours, presence of bacteremia or fungemia, recent chemotherapy administration, and DIC due to other etiologies.

Management

- If suspected, immediate removal of heparin and low molecular weight heparin from all sources.
- If ongoing anticoagulation is needed, use vitamin K antagonist or direct thrombin inhibitor.
- Platelet recovery and disappearance of antibodies can take weeks once heparin is discontinued.

PEARL

- *In cases of suspected HIT, do not delay treatment while awaiting confirmatory testing*

Glucose-6-Phosphate Dehydrogenase Deficiency

Myra Cleary

Background/Definition

- G6PD deficiency is a partial or complete deletion of G6PD, an enzyme that is crucial in aerobic glycolysis. Children who have G6PD-deficient RBCs are susceptible to oxidative damage and hemolysis during certain conditions of stress, exposure to certain medications, foods, or chemicals. Occurs most often in males.

Etiology/Types

- Three forms have been described.
  - Variant 1: G6PD activity is less than 10% of normal, resulting in severe neonatal jaundice or congenital nonspherocytic hemolytic anemia.
  - Variant 2: G6PD activity is typically less than 30% of the normal range, resulting in an asymptomatic steady state. Individuals who carry this mutation are at risk for neonatal jaundice, acute hemolytic anemia, and favism.
  - Variant 3: Enzyme activity is greater than 85% of the normal reference range, resulting in no clinical manifestations. Considered the "wild type" disease.
- X-linked inherited disease that affects primarily men.

Pathophysiology

- G6PD is the first enzyme in the hexose monophosphate shunt. This enzyme is required for the production of the reduced form of nicotinamide adenine dinucleotide phosphate (NADPH).
- NADPH is critical in preventing oxidative damage.

- RBCs are susceptible to oxidative damage since they carry oxygen.
- Reactive oxygen radicals damage the RBC membrane and hemoglobin resulting in hemolysis of the RBC.

Clinical Presentation

- Children with G6PD deficiency are clinically and hematologically normal for the majority of their lifetime.
- Acute exacerbations may occur with the ingestion of fava beans (favism), during the course of an infection, and exposure to oxidative drugs (e.g., antimalarials, sulfa-containing drugs, aspirin, and quinolones).
- Symptoms: fever, nausea, abdominal pain, diarrhea, and occasionally vomiting within 24 to 48 hours after oxidative challenge.
- Findings: Dark brown or black discoloration of the urine is present within 6 to 24 hours after exposure (result of hemolysis); jaundice, pallor, tachycardia, hypovolemic shock, and hepatosplenomegaly may develop.

Diagnostic Evaluation

- Severe anemia with marked variation in the size of the RBCs resulting in an increase in the RBC distribution width. WBC count may be elevated.
- Large polychromatic cells with spherocytic morphology as well as markedly irregular-shaped cells known as poikilocytes on peripheral blood smear.
- Increased reticulocyte count; may reach levels as high as 30%.
- Heinz body stain: As the RBCs circulate through the spleen, Heinz bodies are removed, resulting in classic "bite cells." Heinz bodies are identified with methyl violet staining and are denatured hemoglobin and a manifestation of the oxidative injury to the hemoglobin.
- Hemoglobinuria may be present.

Management

- Blood transfusion is indicated if the child is hemodynamically unstable or the hemoglobin level declines to <7g/dL.
- If the hemoglobin is <9 g/dL with evidence of persistent brisk hemolysis with hemoglobinuria, blood transfusion may be indicated.
- Dialysis may be indicated for acute kidney failure.
- Neonatal jaundice related to G6PD deficiency is managed with observation for mild cases, phototherapy, and hydration for more significant cases, and exchange transfusion may be beneficial for severe cases.

Methemoglobinemia

Christine A. Schindler

Background/Definition

- Methemoglobinemia is an uncommon cause of cyanosis in infants and children that is a result of the heme iron being in the ferric rather than ferrous state. Under these conditions, oxygen binding to hemoglobin is severely impaired. A small amount of methemoglobin is normal (higher baseline levels in smokers); however, when a large portion of methemoglobin is present, cyanosis can result due to the inability of methemoglobin to carry oxygen.

Etiology/Types

- Congenital methemoglobinemia is caused by diminished enzymatic reduction of methemoglobin back to functional hemoglobin. Patients may present with a cyanotic appearance, but may be aysmptomatic.
- Acquired methemoglobinemia is generally caused from exposure to certain medications or agents that cause an increase in the production of methemoglobin.
  - Substances that have been implicated in the formation of methemoglobin include:
    - Oxidant drugs: Sulfonamide antibiotics, Quinones, Phenacetin, Benzocaine.
    - Domestic and environmental substances: foods containing nitrates or nitrites, well water with nitrates, aniline dyes, naphthalene (mothballs), soap enemas, certain industrial compounds (e.g., nitrobenzenes, nitrous gases, organic amines).

Pathophysiology

- Methemoglobin is an altered state of hemoglobin in which the ferrous (Fe^{2+}) irons of heme are oxidized to the ferric (Fe^{3+}) state. The ferric hemes are unable to bind to oxygen, resulting in an inability of the methemoglobin-containing hemoglobin to carry oxygen. The ultimate result is impaired oxygen delivery to the tissues and cyanosis.

Clinical Presentation

- Symptoms depend on the concentration of methemoglobin:
  - 10% to 30% methemoglobin—cyanosis only.
  - 30% to 50% methemoglobin—dyspnea, tachycardia, dizziness, fatigue, headache.
  - 50% to 70% methemoglobin—severe lethargy and stupor.
  - >70% methemoglobin—death.
- Oxygen administration fails to affect the cyanosis.
- "Chocolate"-appearing blood with laboratory sampling.

Diagnostic Evaluation

- Patients with methemoglobinemia and cyanosis may have normal oxygen saturation measurements on pulse oximetry.
- Rapid screening test—A drop of the patient's blood should be placed on filter paper. After the filter paper is waved in the air for 30 to 60 seconds, normal blood appears bright red, while blood from a patient with methemoglobinemia remains reddish-brown.
- Spectrophotometric assays—used for confirmation of methemoglobinemia and for determination of the level of methemoglobin.
- Arterial blood gas with co-oximetry to measure level of methemoglobin.

Management

- Remove the causative substance.

- Depends on clinical severity:
  - Mild symptoms—therapy unnecessary.
  - Severe symptoms—treatment is administration of Methylene blue.
  - Failure of methylene blue therapy may be a result of concomitant G6PD deficiency. Ascorbic acid may be of some value, but if severe symptoms persist, exchange transfusion or hyperbaric oxygen may be required.

Sickle Cell Disease
Nneka Okoye

Background/Definition

- Sickle cell disease (SCD) encompasses a group of hemoglobinopathies in which an abnormal sickle hemoglobin gene is inherited. Sickling of blood cells causes increased hemolysis, anemia, and acute and chronic vasoocclusive complications that affect multiple organs of varying severity.

Etiology/Types

- There are several different types of SCD ranging in severity, listed below from most to least common.
  - Sickle cell anemia (HbSS)—most common, majority of patients, and most severe form of disease.
  - Sickle hemoglobin C disease (HbSC)—typically milder disease.
  - Sickle β^+ thalassemia (HbSβ^+Thal)—typically milder disease.
  - Sickle β^0 thalassemia (HbSβ^0Thal)—typically severe disease.
  - Rare types of SCD—sickle hemoglobin D disease (HbSD), sickle hemoglobin E disease (HbSE), sickle hemoglobin O disease (HbSO). Variable severity.
  - Sickle cell trait (AS)—This is not a type of SCD, but an asymptomatic carrier state affecting 10% of African Americans.

Pathophysiology

- Autosomal recessive inherited disorder.
- Cause of SCD is the substitution of valine for glutamic acid at the sixth position of beta (β) globin. The immediate consequence of the mutation is that deoxygenated hemoglobin S polymerizes and distorts the shape of the RBC into a sickle shape.
- Sickle hemoglobin also has adverse effects on the red cell membrane that causes oxidative damage, cellular dehydration, abnormal phospholipid asymmetry, and increased adherence to endothelial cells.
- The net result of these cellular abnormalities is a shortened red cell lifespan (e.g., hemolysis) and intermittent episodes of vascular occlusion that cause tissue ischemia and acute and chronic organ dysfunction.

Clinical Presentation

- Clinical manifestations are widely variable in all forms of SCD, ranging from asymptomatic, mildly affected, to severely affected.
- See clinical presentation table below (Table 10.1).

TABLE 10.1 **Clinical Presentation and Management of Sickle Cell Disease**

Clinical Manifestation	Description	Signs and Symptoms	Management	Comments
Anemia	Decreased hemoglobin and hematocrit.	Often asymptomatic, fatigue, pallor, dizziness, jaundice.	Transfusion.	Most marked in HbSS and HbSβ Thalassemia.
Vasoocclusive crisis/event	Vascular occlusion by sickled cells causing tissue ischemia. Wide range of pain. Common triggers are cold temperatures, hypoxia, dehydration, acidosis.	Pain and tenderness of affected area, painful area may be edematous. Low-grade fever possible.	Acetaminophen, NSAIDs, opiates, heat, distraction, massage, hydration.	In infants may manifest as dactylitis/hand–foot syndrome.
Infections	Functional asplenia can result in: severe bacterial infections, sepsis, meningitis, osteomyelitis.	Fever, pain, malaise, tachycardia, tachypnea, hypotension, lethargy, weakness, anorexia.	Fevers of 101.5°F or higher: prompt evaluation, bacterial cultures, empiric parenteral broad-spectrum antibiotics. Penicillin prophylaxis until at least 5 y of age.	Can be life-threatening.
Splenic sequestration	Sickled RBCs pool in spleen, causing splenomegaly, severe anemia, and shock.	Splenomegaly, abdominal pain, lethargy, pallor, hypotension, tachycardia, weakness, irritability.	Consult hematology. Blood transfusion, IV fluids, pain management, serial CBC monitoring, for recurrent episodes splenectomy.	Typically occurs in patients <5y. Can be life-threatening. Chronic splenomegaly may be seen in those with HbSC.
Acute chest syndrome	Occlusion of lung vasculature by sickled cells causing tissue ischemia.	New infiltrate on CXR along with one or more of the following: tachypnea, fever, cough, chest pain, shortness of breath or hypoxia. Often associated with significant decrease in hemoglobin.	Antibiotics, oxygen, bronchodilators, pain management, blood transfusion, mechanical ventilation support. Exchange transfusion most often beneficial.	Clinical condition may deteriorate rapidly. Can be life-threatening.
Cerebrovascular accident	Vascular occlusion by sickled cells and/or damage to endothelial cells of blood vessels. Ischemia of brain tissue and neurological deficits. Strokes may be ischemic or hemorrhagic.	Motor or sensory deficits, cognitive deficits, asymptomatic with silent strokes.	Exchange transfusion, followed by chronic transfusions.	Can be life-threatening.
Aplastic crisis	Severe anemia with reticulocytopenia often caused by viral infections.	Lethargy, pallor, malaise, fever, symptoms of upper respiratory infection.	Pain management, pseudoephedrine, hydration, consult urology for penile aspiration.	Common etiology: Parvovirus B19.
Avascular necrosis	Bone ischemia and necrosis due to a lack of blood supply to area.	Joint pain especially with ambulation, bone collapse may occur in late stages.	Surgical emergency.	Commonly affects hips and shoulders. Seen more frequently in HbSC.

TABLE 10.1 **Clinical Presentation and Management of Sickle Cell Disease** (*Continued*)

Clinical Manifestation	Description	Signs and Symptoms	Management	Comments
Priapism	Painful long-lasting erections.	Painful erection.	Pain management, pseudoephedrine, hydration, penile aspiration.	
Retinopathy	Vascular occlusion of the vessels in the eye.	Visual changes, vitreous hemorrhage, retinal detachment.	Ophthalmology.	Seen more frequently in HbSC.
Cholelithiasis/ Cholecystitis	Hemolysis leads to increased buildup of bilirubin, resulting in gallstones.	Abdominal pain, jaundice.	Consult surgery.	Typically seen in older children and adolescents.
Delayed growth and puberty	Shorter stature and delayed puberty.	Late gonadarche, adrenarche, thelarche, menarche.		Will attain normal height with late adolescent growth.

Diagnostic Evaluation

- SCD can be identified through newborn screening in all 50 US states.
- Confirmatory testing is done with hemoglobin electrophoresis.
- Prenatal diagnosis is available via amniocentesis or chorionic villus sampling.

Management

- The only cure for sickle cell anemia is BMT.
- Hydroxyurea is the only disease-modifying medication to treat SCD; increases fetal hemoglobin levels, resulting in decreased incidence of complications.
- Other supportive care includes:
  - Initiation of penicillin prophylaxis by 2 months of age and continued to at least 5 years of age.
  - Additional vaccines (i.e., pneumococcal and meningococcal) given at age 2 and 5 years of age.
  - Blood transfusions, either simple, exchange, or chronic.

Thalassemia

Cathy Haut

Background

- Most common worldwide genetic disorder.
- α-Thalassemia is typically seen in Southeast Asia, people of African descent, China, and Middle East. Greater than 50% of some populations carry the α-thalassemia gene.

- β-Thalassemia is most common in people of Mediterranean descent; 1.7% of the world's population has α- or β-thalassemia trait.
- Must inherit defective genes from both parents to have thalassemia major.
- Thalassemia minor is often found in an asymptomatic carrier.

Definition

- Thalassemia is an autosomal dominant hematologic disorder that results in the production of an abnormal form of hemoglobin that results in destruction of RBCs.

Etiology/Types

- α-Thalassemia major.
- β-Thalassemia major, also called "Cooley Anemia."
- Thalassemia minor.

Pathophysiology

- The thalassemias are classified according to the chain of the hemoglobin molecule that is affected. α-Thalassemia occurs when a gene or genes related to the α-globin protein are missing or changed (mutated). β-Thalassemia occurs when similar gene defects affect production of the β-globin protein. Both types result in excessive destruction of RBCs, causing anemia.

Clinical Presentation

- Typical features: chipmunk facies with prominent frontal bossing, delayed pneumatization of the sinuses, marked overgrowth of maxillae.
- Bones and ribs become "box-like," premature fusion of epiphyses, and thinning of the cortex of the bone.

- Findings: hepatomegaly, splenomegaly, enlarged kidneys with dilated renal tubules, dark urine, cardiac abnormalities, and delayed sexual development.

Diagnostic Evaluation

- Anemia, typically found in the first year of life.
- Hypochromic, microcytic anemia with decreased MCV, basophilic stippling, presence of Hgb A.
- May have hyperuricemia.

Management

- Primary treatment is blood transfusion and folate replacement.
- BMT from a matched sibling donor is the best chance for cure.
- Complications include iron overload from transfusions, congestive heart failure, and early death.

Thromboembolytic Disorders
Christine Guelcher

Background

- Although relatively uncommon in pediatric patients, the incidence of venous thromboembolism is increasing as a result of advances in surgical and medical care for previously fatal illnesses. Thrombotic complications in pediatric patients are often a result of therapies, including central venous catheters.

Definition

- Thrombosis is pathological formation of a blood clot (thrombus) in a blood vessel affecting blood flow. The thrombus may be occlusive or nonocclusive and either provoked or unprovoked. Embolism occurs when the thrombus travels through the blood vessels to the lungs, brain, or elsewhere, causing significant life-threatening acute events.
- Most pediatric thrombotic events are associated with at least one risk factor, which can include genetic (e.g., inherited thrombophilia) or acquired (e.g., sepsis, trauma, dehydration, use of oral contraceptives).

Pathophysiology

- According to Virchow's triad concept, thrombosis is caused by a disruption of one of the three elements in this triad: changes in the vessel wall, alteration in blood flow, or increased coagulability of the blood.

Etiology/Risk Factors

- Acquired risk factors: obesity, smoking, cancer, and medications including L-Asparginase and estrogen-based hormones.
- Increased risk in pregnancy related to elevations of procoagulant factors and relative deficiency of anticoagulant factors.
- Trauma can lead to vessel damage; can be compounded by venous stasis secondary to bed rest during recovery.
- Antiphospholipid antibodies.

- Presence of antiphospholipid antibodies on two occasions (separated by 12 weeks) and a thrombotic event is considered antiphospholipid syndrome.
- Significantly increased risk for recurrent thrombosis.
- Consider indefinite anticoagulation to prevent repeated thrombotic events.
- Inherited risk factors.
  - Factor V Leiden mutation is the most common inherited thrombophilia, affecting 5% of Caucasians; rare in African or Asian populations. Factor V is not cleaved by activated protein C, resulting in resistance to activated protein C.
  - Prothrombin gene mutation is the second-most common inherited thrombophilia, more common in Caucasians, involving point mutation that results in increased levels of prothrombin (factors).
  - Protein S deficiency is rare (0.03%–0.13%).
  - Elevated factor VIII, an acute phase reactant, is increased by stresses to the system (e.g., trauma, surgery).

Presentation

- Symptoms: impaired/absent blood flow in a deep vein. DVT in an extremity results in painful swelling of the extremity; symptoms depend on the location of the clot and the impact on blood flow to the distal vessels.
- VT in the neck vessels can result in superior vena cava syndrome.
- Pulmonary embolus can be life-threatening; symptoms may be more subtle in pediatric patients.
- Cerebral sinus venous thrombosis is a thrombus in the deep veins of the head, resulting in persistent headache, blurred vision, neurologic signs, or seizures.
- Renal vein thrombosis is associated with nephrotic syndrome, presenting with generalized edema.
- Portal vein thrombosis causes splenomegaly with thrombocytopenia and anemia. Esophageal varices can result.
- May–Thurner Syndrome is a vascular anomaly in the pelvis in which the right common iliac artery compresses the left common iliac vein; predisposes patients to left lower extremity DVT.
- Paget–Schroetter syndrome is an upper extremity DVT that results from venous thoracic outlet syndrome, in which the axillary and subclavian veins are compressed at their exit site into the chest. Thrombosis is triggered by repetitive overhead arm motion (e.g., baseball pitching) that exacerbates the compression.

Diagnostic Evaluation

- Imaging.
  - DVT—Doppler ultrasound can document the presence and extent of most DVTs (CT/MRI evaluate extension into the pelvis or head).
  - Pulmonary embolus—Spiral CT or ventilation–perfusion scan.
  - Cerebral sinus venous thrombosis—Contrast-enhanced MRI scan.
  - Renal vein thrombosis, portal vein thrombosis—Doppler US or Contrast CT scan.

Laboratory Evaluation

- Evaluate for prothrombotic risk factors.
- Some laboratory tests (e.g., protein C, protein S, ATIII) may be low with acute thrombosis.
- Other laboratory tests may be elevated (e.g., factor VIII) with acute thrombosis.
- Tests should be repeated if abnormal in the acute phase of disease.
- Anticoagulation monitoring:
  - PTT is an indirect measurement of anticoagulation and should be correlated with patient's anti-Xa level.
  - Anti-Xa is a more direct measure of heparin anticoagulation.
  - Anti-Xa levels for patients receiving low molecular weight heparin (e.g., Enoxaparin).
  - PT for patients receiving vitamin K antagonist (e.g., warfarin).

Management

- The American College of Chest Physicians guidelines (2012) recommend that pediatric patients with a catheter-related thrombotic event undergo removal of a central venous access device within 3 to 5 days of starting anticoagulation. Follow protocols for continued therapy and prophylaxis if catheter is not removed.
- For pediatric patients who have other risk factors that may resolve, the guidelines suggest anticoagulation treatment for at least 3 months or more with consideration of risk factor resolution (Figure 10.1).
- Patients with occlusive thrombosis will develop collateral vessels, and some thrombi will never completely resolve. Anticoagulation therapy is designed to prevent propagation of the thrombus as fibrinolysis will occur to break down clot.

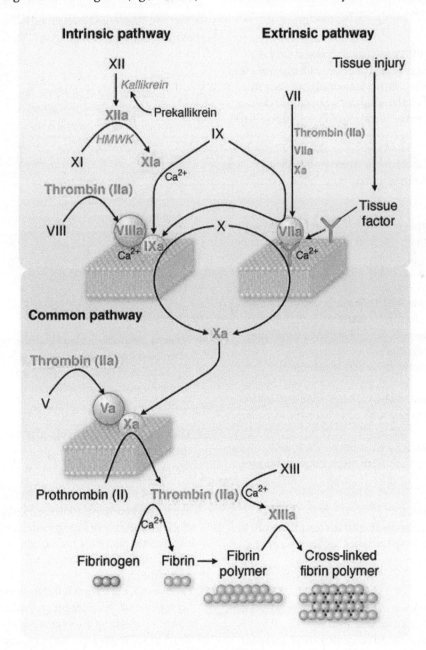

FIGURE 10.1 • **Coagulation Cascade.**

Von Willebrand Disease

Christine Guelcher

Background

- Von Willebrand disease (VWD) was first discussed in 1924 as a bleeding disorder that was associated primarily with mucosal membrane bleeding. Inheritance pattern is autosomal dominant. Affected patients had prolonged bleeding times, but normal clotting times. VWD affects between 0.1% and 1% of the world population.

Definition

- A disease of either a quantitative deficiency or qualitative defect of the von Willebrand protein.

Etiology/Types

- There are three main types of VWD that are characterized by the qualitative or quantitative defects in von Willebrand factor (VWF).

Pathophysiology

- Some VWF is produced in Weibel–Pilade bodies and stored in epithelial cells that line the blood vessels.
- VWF synthesized in macrophages and stored in α-granules
- Binds to factor VIII in circulation.
- Mobilized to site of vessel injury where it adheres to endothelium.
- May be released from endothelial cells in response to injury.
- Interacts with platelets to help with adherence and activation at the site of injury.
- Patients who are deficient or have a defect of VWF are at risk for prolonged bleeding, particularly from the mucous membranes.

Clinical Presentation

- Often diagnosed later in life.
- History of easy bruising, frequent epistaxis (incidence can be 50% to 75%), heavy menstrual bleeding, or bleeding after a surgical/dental procedure.

Diagnostic Evaluation

- Von Willebrand protein levels may fluctuate, so repeated laboratory testing may be needed for diagnosis.
- Other screening tests can be used to identify coagulation factors and assist in diagnosis, but studies are complicated and not always reliable.

Management

- Treatment capitalizes on interactions that occur during times of stress or with hormonal changes.
- Desmopressin acetate (DDAVP).
  - Stimulates release of VWF and factor VIII.
  - Management of prolonged or refractory bleeding and prior to minor elective procedures.
- Antifibrinolytic agents.
  - Used in managing recurrent bleeding in VWD, but do not stop active bleeding; slow the breakdown of clots to preventing rebleeding.
- Aminocaproic acid (Amicar); contraindicated with hematuria.
- Tranexamic acid (Lysteda): FDA-approved for menorrhagia.
- VWF concentrates are derived from human blood donation.
- The von Willebrand containing factors have both von Willebrand antigen and factor VIII.

Transfusion Therapy

Cathy Haut

Background

- Modern methods of blood transfusions began only in 1901, when blood types were discovered.
- Pretransfusion typing is performed to determine the best match for minimal complications.

Definition

- The transfer of blood or blood products from a donor to a recipient.

Physiology

- The main function of blood is facilitation of delivery of oxygen and nutrients to tissues. Oxygen is carried by hemoglobin, an iron-containing protein. Blood also transports electrolytes, nutrients such as glucose, and waste products. The maintenance of immune surveillance is another function of blood.
- FFP is extracted from whole blood and contains coagulation, fibrolytic, and complement systems that assist in the restoration of coagulation disorders such as DIC.
- Platelets are responsible for hemostasis with resulting thrombus formation. Transfusion of platelets is used to restore abnormally low levels.

- Cryoprecipitate is obtained by centrifuging plasma and removing the precipitate. It is not used as commonly as FFP, but can be used to replace low fibrinogen levels and when certain factors are not available for treatment of coagulation disorders.

Clinical Presentation

- Transfusions are performed for a variety of diagnoses, both acute and chronic.
- RBC transfusions are administered to increase oxygen circulation and delivery.
- Guidelines for transfusion vary somewhat, often based on symptomatology, reason for transfusion, underlying disease process, and age and weight of patient.

Diagnostic Evaluation

- Transfusion of PRBCs, platelets, and FFP is based on underlying hematologic profiles and crossmatching.
- Other indices, including presence of antibodies, are also important for matching appropriate products with recipients. This is especially significant in patients that may require stem cell or organ transplantation.
- Management; typically weight based.
  - PRBC 10 to 20 mL/kg per transfusion.
  - Platelets 1 unit per every 10 kg patient weight; expect approximately 50,000/µL rise.
  - FFP 10 to 15 mL/kg per transfusion.
  - Cryoprecipitate 1 unit per every 10 kg patient weight; expect rise of 60 to 100 mg/dL.
    Calculating PRBC transfusion dose—What is the target or goal for the hematocrit?

    $$\text{Volume of PREC required (mLs)} = \frac{\text{HCT (d)} - \text{HCT (i)} \times \text{TBV}}{\text{HCT}_{PRBCs}}$$

    HCT (d) desired HCT.
    HCT (i) initial HCT.
    TBV total body volume: (infant—100 mL/kg, child—80 mL/kg, adult—65 mL/kg).

PEARLS

- *Anemia is possible when children drink large volumes of milk.*
- *Stored PRBC's lack calcium content, so children who receive any type of multiple transfusion require additional calcium.*
- *PRBCs stored >5 days are associated with higher potassium concentrations.*
- *Based on illness severity, infants <4 months of age will not require crossmatching, and in critical, emergent situations, un-crossmatched blood can be used for children of other ages.*
- *Estimating circulating blood volume is based on an average calculation of 80 mL/kg. Adult volumes are 70 mL/kg.*
- *Massive transfusion complications include thrombocytopenia, hypocalcemia, coagulation factor depletion, hyperkalemia, and increased levels of lactic acid, leading to acid–base disorders, hypothermia, and altered or decreased oxygen delivery to tissues.*

Chronic Transfusion Therapy

Cathy Haut

Background/Definition

- Children with transfusion-dependent hemoglobinopathies, including SCD and thalassemia, along with children with other forms of chronic anemia may require frequent or regular transfusions. Children with other forms of chronic anemia may also require chronic transfusions.

Physiology

- The clinical challenge of chronic red cell transfusion therapy is managing the resulting iron overload. Each unit of RBC's contains 200 to 250 mg of iron, with repeated transfusions saturating the patient's transferrin. Accumulation of iron leads to the formation of nontransferrin-bound iron, which is associated with progressive organ damage, primarily liver and heart disease.
- 10 to 20 PRBC transfusions can saturate the transferrin.
- In children, iron accumulation in the anterior pituitary gland will produce systemic endocrine disturbances, including delayed sexual maturation and growth failure.

Presentation

- Congestive heart failure can be present in children as young as 15 years of age as a result of iron overload.

Diagnostic Evaluation

- Serum ferritin levels.
- Liver iron concentrations by biopsy.
- Superconducting quantum interference device.
- Modified MRI for evaluation of cardiac iron overload.

Management

- Routine screening for signs of iron overload (e.g., CHF).
- Iron chelation therapy is often required.
  - Chelation therapies are utilized to treat iron overload by binding metal ions that are then excreted through feces.
  - Deferoxamine, IV chelation agent.
  - Deferasirox, oral chelation agent is administered once daily.

Transfusion Reaction and Evaluation

Danielle Van Damme & Barbara Wise

Background

- Blood transfusion–related adverse events include transfusion-associated infection, transfusion-related acute lung injury, medical error, and transfusion reactions.
- Blood transfusion reactions can be classified as immune or nonimmune, acute or delayed, and then include hemolytic, febrile, allergic, or anaphylactic reactions (Table 10.2).

TABLE 10.2 Common Pediatric Blood Transfusion Reactions

Reaction	Definition and Etiology	Pathophysiology	Clinical Presentation	Diagnostic Evaluation	Management
TRALI: transfusion-related acute lung injury	Acute onset of respiratory distress during or within 6 hr of transfusion. Infusion of FFP. Multiparous donors. Recipient characteristics and sepsis.	Pulmonary endothelial damage from donor HLA class I and II antibodies activated by the patient's antigen positive neutrophils. WBC alloantibody-mediated reaction.	Hypotension, fever, tachycardia, hypoxemia, pulmonary infiltrates, with no evidence of left atrial hypertension during or within 6 hr of transfusion. Physical examination—diffuse rales and respiratory distress.	Chest radiograph, blood gas if indicated.	Oxygen. Supportive ventilation as indicated. Stop blood product transfusion.
Acute hemolytic reaction	ABO-incompatible or other RBC antigen incompatibilities that occur when wrong type is administered. Etiology includes preexisting iso-hemoglutinins.	Transfused red cells react with recipient antibody: intravascular hemolysis.	Fever, chills, rigor, lumbar pain, chest pain, nausea, vomiting, and hematuria. Severe reaction: shock, acute tubular necrosis, and disseminated intravascular coagulation, leading to significant morbidity and mortality.	Repeat ABO typing, CBC, renal and liver studies and evaluation of urine for hemoglobin, coagulation screen, direct antiglobulin test (DAT), lactate dehydrogenase (LDH), haptoglobin, oxygen saturation and chest radiograph.	Immediately stop the transfusion Administer normal saline through a free flowing venous access line. Check the patient for label compatibility and evaluate unit of blood.
Febrile nonhemolytic reaction	Reaction caused by antileukocyte antibodies, often in children who have received multiple blood transfusions. Recipient antibodies directed against the leukocytes in the RBC. Infusion of pyrogenic cytokines or inflammatory mediators in stored blood. Platelet transfusions caused by cytokines in stored products.	Presence of pyogenic cytokines released from donor lymphocytes. Occurs more frequently with platelet transfusions.	Fever and chills occur at any point, up to a few hours after a transfusion. Temperature ≥1°C from pretransfusion temperature, chills, and myalgias. Pruritus, urticaria, maculopapular rash, and bronchospasm that occur after infusion of several mLs of blood. Anaphylactic reactions are systemic and severe characterized by angioedema, respiratory distress, hypotension, erythema, and periorbital edema.	Blood cultures, Direct Antiglobulin Coombs test (DAT).	Immediately stop the transfusion. Administer antipyretics, narcotics for rigors, and administer antibiotics if sepsis suspected. Premedicate with antipyretics. Evaluate for other causes of fever. Leukoreduction to remove WBCs and platelets from product.

TABLE 10.2 Common Pediatric Blood Transfusion Reactions (Continued)

Reaction	Definition and Etiology	Pathophysiology	Clinical Presentation	Diagnostic Evaluation	Management
Allergic transfusion reaction	Most common transfusion reaction. Idiosyncratic related to plasma protein sensitization. Reaction leading to acute urticaria is an IgE-mediated response, which is rarely severe and often self-limiting.	Protein binds to the cell associated with IgA. Mast cell releases cytokines, histamine, and leukotrines. Histamine release causes pruritis, erythema, and urticaria. Anaphylactoid reaction results in bronchospasm and laryngeal edema. Anaphylactic reaction results from an IgG anti-IgA deficiency and causes hypotension and shock.	Pruritis, erythema, bronchospasm, laryngeal edema, hypotension and shock.	Screen patient for anti-IgA for moderate or severe allergic reaction.	May not require termination of blood transfusion and may be managed with antihistamines. Stop transfusion if indicated. Administer IM epinephrine emergently, oral or IV antihistamines and fluid boluses with crystalloid for hydration. Premedicate with antihistamines and/or corticosteroids.
Delayed hemolytic transfusion reaction	"Minor" RBC antigen mismatch. Memory response, IgG response that occurs secondary to prior transfusion or pregnancy.	Destruction of transfused cells by alloantibody through extravascular hemolysis.	Nonspecific symptoms. May occur 7–14 d posttransfusion. Anemia, hyperbilirubinemia, hemoglobinuria, myalgias, unexplained drop in hemoglobin, extravascular hemolysis, chills, pain, transient jaundice, and low-grade fever.	Laboratory evaluation for red cell antibodies — most frequently anti-Kidd or anti-Duffy and bilirubinemia.	Supportive care. Identify alternatives to transfusion.
Anaphylactic transfusion reaction	Occurs in children with IgA deficiency and IgA antibodies, who receive blood transfusion containing IgA. Reaction can be severe and life-threatening after infusion of only a few milliliters of blood.	Pathophysiology mostly unknown. Can be linked to two primary processes: 1. Anti-IgA—Congenital IgA deficiency may develop anti-IgA antibodies; exposure to IgA can lead to anaphylactic reaction. 2. Hypersensitivity to protein in the plasma of the transfused blood.	Symptoms can include chills, flushing, hypertension, followed by hypotension, leading to shock.	Urinalysis for hemoglobin-uria. Serum specimen to evaluate for elevated LDH, hyperbilirubinemia, elevated BUN and creatinine, and coagulopathy. Blood cultures should be sent with a febrile reaction to evaluate for infectious etiology.	Blood products should be washed red blood cells or from an IgA deficient donor. Mild reactions (isolated temperature 38°C and/or rash) restart the transfusion and observe the patient. Moderate reactions (temperature ≥ 39°C & symptoms other than rash) monitor patient more frequently. Acute reactions, administer oxygen, bronchodilators and treat acute symptoms/resuscitation if necessary.

(Continued)

TABLE 10.2 Common Pediatric Blood Transfusion Reactions (*Continued*)

Reaction	Definition and Etiology	Pathophysiology	Clinical Presentation	Diagnostic Evaluation	Management
Antiserum agglutinates to RBC	Alloantibodies to Rh blood group (most common are C, E, and K), resulting in extravascular hemolysis. Frequent transfusions and the disparity in RBC phentoype between the donor and recipient.	Rh(D)-positive RBC exposure or Rh-negative patient. Extravascular hemolysis.	Hyperhemolysis, fever, pain, splenomegaly, and acute respiratory distress syndrome (ARDS).	Pretransfusion testing for RBC antigens by serology and genotyping, CBC, antibody screen and hemoglobin S (for SCD patients).	Stop transfusion. Administer anti-Rh(D) IgG (Rhogam, RhIg) with exposure. Match patient with attention to blood group (C, E, K). Administer fluids, steroids, IVIG, erythropoietin, and RBC transfusion. Administer transfusions from male donors.
Hemolysis	Acute reaction due to ABO incompatibility. Inadvertent transfusion of red cells that are incompatible with recipient antibodies, most severe type is A administered to O recipient.	Immune mediated caused by IgM anti-A, anti-B, resulting in intravascular hemolysis.	Chills, rigors, hypotension, tachycardia, hemoglobinuria, microvascular bleeding, epistaxis, renal failure, disseminated intravascular coagulation (DIC).	Hemoglobinemia, hemoglobinuria, elevated LDH.	Stop transfusion. Direct antiglobulin test (DAT)/Coombs test, repeat patient ABO, visible investigation of posttransfusion sample. Symptom management/ Resuscitation as necessary.

- *Administer blood products (RBC and platelets) through a leukofiltration system to reduce the risk of febrile reactions, platelet alloimmunization, and CMV transmission.*
- *Irradiate blood products to prevent posttransfusion GVHD.*
- *Use leukoreduction for blood products (except granulocytes) to decrease the risk of sensitization, the risk of CMV, and decrease the number of febrile nonhemolytic transfusion reactions. Administer CMV–negative blood.*
- *Washed products reduce the risk of inflammatory markers.*
- *Administer single donor platelets to reduce the exposure to multiple donors, platelet alloimmunization, and septic reactions.*
- *For chronically transfused patients, administer units ≤21 days old.*
- *Use ethnic-/race-matched potential donors.*

Oncologic Disorders

Brain Tumors

Kristi Waddell & Wendy S. Fitzgerald

Background

- Pediatric brain tumors are a heterogeneous mix of tumors with a wide variety of clinical symptoms and treatment modalities. Outcomes vary from 0% to 95% for 5-year event-free survival. They are the most common pediatric solid tumor and the second-most common childhood cancer, accounting for 17% of all childhood malignancies.

Definition

- Malignant lesions/tissue arising in the CNS, including the brain and spinal cord.
- Classification is based on location:
  - Infratentorial (posterior fossa)—cerebellum and brainstem.
  - Supratentorial—cerebrum, basal ganglia, thalamus, hypothalamus and optic chiasm, parasellar, spinal.

Types

- Low-grade glioma (i.e., astrocytoma).
- High-grade glioma (e.g., anaplastic astrocytoma, glioblastoma multiforme).
- Medulloblastoma.
- Ependymoma.
- Germ cell tumor.
- Diffuse intrinsic pontine glioma.
- Primary neuroectodermal tumor.
- Atypical teratoid rhabdoid tumor.

Clinical Presentation

- Dependent on histology, tumor location, patient age, and associated brain function.
- Supratentorial tumors: seizures, hemiparesis, hemisensory loss, hyperreflexia, visual complaints; infratentorial tumors: ataxia, cranial neuropathies.
- Signs and symptoms of increased intracranial pressure (e.g., headaches, early morning emesis) related to obstruction of cerebral spinal fluid (CSF) and resultant hydrocephalus, cranial nerve deficits (e.g., ataxia, dysmetria, difficulty swallowing, esotropia, nystagmus, seizures).
- Infants/toddlers can present with full/bulging fontanelle and loss of milestones, irritability, developmental delay, regression, "setting sun sign."
- Personality/behavior changes, confusion, lethargy are additional signs.
- Spinal cord tumors as a dissemination of brain tumors manifest through sensory deficits, long nerve-tract motor deficits, or both (e.g., back pain, radicular pain, bowel or bladder dysfunction).
- Brain lesions that occupy specific areas of the brain will alter function that is controlled by the area (Table 10.3) (Figure 10.2).

Diagnostic Evaluation

- Suspicion of a brain tumor is a medical emergency.
- History and physical examination with complete neurologic examination.
- CT scan; detects approximately 95% of brain tumors—can be used as a screening tool.
- MRI of brain and spine; more sensitive than CT at determining location and tumor characteristics; neuroimaging standard for brain tumors. Spine imaging is used to determine presence of metastases.

TABLE 10.3	Brain Anatomy and Associated Function	
Location	**Function**
Cerebrum (right and left hemispheres)	Initiation and coordination of movement, vision, hearing, problem solving, reasoning, emotion, touch, temperature.
Brainstem (including midbrain, pons, medulla)	Ocular and oral movements, transmission of sensory messages (e.g., hot, cold, pain), hunger, apneustic/respiratory center, body temperature, sneezing, coughing, vomiting, swallowing; can result in cranial nerve palsies.
Cerebellum	Posture, balance, voluntary muscle movements, equilibrium.

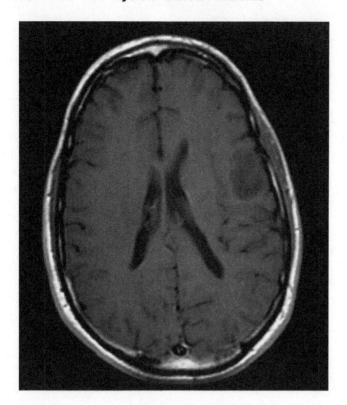

FIGURE 10.2 • **Astrocytoma Head MRI.** Axial T1-weighted MRI showing nonenhancing left frontal astrocytoma.

- Lumbar puncture (LP) for cytologic analysis; measurement of β-human chorionic gonadotropin and α-fetoprotein levels assists in determining diagnosis of germ cell tumor.
- Cerebral angiogram is indicated in some cases.
- Neuroendocrine evaluation (midline tumors, pituitary, suprasellar, optic chiasmal region).

Management

- Dependent on type and location of lesion.
- Surgery:
  - A complete surgical resection is the goal, though may be difficult, depending on location.
  - Biopsy at time of surgery to identify type and direct management strategies.
- Chemotherapy, radiation therapy.
- Steroids to treat and prevent cerebral edema.
- Anticonvulsant therapy; selected patients with seizures or high risk for seizures.
- Ventriculopleural shunt; selected patients with tumor-associated hydrocephalus.

Long-Term Side Effects

- Variable; depending on size, location, metastases, and type of tumor.
- Long-term physical, cognitive, speech therapy as indicated to facilitate return to daily activities.
- Routine neuropsychologic evaluation; some long-term effects may not be noted for years.
- Therapies may result in infertility (e.g., chemotherapy), conversations about fertility preservation may be indicated.

PEARLS
- *Most common types of brain tumors are gliomas.*
- *Peak incidence of brain tumor is 4 to 5 years of age.*
- *Signs of increased intracranial pressure related to tumors may be more subtle in school-age children.*
- *Children with neurofibromatosis have an increased risk of developing benign and malignant brain tumors.*

Leukemia

Jessica L. Diver

Definition

- Cancer of the blood and blood-forming organs, such as the bone marrow, lymph nodes, and spleen.

Etiology/Types

- Classified by the cell line affected and level where differentiation has been interrupted.
- Acute lymphoblastic leukemia (ALL):
  - 75% of childhood cancers, most common between 2 and 5 years of age.
  - Inherited conditions predispose patients to ALL, including Fanconi anemia, trisomy 21, ataxia telangiectasis, Klinefelter syndrome, and Shwachman–Diamond syndrome.
- Acute myeloid leukemia (AML):
  - 15% to 25% of pediatric leukemia.
  - Slightly increased incidence after 10 years of age.
  - Increased incidence with previous exposure to chemotherapy and inherited conditions, including trisomy 21, Diamond–Blackfan anemia, Fanconi anemia, Li–Fraumeni syndrome, paroxysmal nocturnal hemoglobinuria, and neurofibromatosis.
- Chronic myelogenous leukemia (CML).
  - Less than or equal to 5% of childhood leukemias.
  - Associated with chromosomal translocation known as Philadelphia chromosome.
  - Initial phase is "chronic" and associated with leukocytosis, mild anemia, and thrombocytosis.
  - May progress after a variable amount of time to the accelerated phase and blast crisis, which resembles acute leukemia.

Pathophysiology

- Dysregulation of hematopoietic development secondary to genetic abnormalities; stem cells that are malignant do not differentiate or mature properly. These cells, called "blasts," accumulate in the marrow and possibly some solid organs (i.e., thymus, liver, spleen, kidneys, CNS) and cause impairment or failure of bone marrow function.

Clinical Presentation

- Dependent on the amount of bone marrow infiltration and extent of disease outside the bone marrow.
- Symptoms are often vague.

- ALL: Fevers, fatigue, anorexia, weight loss, nonspecific or bone pain, infections that do not resolve, persistent lymphadenopathy. WBC may be elevated; very high WBC may cause leukostasis.
- AML: Tend to appear more ill than patients with ALL, cytopenias more significant, ecchymoses, petechiae, epistaxis, and other bleeding. Collections of tumor cells, called chloromas, may present as masses most commonly located in the orbital or periorbital areas.
- CML: Often asymptomatic, diagnosed incidentally, and identified by abnormal CBC results. Nonspecific symptoms including fever, fatigue, weight loss, and left upper quadrant pain may be present. Patients in blast crisis will resemble those symptomatic with ALL or AML.

Diagnostic Evaluation

- CBC with anemia, thrombocytopenia, and leucopenia or leukocytosis. Blasts present on peripheral blood smear.
- Bone marrow aspirate is diagnostic when blasts comprise >25% of the marrow space.
- Marrow is evaluated for morphology, immunophenotyping, immunohistochemical stains, and cytogenetic abnormalities.
- Metabolic studies for kidney and liver function, as well as complications such as tumor lysis syndrome.
- An LP will determine whether or not the CNS is involved; determines therapy required.

Management

- Prompt evaluation by oncology specialist.
- Patients with elevated WBCs or complications such as hyperleukocytosis (WBC count >100,000 mm³) or tumor lysis syndrome may require admission to the pediatric intensive care unit.
  - Hyperleukocytosis results in increased blood viscosity (may result in neurologic, pulmonary, or cardiac sequelae) and is a medical emergency. Initial therapy includes aggressive hydration, correction of metabolic disturbances, and prevention of tumor lysis syndrome. May require leukopheresis or exchange transfusion.
- Tumor lysis syndrome therapy (see TLS section for additional information).
- Early identification of coagulopathies, sepsis, and leukostasis leads to better outcomes.
- Transfusions may be indicated.
  - Careful consideration for transfusion is required in children with hyperleukocytosis since it may complicate already viscous blood.
- ALL: Treatment in three phases, induction, consolidation, and maintenance, includes chemotherapy and steroids.
  - Chemotherapy agents are determined by risk stratification based on age and WBC at time of presentation; lasts 2 to 3 years depending on risk and gender.
  - CNS therapy is required; either prophylaxis or treatment due to the risk for CNS relapse and failure of systemic chemotherapy to penetrate the blood–brain barrier adequately.
- AML: Short, intense periods of multiagent chemotherapy, causes prolonged marrow hypoplasia and

immunosuppression. May require hematopoietic stem cell transplant (HSCT) from an allogeneic donor.
- CML: Current therapy is tyrosine kinase inhibitor (imatinib mesylate) while in chronic phase. The only curative therapy for CML is HSCT from an allogeneic donor; indicated if the patient does not tolerate or fails to achieve or maintain a remission with imatinib mesylate.

PEARLS

- *Side effects of chemotherapy and radiation, including nausea, vomiting, alopecia, mucositis, anorexia, and pancytopenia, should be addressed with supportive care.*
- *Frequency/type of evaluation for children receiving chemotherapy is dependent on the agents utilized in each patient's care.*
- *Leukopenia, specifically neutropenia, combined with central venous catheters, place patients at especially high risk for infections and serious complications of infections.*

Lymphoma

Jessica L. Diver

Definition

- Malignancy arises from lymph node or lymph tissue; many varieties.

Etiology/Types

- Third most common type of pediatric cancer.
- Hodgkins lymphoma (HL): accounts for 5% of cancers in children less than age 15 years.
  - Four subtypes: lymphocyte predominant, nodular sclerosing, mixed cellularity, and lymphocyte depleted.
  - Typically occurs in adolescents/young adults between 15 and 35 years of age.
  - Ebstein–Barr virus is believed to have an association.
  - Children with immunodeficiencies are at greater risk for HL.
- NHL (non-Hodgkin lymphoma): 6% of childhood cancers occurs most commonly between ages 5 and 15 years.
- Three main types include lymphoblastic lymphoma, mature B-cell lymphoma (i.e., Burkitt lymphoma, diffuse large B-cell, and primary mediastinal large B-cell lymphoma), and anaplastic large cell lymphoma.
- Etiology not fully understood, although geographic, immunologic, viral, and genetic factors are all thought to contribute to the development of NHL.

Pathophysiology

- Lymphocyte is malignant cell of origin; two broad categories: HL and NHL.

- NHL is the result of proliferation of T, B, or indeterminant-cell origin lymphocytes, leads to rapidly multiplying abnormal cells and unpredictable aggressive spread.
- HL spreads more slowly and orderly, typically to adjacent lymph nodes and possibly involving the liver, spleen, bone, bone marrow, lungs, or brain.

Clinical Presentation

- Dependent on sites involved.
  - HL: lymphadenopathy of one or more nodes; systemic symptoms include fatigue, anorexia, weight loss, and pruritis. "B symptoms" include unexplained fevers greater than 38.0°C, unexplained weight loss of at least 10% of body weight in 6 months, and drenching night sweats are of prognostic value.
    - Superior vena cava syndrome may result from significant mediastinal adenopathy.
  - NHL: Lymphadenopathy may be present. If abdomen is involved, palpable mass may be present and associated with pain, nausea, vomiting, abdominal distension, hepatosplenomegaly, changes in bowel habits, or hematochezia. Mediastinal involvement may present as superior vena cava syndrome, facial/neck swelling, snoring, dysphagia, or chest pain. Systemic symptoms may include fatigue, fever, malaise, weight loss, anorexia, and night sweats. Pancytopenia and related complications may be present if the bone marrow is involved.

Diagnostic Evaluation

- Imaging: CT scan—evaluation of lymphadenopathy or palpable mass.
- Staging.
  - Accomplished by measuring the tumor/mass and identifying spread, therapy is indicated based on risk and used to predict survival.
  - Bone scans and bone marrow aspirate.
  - LP is performed if patients have symptoms of CNS disease.
  - Positron emission tomography (PET) scans may be utilized.
- Biopsy determines definitive diagnosis and includes application of immunohistochemical stains, flow cytometry, and cytogenetic analysis.

Management

- Observation for complications of the tumor, such as airway compromise, superior vena cava syndrome, and tumor lysis syndrome, is priority.
- HL: Stratified based on risk to determine treatment regimens, "early response" is associated with better outcomes, multiagent chemotherapy with serial imaging to evaluate for response. Radiation and HSCT for some relapsed or refractory disease, use of antibody therapy for HL are being investigated.
- NHL: Variable depending on type and tumor burden at time of diagnosis. Lymphoblastic lymphoma is treated similarly to ALL with 2 to 3 years of multiagent chemotherapy and CNS prophylaxis or treatment based on disease status. Mature B-cell lymphoma treated with intense chemotherapy

associated with several toxicities, including mucositis, myelosuppression, and typhlitis. Anaplastic large cell lymphoma is treated with combination chemotherapy and limited CNS prophylaxis; radiation is generally not needed.

PEARLS

- *Approximate overall survival for patients with HL is about 90%.*
- *NHL outcomes dependent on the stage at diagnosis; localized disease (stages I or II) have at least 95% survival rates, and stages III and IV have an overall survival of approximately 80% to 90%.*

Neuroblastoma

Jessica L. Diver & Wendy S. Fitzgerald

Background/Definition

- Neoplasm from the sympathetic nervous system, most common extracranial solid tumor of childhood, typically disease of infants and young children.
- Benign counterpart is ganglioneuroma.

Etiology/Types

- Tumors classified as low, intermediate, and high-risk based on extent of spread/metastasis (stages I, II, III, IV, and IVs), and tumor histology.
- Etiology is unclear: favorable versus nonfavorable.
- Biologic features:
  - MYCN gene amplification = poorer prognosis.
  - DNA index of 1 = poorer prognosis.
- Age $\geq$ 12 to 18 months = poorer prognosis.
- Accounts for 7% to 10% of malignancies in children less than 15 years of age.
- Most frequently diagnosed during infancy.

Pathophysiology

- Biology of the tumor dictates the clinical behavior.
- Small, round, blue cell neoplasm from primordial neural crest cells.
- Subtypes of neuroblastoma include neuroblastoma, ganglioneuroblastoma, and ganglioneuroma.
- Neuroblastoma is the most undifferentiated, least mature malignant subtype.

Clinical Presentation

- Primary mass—symptoms depend on location.
- Abdominal mass two third of cases (half arising from adrenal gland). Present with palpable mass, constipation, refusal to walk.
- Thoracic, cervical, or pelvic mass.
- 5% to 15% with spinal cord involvement and neurologic symptoms.
- Patients with bone marrow metastases may present with anemia, thrombocytopenia, and neutropenia, and associated symptoms.

- Commonly found within the chest, abdomen, and pelvis.
- May present anywhere in the sympathetic nervous system; presentation dependent on location of disease.
- Approximately 40% of patients present with localized disease without metastasis.
- Patients with metastatic disease may present with bone pain, malaise, fever, "raccoon eyes" (periorbital ecchymosis), "blueberry muffin spots" (metastasis to subcutaneous tissue).
- 65% of patients are diagnosed with a tumor in the abdomen; at least 50% of tumors arise from the adrenal medulla.
- Signs and symptoms may include abdominal tenderness/distension, hepatomegaly, distal edema. 5% to 15% of tumors are in the paraspinal region, resulting in spinal cord compression. Tumors of the upper thoracic spine can cause mechanical obstruction and superior vena cava syndrome. Horner syndrome may be noted in patients with cervical masses. Hypertension may be present.
- Bone marrow infiltration may cause fatigue, weakness, increased infections, pallor, and bruising.
- Infiltration of the periorbital bones may cause proptosis and periorbital ecchymosis.
- Opsoclonus–myoclonus ataxia (OMA) is present in approximately 2% to 4%; important to note that 50% of patients who present with OMA have neuroblastoma. OMA manifests as myoclonic jerking and random eye movements, with or without cerebellar ataxia.

Diagnostic Evaluation

- Laboratory evaluation: CBC, complete chemistry panel, serum ferritin, liver function tests, and urine for catecholamine metabolites (vanillylmandelic acid [VMA] and homovanillic acid [HVA]).
- Bilateral bone marrow aspirate and biopsy.
- Urine catecholamines HVA and VMA elevated in 90% to 95% of cases.
- Imaging Studies.
  - Include CT, MRI, and meta-iodobenzylguanidine (MIBG) scintiscan (nuclear medicine study).
- Biopsy: Tissue obtained in biopsy will make final diagnosis and evaluate biologic features. Biopsy primary lesion and bone marrow aspirate and biopsy × 2 locations.

Management

- Intensive, multiagent chemotherapy followed by surgical resection and possible local irradiation to achieve local control as part of induction therapy.
- Consolidation therapy includes myeloablative chemotherapy and autologous stem cell rescue.
- Maintenance therapy may include retinoids and, more recently, immunotherapy.
- High-risk patients go on to receive autologous bone marrow transplant followed by radiation therapy and biologic therapy with isotretinoin and monoclonal antibody.

PEARLS
- *Patients with orbital, mediastinal, spinal cord, or extensive abdominal disease may present emergently and require immediate evaluation; risk for superior vena cava syndrome.*
- *Aggressive supportive care, may include anti-infective prophylaxis, transfusion support, pain management, and close monitoring as required.*

Osteosarcoma and Ewing Sarcoma

Jessica L. Diver & Wendy S. Fitzgerald

Background/Definition

- Genetically complex bone tumor.

Etiology/Types

- Tumor arising from primitive mesenchyme/osteoblasts.
- Most common bone malignancy in childhood; 98% of osteosarcoma cases are considered "high-grade."
- Peak incidence around growth spurts, usually arise without any identified cause, and 20% present with metastases, primarily to lungs; less often bone, brain.
- Subtypes of OS, parosteal and periosteal osteosarcoma, are associated with lower risk for metastasis and better prognosis.
- ES—most frequent location is axial skeleton; osteosarcoma more common in long bones.
- ES more commonly arises from diaphyseal as opposed to metaphyseal bone.
- Ewing sarcoma of Bone.
  - Tumor may derive from primordial mesenchymal stem cell.
  - Associated with somatic translocation 22q11—EWS-FLI1 fusion gene.
  - Ewing Sarcoma can be extraosseous in origin.
  - 25% present with metastases to bone, bone marrow, or lungs.
- Bone tumors are staged I, II, III, or IV—stage IV designating distant metastases.

Pathophysiology

- Results from clonal proliferation of osteoblasts, and in half of cases diagnosed, inactivation of tumor pathways is present.

Clinical Presentation

- Pain (constant or intermittent) that may have been present for weeks or months.
- Swelling of joint or bone; usually develops where bone is growing quickly such as at the ends of long bones.
- Patients with metastatic disease may present with fever, night sweats, weight loss, or other systemic complaints.

Diagnostic Evaluation

- "Starburst" or "bone in bone" formation noted in radiographs, lytic lesion, or "Codman triangle" suggests malignancy.

- Imaging.
  - Initial plain radiograph, MRI recommended.
  - Chest radiograph, chest CT, and bone scan to evaluate for metastases.
  - PET scans increasingly used for ES.

Laboratory Evaluation

- Baseline CBC, chemistries, liver function tests. LDH may be elevated in ES.
- Bone marrow aspirates and biopsies for ES.
  - Open biopsy determines diagnosis and management strategies.

Management

- Surgical resection and chemotherapy. Limb-salvage procedures may prevent 90% of amputations.
- Total resection of tumor essential for OS; Radiation is not useful for OS.
- Patients with unresectable ES can receive radiation for local control.

PEARLS

- *Nonmetastatic osteosarcoma cure rates are approximately 65% to 75%.*
- *Survival rates after relapse of osteosarcoma are very low.*
- *Immediate needs after surgical resection include physical therapy and possible prosthesis.*
- *Long-term follow-up should include monitoring for chemotherapy-related toxicities and secondary malignancies (including fertility preservation strategies).*

Rhabdomyosarcoma

Jessica L. Diver

Background/Definition

- Tumor arising from mesenchymal cells, likely skeletal in origin, although may present where skeletal muscle is not otherwise present.
- Third most common solid tumor of childhood; most common soft-tissue sarcoma in children. 50% are Rhabdomyosarcoma—arise from immature striated muscle progenitors.
- Two-thirds of cases occur in children 10 years of age or younger.
- Increased risk for children with RB mutation for retinoblastoma, neurofibromatosis-type 1, and other congenital anomalies.
- Most common variant is the embryonal form, which typically presents in the head, neck, orbits, and genitourinary system.
  - Two subtypes of embryonal form: botryoid (seen in infants, arises from bladder or vagina) and alveolar (develops in extremities or bone marrow, most common in adolescents and young adults).

Etiology

- Unclear; thought to be a result of dysregulation of gene expression leading to neoangiogenesis, autocrine growth, evasion of apoptosis, immortalization, metastasis and invasion, and resistance to growth inhibition.

Pathophysiology

- Arises from the primitive mesenchymal stem cells.
- Tumor is a small, round, blue cell tumor of childhood.

Clinical Presentation

- Varies according to anatomic presentation.
- Physical changes related to growth (e.g., orbits), epistaxis, sinusitis, nasal obstruction, visible masses, facial nerve palsy, drainage from the affected ear, and conductive hearing loss.
- Genitourinary tumors may present with urinary retention, straining to void, hematuria, or unexplained vaginal bleeding.
- Tumors of the extremities are often tender, firm, and fixed upon palpation.

Diagnostic Evaluation

- Imaging of the affected areas and chest, CT, MRI, PET, and ultrasound.
- Evaluation for metastasis should be performed, and a bone marrow aspirate is recommended.
- Open biopsy confirms diagnosis.

Management

- Tumor resection, chemotherapy, and local radiation, determined by grouping and staging classification.

PEARLS

- *Survival rates have improved, largely dependent on the group and stage.*
- *Long-term follow-up to monitor for complications of therapy and possible secondary malignancy.*

Retinoblastoma

Wendy S. Fitzgerald

Definition

- Rare childhood tumor arising from retina.

Background

- Accounts for approximately 3% of childhood cancers; 2/3 of all cases diagnosed before 2 years of age.
- Bilateral disease is always hereditary.

Pathophysiology

- Arises from embryonic retinal cells, may be unilateral or bilateral.

- 25% to 30% cases inheritable form with germline mutation in RB-1 gene.

Etiology/Types

- Trilateral Retinoblastoma—development of midline neuroblastic tumor in pineal/parasellar region of brain—usually presents at approximately 20 months after diagnosis.
- Hereditary and nonhereditary.
  - Patients <1 year of age at diagnosis more likely to have heritable form.

Clinical Presentation

- Often present at birth; 80% diagnosed by age 3 to 4 years of age; 95% diagnosed by age 5.
- Leukocoria—lack of normal red reflex of the eye. Typically, white mass visualized in vitreous during ophthalmic examination.
- Strabismus and Heterochromia.
- Rubeosis iridis.
- Diagnosis may be made by genetic screening if the RB1 oncogene has been detected in families.

Diagnostic Evaluation

- Referral to ophthalmology specialist.
- Diagnosed on fundoscopic examination; may require examination under anesthesia.
- Imaging studies to determine the extent of the tumor using CT and MRI.
- Biopsy.
- LP, as indicated.

Management

- Determined based on staging.
- Goal is prevention of tumor extension and preserving vision.
- May require enucleation (treatment of choice for unilateral disease with orbit or optic nerve involvement), cryotherapy, brachytherapy, laser photocoagulation, radiation, and chemotherapy.

PEARLS

- *Require long-term follow-up due to risk of secondary malignancies.*
- *Children of retinoblastoma survivors should be monitored closely due to the genetic inheritance patterns.*

Wilms Tumor and Other Renal Tumors

Wendy S. Fitzgerald

Background

- Wilms Tumor is the most common abdominal tumor of childhood.

Definition

- Wilms Tumor arises from embryonal nephroblastic cells.

- Can be associated with congenital cancer predisposition syndromes including Beckwith-Wiedemann, WAGR syndrome (Wilms tumor, aniridia, genitourinary abnormalities, and mental retardation).

Etiology/Types

- Prognostic Groups based on histopathology:
  - Favorable, anaplastic, and nephrogenic rests.
- Bilateral (always associated with congenital cancer predisposition).
  - Clear Cell Sarcoma of the Kidney (more prone to metastasis).
  - Rhabdoid Tumor of the Kidney—very poor prognosis.
  - Congenital Mesoblastic Nephroma.
  - Renal Cell Carcinoma.

Clinical Presentation

- Asymptomatic abdominal mass; most common presenting sign.
- Hypertension (due to renal artery compression and possibly increased renin production).
- Gross hematuria.
- Fever.
- Constipation.
- Rare: hypotension, anemia.

Diagnostic Evaluation

- Physical examination.
  - Large palpable flank mass—gentle examination so as not to disrupt the capsule.
  - Evaluate for features of congenital predisposition syndrome—aniridia, hemihypertrophy, macroglossia, urogenital malformations.
- Imaging studies.
  - Ultrasound.
  - CT scan abdomen and chest.
- Laboratory studies.
  - CBC, chemistry (renal function tests, electrolytes, calcium).
  - Urinalysis.
  - Coagulation (preoperative).
  - Pathologic evaluation including histology and cytogenetic testing for 1p and 16q deletion.

Management

- Upfront surgery when possible with nephrectomy for unilateral disease.
- Patients with bilateral disease or unresectable tumor receive preoperative chemotherapy.
- Postoperative chemotherapy given to all but very low-risk patients–regimen determined by staging based on factors such as presence of metastases, rupture of the capsule around tumor, invasion of the renal artery, and presence of positive lymph nodes.
- Radiation therapy for Stages III and IV.

Long-Term Effects

- Reduced kidney function.
- Cardiopulmonary problems, depending on chemotherapeutic/radiation therapy received.

- Slowed or decreased growth.
- Changes in sexual development and fertility issues (especially females that have received abdominal radiation therapy).
- Development of secondary cancers (later in life).

Stem Cell Transplant/Bone Marrow Transplant
Cathy Haut

Background

- HSCT is used as treatment for both malignant and nonmalignant diagnoses. The existence of stem cells was published in 1961, but ethics of the use of human embryos or embryonic cells continues in political discussion.

Definition

- Bone marrow cells from either patient (autograft) or a donor (allograft) are infused or transplanted to engraft and rescue a patient whose marrow is toxic to response of chemotherapy.

Etiology/Types

- There are two different types of stem cell transplants, characterized by the donor:
  - Autologous bone marrow transplant, where the patient receives his or her own cells that were collected at an earlier time frame following a course of high-dose chemotherapy. This type of transplant is often more successful than an allogeneic transplant.
  - Allogeneic bone marrow transplants involve transplanting cells from matched, unrelated donors, volunteers, or partially matched family members with a similar process.

Clinical Presentation

- Malignant indications: leukemia and lymphoma, some solid tumor malignancies.
- Nonmalignant indications:
  - Bone marrow failure: severe aplastic anemia, Fanconi anemia, Diamond–Blackfan anemia.
  - Hemoglobinopathies: SCD, thalassemia.
  - Immunodeficiencies: severe combined immunodeficiency syndrome, Wiskott–Aldrich syndrome, leukocyte adhesion deficiency.
  - Inborn errors of metabolism to include mucopolysaccharidosis, leukodystrophy.

Diagnostic Evaluation/Preparation for Transplant

- Harvesting cells from patient or from donor bone marrow.
  - Performed in operating room under anesthesia.
  - Cells are harvested from bilateral posterior iliac crests.
  - A maximum of 20 mL/kg (of donor weight) is aspirated.

- Or, collection from circulation utilizing a pheresis machine and stimulation via chemotherapy or granulocyte colony-stimulating factor.
- Umbilical cord stem cell collection immediately following delivery of the placenta; poses no risk to donor.
- Preparing the patient.
  - For allogenetic transplant: HLA testing for compatibility of donor cells; major histocompatibility complex encoded genes present on chromosome 6.
  - Chemotherapy, radiation, and immunotherapy are used to prepare the patient to be a stem cell recipient. This process is to eradicate existing malignant cells and to create space for new cells. Recipient immunosuppression reduces the risk of rejection.
  - Pancytopenia, mucositis, and veno-occlusive disease (VOD) are complications of the preparation process. Each should be discussed with the patient/caregivers prior to the procedure.
- Infusion of stem cells: Infused intravenously using a syringe pump or gravity infusion to preserve the integrity of the cells.
  - Frozen products contain preservatives and are not thawed until immediately prior to transfusion, and then rapidly infused. Patients receive antiemetics, diuretics, corticosteroids, and antihistamines during the transplant process.
  - Fresh products are obtained from a donor within 48 hours and are administered similarly to other blood products.

Management

- Prior to transplant:
  - Chemotherapy, biological response modifiers, and antiemetics are administered to patient.
- Peritransplant:
  - Infusion of stem cells is day "0" of transplant (e.g., day after transplant is day "+1"; 2 days prior to transplant is day "−2").
  - Generally, cells are infused in the patient's room through a central venous catheter.
    - Analgesics, infection prophylaxis, and treatment if needed, blood products, nutrition, GVHD prophylaxis (e.g., mycophenolate mofetil), viral prophylaxis (e.g., ganciclovir), *Pneumocystis jiroveci* pneumonia (trimethoprim-sulfamethoxazole).
- Posttransplant.
  - Monitor for complications and side effects.
  - Opportunistic infections.
  - GVHD.
  - Interstitial pneumonitis.
  - Infectious complications and occurrence of specific organism infections are identified by expected time after transplant: first month, 1 to 4 months, 4 to 12 months, and after 12 months.
  - Viral, bacterial, and fungal infections are likely.
  - Preparation of the family for the sequence of events and potential outcomes.

Oncologic Complications/Emergencies

- Can occur at any time during the course of diagnosis, treatment, or relapse.

- Most require vigilant monitoring, emergent care, and intensive care.
- Can result in either negative or positive outcomes; evidence indicates that most are positive.

- Can be severe—may require continuous opioid infusions/PCA, TPN.
- Usually resolves with return of bone marrow activity or with engraftment following HSCT.

Graft Versus Host Disease
Cathy Haut

Background

- Complication of allogeneic stem cell transplant, typically occurring in the first 100 days post–transplant and includes multisystem involvement of problems. GVHD can be either acute or chronic.

Definition

- Transplanted immune cells recognize the host as foreign, and attack host cells.
- Three specific systems are usually involved: skin, mucosal cells (oral and GI tract), and liver.

Etiology/Types

- Can be acute or chronic.
- Risk factors include source of stem cells, with allogeneic transplants higher risk, degree of HLA matching. Also, female cells for male and increased donor age pose risks.
- Rash, staged from grade I with less than 25% of BSA involved to grade IV with bullae and desquamation.
- Liver, measured by total bilirubin levels.
- GI tract; determined by volume of diarrhea.

Pathophysiology

- Three-step process of conditioning-induced tissue damage, donor lymphocyte activation phase, and cellular and inflammatory effector phase.

Clinical Presentation

- Mouth sores and/or ulcerations from esophagus to rectum.
- May cause severe pain, anorexia, dehydration, bleeding, or infection.

Diagnostic Evaluation

- Based on clinical presentation.
- Biopsy for apoptotic bodies, eosinophilic bodies, and lymphocytic infiltration of the skin.
- Hyperbilirubinemia and Transaminasitis noted with liver function testing.
- Endoscopy/colonoscopy with biopsy determines grade of GI involvement.

Management

- Diligent oral care—may decrease severity.
- Mouth rinses such as sodium chloride—may prevent infections.
- Pain management—lidocaine mouth rinses, opioids.

Veno-Occlusive Disease
Cathy Haut

Background/Definition

- VOD of the liver is characterized as an obstructive vasculitis.
- One of the most frequently occurring complications of HSCT, with a reported incidence of 5% to 60%.
- Associated with high morbidity and mortality rates.

Etiology/Types

- The principal cause of VOD is toxicity of the preparatory therapy of BMT.
- VOD also occurs after liver transplantation and radiation to the liver.
- Risk factors for VOD.
  - Pretransplant chemotherapy.
  - Abdominal radiation.
  - Preexisting liver disease, elevated transaminases, viral hepatitis.
  - HLA mismatched or unrelated allogeneic transplant.
  - Osteopetrosis.
  - Second transplant.
  - Conditioning with busulfan, melphalan, or both.
  - Macrophage activating syndromes like HLH.
  - Early onset is within first 20 days posttransplant.
  - Late onset occurs after 20 days.
  - Described as mild, moderate, and severe.
- Severe with unresolved symptoms resulting in death.

Pathophysiology

- Remains unclear.
- The primary injury is most likely a lesion of the sinusoidal endothelial cells of hepatic venules.
- A variety of histologic changes eventually lead to complete venular obliteration, extensive hepatocellular necrosis, and widespread fibrous tissue replacement of normal liver.

Clinical Presentation

- Symptoms include weight gain, increased abdominal circumference, hepatomegaly, right upper quadrant pain, ascites, and elevated total and direct bilirubin levels.
- Transfusion-refractory thrombocytopenia with no detectable cause is noted as an early sign.

Diagnostic Studies

- Ultrasonography of the liver and liver vasculature.
- CBC with differential, electrolytes, bilirubin levels, γ-glutamyltransferase and other transaminases, and alkaline phosphatase, coagulation panel.

Management

- No specific therapy guidelines exist.
- Some therapies include low-dose tissue plasminogen activator (t-PA), ATIII replacement, and ATIII administered in combination with heparin/t-PA, along with other anticoagulants.

Mucositis
Jessica Hoffman Murphy

Background

- Mucositis occurs in children as a side effect of chemotherapy, radiation, or immunotherapy.

Definition

- Inflammation or destruction of mucosal cells of the oral cavity and throughout the GI tract.

Clinical Presentation

- Mouth sores and/or ulcerations from esophagus to rectum.
- May cause severe pain, anorexia, dehydration, bleeding, or infection.

Diagnostic Evaluation

- Based on clinical presentation.

Management

- Diligent oral care; may decrease severity.
- Mouth rinses such as sodium chloride—may prevent infections.
- Pain management; lidocaine mouth rinses, opioids.
- Can be severe; may require continuous opioid infusions/ PCA, TPN.
- Usually resolves with return of bone marrow activity or with engraftment following HSCT.

Hyperleukocytosis
Jessica Hoffman Murphy

Background

- Hyperleukocytosis is an oncological emergency!

Definition

- Elevated WBC, usually seen in new-onset leukemic patients.
- Leads to leukostasis, a clinicopathologic syndrome caused by sludging of circulating blasts into tissues.

Etiology/Types

- WBC $>100,000 \times 10^3\,\mu/L$ = increased risk of leukostasis and subsequent complications.

- Complications more significant in AML; most common complication is stroke.
- Patients with lymphoid leukemias present more often with hyperleukocystosis, but do not generally have symptoms until WBC $>250,000 \times 10^3\,\mu/L$.

Clinical Presentation

- Fever, lethargy, mental status changes, headache, seizure, stroke, coma, dyspnea, tachypnea, hypoxemia, respiratory failure, acidosis, cor pulmonale, hemorrhage, DIC, renal failure.

Diagnostic Evaluation

- WBC count $>100,000 \times 10^3\,\mu/L$.
- CXR—diffuse interstitial infiltrates.
- Head CT—high risk of intracranial hemorrhage.

Management

- Goal is rapid reduction in number of circulating WBCs— exchange transfusion, leukopheresis, cytotoxic therapy initiation.
- Hydration—2–$4 \times$ maintenance, avoid diuretics.
- Allopurinol, rasburicase.
- Serial electrolytes, BUN, uric acid.
- Transfuse platelets, treat coagulopathy, avoid PRBCs (goal $<10\,g/dL$).

PEARL
- *Morbidity and mortality are directly related to decreased blood viscosity.*

Sepsis in Oncology Diagnoses
Cathy Haut

Background

- Occurs as a result of chemotherapy-induced bone marrow suppression, nutritional deficits, and both gram-positive and gram-negative organisms that take advantage of the immuno-compromised host.

Definition

- Systemic inflammatory response to an organism or associated endotoxin in the blood. In children with oncologic diagnoses, can be related to cancer, immunocompromised status, or therapy-related.

Pathophysiology

- The basic pathophysiology of severe sepsis and septic shock includes vasodilatation, myocardial dysfunction leading to multiorgan system dysfunction, and third spacing of fluid as a result of capillary leak.
- Refer to Section 11, Infectious Disease for clinical presentation, diagnostic evaluation, and management.

- *Fever in an immunocompromised host is considered an emergency. After addressing life-threatening issues, administering antibiotics is the mainstay of treatment.*
- *Infectious etiologies in the immunocompromised host include bacterial, fungal, and viral origins. If response is not adequate with antibiotics, look for other sources of infection.*

Superior Vena Cava Syndrome

Cathy Haut

Background/Definition

- Occurs as a result of obstruction of the superior vena cava by malignancies of the vessel wall, mediastinal masses, or other compressive or obstructive processes.

Pathophysiology

- The superior vena cava is usually a low-pressure vessel that can easily become compressed.
- In superior vena cava syndrome, compression occurs as a result of invasion of tumor into the wall of the vessel, lymphadenopathy, intraluminal thrombus, or intravascular thrombosis formation, resulting in increased venous pressure and decreased cardiac output.

Clinical Presentation

- History of cough, fever, dyspnea, chest pain.
- Symptoms: edema/engorgement of the face, neck, and upper torso, dilation of superficial veins, cyanosis or plethora, stridor, dyspnea, anxiety.

Diagnostic Evaluation

- Chest radiograph.
- Chest CT.
- Ultrasound.

Management

- Airway management with relief of obstructive process or underlying cause.
- Emergent management includes oxygen, noninvasive ventilation, heliox therapy, imaging, minimizing pressures by addressing the source of compression.
- Identify and treat underlying cause.
- Elevation of head of the bed may provide some relief.
- Diuretic therapy; some cases.
- Steroids; indicated in some cases associated with malignancy/tumor.
- If etiology is associated with a clot; anticoagulation indicated.

- *It is essential to recognize early signs of superior vena cava syndrome in order to address them prior to complete compression of the vessel, which can be life-threatening.*

Tumor Lysis Syndrome

Jessica Hoffman Murphy

Background

- Tumor Lysis Syndrome is an oncological emergency associated with initial chemotherapy for leukemias, lymphomas, and other tumors with high growth rates.
- Can affect neurological, pulmonary, cardiac, and renal function.

Definition

- Massive tumor cell lysis with the release of large amounts of potassium, phosphate, and uric acid.

Etiology/Types

- Risk factors include high uric acid on presentation, high tumor burden, NHL (especially Burkitt), T-cell leukemia, and hyperleukocytosis.

Clinical Presentation

- Most commonly occurs shortly after initiation of therapy (within 6–48 hours, and up to 7 days after initiation of therapy).
- Symptoms: anorexia, cardiac arrhythmias, heart failure, edema, fluid overload, hematuria, lethargy, muscle cramps, nausea, vomiting, diarrhea, oliguria, seizures, syncope, muscle cramps, tetany, sudden death.
- Can be asymptomatic but with hyperkalemia, hyperphosphatemia, and hyperuricemia.

Diagnostic Evaluation

- Complete metabolic profile—hyperkalemia, hyperphosphotemia, hyperuricemia, hypocalcemia.

Management

- Prevention is key.
- Aggressive hydration—2 to 3 L/m^2/day to enhance uric acid and phosphate excretion, diuretics.
- Urine specific gravity and pH.
- Strict intake and output monitoring.
- Allopurinol, Rasburicase.
- Serial electrolyte monitoring.
- Dialysis—if oliguria, azotemia, dangerously high potassium or phosphorus levels, or refractory hyperuricemia.

Typhlitis (Neutropenic Enterocolitis)

Jacqueline Toia

Background

- A potentially life-threatening disorder, defined by the triad of neutropenia, abdominal pain, and fever.

Definition

- Also referred to as neutropenic enterocolitis, is most commonly inflammation of the cecum, but may also be in the ascending and proximal colon. Inflammation can progress rapidly to gangrene or bowel perforation.

Etiology/Types

- The exact etiology and progression of typhlitis are unknown; neutropenia is the common finding.

Pathophysiology

- Mucosal wall injury from cytotoxic therapy and intramural infection leads to mucosal wall thickening, ischemia, ulceration, hemorrhage, and possible perforation.

Clinical Presentation

- Fever and neutropenia (ANC <500 cells/μL).
- Elevated C-reactive protein (CRP).
- Abdominal pain (right lower quadrant) with distended abdomen.
- Peritoneal signs (e.g., guarding, abdominal wall rigidity, rebound tenderness).
- Nausea/vomiting.
- Diarrhea (may be bloody).
- Poor appetite.
- Range in bowel sounds from high-pitched to diminished or absent.
- Clinical presentation may vary with the severity of the disease.

Diagnostic Evaluation

- Imaging.
  - Computed tomography with PO and IV contrast (preferred): may demonstrate colonic wall thickening, mesenteric fat stranding secondary to inflammation, submucosal bowel wall edema, paralytic ileus, pneumatosis (Figure 10.3).
  - Plain abdominal film: may demonstrate right lower soft tissue mass, paralytic ileus, "thumbprinting" due to bowel wall edema, bowel edema, or intraluminal gas.

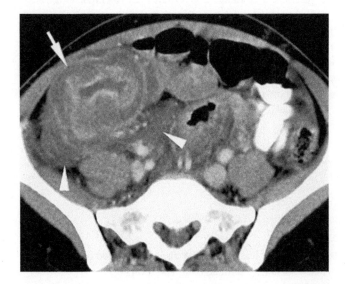

FIGURE 10.3 • **Typhlitis–CT Scan.** Arrow is pointing toward "thickened cecum" in above image.

- Ultrasound: nonspecific findings; may demonstrate thickening of bowel wall, intraluminal fluid, or pericecal fluid.
- Laboratory Evaluation.
  - CBC, coagulation profile, blood and stool cultures, chemistries.

Management

- Broad-spectrum antibiotics with both gram-positive, gram-negative, and anaerobic coverage.
- Bowel rest and abdominal decompression (e.g., nasogastric tube).
- Pain management.
- Granulocyte colony-stimulating factor.
- IV fluids for hydration; parenteral nutrition.
- If pneumatosis, pneumoperitoneum, or pericolic fluid are noted on imaging studies, urgent surgical evaluation is needed.
- Persistent GI bleeding requires surgical evaluation.
- Avoidance or caution with medications such as anticholinergic agents, antidiarrheals, and narcotics.

Diagnostic Testing in Hematology and Oncology

Complete Blood Cell Count

Barbara Wise

Background

- Primarily measures the number of RBCs (RBC = erythrocytes), WBCs, total amount of hemoglobin, and the fraction of blood composed of RBCs. Other components of the CBC are the reticulocyte count, MCV, hematocrit, and platelet count.

Terminology, Definitions, Pathophysiology

- RBCs:
  - Ranges are age- and gender-specific; life span approximately 120 days.
- Hemoglobin measures oxygen carrying potential; Hematocrit measures mass of the RBCs.
- Reticulocyte count—RBC production.
  - Indicates bone marrow response to anemia.
- WBCs: mediators of inflammation.
  - Decreased WBC count—leukopenia.
  - Elevated WBC count—leukocytosis.
  - Granulocytes:
    - Segmented neutrophils (57% to 67% of differential)—primary infectious response.
    - Polys—mature neutrophils.
    - Bands—immature neutrophils.
    - Eosinophils—allergic response.
  - Agranulocytes.
    - Lymphocytes—immune response; T-cell and B-cell lymphocytes.
    - Monocytes—produced by bone marrow, process foreign antigens through phagocytosis.

- Absolute neutrophil count—indicator of patient's ability to fight infection; ANC <500 is concerning.
  - ANC=Total # of WBCs × (% polys + % bands).
- Platelets.
  - Life span: 5 to 9 days; Transfused platelets have a shorter life span.
- Additional Indices:
  - Mean corpuscular hemoglobin concentration (MCHC)—average concentration of hemoglobin of a given volume of PRBC, calculated by dividing the hemoglobin by the hematocrit.
  - Mean corpuscular hemoglobin (MCH)—average quantity of hemoglobin.
  - MCV—index of the size of RBC.
  - Blasts—abnormal WBCs.
- Peripheral smear—evaluates function of the bone marrow, especially to assess cytopenia states; in thrombocytopenia used to differentiate increased platelet consumption from reduced platelet production, morphology (e.g., cell size, color, and shape) and color of RBC (e.g., micro, macro, or normal).

Coagulation Studies

Background

- Initially developed to monitor anticoagulation therapy.
- Coagulation status changes rapidly in bleeding patients.
- Malignancy affects the hemostatic system, increasing the risk of developing thrombosis and hemorrhage.

Terminology/Definition

- Prothrombin time (PT) indicates the time for plasma to clot in the presence of thromboplastin (extrinsic pathway), altered in vitamin K deficiency.
- Activated partial thromboplastin time measures clotting time after the addition of excessive phospholipid (intrinsic pathway).
- Thrombin time (TT) measures conversion of fibrinogen to fibrin, the last step in the clotting process.

Pathophysiology

- The imbalance in the coagulation system is caused by clinical factors (immobility, dehydration, infection, inherited thrombophilia, obesity, leukocytosis) and biologic factors (coagulation activation that relates to tumor progression).

PEARLS
- *Activated partial thromboplastin time is most accurate if results obtained within 4 hours of specimen collection.*
- *Tests results affected by high hematocrit and time between specimen collection and assay.*

Ferritin and Iron Indices

Background

- Iron is stored in tissue as ferritin.

Terminology/Definition

- Transferrin saturation is expressed as percentage of transferrin saturated with iron, which indicates capacity of blood to transport iron.
- Total iron binding capacity (TIBC) measures reserve capacity of transferrin.

Other Laboratory Studies

- LDH—lactic acid dehydrogenase.
  - Isoenzyme used as a marker of tissue breakdown or damage and hemolysis.
- Uric Acid.
  - Product of the metabolic breakdown of purine nucleotides. Some cancers and chemotherapy increase cell death, resulting in hyperuricemia. High uric acid levels contribute to renal failure.

PET Scan
Christina Graham & Barbara Wise

Background

- Standard imaging component of diagnosis and staging in pediatric oncology.
- Performed in combination with anatomic imaging such as CT scan.
- Advantages: Ability to up- and downstage disease and evaluate response to chemotherapy.
- Disadvantages: Results are not specific to a cancer diagnosis; patients are exposed to significant radiation and lower sensitivity in brain and lungs.

Definition

- Nuclear medicine imaging technique that uses a radiolabeled glucose analog (FDG) to evaluate glycolytic activity, and combines anatomic and metabolic information to evaluate pediatric tumors. A PET scan provides information about metabolic activity and the proliferative potential of a residual tumor.

Clinical Indications

- Baseline staging, disease response, and follow-up for disease surveillance.
- Evaluation tool for investigational drugs that achieve therapeutic response without manifestations of change in tumor size.
- PET-CT fuses metabolic activity with anatomical structures.
- PET-CT is superior to a bone scan in detecting bone marrow and bony sites of disease in rhabdomyosarcoma.

Clinical Application

- FDG uptake is measured as standardized uptake value (SUV) and has a large degree of variability due to physical and biologic sources.

- When performed in a standard manner, PET studies provide a robust value for image comparison.
- A 35% reduction in SUV from baseline is considered predictive of a histologic response.
- Radiopharmaceutical doses vary in children, and estimating doses is dependent on the child's body habitus, younger children being at highest risk from ionizing radiation because actively growing and longer life span.

Patient Education

- Blood glucose levels inversely affect SUV; patients must strictly adhere to institutional NPO guidelines.

PEARLS

- *Pediatric challenges include need for sedation, pregnancy screening, and potential artifact caused by normal physiologic uptake.*
- *Correct weight measurement is critical in ensuring accurate imaging measurements.*

Bone Marrow Aspiration and Biopsy

Danielle Van Damme

Background

- Provides qualitative and quantitative information about cell lines and is performed to evaluate hematopoietic and nonhematopoietic diseases. It is used to evaluate and stratify response to therapy, extent of marrow damage, and prognosis.
- Results describe the appearance of three types of stem cells: hematopoietic system, mesenchymal stem cells, and endothelial stem cells.
- Immature cells are increased in hyperplastic conditions such as leukemia.
- Atypical cells are increased in vitamin B_{12} or folate deficiency, myelodysplastic syndromes, drug toxins or infectious problems. The results of BM examination are compared with peripheral blood findings.

Diagnostic Indication

- Staging and evaluation for abnormal peripheral blood findings, inherited bone marrow failure syndromes, microbiologic cultures in fever of unknown origin, and for follow-up of minimal residual disease (MRD) after chemotherapy or BMT.

Pathophysiology

- Bone marrow (BM) occupies the cavity of 85% of the skeletal system and is the major site of blood cell formation in the body.
- BM produces 2.5 million RBC, 1 billion granulocytes, and 2.5 billion platelets per kilogram of body weight. Components of the BM are bone, stroma cells, fibroblasts, adipose tissue,

and hematopoietic tissue. Red marrow is widespread in the bones of children.
- Cellularity of the BM is defined as the proportion of cellular elements relative to adipose tissue. Cellularity is variable, decreases with age, and changes in response to stress, infection, and disease. The BM is a major site for iron storage.
- Blood cells produced in the BM are continuously renewed and derived from progenitors of primitive mesenchymal cells called pleuripotent hematopoietic stem cells.

Diagnostic Evaluation

- BM aspiration is obtained from the anterior and posterior iliac crest and sternal sites for morphology and flow.
- BM aspirate assesses cellularity, the proportion of each cell type, the morphology of each cell type, and the presence or absence of malignant cells.

Other Testing

- Flow cytometry.
  - Demonstrates and enumerates the abnormal blast population, demonstrates abnormal patterns of antigen expression in clinical cell analyses, identification of markers on the cell surface.
- Cell-based analysis of phenotypic and functional markers, immunophenotypic analysis culture.
  - Polymerase chain reaction—a quantitative method to amplify a targeted DNA molecule—detects nucleic acids that are diagnostic in cancer, examines T and/or B-cell gene rearrangement studies. Limitations include potential false positive results and inadequate tissue at initial biopsy.
  - Fluorescent in situ hybridization—molecular test to detect chromosomal abnormalities, translocations, can be performed on peripheral blood and BM samples.

Management/Procedure

- Position the child prone, lateral decubitus position, for a posterior iliac site, or supine for an anterior exposure.
- Clean the site according to institutional policy, and use local anesthetic.
- Puncture the skin with the bone marrow aspiration needle (16G or 18G, variety of lengths), and advance to the periosteum using a twisting motion until the needle is anchored in the bone.
- Remove the stylet, attach a 5- or 10-mL syringe to the needle, and aspirate 0.3 to 1 mL of marrow.
- Prepare a smear, and confirm the presence of spicules, bony particles. Using a different syringe, obtain the necessary samples.
- If a biopsy is required, insert the appropriate needle into the iliac crest.
- Remove the stylet, and advance the needle 2 to 10 mm until an adequate specimen can be obtained. Rotate the needle to clockwise and counterclockwise without advancing further. Remove the needle and push the specimen from the distal end of the biopsy needle by using a probe.
- Apply a pressure dressing, and leave intact for 24 hours.

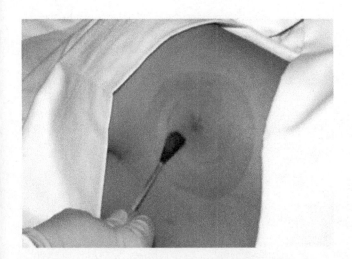

FIGURE 10.4 • **Bone Marrow Aspirate Skin Preparation.** Photo Courtesy of Danielle Van Damme.

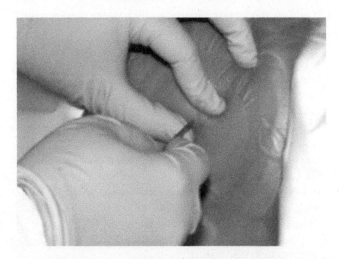

FIGURE 10.5 • **Bone Marrow Aspirate Puncture Site.** Photo Courtesy of Danielle Van Damme.

PEARLS
- *Maintaining a platelet count >15 × 10⁹/L is advised.*
- *The needle should be reoriented to a different site between the aspiration and biopsy procedures.*
- *The anterior iliac crest is the preferred site in obese patients.*
- *Bone marrow biopsies should not be obtained from the sternal site.*
- *Bilateral aspirates and biopsies may be required in certain diseases such as neuroblastoma, lymphoproliferative disease, sarcomas, and non-Hodgkin lymphoma (Figures 10.4–10.6).*

Lumbar Puncture and Administration of Intrathecal Chemotherapy

Barbara Wise & Shannon Konieczki

Background

- Purpose is to obtain cerebrospinal fluid for diagnostic testing, measuring opening and closing pressures, and administration of intrathecal chemotherapy.
- Intrathecal administration of antitumor drugs allows for consistent CSF concentration with a smaller dose and a longer drug half-life compared with systemic administration. Blood–brain barrier limits the availability of systemic chemotherapeutic agents to brain tumors.

Diagnostic Evaluation

- CSF fluid is dynamic; normal appearance clear and colorless.
- Cultures to evaluate for presence of bacterial, viral, and fungal pathogens. Normal is no growth.
- Differential cell counts—0 to 5 WBCs (all mononuclear), no RBCs, increased with infection, bleeding.
- Cytology—presence of suspicious cells may be insufficient to confirm diagnosis of leptomeningeal disease.

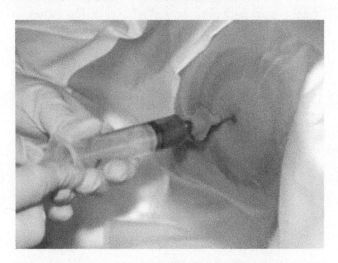

FIGURE 10.6 • **Bone Marrow Aspirate Specimen.** Photo courtesy of Danielle Van Damme.

- Flow cytometry—more sensitive when compared with cytology in detecting leptomeningeal disease.
- Elevated protein levels indicate CNS tumor, infection, bleeding, or inflammation.
- Abnormal glucose levels indicate CNS tumor, infection, or inflammation.

Management/Procedure

- Subcutaneously infiltrate the insertion site with local anesthetic.
- Insert 20G to 22G needle at the superior aspect of the spinous process and inferior to the space entered.
- Insert the needle at the L3/L4 or L4/L5 interspace, the area where the iliac crests intersect the midline.
- Pass the needle through the supraspinous ligament and the ligamentum flavum. At this point, the clinician may feel a "give" or "pop".
- Continue to gently advance the needle, and remove the stylet at 2-mm intervals to assess for free flow of CSF.

- If bone is encountered, partially withdraw the needle to the subcutaneous tissue, repalpate the back and try again.
- Rotate the needle at a 90 degree angle; if CSF is not free flowing, the needle may be obstructed.
- Return the stylet to the catheter before removing the needle to reduce post-LP CSF leakage and headache.
- Encourage the child to lie on their back for approximately 2 hours after the procedure, monitor for neurological changes.
- Obtaining opening and closing pressures: Attach stopcock to measure height of fluid flow prior to and following obtaining fluid samples.
- Intrathecal Medication: Connect medication syringe to stopcock, and infuse. After giving chemotherapy, do not reattach stylet because of risk of chemotherapy spill.

Potential Complications

- Headache is a potential complication, but uncommon in children <13 years of age. Associated symptoms include nausea, vomiting, low back pain, vertigo, and tinnitus. Risk factors for headache are female gender, lower BMI, large needle size, and type of needle (beveled vs. pencil point).
- Traumatic tap presents with macroscopic blood in the CSF. The fluid will generally clear after the first and second tubes are collected. A traumatic LP may alter the cell count in the CSF, increase the CSF protein level, and alter culture and cytology results.
- Neurologic complications associated with intrathecal chemotherapy such as cauda equina syndrome (urinary retention, fecal incontinence), transient communicating hydrocephalus, sacral nerve injury, and arachnoiditis.

PEARLS

- *Fluoroscopic guidance may be used for difficult or failed LP attempts. Restrict the CSF collection to the smallest volume necessary for diagnostic purposes.*
- *If the child complains of shooting pain down their leg during the procedure, withdraw the needle (a nerve root may have inadvertently hit), and start again.*

1. A 3-year-old patient with newly diagnosed ALL is being prepped for a LP. Which landmarks are used to find the L4-L5 intervertebral space?
   a. Measure ¾ of the way down from shoulders to hips.
   b. The space between right and left bilateral posterior iliac crests.
   c. The space between bilateral femoral heads.
   d. The top of the sacrum.

Answer: **B**

The L4-L5 interspace is most easily found by measuring between the tops of the bilateral iliac crests, whether the child is positioned in the recumbent or sitting position.

2. A 14-year-old male patient is currently being treated in PICU with newly diagnosed Burkitt lymphoma and respiratory distress secondary to large mediastinal mass. On physical examination, it is noted that he has increasing facial edema with jugular vein distension and tachycardia. Vital signs are within normal limits. The patient is easily arousable, but complains of headache. These findings most likely represent:
   a. Chest pain secondary to malignancy and mediastinal mass.
   b. Superior vena cava syndrome secondary to tumor compression.
   c. Generalized edema from IV fluids and immobilization.
   d. Congestive heart failure due to cardiotoxicity of the chemotherapy.

Answer: **B**

Superior vena cava syndrome results from compromised venous drainage to the thrombus, which manifests with facial swelling, jugular vein distension, dyspnea, severe headache, visual disturbances, dysphagia, tachycardia, and hypotension.

3. A 5-month-old female infant recently adopted from Southeast Asia presents to the Emergency Department (ED) with pallor, failure to thrive, frontal bossing, hepatosplenomegaly, and jaundice. In considering differential diagnoses, the most helpful diagnostic study results to indicate β-thalassemia would be:
   a. Absence of hemoglobin A on electrophoresis and microcytic anemia.
   b. Presence of hemoglobin SS on electrophoresis with normal RBC indices.
   c. Normal hemoglobin electrophoresis with hypochromic/microcytic anemia.
   d. Presence of fetal hemoglobin on electrophoresis with normal MCV.

Answer: **A**

A hallmark finding of β-thalassemia is absence of hemoglobin A on electrophoresis, which is the study of choice for diagnosis along with microcytic anemia.

4. A 3-year-old presents to the ED with tachycardia, pallor, and petechial rash distributed on his trunk and face. Initial CBC reveals Hgb 3 g/dL, platelet count 19 K/uL, and WBC 1 K/uL. Which of the following diagnoses is highest on the differential list?
   a. Diamond–Blackfan Anemia.
   b. Aplastic Anemia.
   c. β-Thalassemia.
   d. DIC.

Answer: **B**

Aplastic anemia is a life-threatening disease of bone marrow failure resulting in decreased production of hematopoietic stem cells that results in peripheral pancytopenia.

5. A 2-year-old is fatigued easily, and has generalized bruising and bleeding gums when his teeth are brushed. CBC reveals pancytopenia with depressed reticulocytes. Which test will help differentiate between aplastic and infiltrative or dysplastic causes of anemia?
   a. Peripheral blood smear.
   b. D-Dimers.
   c. Protein S.
   d. Total bilirubin.

Answer: **A**

In aplastic anemia, the peripheral blood smear reveals RBCs that are normocytic or macrocytic, and the remaining cellular elements are reduced in number, but morphologically normal. In an infiltrative or dysplastic disease, abnormal cells would be present (i.e., myeloblasts, atypical lymphoid cells).

The next two questions refer to this scenario:
A 10-year-old with ALL, who received chemotherapy 8 days ago, presents with diffuse abdominal pain, intermittent vomiting, poor PO intake, and a fever of 38.7°C.

6. Which of the following diagnoses is the highest on the differential list?
   a. Appendicitis.
   b. Ileus.
   c. Lower lobe pneumonia.
   d. Typhlitis.

Answer: **D**

(continues on page 292)

Historically, patients with typhlitis have received chemotherapy in the previous 2 weeks. Neutropenia is likely to occur 7 to 14 days post–chemotherapy. The classic triad of symptoms for typhlitis is neutropenia, RLQ pain, and fever. In immunocompromised patients, RLQ pain and tenderness usually indicate typhlitis and not appendicitis.

7. A CBC confirms an ANC of 200, with a platelet count of $50,000 \times 10^3/\mu L$ and a hemoglobin of 9.0 g/dL. During the evaluation in the emergency department, symptoms progress in this child to include worsening abdominal pain, bloody diarrhea, pallor, and hypotension. The most appropriate initial management will be to:
   a. Order a PRBC infusion.
   b. Order broad-spectrum antibiotics.
   c. Obtain a surgical consult.
   d. Call for a pain consult.

Answer: **C**

Survival for a child with typhlitis depends on early suspicion in at-risk patients. Surgery is indicated when the patient has persistent bleeding, bowel perforation, or clinical deterioration. Involve surgical specialists early in plan of care.

8. A 9-year-old patient is referred to the ED for fatigue, pallor, and petechiae. She is clinically stable; however, a complete blood count reveals pancytopenia. The priority intervention for this patient is:
   a. Blood transfusion with PRBCs and platelets.
   b. Immediate consult to hematology.
   c. Administration of rasburicase and initiation of IVF at 1.5 times maintenance.
   d. Placement of a central venous catheter for administration of chemotherapy.

Answer: **B**

Early evaluation of a patient with pancytopenia by pediatric oncology will allow for timely diagnosis and intervention. Although transfusion may be necessary, the consult is a priority as this patient is described as clinically stable.

9. A 12-year-old male presents to the ED with complaints of unilateral swelling just below his knee and intermittent pain. A radiograph is obtained that reveals a "starburst" mass in the proximal tibia. This is most concerning for:
   a. Ewing sarcoma.
   b. AML with chloroma formation.
   c. Hodgkin Lymphoma.
   d. Osteosarcoma.

Answer: **D**

Although intermittent pain and soft tissue swelling may occur with Ewing sarcoma, the radiographic finding of a "starburst" mass makes the diagnosis of osteosarcoma more likely, compared with the "moth-eaten" or "onion-skin" appearance described in Ewing sarcoma. This is a less likely site for a chloroma associated with AML, and other symptoms are not described in this patient.

10. Which orders are most appropriate for a 7-year-old with an unremarkable physical examination and a diagnosis of Burkitt lymphoma prior to receiving chemotherapy today?
   a. CBC and complete metabolic profile every 6 hours.
   b. IV fluids at 2 to 3 L/m²/day.
   c. Urine specific gravity checks every 2 hours.
   d. Daily CXR.

Answer: **B**

A child with a newly diagnosed tumor is at an increased risk for tumor lysis syndrome, because of the breakdown of dying cells. Aggressive hydration is the most important preventive measure for tumor lysis syndrome.

11. A 16-year-old with osteosarcoma of the left distal femur has the following laboratory results 6 hours after initiation of chemotherapy:
   Hgb 7.8 g/dL, HCT 22 g/dL, WBC 77,000 mm, Platelets 19,000.
   Na 136 mmol/L, K 6.2 mmol/L, Cl 106 mmol/L, CO_2 18 mmol/L, BUN 33 mg/dL, creat 1.0 mg/dL, glucose 95 mg/dL, calcium 7.5 mg/dL, phos 11 mg/dL.
   Uric acid 8 mg/dL.

   The urine output is currently 1.8 cc/kg/hour. Which of the following would be the next appropriate action?
   a. Administer PRBCs.
   b. Initiate Dialysis.
   c. Administer Allopurinol and Rasburicase.
   d. Administer Calcium Gluconate.

Answer: **C**

Elevated potassium, phosphorous, and uric acid levels are indicative of tumor lysis syndrome. Rasburicase and/or Allopurinol are antihyperuricemic agents used in prevention and treatment of tumor lysis syndrome.

12. A noninvasive test that can be ordered to confirm a suspicion of Neuroblastoma is:
   a. Bone marrow flow cytometry.
   b. Urine for HVA and VMA (catecholamines).
   c. Serum for p53 mutational testing.
   d. Ultrasound of the abdomen.

Answer: **B**

Elevated urine catecholamines are a finding specific to the diagnosis of Neuroblastoma and can be obtained by 24-hour or random urine specimen.

13. The parents of a 4-month-old are concerned that they noticed a white spot in their child's eye. On examination, there is absence of a red reflex in the right eye. This is most likely:
   a. Retinoblastoma.
   b. Periorbital ecchymoses.
   c. Congenital neuroblastoma.
   d. Opsoclonus.

Answer: **A**

Findings of leukocoria, which appears as an abnormal white reflection, in a young infant is most often indicative of a retinoblastoma. An ophthalmology consult should be obtained immediately.

14. A 2-year-old previously healthy child presents to the ED with a report of extreme fatigue, dyspnea on exertion, and pale skin just noticeable today. On examination, the child has marked pallor, tachycardia, and a flow murmur. The child has also had diarrhea over the past few days. The most important initial test to obtain is which of the following.
a. CBC.
b. Stool Culture.
c. Blood Culture.
d. Chest X-Ray.

Answer: **A**

Tachycardia, pallor, and a flow murmur in a child who is fatigued are indications of acute anemia that can occur as a result of many factors, including a recent viral illness.

15. Jaundice is associated with anemia in which of the following conditions?
a. Increased red cell destruction (hemolysis).
b. Excessive blood loss (hemorrhage).
c. Deficient red cell production (ineffective hematopoiesis).
d. Infectious process of hepatitis.

Answer: **A**

Increased rate of RBC destruction may result in an unconjugated hyperbilirubinemia secondary to the liver's inability to conjugate and remove the destroyed RBCs as quickly as they are being hemolyzed.

16. A 7-year-old has been increasingly more irritable over the past 2 weeks. She has also been waking up each morning for the last week with complaints of headache and then vomits. Initial vital signs include BP of 135/88 mmHg and heart rate of 68 beats per minute. The most important initial diagnostic test is:
a. Complete metabolic panel to evaluate liver function.
b. Serum renin test to evaluate hypertension.
c. Echocardiogram to evaluate for left ventricular hypertrophy.
d. CT scan to evaluate for increased intracranial pressure and/or hemorrhage.

Answer: **D**

Headache with emesis on arising can indicate increased intracranial pressure, and without other known etiologies such as trauma, a head CT is the most important initial test, especially to determine the presence of a brain lesion.

17. A four-year old presents to the emergency room (ED) with constipation, abdominal pain and distension, and general malaise. Of note, she also has periorbital ecchymosis, although her caregiver does not recall trauma. The child is hypertensive and ill appearing on initial examination. Which of the following is highest on the differential diagnosis?
a. Wilm tumor.
b. Ewing sarcoma.
c. Hodgkin Lymphoma.
d. Neuroblastoma.

Answer: **D**

Although this patient could have Wilm tumor, the description portrays an ill child with a mass that is impairing her bowel habits. Additionally, she has periorbital ecchymosis, which is likely secondary to metastasis. The hypertension is the result of a sympathetic nervous system tumor arising from the adrenal medulla. Based on this patient's age and the description of her clinically, Ewing sarcoma and Hodgkin Lymphoma are less likely.

18. Children receiving anticoagulation with unfractionated heparin should be monitored:
a. Using PT/INR with a goal of 2 to 3.
b. With Factor X level with a goal of 0.5 to 1.
c. For heparin-induced thrombocytopenia.
d. With Anti-Xa with a goal of 0.5.

Answer: **D**

Unfractionated heparin such as Enoxaparin is used for anticoagulation in many instances instead of heparin or warfarin as it is just as effective with consistent therapy. Factor Xa level is the monitor for effect, but is not always warranted for every patient.

19. A 14-year-old with known sickle cell disease has a history of avascular necrosis of his shoulder a year ago. His current hemoglobin is 11.8 g/dL. Which type of SCD does the patient most likely have?
a. HbSS.
b. HbSC.
c. HbSβ⁰ Thal.
d. Sickle cell trait.

Answer: **B**

Patients with HbSC typically have milder disease, mild anemia, or normal hemoglobin levels. They are also more commonly affected by vascular necrosis than the other types of SCD.

20. The parents of an 18-month-old female are concerned that her abdomen was distended while bathing her last night. She has no other signs or symptoms. On examination, a large right-sided abdominal mass is palpated. Which of the following findings would lead to a higher suspicion of Wilms' Tumor?
a. Multiple café-au-lait lesions.
b. Hemihypertrophy.
c. Ptosis of the right eye.
d. Multiple petechiae and ecchymoses.

Answer: **B**

(continues on page 294)

Congenital hemihypertrophy is a condition of unknown etiology characterized by unilateral overgrowth of part or all of one side of the body, including limbs. Hemihypertrophy is a finding associated with Beckwith–Weidemann Syndrome (BWS). Patients with BWS have a higher risk of developing WIlms' tumor.

21. In a child who is suspected of experiencing a transfusion reaction, the first action is to
    a. Contact the transfusion service to report the reaction.
    b. Administer diphenhydramine and corticosteroids.
    c. Stop the transfusion and administer normal saline.
    d. Administer oxygen via face mask.

Answer: **C**

In a child with a suspected transfusion reaction, the first plan of management is to discontinue the transfusion and closely monitor the patient. The child should receive IV fluids as normal saline to prevent compromise of hemodynamic status.

22. An 8-year-old with HbSS disease presents to the ED with fever, tachypnea, cough, chest pain, and hypoxia. Which disease process are you most concerned about?
    a. Splenic sequestration.
    b. Asthma exacerbation.
    c. Acute chest syndrome.
    d. Pneumonia.

Answer: **C**

While tachypnea, cough, chest pain, hypoxia, and fever may be seen in pneumonia asthma, and acute chest syndrome, the patient with acute chest syndrome can deteriorate rapidly, and this process can be life-threatening. Splenic sequestration typically does not present with hypoxia or chest pain. An 8-year-old patient with HbSS usually will not have splenic sequestration, as the spleen tends to auto-infarct by 5 years of age.

23. Which of the following therapies is most effective in managing vasoocclusive crisis in sickle cell disease?
    a. NSAIDs.
    b. Blood transfusion.
    c. Antibiotics.
    d. Cold packs.

Answer: **A**

NSAIDs are used to manage vasoocclusive crisis. Other ways to manage vasoocclusive crisis include acetaminophen, opiates, heat, distraction, massage, hydration. Cold can trigger vasoocclusive crisis. Blood transfusions are used to treat other complications such as acute chest syndrome, splenic sequestration, and aplastic crisis.

24. A 16-year-old presents to the ED with profound cyanosis, dyspnea, and tachycardia. She has no significant health history, but is currently being treated with Bactrim (Sulfamethoxazole-Trimethoprim) for a urinary tract infection. Despite cyanosis, her pulse oximetry reads 100%, and supplemental oxygen delivered via nonrebreather mask does not improve her cyanosis. Which of the following diagnoses is highest on the differential list?
    a. G6PD deficiency.
    b. Aplastic anemia.
    c. Autoimmune Hemolytic Anemia.
    d. Methemoglobinemia.

Answer: **D**

Methemoglobinemia may develop after exposure to an oxidant drug such as sulfonamide antibiotics, resulting in an altered state of hemoglobin in which the ferrous ($Fe2^+$) irons of heme are oxidized to the ferric ($Fe3^+$) state. Methemoglobin-containing hemoglobin is unable to carry oxygen, ultimately resulting in impaired oxygen delivery to the tissues and cyanosis. Patients with methemoglobinemia and cyanosis may have normal oxygen saturation as measured by pulse oximetry as these devices measure oxygen saturation of only the hemoglobin that is available for saturation. Hallmark clinical finding is that supplemental oxygen does not improve the degree of cyanosis because the oxygen cannot bind to the methemoglobin.

25. Hyperleukocytosis is most likely to occur in which of the following patients?
    a. 2-year-old boy with Wilm tumor.
    b. 13-year-old girl with Osteosarcoma of the left tibia.
    c. 10-year-old boy with newly diagnosed AML.
    d. 11-year-old girl in maintenance therapy for ALL.

Answer: **C**

Hyperleukocytosis, which typically refers to a WBC count of greater than $50 \times 10^9/L$ (50,000/μL) or $100 \times 10^9/L$ (100,000/μL), is often seen in new-onset leukemia. Obtaining a CBC with suspicion of a hematologic illness is a most important diagnostic key in order to identify the diagnosis and begin management.

26. Which test provides the most accurate diagnosis of methemoglobinemia?
    a. Spectrophotometric assay.
    b. CBC.
    c. Peripheral Blood Smear.
    d. Reticulocyte Count.

Answer: **A**

Spectrophotometric assays are used to confirm the presence of methemoglobinemia and to determine the level of methemoglobin. Typically, methemoglobinemia occurs when there is a higher than 1% content in the RBCs.

27. An afebrile 1-year-old male, weighing 11 kg, presents to the pediatric emergency room with significant swelling to both knees after sustaining a fall in the driveway of their home. He has various bruises scattered over his extremities and forehead. Vital signs are stable, but the child is irritable and has been since his fall. What is the most appropriate next step in management?
    a. Obtain CBC with differential and coagulation panel.
    b. Notify child protective services.

c. Obtain bilateral CT scan of his knees.

d. Obtain hemoglobin electrophoresis and coagulation panel.

Answer: **A**

A full hematologic workup is indicated to evaluate for coagulopathy before making assumptions regarding nonaccidental trauma. Radiation exposure is a concern of a CT scan, so the initial laboratory results need review prior to determining imaging studies.

28. A child with cyanosis, dyspnea, and tachycardia was diagnosed with methemoglobinemia secondary to sulfonamide antibiotics. The antibiotics were discontinued. The most appropriate next intervention is:

a. Supportive care.

b. Vitamin K administration.

c. Blood transfusion.

d. Methylene blue administration.

Answer: **D**

Once the causative agent is removed or addressed, Methylene blue administration is the treatment of choice for children with methemoglobinemia who are symptomatic.

29. A 12-year-old, 50 kg female was admitted to the PICU 5 days ago following a motor vehicle crash in which she sustained a crushed pelvis and grade III liver laceration, requiring multiple blood transfusions and significant fluid resuscitation. She underwent an emergency exploratory laparotomy with splenectomy on the day of admission. She has remained sedated, intubated, and ventilated due to bilateral pulmonary contusions. She had an episode of epistaxis last night; today, she has developed blood-tinged secretions from her endotracheal tube (ETT) and has gross hematuria. Which of the following is the highest on the differential list?

a. Pulmonary embolus.

b. DIC.

c. Acute tubular necrosis.

d. Mismatched blood transfusion.

Answer: **B**

The incidence of bleeding is highly suspicious for DIC, especially considering the extent of injuries and support along with the timing. Transfusion reactions would not occur at 5 days following the transfusion.

30. A 20-month-old female presents to the ED with concerns of watery diarrhea for the past 3 days and a new-onset fever. She has been lethargic and listless since the fever started, has had loss of appetite and decreased wet diapers. Her exam is significant for periorbital edema with fine scattered petechiae over her face, upper arms, and legs. Laboratory evaluation indicates normal coagulation studies with elevated BUN and creatinine, anemia, and reticulocytosis. The most likely diagnosis is:

a. HUS.

b. Henoch–Schönlein purpura.

c. Diamond–Blackfan anemia.

d. Septic shock.

Answer: **A**

HUS typically presents with bloody diarrhea and fever. Laboratory studies usually include normal coagulation profile and azotemia. Hemolysis of RBC's occurs secondary to toxin-mediated microangiopathy causing anemia and reticulocytosis.

31. A 9-month-old with a history of prematurity and chronic lung disease was admitted for acute respiratory failure due to RSV bronchiolitis. History includes a 1-month NICU stay with a diagnosis of heparin induced thrombocytopenia during that time. An ultrasound for edema of one lower extremity confirmed an acute nonocclusive thrombus in the left common femoral vein. Best choice for anticoagulation will be:

a. Heparin infusion.

b. Enoxaparin.

c. Aspirin.

d. Bivalirudin.

Answer: **D**

Bivalirudin is a direct thrombin inhibitor and preferred choice of anticoagulation in a patient with a history of HIT. Enoxaparin is a low molecular weight heparin, and aspirin would not be an appropriate anticoagulant for deep vein thrombosis.

32. Analysis of a bone marrow aspirate specimen to identify chromosomal abnormalities is known as

a. Cytogenetics.

b. Flow cytometry.

c. Polymerase chain reaction.

d. Fluorescent in situ hybridization.

Answer: **A**

Cytogenetics is the part of genetics that is involved with the study of the cell. Bone marrow aspirate can be evaluated for chromosomal abnormalities through this process.

33. Type 1 Von Willebrand Disease is inherited as a

a. X-linked disorder.

b. Recessive disorder.

c. Autosomal disorder.

d. Y-linked disorder.

Answer: **C**

Type 1 VWD is a quantitative disorder affecting 75% of patients with VWD. It is inherited as an autosomal dominant disorder. Multimers are normal, but reduced in number and faded on gel with the VWF normal, but present in smaller amounts.

34. An irritable 6-month-old presents with a history of fatigue with feeds, pallor, and low tone. The physical examination indicates that the infant is less than the 3rd percentile for weight and height, tachycardic, and difficult to console. The initial CBC

(continues on page 296)

shows a profound macrocytic anemia, normal WBC, and normal platelet count. The reticulocyte count is very low. Which of the following diagnoses is highest on the differential list?
a. Diamond–Blackfan Anemia.
b. Aplastic Anemia.
c. β-Thalassemia.
d. DIC.

Answer: **A**

Diamond–Blackfan anemia is a rare congenital hypoplastic anemia resulting in constitutional bone marrow failure characterized by a macrocytic anemia, normal WBC count, and normal platelet count. It is associated with an inadequate reticulocyte response.

35. A child with β-thalassemia receives frequent blood transfusions. What is the best way to evaluate the need for iron chelation therapy?
a. Serum ferritin levels and abdominal CT.
b. Serum ferritin levels, superconducting quantum interference device and MRI.
c. Serum iron levels and brain MRI.
d. Serum iron levels and superconducting quantum interference device and CT.

Answer: **B**

Body iron burdens need to be assessed in children who receive frequent blood transfusions. Even though ferritin levels are an appropriate method of evaluation, levels may not reliably indicate total body iron stores. Superconducting quantum interference device and modified MRI is a noninvasive and effective method of determining iron overload.

> **CASE STUDY: THE NEXT TWO QUESTIONS ARE RELATED TO THIS PATIENT**
> *A 4-year-old female is suspected to have Hemophagocytic Lymphohistiocytosis (HLH). In eliciting the family history, it is discovered that the patient had a younger sibling who died as a newborn from "some massive inflammatory disorder, but we are not sure which one." There is also a strong family history of autoimmune disease.*

36. Which of the following tests would be reasonable to perform in the *initial* diagnostic evaluation HLH of this patient?
a. Karyotype of the patient.
b. Genetic testing for gene defects associated HLH, such as Perforin and Syntaxin-11.
c. HLA typing of the patient.
d. Bone marrow biopsy.

Answer: **C**

This patient has a family history suspicious for a genetic/familial predisposition to HLH. It is reasonable to assume that this patient will ultimately proceed to a stem cell transplantation, in which case obtaining HLA typing early is critical in order to have time to find a proper HLA match. Genetic testing for gene defects in Perforin, Syntaxin-11 are appropriate, but not in the initial evaluation, and should be performed with the guidance of a pediatric hematologist/oncologist. Karyotype of the patient is not indicated in the evaluation for HLH.

37. The patient in question #2 (above) is started on HLH therapy. The caregivers ask which therapy will be used, and what the following steps will be? Which of the following is the correct response to these questions?
a. Therapy will be with dexamethasone for 1 month, followed by etoposide for another month, then reevaluation.
b. Therapy will be with dexamethasone and etoposide for 2 months, then if in remission, will likely proceed to a stem cell transplantation if a donor is available.
c. As soon as the patient is stable, a stem cell transplantation with a HLA-matched donor is the next step.
d. The patient's underlying infection will be treated, and then the body will be allowed to "correct itself."

Answer: **B**

Steroids are seldom used alone in treating HLH. Treatment duration is 8 weeks of upfront therapy, with stem cell transplantation as an option to those with a high risk of HLH recurrence. Treating any concurrent infection will seldom make the immune activation in HLH completely "correct itself."

Recommended Readings

Am, S. (2011). PET/CT in pediatric oncology. *Indian Journal of Cancer, 47,* 360–370.

Athale, U., Cox, S., Siciliano, S., & Chan, A. K. (2007). Thromboembolism in children with sarcoma. *Pediatric Blood Cancer, 49*(2), 171–176.

Baggott, C., Fochtman, D., Foley, G., & Kelly, K. (Eds.). (2011). *Nursing care of children and adolescents with cancer and blood disorders* (4th ed.). Glenview, IL: Association of Pediatric Oncology Nurses.

Bain, B. J. (2011). The peripheral smear. In L. Goldman & A. I. Schafer (Eds.), *Cecil medicine* (24th ed., chap 160). Philadelphia, PA: Saunders Elsevier.

Bakhshi, S., Meel, R., Kashyap, S., & Sharma, S. (2011). Bone marrow aspirations and lumbar punctures in retinoblastoma at diagnosis: Correlation with IRSS staging. *Journal of Pediatric Hematology Oncology, 33*(5), 182–185.

Bruccoleri, R. E., & Chen, L. (2012). Needle-entry for lumbar puncture in children as determined by using ultrasonography. *Pediatrics, 127,* 921–926.

Bunn, H. F. (2011). Approach to anemias. In L. Goldman & A. I. Schafer (Eds.), *Cecil medicine* (24th ed., chap 161). Philadelphia PA: Saunders Elsevier.

Castaman, G., Montgomery, R. R., Meschengieser, S. S., Haberichter, S. L., Woods, A. I., & Lazzari, M. A. (2010). Von Willebrand disease diagnosis and laboratory issues. *Haemophilia, 16*(Suppl. 5), 67–73.

Cessna, C., Klersy, C., Scarpati, B., Brando, B., Faleri, M., Bertani, G., . . . Cairoli, R. (2011). Flow cytometry and cytomorphology evaluation of hematologic malignancy in cerebrospinal fluids: Comparison with retrospective clinical data. *Annals of Hematology, 90,* 827–835.

Chi, C., Pollard, D., Tuddenham, E. G., & Kadir, R. A. (2010). Menorrhagia in adolescents with inherited bleeding disorders. *Journal of Pediatric Adolescent Gynecology, 23,* 215–222.

Donelan, K. J., & Anderson, K. A. (2011). Transfusion-related acute lung injury (TRALI) a case report and literature review. *South Dakota Medicine, 64*(3), 85–88.

Eary, J., & Conrad, E. (2011). Imaging in sarcoma. *Journal of Nuclear Medicine, 52,* 1903–1913.

Eng, J., & Fish, J. D. (2011). Insidious iron burden in pediatric patients with acute lymphoblastic leukemia. *Pediatric Blood & Cancer, 56,* 368–371.

Fahey, F. H., Treves, S. T., & Adelstein, S. J. (2012). Minimizing and communicating radiation risk in pediatric nuclear medicine. *Journal of Nuclear Medicine Technology, 40,* 13–24.

Falanga, A., Marchetti, M., & Vignoli, A. (2012). Caaogulation and cancer: biological and clinical aspects. *Journal of Thrombosis & Haemostasis, 11,* 223–233.

Franzius, C. (2010). FDG-PET/CT in pediatric solid tumors. *The Quarterly Journal of Nuclear Medicine and Molecular Imaging, 54,* 401–409.

Frederica, S. M., Spunt, S. L., Krasin, M. J., Billup, C. A., Wu, J., Shulkin, B., . . . McCarville, M. B. (2012). Comparison of PET-CT and conventional imaging in staging pediatric rhabdomyosarcoma. *Pediatric Blood Cancer, 60*(7), 1128–1134.

Gelfand, M. J., Parisi, M. T., & Treves, S. T. (2011). Pediatric radiopharmaceutical administered doses: 2010 North American consensus guidelines. *Journal of Nuclear Medicine, 52,* 318–322.

Gurram, M. K., Newman, W., & Kobrinsky, N. (2012). Prevalence of iron overload in pediatric oncology patients after blood transfusion. *Clinical Advances in Hematology & Oncology, 10,* 363–365.

Goldenberg, N. A., & Bernard, T. J. (2010). Venous thromboembolism in children. *Hematology Oncology Clinics of North America, 24,* 151–166.

Hasegawa, D., Manabe, A., & Ohara, A. (2012). The utility of performing the initial lumbar puncture on D8 in remission induction therapy for childhood acute lymphoblastic leukemia: TCCSG L99-15 study. *Pediatric Blood Cancer, 58,* 23–30.

Helgestad, J., Rosthoj, S., Johansen, P., Varming, K., & Ostergaard, E. (2011). Bone marrow aspiration technique may have an impact on therapy stratification in children with acute lymphoblastic leukemia. *Pediatric Blood Cancer, 57,* 224–226.

Hesselgrave, J. (2011). Oncologic emergencies. In C. Baggott, D. Fochtman, G. Foley & K. P. Kelly (Eds.), *Nursing care of children and adolescents with cancer and blood disorders* (4th ed., pp. 676–677). Philadelphia, PA: Saunders.

Holzhauer, S., Goldenberg, N. A., Junker, R., Heller, C., Stoll, M., Manner, D., . . . Nowak-Göttl, U. (2012). Inherited thrombophilia in children with venous thromboembolism and the familial risk of thromboembolism: An observational study. *Blood, 120,* 1353–1355.

Istaphanous, G. K., Wheeler, D. S., Lisco, S. J., & Shander, A. (2011). Red blood cell transfusion in critically ill children: A narrative review. *Pediatric Critical Care Medicine, 12,* 174–183.

Jordan, M. B., Allen, C. E., Weitzman, S., Filipovich, A. H., & McClain, K. L. (2011). How I treat hemophagocytic lymphohistiocytosis. *Blood, 118*(15), 4041–4052.

Kaste, S. (2011). PET-CT in children: Where is it appropriate? *Pediatric Radiology, 41*(Suppl. 2), S509–S513.

Landier, W., Armenian, S. H., Lee, J., Thomas, O., Wong, F. L., Francisco, L., . . . Bhatia S. (2012). Yield of screening for long-term complications using the Children's Oncology Group long-term follow-up guidelines. *Journal of Clinical Oncology, 30,* 4401–4408.

Lavole, J. (2011). Blood transfusion risks and alternative strategies in pediatric patients. *Pediatric Anesthesia, 21,* 14–24.

Linkins, L. A., Dans, A. L., Moores, L. K., Bona, R., Davidson, B. L., Schulman, S., . . . American College of Chest Physicians. (2012). Treatment and prevention of heparin-induced thrombocytopenia: Antithrombotic therapy and prevention of thrombosis, 9th ed: American college of chest physicians evidence-based clinical practice guidelines. *Chest, 141*(2 Suppl), e495s–e530s.

Mikhail, S., & Kouides, P. (2010). Von Willebrand disease in the pediatric and adolescent population. *Journal of Pediatric Adolescent Gynecology, 23,* S3–S10.

Monagle, P., Chan, A. K., Goldenberg, N. A., Ichord, R. N., Journeycake, J. M., Nowak-Gᾶkttl, U., . . . American College of Chest Physicians. (2012). Antithrombotic therapy in neonates and children: Antithrombotic therapy and prevention of thrombosis, 9th ed: American college of chest physicians evidence-based clinical practice guidelines. *Chest, 141*(2 Suppl.), e737S–e801S.

Nakatani, K., Nakamoto, Y., & Watanabe, K. (2012). Roles and limitations of FDG PET in pediatric non-hodgkin lymphoma. *Clinical Nuclear Medicine, 37,* 656–662.

National Cancer Institute. (n.d.). *Childhood cancers.* Retrieved from http://www .cancer.gov/cancertopics/types/childhoodcancers

National Institutes of Health, National Cancer Institute. (2014a). *Childhood brain and spinal cord tumors treatment overview (PDQ®).* Retrieved from http://cancer.gov/cancertopics/pdq/treatment/childbrain/healthprofessional

National Institutes of Health, National Cancer Institute. (2014). *Childhood rhabdomyosarcoma treatment (PDQ®).* Retrieved from http://cancer.gov/cancertopics/pdq/treatment/childrhabdomyosarcoma/HealthProfessional

National Institutes of Health, National Cancer Institute. (2014). *Osteosarcoma and malignant fibrous histiocytoma of bone treatment (PDQ®).* Retrieved from http://cancer.gov/cancertopics/pdq/treatment/osteosarcoma/HealthProfessional

National Institutes of Health, National Cancer Institute.(2015). *Retinoblastoma treatment (PDQ®).* Retrieved from http://cancer.gov/cancertopics/pdq/treatment/retinoblastoma/HealthProfessional

National Institutes of Health, National Cancer Institute. (2015). *Childhood soft tissue sarcoma treatment (PDQ®).* Retrieved from http://cancer.gov/cancertopics/pdq/treatment/child-soft-tissue-sarcoma/HealthProfessional

Parker, H. (2012). Lumbar puncture. In K. Reuter-Rice & B. Bolick (Eds.), *Pediatric acute care: A guide for interprofessional practice* (pp. 1278–1284). Burlington, MA: Jones & Bartlett Learning.

Pizzo, P. A., & Poplack, D. G. (Eds.). (2011). *Principles and practice of pediatric oncology* (6th ed.). Philadelphia, PA: Lippincott Williams & Wilkins.

Ruccione, K. S. (2012). Association of projected transfusional iron burden with treatment intensity in childhood cancer survivors. *Pediatric Blood Cancer, 59,* 697–702.

Vakil, N. H., Kanaan, A. O., & Donovan, J. L. (2012). Heparin-induced thrombocytopenia in the pediatric population: A review of the current literature. *Journal of Pediatric Pharmacology & Therapeutics, 17*(1), 12–30.

Voss, S. D., Chen, L., Constine, L. S., Chauvenet, A., Fitzgerald, T. J., Kaste, S. C., . . . Schwartz, C. L. (2012). Surveillance computed tomography imaging and detection of relapse in intermediate and advanced stage pediatric Hodgkin's lymphoma: A report from the Children's Oncology Group. *American Society of Clinical Oncology, 30,* 2635–2640.

Walter, F., Czernin, J., Hall, T., Allen-Auerbach, M., Walter, M. A., Dunkelmann, S., & Federman, N. (2012). Is there a need for dedicated bone imaging in addition to F-FDG PET/CT imaging in pediatric sarcoma patients? *Journal of Pediatric Hematology Oncology, 34,* 131–136.

Infectious Disorders

Fever

Background

- Elevation in body temperature as a result of cytokine-induced displacement of the hypothalamic set point.
- Regulated through the hypothalamus.
- Pyrogens can be exogenous or endogenous substances.
  - Endogenous pyrogens: interleukin 1 (IL-1), interleukin 6 (IL-6), tumor necrosis factor α (TNF-α).
  - Exogenous cytokines: derived from bacterial toxins, bacterial products, or microorganisms.
- Results in elevated core temperature, shivering, and core vasoconstriction.

Definitions (Rectal)

- Neonate (0–28 days): ≥38.0°F/100.4°C.
- Young infant (29–90 days): ≥38.0°F/100.4°C.
- Older infant and toddler: ≥39.0°F/102.2°C.

Fever in Neonate

Andrea M. Kline-Tilford

- Temperature ≥38.0°C (100.4°F); rectal.
- Neonates, birth to 28 days, are at greater risk for significant bacterial infection (SBI).
- At birth, presence of maternal IgG cells; however, absence of immunologic memory and adaptive immunity.
- B and T cells are at normal levels, but are less efficient than adult cells.
- Complete evaluation required when a neonate develops fever (e.g., full septic workup/evaluation).
  - Complete blood count (CBC) with differential, blood culture, urinalysis (UA), and urine culture (specimen obtained through catheterization).
  - Lumbar puncture.
- Immune system rapidly develops in the first 3 months of life.

- Neonates often lack focal examination findings in the presence of an SBI.
- Most commonly, SBI in neonates results from bacteremia, meningitis, pneumonia, or urinary tract infection (UTI).
- Common SBI pathogens in neonates:
  - Group B streptococcus.
  - *Listeria monocytogenes.*
  - *Salmonella.*
  - *Escherichia coli.*
  - *Neisseria meningitides.*
  - *Streptococcus pneumoniae.*
  - *Haemophilus influenzae* type B.
  - *Staphylococcus aureus.*
- Other common pathogens resulting in serious infection/illness in the neonate:
  - Respiratory syncytial virus (RSV).
  - Varicella-zoster virus.
  - *Candida* species.
- If nasal congestion, evaluation is needed for RSV, parainfluenza, and influenza.
- Plan is individualized; however, admission indicated in negative evaluation.
- If nontoxic, empiric antibiotics may be delayed until laboratory evaluation is collected and results are available.
- Recommended empiric antibiotic coverage in neonates includes ampicillin and gentamicin or ampicillin and cefotaxime.
- Acyclovir, in addition to empiric antibiotics, if one of the following: seizures, cerebrospinal fluid (CSF) pleocytosis, primary maternal herpes simplex virus (HSV) infection, prolonged maternal rupture of membranes, mucocutaneous lesion, or fetal scalp electrode use.
  - Continue until CSF HSV polymerase chain reaction (PCR) results are available.
  - Recent evidence suggests acyclovir therapy for any infant <4 weeks of age with fever.
- If laboratory evaluation is suggestive of UTI, full laboratory evaluation is still warranted. Admission and initiation of ampicillin and gentamicin are indicated.

- Discharge if cultures are negative at 48 to 72 hours and the neonate is stable and afebrile. Close with primary care provider is needed, typically 48 hours after discharge.

PEARLS
- *Normal white blood cell (WBC) count does not exclude infection.*
- *If CSF pleocytosis, send CSF sample for HSV PCR.*
- *If RSV positive, risk for SBI does not change and full evaluation for SBI is indicated.*
- *An identifiable source is not found in most neonates with fever.*

Fever without a Source

Andrea M. Kline-Tilford

Definition

- Presence of fever when history and physical examination are unable to identify a specific etiology / cause in an acutely ill nontoxic-appearing infant / child <3 years of age.
- Also called "fever without localizing signs" or "fever without a focus."
- Risk of SBI is higher in younger infants / children.
- Most infants / children with fever without a source (FWS) will have an underlying self-limiting viral infection.
- Etiology has changed significantly since the advancement in vaccination (e.g., use of *H. influenzae* [Hib] vaccine has reduced the incidence of invasive infection by 90% in developed countries).
- Bacteremia, UTIs, and pneumonia may not be associated with clinical symptoms.
- If toxic-appearing, hospital admission, empiric antibiotics, and full diagnostic evaluation are indicated. If well-appearing, hospital admission and empiric antibiotic therapy are determined based on patient age and laboratory evaluation results.
- Physical examination in young infants cannot be relied on, solely, and a more detailed diagnostic evaluation is needed.
  - Higher fever in older infants / toddlers is associated with increased incidence of occult bacteremia.
- If toxic in appearance (any age infant / child), evaluation includes CBC, UA, urine culture, and lumbar puncture. Chest radiography if respiratory signs / symptoms, temperature >40°C, or pulse oximetry value <95% on room air; stool evaluation for WBCs if presence of diarrhea.
- Common bacterial infection in older infants and children:
  - *Staph. aureus* and *Mycoplasma pneumoniae*
  - *N. meningitides.*
  - *Salmonella.*
- Empiric antibiotic coverage in young infants often includes ampicillin, ceftriaxone, or cefotaxime and vancomycin. In older toxic-appearing infants and children, ceftriaxone or cefotaxime and vancomycin are often selected.
  - Tailor antibiotics when organism and sensitivities are available.

- If an older infant is well-appearing and able to tolerate oral medications, consider a dose of intramuscular ceftriaxone, followed by oral antibiotics and with primary health care provider in 1 to 2 days.
- Three most common approaches with FWS are summarized by Rochester, Milwaukee, Boston, and Philadelphia Criteria (see Table 11.1).

PEARLS
- *Approach to FWS is greatly impacted by infant/ child's immunization status.*
- *Fever >38.5°C is not typically associated with teething.*
- *In older toddlers and children, incidence of occult bacteremia increases with height of temperature.*
- *Normal CBC and physical examination do not exclude meningitis.*
- *UTI is the most common cause of SBI in febrile infants.*

Fever of Unknown Origin

Meghan Shackelford

Definition

- Fever >101°F or >38.3°C lasting for at least 8 days and up to 3 weeks with no apparent clinical diagnosis.

Etiology

- Most common causes of fever of unknown origin (FUO) are infectious disease and connective tissue disorders.
- Neoplastic disorders are less common and typically have manifestations other than fever.
- Generally caused by a common disorder with an unusual presentation.
  - Sepsis, meningitis, urosepsis, toxic shock syndrome (TSS), and pneumonia should be considered during investigation of fever.
  - Meningitis should always be considered when evaluating an infant / child with FUO. See Table 11.2 for common pathogens in meningitis.

Pathophysiology

- Variable, depending on fever source.

Evaluation

- History.
  - Fever identification: touch, thermometry device, and site of temperature measurement.
  - Fever history is an important consideration.
  - Presentation of fever with sweating could indicate heat intolerance or hyperthyroid disease.
  - Lack of response to nonsteroidal anti-inflammatory drugs (NSAIDs) can indicate a noninflammatory condition causing the FUO (e.g., dysautonomia, ectodermal dysplasia).

TABLE 11.1 Examples of Criteria Approaches to FWS

	Boston	Milwaukee	Philadelphia	Rochester
Age	28–89 d	28–56 d	29–60 d	≤60 d
Temperature	≥38.0°C	≥38.0°C	≥38.2°C	≥38.0°C
History	No immunizations or antibiotics in prior 48 hr. No evidence of dehydration.	Not defined.	Not defined.	Term infant. No perinatal antibiotic administration. Absence of underlying disease. Not hospitalized longer than mother.
Appearance/ Physical Examination	Well-appearing. No signs of focal infection (e.g., otitis media, soft tissue).	Well-appearing. No evidence of dehydration. No signs of focal infection (e.g., otitis media, soft tissue).	Well-appearing. Unremarkable physical examination.	Well-appearing. No signs of focal infection (e.g., otitis media, soft tissue).
Laboratory Results	Serum WBC <20,000/mm^3. CSF <10 WBC/mm^3. UA <10 WBC/hpf. Chest radiograph: no focal infiltrate (if obtained).	Serum WBC <15,000/mm^3. CSF <10 WBC/mm^3. UA <5–10 WBC/hpf; no bacteria, leukocyte, and nitrite negative. Chest radiograph: no focal infiltrate (if obtained).	Serum WBC <15,000 /mm^3. Band to neutrophil ratio <0.2. CSF <8 WBC/mm^3. CSF Gram stain negative. UA <10 WBC/hpf. Urine Gram stain negative. Chest radiograph: no focal infiltrate. Stool: no blood, few or no WBCs on smear (if obtained).	Serum WBC <5,000/mm^3 >15,000/mm^3. Band neutrophils <1,500/mm^3. CSF: not applicable; no lumbar puncture indicated. UA <10 WBC/hpf Stool WBC ≤5/hpf (if obtained).
Low-Risk Management Strategy	Home/outpatient. Empiric antibiotics. Follow-up evaluation required.	Home with reliable caretaker. Follow-up evaluation required. Ceftriaxone 50 mg/kg IM with reevaluation in 24 hr.	Home/outpatient. No antibiotics. Follow-up evaluation required.	Home/outpatient. No antibiotics. Follow-up evaluation required.
High-Risk Management Strategy	Hospitalize. Antibiotic therapy.	Not defined.	Hospitalize. Antibiotic therapy.	Hospitalize. Antibiotic therapy.

hpf, high-powered field; WBC, white blood cell; IM, intramuscular

TABLE 11.2 Most Common Pathogens in Meningitis by Age Group

Age	Pathogens	Symptoms
Neonates–28 d of life	Group B streptococcus *E. coli.* *L. monocytogenes* *Strep. pneumoniae* *H. influenzae type b* *Staph. aureus* *Herpes simplex virus (HSV)* Also consider viral etiology.	Lethargy Poor feeding Fever or hypothermia Vomiting Apnea
1–3 mo of age	*C. trachomatis* *Strep. pneumoniae* *N. meningitidis* Group B streptococcus (late-onset GBS infection) Pertussis Consider viral etiology.	Fever Nuchal rigidity Change in mental status Change in LOC + Kernig sign + Brudzinski sign
3 mo–2 y of age	*N. meningitidis* *Strep. pneumoniae* *Moraxella catarrhalis* Group A streptococcus *Salmonella* *Mycoplasma pneumoniae* *M. tuberculosis* Mostly bacterial; low incidence of viral.	Fever Headache Nuchal rigidity Change in LOC + Kernig sign + Brudzinski sign Erythematous rash, if toxic shock syndrome present.
2–18 y of age	*N. meningitidis* *Strep. pneumoniae* *Chlamydia* *M. tuberculosis* Mostly bacterial; low incidence of *H. influenzae.*	Fever Headache Nuchal rigidity Change in LOC + Kernig sign + Brudzinski sign Erythematous rash if toxic shock syndrome present.

LOC, loss of consciousness

- Evaluate other clinical manifestations that accompany the fever, such as urine output, feeding intolerance, vomiting, pain, headache.
- Diagnostic evaluation.
  - CBC, blood culture, UA and urine culture, erythrocyte sedimentation rate (ESR), C-reactive protein (CRP), complete metabolic panel (CMP); consider lactate if the child appears septic.
  - Consider chest radiography.
  - Tuberculosis testing, human immunodeficiency virus (HIV) evaluation, or immune evaluation.

Management

- Based on age and presentation at time of fever.
- If a child is ill-appearing or in septic shock, the evaluation is more comprehensive.
- *Neonates to 28 days* with temperature >38.0°C rectal (see "Fever in Neonate" for more detail).
- *Infants 1 to 3 months of age:*
  - The most common differential for this age group includes bacteremia, meningitis, and UTI.
  - In the ill-appearing infant, cultures should be obtained, including blood, urine, and CSF culture. A WBC count with differential should also be obtained. IV antibiotics should be started and the child is admitted to the hospital. A chest radiography is optional in this age group.
  - If meningitis is suspected, ampicillin and cefotaxime are indicated with acyclovir.
- *Infant >3 months of age:*
  - Vancomycin and ceftriaxone are antibiotics of choice.
  - If treating pneumonia, cefotaxime and ampicillin or clindamycin are recommended.
- *Children 3 months to 2 years of age:*
  - This age group has fever typically related to a bacterial etiology.
  - Differential diagnosis: meningitis, pneumonia, toxic shock, and urosepsis. Toxic shock typically presents with an erythematous rash.
  - In the ill-appearing child, cultures should be sent in addition to WBC count with differential and hospital admission is warranted.
  - Antibiotic choices for meningitis include vancomycin and ceftriaxone.
  - If treating pneumonia, ampicillin, cefuroxime, or ceftriaxone can be used with clindamycin or vancomycin for empiric treatment.
  - If the child is well-appearing, discharge home with outpatient follow-up.
- *Children 2 to 18 years of age:*
  - Toxic shock, meningitis, and pneumonia are common etiologies.
  - If the child is ill-appearing and hemodynamically unstable, blood, urine, and CSF cultures should be obtained, along with CBC count and differential. IV antibiotics should be started and hospital admission is warranted.
  - If treating pneumonia, azithromycin with cefuroxime or ceftriaxone, and clindamycin or vancomycin are antibiotics of choice.
  - If meningitis is suspected, ceftriaxone and vancomycin are initiated.
- See Table 11.3 for common infectious diseases by body system.
- See Table 11.4 for examples of cephalosporin coverage.
- See Box 11.1 for helpful cephalosporin mnemonics.

TABLE 11.3 Common Infectious Organisms and Disease/System Involved

Organism	Disease/System Process
Gram-positive cocci (aerobic): *Staph. aureus* *Staph. epidermis* Other *Staphylococcus* species	Nosocomial: wound, ventilator Neonatal UTI (typically hospital-associated infections)
Gram-positive enterococcus (aerobic): *Strep. gordoni* *Strep. pneumoniae* *Strep. mutans* *Strep. viridans*	Endocarditis Sepsis Meningitis Urinary tract infection
Gram-positive enterococcus (aerobic): *Staph. pyogenes*	Toxic shock syndrome Necrotizing fasciitis
Gram-positive cocci (anaerobic): *Peptostreptococcus*	Peritonitis; can occur anywhere (e.g., soft tissue, CNS, chest, bone)
Gram-negative cocci: *N. meningiditis* *M. cattarhalis*	Meningitis Myocarditis Otitis media Sinusitis
Gram-positive bacilli: *L. monocytogenes* *C. difficile* *C. botulinum*	Sepsis (*L. monocytogenes*); primarily <2 mo of age Meningitis (*L. monocytogenes*); primarily <2 mo of age Antibiotic or hospital-acquired diarrhea (*C. difficile*) Flaccid paralysis (*C. botulinum*)
Gram-negative bacilli: *E. coli* *Enterobacter* *P. mirabilis* *K. pneumoniae*	Wound infection UTI Meningitis Bacteremia Health care–associated infections (especially Klebsiella; increasing resistance also)
Gram-negative bacilli: *P. aeruginosa*	Bacteremia Sepsis Health care–associated infections Encephalitis Meningitis Pneumonia

---

Box 11.1 First- and Second-Generation Cephalosporin Coverage Mnemonic

First-Generation Cephalosporin Coverage:

"PEcK"

Proteus

E. coli

Klebsiella.

In addition, first-generation cephalosporins cover gram-positive cocci, including methicillin-sensitive *Staph. aureus*, *Staph. epidermis*, *Strep. agalactiae*, *Strep. pneumoniae*, and *Strep. pyogenes*.

Second-Generation Cephalosporin Coverage:

"HENPEcKS"

H. influenzae

Enterobacter aerogenes

N. meningitidis

Proteus

E. coli

Klebsiella

Serratia marcescens

In addition, second-generation cephalosporins are active against gram-positive cocci, including methicillin-sensitive *Staph. aureus*, *Staph. epidermidis*, *Strep.* species (excluding *Strep. faecalis*). Activity against gram-positive cocci is not as strong as first-generation cephalosporins.

- See Box 11.2 for examples of organisms requiring double antibiotic coverage.

Box 11.2 Pathogens Requiring "Double" Antimicrobial Coverage*

"SPACE" Mnemonic

S—Serratia

P—Pseudomonas

A—Acinetobacter

C—Citrobacter

E—Enterobacter

*These are examples of pathogens requiring double coverage with antibiotics. Additional pathogens may require double coverage, depending on local antibiotic resistance patterns.

- Refer to an antimicrobial reference (e.g., Sanford Guide) for additional information on appropriate antibiotic coverage for pathogens (Tables 11.5 and 11.6).

TABLE 11.4 Examples of Cephalosporin Generations

First Generation	Second Generation	Third Generation	Fourth Generation
Cefazolin Cephalexin Cefadroxil Cephradine	Cefaclor Cefuroxime Cefprozil Loracarbef Cephamycins; give resistance to β-lactamases. Different from other second-generation cephalosporins. Similar activity, though, have activity against anaerobic bacteroides.	Cefdinir Cefixime Cefotaxime Ceftriaxone Cefpiramide	Cefepime Cefluprenam Cefozopran Cefpirome

Spectrum of Activity

Good gram-positive cocci coverage (e.g., *Streptococci*, *Staphylococci, Enterococci*). Not effective against methicillin-resistant *Staph. aureus* or penicillin-resistant *Strep. pneumoniae*. Some gram-negative coverage (e.g., *E. coli, P. mirabilis*, and *K. pneumoniae*). Poor activity *H. influenzae* and *M. catarrhalis*.	Almost comparable to first-generation agents against *Streptococci*; slight loss of activity against *Staphylococcus*. Do not provide coverage against MRSA. Gram-negative aerobe coverage: *M. catarrhalis, P. mirabilis, H. influenzae, Klebsiella, N. gonorrheae*. No coverage against *Enterococci* or *Pseudomonas*.	Limited gram-positive coverage. Cefotaxime, ceftriaxone, and ceftizoxime have the best gram-positive coverage of third generation cephalosporins including *Staph. aureus* (methicillin-sensitive), group A and B streptococci, viridans streptococci. Enhanced β-lactamase stability; activity against gram-negative bacteria. Known to induce gram-negative bacteria resistance. Gram-negative bacteria: *H. influenzae, M. catarrhalis, N. meningitidis, Proteus, Klebsiella, Serratia, Providencia, Citrobacter, E. coli*. None are effective against *Listeria*, or methicillin-resistant *Staphylococci* or *Enterococci*. No coverage for *Pseudomonas*. Cefotaxime and ceftriaxone have coverage against oral anaerobes.	Broadest spectrum of activity. Similar gram-positive coverage as first-generation cephalosporins. Gram-positive cocci: group A and B streptococci, *Strep. pneumoniae, Staph. aureus* (methicillin susceptible). Gram-negative bacteria: improved activity compared with third generation. Excellent coverage for *Pseudomonas* and Enterobacteriaceae. Limited anaerobic coverage.

Uses

Uncomplicated skin/ soft tissue infections, uncomplicated UTIs, group A streptococcal pharyngitis, surgical prophylaxis. Does NOT provide good coverage for acute otitis media. Do *not* cross the blood–brain barrier; NOT a good choice for CNS infections (e.g., meningitis). Cefazolin is used most frequently.	Otitis media, acute sinusitis, upper and lower respiratory tract infections, uncomplicated UTIs. Do *not* cross blood–brain barrier; *not* a good choice for CNS infections.	Meningitis: gram-negative bacilli; upper respiratory tract infections, otitis media, pyelonephritis, skin and soft tissue infections. Lyme disease (Ceftriaxone). Gonorrhea (Ceftriaxone). Good penetration into CSF (cefotaxime, ceftazadime, ceftriaxone). Antipseudomonal cephalosporin; ceftazadime.	Nosocomial pathogens; especially cefepime and cefpirome. Crosses blood–brain barrier/CNS penetration: cefepime.

Fever and Neutropenia

Meghan Shackelford

Definition

- Fever with neutropenia can present in a patient with cancer diagnosis secondary to chemotherapy or secondary to hematologic disease.
- One third of children treated with chemotherapy or stem cell transplant develop fever.
- Fever in a neutropenic patient is defined as a single temperature >38.3°C or >38.0°C for >1 hour with an absolute neutrophil count (ANC) <500 cells/μL or an ANC that is expected to decrease <500 cells/μL within the next 48 hours.

Etiology

- Bacteremia is the most common etiology.
- Common sites of infection include the gastrointestinal (GI) tract (e.g., oral and intestinal mucositis, diarrhea), upper and lower respiratory tracts, urinary tract, skin, and soft tissues.
- Diarrhea is most commonly caused by *Clostridium difficile* and *Salmonella*.
- Gram-positive and gram-negative organisms must be considered.
  - Gram-positive pathogens are coagulase-negative staphylococci, viridans streptococci, and *Staph. aureus* (including MRSA).
  - Gram-negative organisms are gram-negative bacilli, *E. coli*, *Klebsiella*, *Pseudomonas*, *Acinetobacter*, and *Enterobacter*.
- Candida and other fungal species can develop after prolonged use of broad-spectrum antibiotic therapy.
  - Other opportunistic fungi include *Aspergillus*, *Phycomycetes*, and *Cryptococcus*.
- Viral etiologies in these children include HSV, varicella-zoster virus, as well as respiratory viruses.

Pathophysiology

- Neutropenia is defined as a decrease in neutrophils with a circulating count of <1,500 cells/μL.
- Occurs secondary to the damage of the precursor cells and depression of bone marrow function or can be linked to an autoimmune reaction.

Clinical Presentation

- A complete history is essential in determining whether neutropenia and fever are linked to chemotherapy and an infectious process or are of a hemolytic etiology.
- Important history includes antimicrobial prophylaxis, infectious exposures, chronic steroid therapy, history of infections or bacterial colonization, fever-causing medications, type of chemotherapeutic agents received, recent blood product transfusion, presence of invasive lines/devices, previous chemotherapy.
- Skin breakdown is a portal of infection for an immunocompromised patient.
- Monitoring for pancreatitis and pneumonia and evaluation of subtle vital sign changes such as tachycardia assist in diagnosis and prompt, accurate treatment.

Diagnostic Evaluation

- Laboratory evaluation: CBC with differential and platelet count, CMP, including BUN (blood urea nitrogen)/creatinine, AST (aspartate aminotransferase)/ALT (alanine transaminase), and total bilirubin; blood, urine, body fluid, and, sometimes, CSF cultures.
- Imaging may be indicated: computed tomography (CT) or ultrasound if concern for fluid collections, effusions, or acute changes; chest radiography if respiratory symptoms.
- If a central venous catheter is present, a blood culture should be obtained and sent from each lumen.
  - Removal of the central line may be indicated.
- In the absence of a central venous catheter, a peripheral culture should be obtained using sterile technique.
- Lumbar puncture if altered mental status.
- *C. difficile* toxin assay if diarrhea is present.

Management

- Broad-spectrum antibiotics are administered quickly to the neutropenic patient with fever. Treatment varies according to individual patient according to specific guidelines.
- Two categories: high-risk and low-risk.
  - High-risk patients have neutropenia expected to last >7 days, are clinically unstable, and have comorbidities.
  - Low-risk patients have neutropenia expected to last <7 days and are clinically stable with no comorbidities.
- Low-risk outpatient: Ciprofloxacin and amoxicillin–clavulanate PO are recommendations for treatment, followed by observation for 4 to 24 hours after initiation of antibiotics.
- Low-risk inpatient: Zosyn, carbapenem, ceftazidime, or cefepime based on suspected organism, severity of infection, and preference.
- High-risk patient: hospital admission and antibiotic therapy with Zosyn, carbapenem, ceftazidime, or cefepime. For patients with minimal response or signs of decline, therapy should be adjusted for clinical, radiographic, and/or culture data. Vancomycin or linezolid should be used for cellulitis or pneumonia. An aminoglycoside and carbapenem should be used for pneumonia or a gram-negative bacteremia. Flagyl should be used if the patient has abdominal symptoms or suspected *C. difficile* infection.

- Infectious disease consult is warranted for the high-risk patient, especially if not responsive to therapy.
- Antifungal therapy is reserved for neutropenic patients with fever persisting for 4 to 7 days after starting broad-spectrum antibiotics.
  - Amphotericin B is often the initial recommendation; however, should be considered with caution because of significant toxicity risk.

PEARLS
- *Prompt treatment in the neutropenic patient with a fever is essential to decreasing mortality.*
- *High-risk and low-risk patient classifications guide therapy.*
- *The gold standard is to treat with a broad-spectrum antibiotic as quickly as possible and to obtain cultures prior to the start of antibiotic therapy.*

Health Care Associated Infections
Jill S. Thomas

Central Line-Associated Bloodstream Infections

Background

- A health care–associated infection is an infection that is not present upon hospital admission but develops within 48 hours of admission in an acute care setting.
- Infections not present at discharge but apparent within 10 days after discharge are also considered to be of nosocomial origin.

Definition

- Central line–associated bloodstream infection: a primary bloodstream infection (BSI) in a patient who had a central line infection within the 48-hour period before the development of a BSI and the BSI is not related to another infected site.

Etiology/Types

- Migration of skin organisms at the insertion site, leading to colonization of the catheter tip.
- Direct catheter or catheter hub contamination; infusate contamination.
- Hematogenous seeding of catheters by other sites of infection.
- Common causative organisms include coagulase-negative staphylococci, gram-negative bacteria, *Staph. aureus*, and *Candida* species.

Clinical Presentation

- Fever, chills, hypotension: neonates/infants may present with hypothermia, apnea, and bradycardia.
- See http://www.cdc.gov/nhsn/PDFs/pscManual/17pscNosInfDef_current.pdf for delineation of Center for Disease Control and Prevention (CDC) CLABSI criteria.

Diagnostic Evaluation

- Two quantitative blood cultures, with at least one drawn peripherally.
- Qualitative blood cultures can be used with continuously monitored differential time to positivity.
- Catheter tip cultures, CBC with differential, CRP, ESR.
- Urine, sputum, respiratory viral cultures as indicated to evaluate for other infectious sources.

Management

- Empiric antibiotic coverage with broad-spectrum gram-positive and gram-negative bacterial coverage with adjustment of coverage on determination of isolate's sensitivities.
- Consideration of central line removal with subsequent replacement of intravenous access.

Ventilator-Associated Events, Including Pneumonia

Definitions

- Ventilator-associated events: include a surveillance algorithm to identify a broad range of conditions and complications occurring during mechanical ventilation.
- Ventilator-associated condition: period of baseline stability or improvement on mechanical ventilation; ≥ 2 calendar days of stable or decreasing Fio_2 or positive end-expiratory pressure (PEEP) values, followed by at least one of the following indicators of deteriorating status.
  - Increase in Fio_2 ≥ 0.20 from baseline period, sustained for ≥ 2 calendar days.
  - Increase in PEEP level of ≥ 3 cm H_2O from baseline period, sustained for ≥ 2 calendar days.
  - PEEP values of 0 to 5 cm H_2O are considered equivalent in ventilator-associated pneumonia (VAP) surveillance.
- Infection-related ventilator-associated complication (IVAC).
  - $\geq$ Calendar day 3 of mechanical ventilation and within 2 days before or after the deterioration in oxygenation, *both* of the following criteria are met.
    - Temperature $>38\,^{\circ}$C or $<36\,^{\circ}$C, or WBC count $\geq 12,000$ cells/mm^3 or $\leq 4,000$ cells/mm^3.
    - New antimicrobial(s) initiated and continued for ≥ 4 calendar days.
- VAP.
  - Pediatric VAP surveillance guidelines were published by the CDC in January 2015. Specific guidelines for diagnosis of pediatric VAP are not yet available. Refer to CDC website: http://www.cdc.gov/HAI/vap/vap.html
  - Guidelines for surveillance and diagnosis are based on changes in ventilation requirements, presence of purulent or increased secretions, fever, and results of laboratory testing to include culture of bronchial aspiration.
- Typical organisms responsible for VAP in children include coagulase-negative staphylococcus, enterococcus, *Pseudomonas aeruginosa*, *E. coli*, *Klebsiella pneumoniae*, *Staph. aureus*, *Staph. epidermidis*.

- Typical viral causes: influenza virus, RSV, adenovirus, parainfluenza virus, rhinovirus, human metapneumovirus, coronavirus.

Clinical Presentation

- Fever, leukopenia, or leukocytosis.
- Increased respiratory secretions or change in sputum character.
- New-onset or worsening apnea, tachypnea, dyspnea, wheezing, rales, rhonchi, cough, bradycardia, oxygenation.
- Two or more serial chest radiographs with new or progressive and persistent infiltrate, consolidation, cavitation, or pneumatoceles (in infants <1 year of age).
- See http://www.cdc.gov/nhsn/PDFs/pscManual/17pscNosInfDef_current.pdf and http://www.cdc.gov/nhsn/PDFs/pscManual/10-VAE_FINAL.pdf for delineation of CDC VAE and VAE criteria.

Diagnostic Evaluation

- Chest radiography.
- CBC with differential, CRP, ESR.
- Blood and bacterial cultures, and Gram staining from endotracheal aspirate.
- Bronchoalveolar lavage, using protected-specimen brush collection specimen.
- Pleural fluid or lung biopsy.
- Evaluation for viral etiology with respiratory viral culture/viral panel.

Management

- Increase oxygen and other ventilator settings.
- Hemodynamic support, as indicated support.
- Broad-spectrum antibiotic administration.

Catheter-Associated Urinary Tract Infection

Definition

- A UTI in which an indwelling urinary catheter was in place for >2 calendar days when all elements of the CDC UTI infection criteria were present.
- The indwelling urinary catheter must be in place on the day of, or the day prior to, diagnosis.

Etiology/Types

- Symptomatic UTI; asymptomatic bacteriuria.

Common Causative Organisms

- *E. coli, P. aeruginosa, Candida* species, *Enterococcus* species, *K. pneumoniae.*

Clinical Presentation

- Fever.
- Urinary urgency, frequency, dysuria.
- Costovertebral pain or suprapubic tenderness.
- Associated with a positive urine culture, pyuria, positive dipstick for leukocyte esterase band/or nitrate.

- Infants may present with hypothermia, apnea, bradycardia, lethargy, vomiting.
- See http://www.cdc.gov/nhsn/PDFs/pscManual/17pscNosInfDef_current.pdf for delineation of CDC catheter-associated urinary tract infection criteria.

Diagnostic Evaluation

- UA and urine culture with Gram stain.
- CBC with differential, CRP.

Management

- Antibiotic administration.
- Analgesia and higher-level support if urosepsis.

Nosocomial Respiratory Syncytial Virus

Definition

- Symptoms of lower respiratory tract infection and RSV antigen >72 hours after hospital admission.

Background

- RSV is one of the most common etiologies of pediatric nosocomial respiratory tract infections in the pediatric intensive care unit (PICU) and is the most common nosocomial infection overall on pediatric wards.
- Incubation period ranges from 2 to 8 days; median hospitalization for RSV disease is approximately 5 days; 10 days for nosocomial RSV disease.
- Children with underlying morbidities and risk for severe disease, increased risk for prolonged hospitalization, and risk for mortality.
- Hand washing and barrier devices are greatest tools in disease transmission prevention.
- For more information, see RSV bronchiolitis in Section 3.

Surgical Site Infection

Definition

- An infection occurring within 30 or 90 days after an operative procedure involving the skin, subcutaneous tissue, or deep soft tissues of the incision; associated with clinical signs of infection or associated positive wound culture.
- Organ/space SSI: An infection that occurs 30 or 90 days after an operative procedure involving any part of the body, excluding the skin incision, fascia, or muscle layers, which was opened or manipulated during an operation.

Etiology/Types

- Superficial incisional primary or secondary SSI.
- Deep incisional primary or secondary SSI.
- Organ/space SSI.

Common Causative Organisms (Pediatrics)

- *Staph. aureus*, coagulase-negative staphylococci, *P. aeruginosa.*

Clinical Presentation

- Purulent incisional drainage; wound dehiscence or abscess.

- Incisional pain or tenderness, localized swelling, redness or heat.
- Fever, leukocytosis.
- See http://www.cdc.gov/nhsn/PDFs/pscManual/17pscNosInfDef_current.pdf for delineation of CDC SSI criteria.

Diagnostic Evaluation

- Wound culture or tissue biopsy.
- CBC with differential, ESR, CRP.
- Radiography, magnetic resonance imaging (MRI), CT, as indicated.

Management

- Antibiotic administration.
- Surgical drainage (include cultures).
- Implant removal, as indicated.

Invasive Fungal Infections in Pediatric Patients: Aspergillus, Mucor, and Pneumocystis

Daniel K. Choi

Background/Definition

- Nonacute fungal infections, such as tinea infections (e.g., tinea capitis, tinea pedis), are quite common.
- Invasive fungal infections are overall rare, usually seen in patients who are immunocompromised, such as children with malignancies, on chronic immunosuppression after a solid organ transplant, patients in the PICU/NICU setting, and children with primary immunodeficiencies (including children with HIV).
- Overall incidence of invasive fungal disease in children is hard to determine, but mortality is quite high, with estimates for mortality by *Aspergillus* alone to be 68% to 77%.

Etiology/Types

- Three major groups of fungus.
  - Yeasts: round/oval, unicellular, and reproduce via budding. Examples include the *Candida* species.
  - Molds: long, floppy, fluffy colonies that have long tubular structures called hyphae. Reproduce by forming spore-forming structures called conidia. Examples include *Aspergillus* and *Mucor* species.
  - Dimorphs: change from yeast to mold and back, and grow in environment as molds.
- Fungus is ubiquitous in the environment, preferring warm/damp environments to grow/reproduce (e.g., respiratory tract, endotracheal tubes, plastic in central venous catheters).

Pathophysiology

- Inhalation of fungal spores is the most common route of infection.
- Fungi then disseminate in the bloodstream to various organs.

- Although fungal infection can occur anywhere, most common organs involved are respiratory tract (sinuses, lungs in particular), skin, kidney/bladder, and CNS.

Clinical Presentation

- Skin rashes.
- Persistent fever in an immunocompromised patient.
- In the oncology population, fever for >4 days in a neutropenic patient is suggestive of fungal infection.
- Persistent cough and/or other sinopulmonary symptoms.
- Purulent sinusitis/sinus pain is suggestive of *Mucor* infection.
- Persistent tachypnea and lower oxygen saturations are suggestive of *Pneumocystis jirovecii* pneumonia (formerly known as *Pneumocystis carinii* pneumonia [PCP]) infection.
- Patients often appear asymptomatic.

Diagnostic Evaluation

- Blood culture, urine culture; specify the specimen for fungal culture as well, as it is not universal across institutions.
  - Note that fungal cultures often take days to start growing.
- Samples should have calcofluor white testing (formerly ordered as KOH) to test for yeast elements.
- Suspicion for *Pneumocystis jirovecii/P. carinii* pneumonia can be tested via silver staining, confirmed by PCR testing.
- Biopsy-proven infection is the gold standard, but is often difficult to obtain (except for skin biopsies).
  - Respiratory tract biopsies can be done via bronchoalveolar lavage, surgical biopsy, induced sputum culture, endotracheal tube culture.
- *Candida* species will grow from urine and blood cultures.
- Chest radiograph with diffuse "fluffy" infiltrates is suggestive of *Pneumocystis jirovecii/P.carinii* pneumonia.
- CT of the sinuses/chest/abdomen/pelvis with contrast often indicated.
  - Fungal imaging varies widely, from single nodules to diffuse/necrotic tissue.
- In some instances, MRI of the soft tissue is indicated.
- Galactomannan antigen testing is helpful for *Aspergillus* species, but has variable sensitivity and specificity; must be interpreted with caution.

Management

- Consultation with a pediatric infectious disease specialist is indicated.
- Broad-spectrum coverage for invasive fungal infections is usually with an IV formulation of an echinocandin (e.g., micafungin) or polyene class (e.g., amphotericin B).
- Azoles (e.g., voriconazole) do have activity against invasive species, although often have multiple drug interactions.
- In localized *Mucor* infection, aggressive debridement (particularly in the sinuses) is indicated to prevent CNS extension.
- For confirmed PCP infection, treatment with IV trimethoprim–sulfamethoxazole (i.e., Bactrim). For patients who cannot tolerate trimethoprim–sulfamethoxazole, IV pentamidine is another option.
- Treatments are often for a minimum of 6 to 8 weeks, and longer as needed under the supervision of pediatric infectious disease specialist.

- Trimethoprim–sulfamethoxazole prophylaxis should strongly be considered for patients who are at risk for continued immunosuppression.

Viral and Bacterial Infections

Jill S. Thomas

Multidrug-Resistant Organisms

- Increased prevalence of microorganisms resistant to one or more antimicrobial agents in the acute care setting leads to increased length of stay, mortality, and hospital costs.
- Have created management challenges due to limited antibiotic selection and limited new antibiotic development.
- Requires commitment to antibiotic stewardship by health care providers (Table 11.5).

Meningococcemia

Elizabeth Rosner

Definition

- Bacteremia and sepsis caused by the bacteria *N. meningitidis*, also referred to as meningococcus.

Etiology

- *N. meningitidis* is an encapsulated, gram-negative, oxidase-positive diplococcus.
- Five clinically important serotypes are A, B, C, W-135, and Y.
  - W-135 accounts for approximately 75% of invasive disease in the United States.
  - Serotype B accounts for the majority of disease in infants <1 year of age.

TABLE 11.5 Multiresistant Organisms

Name	Definition	Clinical Presentation	Diagnoses	Management
Methicillin-resistant *Staph. aureus* (MRSA)	Strains of *Staph. aureus* resistant to β-lactams, found in community and health care settings.	Skin and soft tissue infections, wounds, bacteremia, pneumonia, osteomyelitis, and sepsis.	Blood and/or fluid culture.	Vancomycin, clindamycin, trimethoprim–sulfamethoxazole, linezolid.
Drug-resistant *Strep. pneumoniae* (DRSP)	Pneumococcal infections resistant to β-lactams; found in community and health care settings.	Otitis media, sinusitis, pneumonia, and bacteremia.	Culture of primary site and blood culture.	Vancomycin, clindamycin, high-dose β-lactam, and fluoroquinolones.
Vancomycin-resistant enterococcus (VRE)	Any bacteria belonging to the genus *Enterococcus* resistant to vancomycin and often resistant to ampicillin.	UTI, intra-abdominal infections, and nosocomial infections.	Culture of primary site and blood culture with Gram stain.	Linezolid or daptomycin.
H. influenzae, nontypable	Community-acquired pathogen. Intrinsic efflux resistance mechanisms of the nontypable strain limit the activity of macrolides, azolides, and ketolides.	Otitis media, sinusitis, pneumonia.	Culture of primary site, blood culture with Gram stain.	Amoxicillin–clavulanate, extended-spectrum cephalosporins.
Extended-spectrum β-lactamase (ESBL) producing *E. coli* and *K. pneumoniae*	Plasmid mediated enzymes capable of inactivating a variety of β-lactams, including penicillins, third-generation cephalosporins, and aztreonam. ESBLs are commonly found in *E. coli* and *K. pneumoniae*; however, may be found in other gram-negative pathogens.	UTIs, nosocomial infections.	Culture of primary site and blood culture with susceptibility.	Broad-spectrum antibiotics. Treatment options include carbapenems.

Pathophysiology

- Acquired primarily through respiratory tract.
- The bacteria attach to epithelial cells and gain access to the bloodstream.
- Survival of meningococcus is enhanced by its polysaccharide capsule and acquisition of iron from human transferrin.
- Growth and lysis of the bacteria lead to release of endotoxin.
- The endotoxin has an important role in stimulating cytokine release through activation of toll-like receptors, especially TLR4.
- The inflammation produced by the cytokines, TNFα, IL-β, IL-6, and IL-8, causes capillary leak, shock, and multiorgan failure.
- Endotoxin also causes activation of the clotting cascade, which can lead to disseminated intravascular coagulopathy (DIC).

Clinical Presentation

- Initially may present with nonspecific symptoms of fever, malaise, vomiting, diarrhea, headache, and myalgias.
- Later symptoms include limb pain, difficulty walking, maculopapular rash, signs of meningitis, including photophobia, nuchal rigidity, lethargy, and seizures.
- In fulminant meningococcemia, purpura, limb ischemia, shock, coma, and death can occur in as little as a few hours (Figure 11.1).

Diagnostic Evaluation

- Blood and CSF cultures identifying *N. meningitidis* are the definitive diagnosis.
  - May not be able to obtain CSF in unstable patients.
- PCR from the blood and CSF can also be used to detect the organism.
- CBC, coagulation studies, and blood gas analysis should also be obtained.

Management

- Intravenous ceftriaxone at meningitic doses (100 mg/kg/day) as soon as possible for 5 to 7 days.
  - Cefotaxime is also acceptable.
  - Once the organism has been identified, it may be acceptable to switch to penicillin G.
  - In a penicillin-allergic patient, use either chloramphenicol or meropenem.
- Fluid resuscitation up to and beyond 60 mL/kg as fast as possible until perfusion improves.
- Hemodynamic support with agents such as dopamine, epinephrine, and/or norepinephrine may be necessary for fluid-refractory shock.
- Correct for metabolic and electrolyte derangements.
- Intubation and mechanical ventilation for severe shock, sepsis, and subsequent multiple organ dysfunction, especially acute respiratory distress syndrome (ARDS).
- Treatment of seizures with antiepileptics, as indicated.

Prevention

- Patients should be placed on droplet precautions for the first 24 hours of antibiotic therapy.
- Close contacts should be given prophylactic antibiotics within 24 hours.
  - Ciprofloxacin 500 mg by mouth × 1 dose.
  - Ceftriaxone and rifampin are other options.
- All adolescents and those at risk for invasive disease should receive a meningococcal conjugate vaccine, (e.g. Menactra, MenHibrix, Menveo).
  - Serotype B is not covered by the vaccine.
- Find latest immunization recommendations on the CDC website http://www.cdc.gov/vaccines/schedules/hcp/child-adolescent.html

Sexually Transmitted Infections

Jill S. Thomas

Sexually Transmitted Infections

- Sexually transmitted infections (STIs) refer to a variety of clinical syndromes caused by pathogens that can be acquired and transmitted through sexual activity.
- Part of the management of any patient with an STI is counseling about prevention and referral of partner.

Human Papillomavirus

Definition

- A double-stranded DNA virus belonging to the family Papovaviridae.
- STIs are most prevalent in individuals <24 years of age.

Etiology/Types

- Genital.
- Recurrent respiratory papillomatosis.

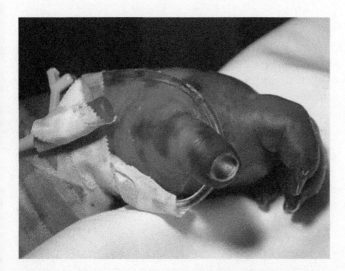

FIGURE 11.1 • Meningococcemia. Gangrene in a child with sepsis from acute meningococcemia.

- Illness caused by various subtypes of human papillomavirus (HPV).

Clinical Presentation

- Typically asymptomatic, may present with genital warts occurring on the vulva, perianal area, vaginal walls, or cervix.
- Recurrent respiratory papillomatosis presents with warts occurring in the throat.

Diagnostic Evaluation

- Visual inspection.
- Pap test with HPV test detecting viral nucleic acid or capsid protein.

Management

- No pharmacologic treatment recommended in the absence of genital warts.
- For external warts, antibiotic therapy includes podofilox 0.5% solution or imiquimod 5% cream, podophyllin resin, or trichloroacetic acid.
- Cryotherapy and/or surgical removal.
- Intralesional interferon, laser surgery.

PEARLS

- *Two vaccines are available for vaccination against HPV with a 9-valent vaccine; routine vaccination has been recommended for males and females beginning at approximately 11 years of age.*
- *Follow the latest immunization recommendations on the CDC website http://www.cdc.gov/vaccines/schedules/hcp/child-adolescent.html*

Herpes Simplex Virus (HSV)

Definition

- An enveloped, double-stranded DNA virus belonging to the family Herpesviridae.
- Genital herpes is a chronic, lifelong viral infection caused by the HSV.

Etiology/Types

- HSV-1.
- HSV-2: believed to cause the majority of genital HSV infections.

Clinical Presentation

- Asymptomatic or may have vesicular lesions, ulcers, leucorrhea, dysuria, inguinal adenopathy.

Diagnostic Evaluation

- Viral cell culture.
- PCR (greater sensitivity than viral cultures).
- HSV type-specific serological assay.

Management

- Antiviral therapy with acyclovir, famciclovir, or valacyclovir.
- Length of therapy dependent on initial presentation or recurrence of infection.

Gonorrhea

Definition

- The second most common STI in the United States.
- Caused by *N. gonorrhoeae*, gram-negative, oxidase-positive diplococcus.

Clinical Presentation

- General: urinary frequency, urgency, and burning with urination.
- Females: may have inflammation of the Bartholin and Skene glands, cervical mucoid discharge, or may remain asymptomatic until complications occur.
- Males: penile discharge.

Diagnostic Evaluation

- Test endocervical, vaginal, urethral (male only), and urine specimens.
- Bacterial culture with Gram stain, nucleic acid hybridization tests, and nucleic acid amplification tests (NAATs) detect *N. gonorrhoeae*.
- Culture and antimicrobial susceptibility testing if treatment failure is suspected.
- Evaluate for other STIs, including chlamydia, syphilis, and HIV.

Management

- Intramuscular ceftriaxone plus azithromycin or doxycycline.

PEARL

- *Major cause of cervicitis, pelvic inflammatory disease (PID), ectopic pregnancy, and infertility.*

Chlamydia

Definition

- The most common reportable STI in the United States.
- Obligate intracellular bacteria.

Etiology/Types

- *Chlamydia trachomatis.*

Clinical Presentation

- Asymptomatic infection common among men and women.
- Women may present with vaginitis, urethritis, cervicitis, endometriosis, salpingitis, PID. May experience vaginal discharge or dysuria.

Diagnostic Evaluation

- Urine, endocervical, vaginal, urethral (men), rectal, and oropharyngeal swabs.
- NAATs are the test of choice.
- Cell culture, direct immunofluorescence, enzyme immunoassay (EIA), and nucleic acid hybridization tests available for endocervical specimens.
- Urethral swab specimens from men.
- U.S. Preventive Services Task Force recommends routine chlamydia screening for all women ≤25 years of age who are sexually active.

Management

- Azithromycin or doxycycline as per CDC recommendations.

- *Leading cause of PID, which can lead to infertility and chronic pelvic pain, often associated with gonorrhea.*

Syphilis

Definition

- A systemic STI caused by the spirochete *Treponema pallidum*.

Etiology/Types

- Primary: develops 10 to 90 days after exposure.
- Secondary: develops 4 to 10 weeks after primary infection.
- Tertiary: develops 2 to 19 years after primary infection in untreated individuals.

Clinical Presentation

- Primary: presents with an ulcer or painless chancre at the infected site.
- Secondary: myalgias, mucocutaneous lesions, lymphadenopathy, influenza-like symptoms, cranial nerve dysfunction, altered mental status, or skin rash involving soles of the feet and palms of the hands.
- Tertiary: cardiac or gummatous lesions.
- Latent infections lack clinical symptoms.

Diagnostic Evaluation

- Darkfield examinations and direct fluorescent antibody (DFA) detection of *T. pallidum* in lesion exudate or tissue are the definitive methods for diagnosing early syphilis.
- Dual serological testing using a nontreponemal test (Venereal Disease Research Laboratory and rapid plasma reagin tests) and treponemal test (fluorescent treponemal antibody absorption tests, the *Treponema pallidum* passive particle agglutination assay, EIA), study of choice for latent, secondary, and tertiary syphilis.

Management

- Benzathine penicillin G.

- *Maternal–fetal transmission of syphilis can result in premature labor, congenital syphilis, or fetal demise.*

Vaginitis

Background

- Some vaginal infections are transmitted sexually, while others occur due to vaginal bacterial flora overgrowth or disruption.

Definition

- Vaginal inflammation, most commonly caused by *Candida albicans*, *Trichomonas vaginalis*, and/or bacterial vaginosis.

Etiology/Types

- Vulvovaginal candidiasis: caused by *Candida albicans*.
- Trichomonas vaginalis: caused by *Trichomonas vaginalis*.
- Bacterial vaginosis: Polymicrobial clinical syndrome resulting from replacement of the normal *Lactobacillus* species in the vagina with anaerobic bacteria (e.g. *Prevotella* species and *Mobiluncus* species), *Gardnerella vaginalis*, and *Mycoplasma hominis*.

Clinical Presentation

- Vulvovaginal candidiasis: vaginal discharge with cottage cheese–like appearance, intense vaginal irritation or pruritus, vulvar and vaginal inflammation.
- Trichomonas vaginalis: vulvar irritation, dyspareunia, dysuria, urinary frequency, vaginal odor, green/yellow vaginal discharge.
- Bacterial vaginosis: vaginal discharge or malodor; may be asymptomatic.

Diagnostic Evaluation

- Vulvovaginal candidiasis: microscopic evaluation of vaginal discharge via wet prep or Gram staining looking for hyphae, pseudohyphae, or budding yeast, vaginal discharge culture.
- *Trichomonas vaginalis*: Women—microscopic evaluation of vaginal discharge via wet prep looking for mobile trichomonads, vaginal discharge culture, OSOM Trichomonas Rapid Test, Affirm VP III nucleic acid probe test. Men—NAATs, culture testing of urethral swab, urine, or semen.
- Bacterial vaginosis: Gram staining, or clinical diagnosis using Amsel's Diagnostic Criteria—must meet three of the following four criteria: homogeneous, thin, white discharge that smoothly coats the vaginal wall, presence of clue cells on microscopic examination, vaginal fluid pH >4.5, "fishy" odor of vaginal discharge before or after addition of 10% potassium hydroxide, known as the "whiff" test.

Management

- Vulvovaginal candidiasis: oral fluconazole or over-the-counter intravaginal antifungal creams or suppositories.
- Trichomonas vaginalis: oral metronidazole.
- Bacterial vaginalis: oral metronidazole or intravaginal metronidazole or clindamycin.

Pelvic Inflammatory Disease

Definition

- A polymicrobial infection of the upper female genital tract.
- Used to describe any combination of endometriosis, salpingitis, tubo-ovarian abscess, and pelvic peritonitis.
- The most common sexually transmitted infectious agents causing PID are *N. gonorrhoeae* and *Chlamydia trachomatis*; however, PID can be caused by other bacterial or viral etiologies.

Clinical Presentation

- Fever with pelvic or abdominal pain, dyspareunia.
- Mucopurulent cervical or vaginal discharge, abnormal vaginal bleeding.

- Cervical motion tenderness, uterine tenderness, adnexal tenderness.
- Symptoms may be mild and nonspecific, making clinical diagnosis difficult.

Diagnostic Evaluation

- CBC with differential, ESR, CRP, culture.
- Endometrial biopsy.
- Radiographic evaluation: transvaginal sonography, MRI, pelvic Doppler studies.
- Laparoscopy evaluation for concomitant infections with a microscopic evaluation of vaginal discharge via wet prep.

Management

- STI prevention counseling.
- Evaluate and treat sexual partners if indicated.
- Inpatient or outpatient parenteral and/or enteral pharmacotherapy regimens vary based on patient risk factors and disease severity. Initiate treatment as soon as a presumptive diagnosis is made to prevent long-term sequelae.

Tubo-Ovarian Abscess

Definition

- An infected ovary with purulent material from the fallopian tube most commonly following exposure to an STI or PID.

Etiology/Types

- Arises from untreated or inadequately treated salpingo-oophoritis or PID.

Clinical Presentation

- Ill-appearing female with severe abdominal-pelvic pain, peritoneal signs.
- Fever, nausea, vomiting.
- Mucopurulent cervical discharge.

Diagnostic Evaluation

- Radiographic evaluation: pelvic or transvaginal ultrasound, MRI of abdomen and pelvis, or CT of abdomen and pelvis.
- CBC with differential, ESR, CRP.
- Cervical cultures (Figure 11.2).

Management

- Hospitalization with administration of parenteral antibiotics.
- Abscess aspiration or surgical excision.
- A ruptured *tubo-ovarian abscess* is a life-threatening condition and requires emergent surgery.

Sepsis

Background

- Bacterial, viral, and fungal infections can progress along a clinical continuum, leading to systemic inflammatory response syndrome (SIRS), sepsis, severe sepsis, and septic shock.

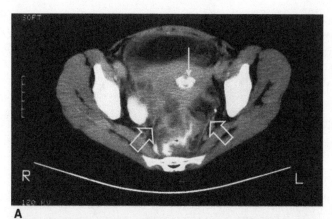

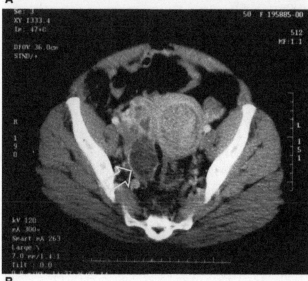

FIGURE 11.2 • **Tubo-Ovarian Abscess. A:** CT of tubo-ovarian abscess (*open arrows*) with Dalkon Shield (*arrow*). **B:** MRI of tubo-ovarian abscess (*open arrow*).

- Risk factors include prematurity, compromised immune status, neurologic or musculoskeletal disease, congenital or chromosomal disease.
- Impacted by increased incidence of drug-resistant organisms.

Definitions

- SIRS: The presence of ≥2 of the following four criteria (one including criterion must be abnormal temperature or leukocyte count).
  - Hyperthermia or hypothermia.
  - Tachycardia or bradycardia.
  - Tachypnea.
  - Leukocytosis or leukopenia.
- Sepsis.
  - SIRS in the presence of or as a result of a suspected or proven infection.
- Severe sepsis.
  - Sepsis plus cardiovascular organ dysfunction or ARDS or two or more other organ dysfunctions.

- Septic shock.
  - Sepsis and cardiovascular organ dysfunction.

Etiology/Types

- Gram-positive bacteria.
  - Cellular structure allows for production of exotoxins that function as superantigens, causing a massive activation of T cells, leading to cytokine release and symptoms of organ dysfunction.
  - Common types include:
    - *Staph. aureus, Strep. pyogenes, Strep. pneumoniae, Staph. epidermidis* (coagulase-negative staphylococci), *Enterococcus* species.
- Gram-negative bacteria.
  - Release endotoxins upon destruction, leading to manifestations of septic shock.
  - Common types include:
    - *P. aeruginosa, E. coli, Acinetobacter* species, *Bacteroides fragilis, N. meningitides.*
- Viruses.
  - Small infectious agents that can replicate only inside living cells; mechanism of disease production varies per virus.
- Fungi.
  - Mycoses virulence patterns vary per fungus and involve a complex interplay of host and fungal factors.
  - Common types include:
    - *Candida* species, *Aspergillus* species.

Clinical Presentation

- General: fever, malaise.
- Neurologic: irritability, lethargy, anxiety.
- Respiratory: tachypnea, nasal flaring, grunting, subcostal or suprasternal retractions, rales, wheezing, crackles.
- Cardiovascular: tachycardia, hypotension, gallop rhythm, hepatosplenomegaly, jugular venous distension.
- Renal: oliguria.
- Dermatologic: presence of rash (type varies per etiology of sepsis).

Diagnostic Evaluation

- Initial studies include CBC with differential, CMP, DIC panel, CRP, blood and bacterial cultures with Gram stain, respiratory viral panel.
- CSF cultures with cell count, protein and glucose levels, CSF viral-specific PCRs, sputum culture with Gram stain, abscess or skin lesion cultures, arterial blood gas analysis as indicated by clinical presentation.
- If possible, obtain cultures prior to antibiotic administration.
- Chest radiography, ultrasound, or CT as indicated to locate infectious source.

Management

- Early goal-directed therapy as recommended by the Surviving Sepsis Campaign. See http://www.survivingsepsis.org/Pages/default.aspx for more information
- Initial management: oxygen administration, respiratory support with intubation and mechanical ventilation as needed, early establishment of vascular access, fluid resuscitation up to and over 60 mL/kg within 15 minutes, correction

of hypoglycemia and hypocalcemia, prompt antibiotic administration.
- For fluid-resistant shock, initiate vasopressor support with titration according to therapeutic endpoints and central venous oxygen saturation $S_{CV}O_2$ saturation, obtain central venous access.
- For catecholamine-resistant shock, administer hydrocortisone if risk of adrenal insufficiency.
- Subsequent therapy guided by delineation of warm versus cold shock.
- Consider extracorporeal membrane oxygenation (ECMO) in resistant shock.
- Therapeutic endpoints of pediatric shock include capillary refill time <2 seconds, normal pulses with no differentiation between central and peripheral pulses, warm extremities, normal blood pressure for age, urine output >1 mL/kg/hour, and normal mental status.

PEARLS
- *Although not specific for bacterial infections, leukocytosis with a left shifted differential classically suggests a bacterial infectious etiology.*
- *Leukocytosis with a lymphocyte predominance is indicative of a viral infectious etiology.*

Viral Illness

Jill S. Thomas

Background

- Viral illnesses are common among pediatric patients, often presenting with diverse, generalized, non–life-threatening symptoms.
- Viral infections rarely manifest as severe systemic diseases.

Adenovirus

Background

- A double-stranded, nonenveloped DNA virus belonging to the family Adenoviridae.
- Incubation period is typically 2 to 14 days for respiratory illnesses and 3 to 10 days for gastroenteritis.

Etiology

- 51 serotypes.
- Transmission occurs via respiratory tract secretions through person-to-person contact, airborne droplets, and fomites.

Clinical Presentation

- Majority of infections involve the respiratory tract, eyes, or GI system, manifesting as common cold, pharyngitis, pneumonia, conjunctivitis, and gastroenteritis.
- Symptoms include cough, rhinorrhea, exudative tonsillitis, cervical lymphadenopathy, fever, conjunctivitis, emesis, abdominal pain, diarrhea, cystitis, and erythematous maculopapular rash.

- Infection less often results in cardiac, neurologic, genitourinary, and systemic compromise.

Diagnostic Evaluation

- Viral cell culture of blood, pleural fluid, pericardial fluid, CSF, nasopharyngeal and throat swabs, urine or stool; bacterial culture and Gram stain.
- PCR, DFA testing, ELISA, or latex agglutination used for rapid detection.
- CBC and differential; manual differential evaluation demonstrates lymphocytic predominance.

Management

- Supportive care, antipyretics, hydration, and rest.
- Oxygen, respiratory support, and vasopressor support as needed for respiratory or cardiovascular compromise.
- Contact precautions with conjunctivitis or gastroenteritis, contact and droplet precautions for respiratory tract infections.

Cytomegalovirus

Definition

- A double-stranded DNA virus of the family Herpesviridae.
- Incubation period is typically 3 to 12 weeks after acquisition via blood transfusion or 1 to 4 months after acquisition via tissue transplantation.

Etiology/Types

- Vertical transmission: occurs during intrauterine life or during perinatal exposure.
- Horizontal transmission: occurs from direct contact with contaminated bodily fluids, tissues, or fomites.
- May occur from blood transfusions or organ transplant.

Clinical Presentation

- Congenital infection.
  - Most asymptomatic at birth; may have hearing loss, microcephaly, seizures, hypotonia, retinitis, cognitive and motor deficits (Figure 11.3).
- Postnatal infection.
  - Infected patients may be asymptomatic.
  - Common presentations include mononucleosis, pneumonia, gastroenteritis, encephalitis, and myelitis.
  - Symptoms include fever, malaise, arthralgias, maculopapular rash, headache, cough, respiratory distress, abdominal pain, nausea, vomiting, diarrhea, photophobia, and nuchal rigidity.

Diagnostic Evaluation

- Viral cell culture with or without shell viral assay of bodily fluids, including blood, urine, saliva, nasopharyngeal wash, conjunctiva, human milk, CSF, and tissue biopsy.
- PCR, antigen identification by ELISA, DFA, or latex agglutination.
- Serologic antibody testing, CBC and differential, CMP, ESR, CRP.
- Bacterial culture and Gram stain to evaluate for bacterial etiologies of illness.

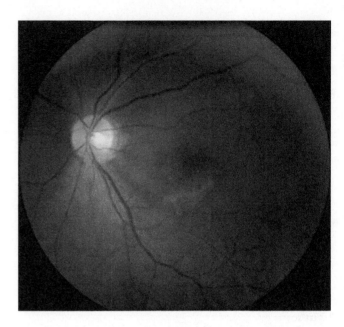

FIGURE 11.3 • **CMV Retinitis.** CMV retinitis in this case is limited to perimacular area with necrotizing retinitis along the inferior arcade, intraretinal hemorrhage, and granularity surrounding fovea.

- Manual differential evaluation demonstrates lymphocytic predominance.

Management

- Antiviral therapy indicated in certain manifestations.
- Management largely supportive with oxygen, fluid resuscitation, respiratory support, and vasopressor support as needed.

PEARLS

- *Significant cause of morbidity and mortality in immunocompromised patients.*
- *Antiviral therapy indicated in mild-to-severe infections.*
- *Infants with congenital cytomegalovirus should receive regular neurologic evaluation with serial hearing and vision screening.*

Epstein-Barr Virus

Definition

- A double-stranded DNA virus of the family Herpesviridae.
- Typical incubation period is approximately 30 to 50 days.

Etiology/Types

- Transmission occurs via intimate contact with sharing of oral secretions.

Clinical Presentation

- Classic cause of infectious mononucleosis: fever, pharyngitis, malaise, lymphadenopathy, splenomegaly.
- Majority of individuals are asymptomatic.

- Multisystemic presentations include tonsillopharyngitis, cervical or peritonsillar abscess, meningitis, encephalitis, and may be associated with malignancy.

Diagnostic Evaluation

- Rapid assays testing for Paul-Bunnell heterophile antibodies, including Monospot, Mono-test, or Mono-Diff test.
- Serologic antibody testing.
- CBC with differential demonstrating atypical lymphocyte counts of >10% of the total leukocyte count, serologic viral antigen and antibody detection, and viral DNA and RNA detection.
- Send bacterial culture and Gram stain to evaluate for bacterial etiologies of illness.

Management

- Supportive care, antipyretics, hydration, and rest.
- Manage respiratory and cardiovascular complications with respiratory support and fluid resuscitation as clinically indicated.

PEARLS

- *Symptoms of mononucleosis may last as long as 3 to 4 weeks with organomegaly persisting for up to 3 months.*
- *Temporary cessation of contact and wheeled sports is required.*

Enterovirus

Definition

- Broad group of single-stranded RNA viruses belonging to the family Picornaviridae.
- Incubation period is typically 3 to 6 days.

Etiology/Types

- Poliovirus, group A coxsackievirus, group B coxsackievirus, Echovirus, Enterovirus, and other viruses.
- Transmission via contaminated respiratory secretions, stool, and infected fomites.

Clinical Presentation

- Wide clinical presentation due to large number of virus within enterovirus class.
- Majority of infections asymptomatic or feature a nonspecific febrile illness.
- May involve respiratory, GI, cardiac, neurologic, and dermatologic systems.
- Specific infections include:
  - Poliovirus infection: pharyngitis with a low-grade fever.
  - Paralytic poliomyelitis: fever, malaise, asymmetric paralysis.
  - Coxsackievirus A16 (hand-foot-and-mouth disease): mild fever, malaise, intraoral ulcers on tongue and buccal mucosa, lesions on hands and feet.
  - Group B coxsackievirus: pericarditis and myocarditis manifesting as congestive heart failure, tachypnea, tachycardia, shortness of breath, hypotension.

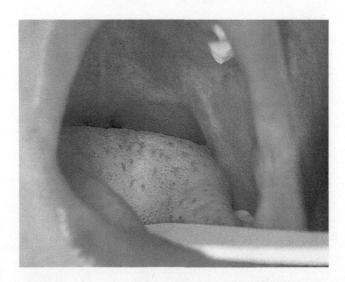

FIGURE 11.4 • **Coxsackievirus Oral Lesions.** Coxsackie hand-foot-and-mouth disease. Scattered petechiae appear centrally, and there is a vesicle posteriorly at the junction of the hard and soft palates. Coxsackievirus produces lesions toward the posterior of the oropharynx, whereas herpes simplex virus appears anteriorly.

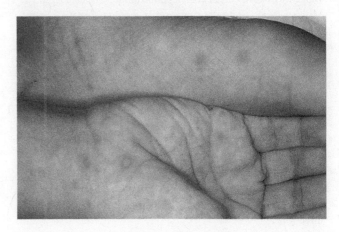

FIGURE 11.5 • **Coxsackievirus Skin Lesions.** Coxsackie hand-foot-and-mouth disease. A hand and a foot of this child show isolated vesicles.

  - Coxsackievirus: gastroenteritis with vomiting, diarrhea, abdominal pain.
  - Echovirus: encephalitis manifesting as seizures, ataxia, altered mental status. Gastroenteritis with vomiting, diarrhea, abdominal pain (Figures 11.4 and 11.5).

Diagnostic Evaluation

- Viral cell cultures of stool, rectal and oropharyngeal swabs, blood, urine, or CSF (if possible send from several sites or fluids simultaneously).
- Reverse-transcriptase PCR, CBC with differential, ESR, CRP.
- Bacterial culture and Gram staining to evaluate for bacterial etiologies of illnesses.

Management

- Supportive care, hydration, analgesia; oxygen, respiratory support, and airway management for respiratory failure, echocardiogram diuretics, or vasopressor support for cardiovascular decompensation.
- Intravenous immunoglobulin (IVIG) may be indicated in life-threatening illnesses.

Herpes Simplex Virus

Definition

- An enveloped double-stranded DNA virus belonging to the family Herpesviridae.
- The incubation period is 2 days to 2 weeks.

Etiology/Types

- HSV-1 and HSV-2.
- Transmission occurs via direct contact with HSV lesions or contaminated secretions.

Clinical Presentation

- Symptoms include fever, oral mucosal vesicles submandibular lymphadenopathy, malodorous breath, corneal injection, ocular watering or pruritus, headache, photophobia, nuchal rigidity.
- Multisystemic presentations include gingivostomatitis, keratoconjunctivitis, and meningitis.
- Neonatal HSV infection may manifest as severe, disseminated disease.

Diagnostic Evaluation

- Viral cell culture obtained from aspirated lesion, blood, urine, stool, CSF, conjunctiva, mouth, nasopharynx, and rectum.
- PCR, DFA, HSV type-specific serological assay.
- CBC with differential, ESR, CRP.
- Bacterial cultures and Gram staining of selected fluids, with CSF cellular analysis, to evaluate for bacterial etiologies of illnesses.
- Lumbar puncture, MRI, and EEG for suspected neurologic infection.

Management

- Acyclovir is the first-line therapy.
- Supportive care, hydration, analgesia.
- Oxygen, respiratory support, airway management, fluid resuscitation, seizure control, and cardiovascular support as needed for severe infections.
- Contact precautions for infants born to mothers with active HSV lesions and individuals with mucocutaneous lesions.

PEARLS

- *In HSV encephalitis, CSF analysis shows a lymphocytic pleocytosis, elevated protein level, and increased number of erythrocytes with an RBC count >1,000/mm³.*
- *MRI demonstrates temporal lobe enhancement.*
- *Electroencephalography may show paroxysmal lateral epileptiform discharges (PLEDs).*

Human Metapneumovirus

Definition

- A single-stranded RNA virus belonging to the family Paramyxoviridae.
- Incubation period is 3 to 5 days.

Etiology/Types

- Human metapneumovirus A and B.
- Transmission mode yet to be identified, though thought to occur via respiratory secretions through person-to-person contact, large-particle respiratory droplets, and contaminated fomites.

Clinical Presentation

- Commonly affects respiratory system, manifesting as otitis media, upper respiratory tract infection, croup, bronchiolitis, asthma exacerbation, pneumonia.
- Uncommonly, causes encephalitis and encephalopathy.

Diagnostic Evaluation

- DFA, reverse-transcriptase PCR, CBC with differential.
- Chest radiography.

Management

- Supportive care, hydration, oxygen, respiratory support, and mechanical ventilation as needed.
- Contact and droplet precautions to prevent spread.

Influenza

Definition

- A single-stranded RNA virus belonging to the family Orthomyxoviridae.
- The incubation period is typically 2 days, but can range between 1 and 4 days.

Etiology/Types

- Influenza A, B, or C.
- Transmission occurs via large-particle respiratory droplets and contact with contaminated individuals or fomites.

Clinical Presentation

- "Classic" influenza: fever, myalgia, headache, malaise, nonproductive cough, sore throat, nasal congestion.
- Multisystemic presentations include acute otitis media, asthma exacerbation, croup, bronchiolitis, pneumonia, ARDS, myocarditis, abdominal pain, nausea, vomiting, diarrhea, seizures, encephalopathy, encephalitis.
- A systemic, sepsis-like syndrome can be seen in infants.

Diagnostic Evaluation

- Viral cell culture (diagnostic study of choice), rapid cell culture via shell vial method.
- DFA, PCR, rapid detection tests.
- Acceptable specimens vary per test and include nasopharyngeal swab, wash, or aspirate; lower respiratory tract samples can be used for viral cell culture, rapid cell culture, or PCR.

- Chest radiography.
- CBC with differential, bacterial culture, and Gram staining of endotracheal aspirate or sputum indicated to evaluate for bacterial etiology of illness.

Management

- Supportive care, hydration, rest, analgesia, and antipyretics with acetaminophen.
- Complicated infections may require oxygen, respiratory support (including mechanical ventilation), fluid resuscitation.
- Antiviral agents are considered based on patient age, illness severity, and time of presentation.

PEARLS

- *Risk for mortality and morbidity is highest in patients with chronic pulmonary, cardiac, neurologic, hepatic, renal, neuromuscular, hematologic, or metabolic disorders.*
- *Seasonal epidemics can be seen from November to May in the United States.*
- *Yearly vaccination is recommended for infants/children >6 months of age.*
- *See CDC website for most current immunization recommendations.*

Parvovirus B19

Definition

- A nonenveloped, single-stranded DNA virus of the family Parvoviridae.
- The usual incubation period is 4 to 14 days, but can last up to 21 days.

Etiology/Types

- Transmission occurs via contact with contaminated respiratory secretions, percutaneous exposure to blood and blood products, and the transplacental route.

Clinical Presentation

- Erythema infectiosum (fifth disease): intensely erythematous exanthem on cheeks with circumoral pallor ("slap cheek rash") (Figure 11.6), diffuse maculopapular rash that fades to a lacy erythematous rash, fever, headache, myalgias, malaise. Arthralgias are more common in adults.
- Multisystemic presentations include anemia, transient aplastic crisis, arthralgias, polyarthropathy syndrome, myocarditis, glomerulonephritis, encephalitis, hydrops fetalis.

Diagnostic Evaluation

- PCR, DNA hybridization, serologic antibody testing.
- CBC with differential, reticulocyte count, CMP, cardiac enzymes.
- Viral and bacterial cultures with Gram stain, virus-specific antibody testing to evaluate for additional infectious causes of severe disease.
- EKG.

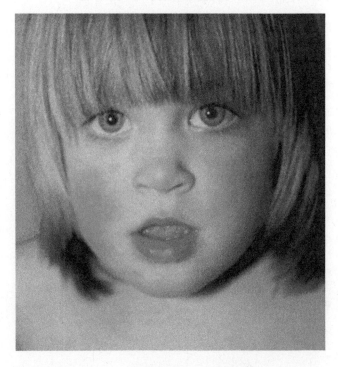

FIGURE 11.6 • **Parvovirus B19 Slap Cheek Rash.** Typical "slapped cheek" appearance of a child infected with parvovirus B19 ("fifth disease").

- Chest radiography.
- EEG as indicated by symptomatology.

Management

- Supportive care, hydration, rest, analgesia.
- Blood product transfusion, IVIG, oxygen, respiratory and cardiovascular support as needed.

Selected Infections

Lemierre Syndrome

Valarie D. Eichler

Background

- Lemierre syndrome (LS) is also known as suppurative jugular thrombophlebitis or postanginal sepsis.
- A rare infection most commonly caused by the gram-negative anaerobic bacteria *Fusobacterium necrophorum*. However, there are case reports of LS caused by other infectious agents, namely, community-acquired methicillin-resistant *Staph. aureus* (CA-MRSA).
- Unrecognized or untreated, LS can have significant mortality and morbidity including death.

Definition

- Well-defined syndrome that affects previously healthy children and most often involves an antecedent pharyngitis, septic pulmonary emboli, and persistent fever despite antimicrobial therapy.

Etiology/Epidemiology

- Rare gram-negative bacteria that normally reside in the oropharynx.
- Typically follows an oropharyngeal infection; however, can arise from an otitis media or mastoiditis.
- Growing incidence of 0.8 to 1.5 per million per year.
- Prior to antibiotic use the mortality was >90%, now <15%.

Pathophysiology

- Hematogenous spread of bacteria after passing through the oral mucosa either by direct tissue contact or via the tonsillar vessels.
- Results in septic thromboemboli in the internal jugular vein.
- Microemboli circulate throughout the body developing abscesses and infarctions.
- Lungs are the primary site for septic emboli to lodge (~85% of patients) followed by large joints such as hips, knees, and elbows.

Clinical Presentation

- Symptoms vary, but most common presentation consists of pharyngitis, fever, and general weakness in a previously healthy child or adolescent who has experienced an antecedent streptococcal infection.
- Generally, patients are toxic or ill-appearing.
- Other symptoms usually appear within 1 to 2 weeks and may include unilateral neck edema, with or without tenderness, headache, fever, altered level of consciousness, sepsis, trismus.
- Pulmonary involvement may include cough, pleuritic chest pain, and shortness of breath.
- Cranial nerve involvement and pericarditis (rare).

Diagnostic Imaging

- Modality of imaging will vary based on history and presentation.
- CT or MRI:
  - Sensitive diagnostic tools when screening for an intravascular thrombus. However, depending on the age of the child, an MRI may be more difficult since it typically requires sedation.
  - CT will reveal a dilated internal jugular vein with low-density intraluminal material and enhancement of the vessel wall and surrounding tissue.
- Ultrasound.
  - May be helpful in an organized thrombus; however, caution should be taken if the ultrasound is deemed normal. Early formations of clots have low echogenicity and may not be noted on ultrasound, resulting in a false-negative study.
- Soft tissue neck radiography is not as helpful, but can assist in evaluating for epiglottitis or retropharyngeal space edema.
- Chest radiography.
  - May reveal abscesses, cavitations, pleural effusions, infiltrates, or nodules.

Laboratory Evaluation

- CBC with differential and platelets, CRP, ESR.
- Blood culture, fluid culture (if available).
- Renal and hepatic functions panel.

Management

- Intravenous antibiotics, including anaerobic coverage.
  - β-Lactams, clindamycin, third-generation cephalosporins, vancomycin, metronidazole, and linezolid.
  - Duration of therapy is tailored for each patient; typically continued until resolution of symptoms (often 4–6 weeks), or resolution of the clot.
- Depending on the degree of edema and risk of airway occlusion, securing the airway by intubation should be initiated early.
  - In extreme cases, tracheostomy may be required.
- Anticoagulation.
  - Controversial.
  - Dependent on invasiveness of the thrombus and organ system involvement, especially if the thrombus extends into the cavernous sinus or the continued presence of septic emboli despite antibiotic therapy.
  - Strongly consider if a family history of hypercoagulability.
  - Initially, treatment with heparin is the therapy of choice; changed to warfarin or enoxaparin for outpatient therapy.
  - Hematologist consult to assist with extended anticoagulation administration.
  - Duration of therapy: median of 3 months.
- Surgical intervention.
  - Incision and drainage (I&D) depends on the size and extent of the fluid collection, impingement on the airway, and structures involved.
  - Thrombectomy, or vessel ligation, is rarely used and is reserved for those patients in whom antibiotic therapy has failed or who have recurrent thrombi. It is associated with increased length of stay and morbidity.

Prognosis/Morbidity and Mortality

- Full recovery in majority of patients.
- Potentially fatal disease if not identified and treated early, mortality of about 5%.

PEARLS

- *Broad-spectrum antimicrobial coverage, including anaerobic coverage, should be initiated early in an effort to decrease morbidity and mortality.*
- *Although the most common cause of LS is the anaerobic bacteria Fusobacterium necrophorum, other bacteria such as Staph. aureus have become more prevalent in the last decade.*
- *Increase in reported cases of LS is unknown if this is related to antibiotic resistance or the judicious antibiotic prescribing patterns.*

Toxic Shock Syndrome

Bradley D. Tilford

Definition

- Toxin-mediated, multisystem febrile illnesses caused by the bacteria *Staph. aureus* and *Strep. pyogenes* (group A streptococcus [GAS]).
- An epidemic of TSS caused by *Staph. aureus* occurred in the late 1970s and early 1980s associated with the use of superabsorbent tampons by menstruating women. Although significantly decreased in number, about 50% of reported cases of staphylococcal TSS are associated with tampon use.
- Streptococcal TSS (STSS) was reported in the late 1980s associated with invasive GAS infections.
- The case fatality rate for STSS is reported to be 5% to 10% in children and may exceed 50% in adults.

Etiology

- *Staph. aureus* is the most common cause of skin and soft tissue infections such as impetigo, cellulitis, abscess, and wound infection.
- *Staph. aureus* colonizes the skin and mucous membranes of 30% to 50% of children and adults.
- Toxins produced by various strains of *Staph. aureus* cause food poisoning, staphylococcal scarlet fever, scalded skin syndrome, and TSS.
- *Strep. pyogenes* (GAS) is a common cause of pharyngitis and impetigo, as well as invasive infections such as necrotizing fasciitis.
- GAS produce a variety of toxins that have been associated with scarlet fever and STSS.

Pathophysiology

- Bacterial toxin production by *Staph. aureus* and GAS triggers massive activation of the host cellular immune response.
- Toxins act as superantigens, binding simultaneously to antigen-presenting cells and helper T cells of the host immune system.
- Superantigens are able to activate 20% to 30% of host T cells simultaneously (typical antigen activates less than 1% of host T cells).
- T-cell activation results in massive production of inflammatory cytokines.
- Since the toxins can be absorbed across mucous membranes, invasive bacterial infection is not required for the illness.
- TSS toxin-1 (TSST-1) and enterotoxins A and B are associated with TSS caused by *Staph. aureus*.
- Exotoxins A, B, and C are associated with streptococcal TSS.

Clinical Presentation

- Both TSS and STSS may begin with nonspecific symptoms of lethargy, myalgia, sore throat, abdominal pain, diarrhea, and rash.
- Patients quickly develop fever and hypotension that can result in severe organ dysfunction.

- Clinical criteria for TSS (from the 2011 CDC case definition).
  - Fever: $\geq 102°F$ ($38.9°C$).
  - Rash: diffuse macular erythroderma.
  - Desquamation: 1 to 2 weeks following onset of rash.
  - Hypotension: systolic blood pressure <90 mmHg for adults or less than the 5th percentile for patients <16 years of age.
  - Multisystem involvement (three or more organ systems):
    - GI: vomiting or diarrhea.
    - Muscular: severe myalgias or creatinine phosphokinase at least twice the upper limit of normal.
    - Mucous membranes: hyperemia of the conjunctiva, oropharynx, or vagina.
    - Renal: BUN or creatinine at least twice the upper limit of normal; urinary sediment with pyuria.
    - Hepatic: total bilirubin, AST, or ALT at least twice the upper limit of normal.
    - Hematologic: platelet count <100,000/mm^3.
    - Neurologic: altered mental status without focal neurologic signs in the absence of fever or hypotension.
- A probable case of TSS caused by *Staph. aureus* fulfills four of the five clinical criteria just listed (Figure 11.7).
- Clinical criteria for STSS (from the 2010 CDC case definition).
  - Hypotension: systolic blood pressure <90 mmHg for adults or less than the 5th percentile for patients <16 years of age.
  - Multisystem involvement (two or more of the following):
    - Renal: creatinine >2 mg/dL for adults or twice the upper limit of normal for age.
    - Hematologic: platelet count <100,000/mm^3 or evidence of disseminated intravascular coagulation.
    - Hepatic: ALT, AST, or total bilirubin more than twice the upper limit for age.
    - Pulmonary: ARDS.
    - Skin: generalized erythematous macular rash that may desquamate.
    - Musculoskeletal: necrotizing fasciitis, myositis, or gangrene.
- A probable case of STSS meets the clinical criteria along with the isolation of GAS from a nonsterile site.

Diagnostic Evaluation

- Diagnosis requires a high index of suspicion and is based on the characteristic clinical presentation.
- Blood cultures; CSF, urine, sputum, throat swab culture, and vaginal culture can be obtained as clinically indicated.
- Antibiotic therapy should not be delayed to obtain cultures or results.
- Blood cultures are positive for *Staph. aureus* in only approximately 10% of cases of TSS.
- Blood cultures are positive for GAS in >70% of cases of streptococcal TSS.
- The differential diagnosis of both TSS and STSS includes sepsis, acute viral infection, bacterial meningitis, meningococcemia, and Rocky Mountain spotted fever (RMSF) (in endemic areas).

Management

- Essentials to the management of patient with TSS include aggressive hemodynamic and respiratory support,

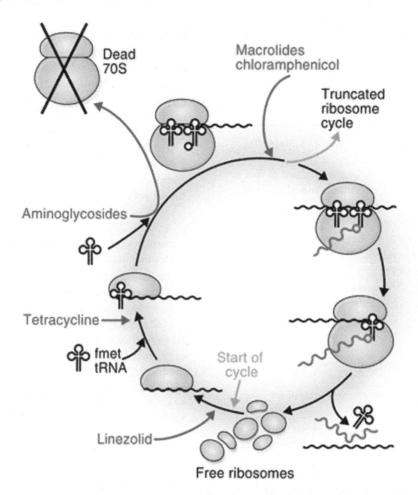

Dead
70S

Macrolides
chloramphenicol

Truncated
ribosome
cycle

Aminoglycosides

Tetracycline

fmet
tRNA

Start of
cycle

Linezolid

Free ribosomes

FIGURE 11.7 • **Toxic Shock Syndrome. A:** Appearance of the rash associated with staphylococcal toxic shock syndrome (TSS). **B:** Gangrenous toes associated with prolonged hypotension in TSS. **C:** Desquamation of the skin that occurs during the resolution of TSS.

removal/debridement of a localized site of infection if present, and antibiotic therapy directed at killing the causative organism and neutralizing the toxin.

- Resuscitation.
  - Patients presenting with signs of shock should receive supplemental oxygen and fluid resuscitation with IV crystalloid.
  - If shock persists despite 40 to 60 mL/kg of isotonic fluid, hemodynamic support should be started with dopamine, epinephrine, or similar agents.
  - Inotropic support should not be delayed while waiting to obtain central venous access.
  - Noninvasive positive pressure ventilation or intubation and mechanical ventilation may be necessary for respiratory distress and hypoxia.
  - The child will require care in a PICU, and arrangements should be made to transfer the patient if those resources are not available at the presenting hospital.
- Removal/debridement of localized site of infection.
  - Tampons, wound packing, and other foreign bodies should be removed, if present.

- A pediatric surgeon should evaluate skin and soft tissue infections for drainage or debridement.
- Failure to remove foreign bodies and/or debride soft tissue infections may result in continued bacterial toxin production.
- Antibiotic therapy and toxin neutralization.
  - Broad-spectrum parenteral antibiotics should be initiated as soon as possible, preferably within the first hour of presentation.
  - A third-generation cephalosporin (e.g., ceftriaxone) and vancomycin are the reasonable empiric regimen.
  - If suspicion for TSS is high, clindamycin should be added, as it may reduce bacterial toxin production.
  - Intravenous pooled human immune globulin (IVIG) has postulated benefit in TSS, presumably due to bacterial toxin neutralization and attenuation of the host inflammatory response.
  - American Academy of Pediatrics recommends considering IVIG therapy in staphylococcal or streptococcal TSS if child is refractory to several hours of aggressive therapy or has an undrainable focus of infection.

- Recent retrospective study in children described increased cost of hospitalization, but no difference in mortality when IVIG was given for STSS.

Vector-Borne Infections

Jill C. Kuester

Vector-Borne Infections

Background

- A worldwide health issue, vector-borne illnesses are caused by bacteria or viruses transmitted to humans from arthropods such as ticks, mosquitoes, or fleas.
- Strategies to prevent and control vector-borne illnesses focus on the complex interplay of host, vector, and environmental factors that affect vector population dynamics and disease transmission.

West Nile Virus

Definition

- West Nile virus: an RNA arthropod-borne virus (arbovirus) belonging to the family Flaviviridae.
- The incubation period ranges from 2 to 14 days.

Etiology/Types

- Transmitted primarily by mosquitoes and birds and less commonly through blood transfusion, organ transplantation intrauterine exposure, and breast-feeding.

Clinical Presentation

- Most are asymptomatic.
- Abrupt fever, headache, malaise, myalgias, diarrhea, maculopapular rash.
- Neuroinvasive disease is rare.

Diagnostic Evaluation

- Anti–West Nile virus IgM antibodies in serum or CSF, NAAT, immunohistochemistry.
- Viral cultures may be performed during the acute phase.
- CBC with manual differential, ESR, CRP.
- CSF bacterial culture with Gram stain, viral-specific CSF PCRs.
- Head CT/MRI to evaluate for alternate differential diagnoses.

Management

- Supportive care, hydration, analgesia, rest.

Lyme Disease

Definition

- A multisystemic tick-borne illness acquired from *Ixodes* ticks with *Borrelia burgdorferi*; most common vector-borne illness in the United States.

Etiology/Types

- Early localized: 3 to 30 days after tick bite.
- Early disseminated: 3 to 12 weeks after tick bite.
- Late disease: >2 months after tick bite.

Clinical Presentation

- Early localized: rash starting as an erythematous macule or papule which expands to form an annular erythematous lesion with a central unaffected one at the site of tick bite (erythema migrans), myalgia, arthralgia, fever, fatigue, headache.
- Early disseminated: erythema migrans, neck pain, facial palsy, myalgia, arthralgia, fever, fatigue, headache. May manifest as meningitis, radiculitis, cranial neuritis, carditis.
- Late disease: arthritis, peripheral neuropathy, and CNS manifestations (Figure 11.8).

Diagnostic Evaluation

- Two-step approach recommended for diagnosis: screening serologic assays (immunofluorescent antibody assay or EIA) confirmed with Western blot testing.

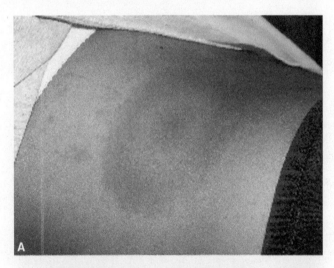

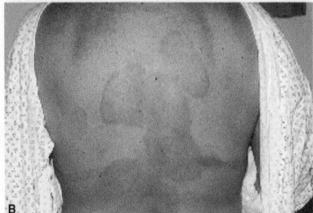

FIGURE 11.8 • **Erythema Migrans.** Erythema migrans rash of Lyme disease. **A:** Erythema migrans lesion on the torso. Note the target-like concentric rings with no scale. **B:** Erythema migrans lesions on the back. The rash may expand rapidly and cover a large area.

- May perform CSF antibody testing.
- CBC, ESR, CRP.
- Blood culture, CSF bacterial cultures with Gram stain, and disease-specific viral PCRs, depending on illness manifestation, may be indicated.

Management

- Antibiotic therapy varies per age, disease stage, and systemic manifestation; options include doxycycline, amoxicillin, or cefuroxime.

PEARL

- *Diagnosis is best made clinically in the early stages of Lyme disease based on the presence of erythema migrans.*

Tularemia

Definition

- Primarily a tick-borne illness caused by *Francisella tularensis*, a gram-negative coccobacillus.

Etiology/Types

- Ulceroglandular tularemia (most common), glandular, oculoglandular, oropharyngeal, pneumonic, typhoidal (septicemic) tularemia.
- Transmitted by ticks, wild rodents, or rabbits carrying *F. tularensis*.

Clinical Presentation

- General: abrupt fever, chills, headache, myalgias, maculopapular lesions, painful lymphadenopathy with or without ulceration.
- Clinical symptoms correspond to the type of tularemia; can include unilateral purulent conjunctivitis, cough, dyspnea, pleuritic chest pain, hilar lymphadenopathy, weight loss.

Diagnostic Evaluation

- Serologic assays above a diagnostic cut-off or with a fourfold rise in serologies between acute and convalescent stages.
- DFA, PCR, culture with cysteine-enriched media.
- CBC with differential, ESR, CRP, CMP, CPK, UA.
- Urine, blood, CSF, and sputum cultures to evaluate for alternate differential diagnoses.

Management

- Streptomycin, gentamicin, or doxycycline.
- Symptomatic and supportive care as clinically indicated.

Rocky Mountain Spotted Fever

Definition

- A tick-borne illness caused by the bacterium *Rickettsia rickettsii*.
- A gram-negative coccobacillus causing systemic vasculitis.

Clinical Presentation

- Fever, headache, myalgias, abdominal pain, emesis, conjunctival injection, macular erythematous rash on wrists, ankles,

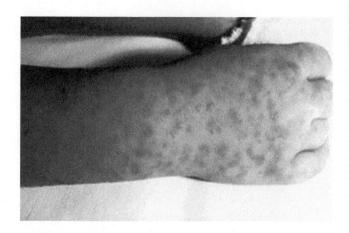

FIGURE 11.9 • **Rocky Mountain Spotted Fever Skin Lesions.** Child's right hand and wrist displaying the characteristic spotted rash with raised or palpable purpura, which is pathognomonic of the lesions of Rocky Mountain spotted fever.

palms, and soles which may spread to trunk; rash may progress to petechial rash (Figure 11.9).

Diagnostic Evaluation

- Indirect immunofluorescent assay (gold standard), serologic antibody testing (may not appear positive for 7–10 days after illness onset), PCR, or immunohistochemistry of skin biopsy.
- CBC with differential, ESR, CRP, comprehensive metabolic panel; hyponatremia and thrombocytopenia are common.
- Chest radiography.
- Blood, urine, CSF cultures and Gram staining to evaluate for alternate differential diagnosis.

Management

- Doxycycline.
- Diagnosis made on clinical signs and symptoms; do not wait for serologic confirmation to start doxycycline.
- Symptomatic and supportive care as clinically indicated.

Plague

Definition

- Primarily a flea-borne zoonotic illness caused by *Yersinia pestis*.
- A gram-negative coccobacillus causing an invasive systemic disease responsible for numerous high-mortality epidemics throughout history.

Etiology/Types

- Bubonic, septicemic, and/or pneumonic plague.
- Transmitted by fleas or rodents carrying *Y. pestis*.

Clinical Presentation

- Clinical symptoms correspond to type of plague.
- Bubonic: acute fever, large, painful lymphadenopathy (buboes) in groin, axilla, or neck, headache, malaise.
- Septicemia: fever, hypotension, shock, chills, headache, malaise, abdominal pain. May lead to DIC, ARDS, multisystem organ failure.

- Pneumonic: fever, cough, dyspnea, chest pain, hemoptysis, hypoxia, headache, malaise.

Diagnostic Evaluation

- Bacterial culture and Gram staining of lymph node aspirate, blood, urine, sputum, or CSF; lumbar puncture as indicated by symptomatology.
- Immunofluorescent antibody tests, PCR, serologic assays, immunohistochemistry.
- CBC with differential, ESR, CRP, CMP.
- Chest radiography.

Management

- Antibiotics.
- Surgical drainage of buboes if needed.
- Hydration, oxygen, respiratory and hemodynamic support as clinically indicated.

Travel Infections
Leah Molloy

Malaria

Background

- Endemic throughout topical regions.
- Highest travel-related risks in sub-Saharan Africa, Vanuatu, Papua New Guinea, the Solomon Islands, Indian subcontinent.
- Almost all cases in the United States are among emigrants or travelers returning from endemic areas.

Definition

- Mosquito-transmitted parasitic infection.
- Working primary diagnosis of all febrile patients with recent travel to endemic areas until proven otherwise.

Etiology/Types

- Five *Plasmodium* species cause malaria: *P. falciparum*, *P. knowlesi*, *P. malariae*, *P. ovale*, and *P. vivax*.

Pathophysiology

- Infective sporozoite transmitted via *Anopheles* mosquito bite.
- Parasites travel to the liver, where they develop and multiply over the next 7 to 14 days, depending on the species.
- The parasites, now termed *merozoites*, then infect erythrocytes to start the symptomatic phase of infection.
- *P. vivax* and *P. ovale* are able to enter a latent phase and remain in the liver, enabling possible future relapses.
- Parasites undergoing mitosis, during which time they are named schizonts, often follow a synchronized cycle of reproduction.

Clinical Presentation

- Paroxysmal fever, owing to the synchronicity of the reproductive cycles, is the characteristic sign of malaria.

- Chills, headache, malaise, cough.
- Normocytic, hemolytic anemia with thrombocytopenia is common, particularly among patients with hyperparasitemia.
- Proteinuria and hemoglobinuria may be seen during times of fever or in the presence of rapid hemolysis.
- *P. falciparum* has greatest proclivity to travel to the CNS and cause cerebral malaria: confusion and delirium progressing to seizures and coma.
- Patients with severe malaria may present with additional systemic signs of illness, including hypotension, renal dysfunction, metabolic acidosis, or hypoglycemia.

Diagnostic Evaluation

- Thick and thin blood smears to identify parasites.
  - Repeated every 12 to 24 hours in cases in which the smear was negative, but the suspicion of malaria remains high.
- Rapid antigen detection test is available but with several limitations, particularly among patients with low levels of parasitemia, necessitating use in combination with microscopy only.
- Clinical presentation and laboratory abnormalities as described above are also important to diagnosis.

Management

- Severe malaria should be treated with intravenous artesunate monotherapy (available through the CDC) or quinidine in combination with doxycycline, tetracycline, or clindamycin.
- Uncomplicated cases may be treated with oral therapy, and medication selection should be guided per species, geographical regions of drug resistance, and in consultation with CDC/WHO guidelines.
- Chloroquine or hydroxychloroquine is preferred for chloroquine-susceptible strains.
- Atovaquone–proguanil alone or quinine in combination with doxycycline, tetracycline, or clindamycin may be used for suspected or confirmed chloroquine-resistant strains.
  - Avoid doxycycline and tetracycline in children <8 years of age.
- Mefloquine may also be used for the treatment of chloroquine-resistant malaria, but should be reserved for intolerance of the options listed above per higher incidence of neuropsychiatric reactions.
- Primaquine must be added for malaria caused by *P. vivax* or *P. ovale* to eradicate latent forms present in the liver, thus preventing relapses.
  - Confirm absence of glucose-6-phosphate dehydrogenase deficiency prior to initiating primaquine.
- Prophylaxis recommended prior to travel per CDC guidelines and must be tailored to patient risk factors and area of travel.
  - Most U.S. cases of malaria occur among travelers who did not follow CDC-recommended prophylaxis recommendations.

Dengue

Background

- Primarily present in tropics and subtropics.
  - USA endemic areas: Puerto Rico, Virgin Islands, American Samoa.
  - USA areas of previous outbreaks: Texas, Hawaii, Florida.

Definition

- Mosquito-transmitted viral illness typically presenting as mild and self-limited febrile illness which may, however, progress to severe shock.

Etiology/Types

- Caused by one of four dengue viruses (DEN 1, 2, 3, 4) and all members of the *Flavivirus* genus.
- Virus is transmitted to humans through bites from infected *Aedes* mosquitoes.
- Humans remain viremic for approximately 7 days, during which time the virus may be transmitted via blood products.

Pathophysiology

- Extrinsic incubation in mosquitoes: 8 to 12 days.
- Intrinsic incubation in humans: 3 to 14 days between bite and symptom onset.

Clinical Presentation

- Acute phase: nonspecific febrile phase, often with retro-orbital headache pain, myalgias, maculopapular rash.
- Critical phase: defervescence within 2 to 7 days after onset; most patients will improve with resolution of illness, but some may progress into severe dengue.
  - Vomiting, mucosal bleeding, leukopenia, thrombocytopenia, elevated hematocrit, difficulty breathing, shock.
  - Plasma leakage including disseminated intravascular coagulation, pleural effusion, ascites.
- Recovery phase: resolution within 2 days of appropriate treatment of severe dengue marked by reabsorption of extravascular fluid, with some patients developing confluent erythematous rash.

Diagnostic Evaluation

- CBC with differential.
  - Leukopenia with thrombocytopenia and elevated hematocrit should raise suspicion.
- Serologic tests including ELISA for anti-dengue IgM and IgG antibodies.

Management

- No specific antiviral therapy exists.
- Supportive care including good hydration is best.
- Avoid agents likely to contribute to coagulopathy, such as aspirin and nonsteroidal anti-inflammatory drugs.
  - Instead use acetaminophen for pain and fever management.

Typhoid

Background

- Most common in tropics, subcontinental India, southeast Asia, southern Africa.

Definition

- Typhoid fever is acquired through ingestion.

Etiology/Types

- Bacterial infection with *Salmonella enterica* serotype Typhi.

Pathophysiology

- Bacterial spread to small intestine and bloodstream after sufficient ingestion.
- Invasion of lymphatic tissues, liver, spleen.

Clinical Presentation

- Enteric fever: fever, headache, lethargy, malaise, abdominal pain with diarrhea or constipation, hepatosplenomegaly, and stupor.
- Minority of patients: rose spots (blanching erythematous macules).
- CNS involvement: confusion, delirium, convulsions, obtundation.
- Most important life-threatening complication: intestinal perforation.

Diagnostic Evaluation

- Blood culture: large volumes (1–15 mL) depending on child size.
- Bone marrow harbors higher bacterial load, best source for culture.
- Stool cultures positive in fewer than half of patients.
- Normal-to-low WBC count, elevated liver function tests.

Management

- Empiric therapy with either ceftriaxone or ciprofloxacin.
  - Resistance emerging: confirm susceptibility.
- Alternative agents: ampicillin, azithromycin, trimethoprim–sulfamethoxazole.
- Fevers may persist for up to 7 days on appropriate therapy.
- Corticosteroids may be of value in severe enteric fever causing altered mental status or shock.
- Vaccination against *S. typhi* for travelers.
  - Vi capsular polysaccharide (Typhim Vi): polysaccharide intramuscular injection for ages ≥2 years.
    - Single dose for primary immunization.
    - Give at least 2 weeks prior to possible exposure.
  - Ty21a (Vivotif): live attenuated oral vaccine for ages ≥6 years.
    - Four doses for primary immunization.
    - Doses taken every other day.
    - Complete at least 1 week prior to possible exposure.
  - Neither vaccine provides reliable protection against *Salmonella* serotype Paratyphi A.

Leptospirosis

Background

- Widespread throughout the United States; more common in southern states.

Definition

- Bacterial spirochete infection.

Etiology/Types

- *Leptospira biflexa*: does not infect humans.
- *Leptospira interrogans*: causes disease in humans.

Pathophysiology

- Transmitted from rodents and domesticated dogs, cows, pigs.
  - Through direct contact, urine, water, or soil.
  - Increased risk among farmers, veterinarians, field workers.
  - Exposure to contaminated water: swimming, boating, floods.
- Enters through intact mucous membranes or skin disruptions.
- 7- to 14-day incubation period.
- Direct toxicity to human tissues permits establishment of invasive disease.

Clinical Presentation

- Septicemic phase: caused by direct effects of pathogen.
  - One week duration: fever, chills, headache, vomiting, rash.
  - Calf and lumbar myalgias.
  - Conjunctival suffusion.
- Immune phase: caused by immune-mediated inflammation.
  - Fever, aseptic meningitis, conjunctival suffusion, uveitis, muscle pain, rash, adenopathy.
- Severe disease attacks liver and kidney.
  - In about 10% of patients.
  - Weil syndrome: hepatic and renal insufficiency, hemorrhage, jaundice, azotemia.
  - Hemorrhagic pneumonitis, cardiac arrhythmias, circulatory collapse.
  - 5% to 15% mortality.

Diagnostic Evaluation

- Cultured on special media from blood or CSF during septicemic phase, or from urine during immune phase.
- Serology: agglutination test to identify antibodies.
  - Do not become positive until after 7 to 10 days into infection.

Management

- Generally self-limited.
- Patients requiring hospitalization: intravenous penicillin G.
  - Serologic confirmation should not delay antibiotic therapy.
- Other treatment options: cefotaxime, ceftriaxone, doxycycline, azithromycin.
- Additional supportive care, including dialysis for fluid and electrolyte management, may be required in severe illness.

Tetanus

Background

- Owing to immunization efforts, U.S. incidence is <0.1 per 100,000.
- Most commonly seen in warmer climates.

Definition

- Spasmic muscle disorder caused by neurotoxin produced by *Clostridium tetani* found in contaminated wounds.

Etiology/Types

- *C. tetani* is an anaerobic gram-positive bacillus that cycles between spore and vegetative states.

- Vegetative form produces an exotoxin called tetanospasmin.
- *C. tetani* is an environmental pathogen commonly found in soil that is most likely to flourish in wounds providing anaerobic conditions, such as necrotic tissue or deep puncture wounds.
  - Common after injuries during farming or gardening with increased likelihood of exposure to soil.

Pathophysiology

- Noninvasive, does not cause systemic inflammation or tissue destruction.
- Tetanospasmin thought to prevent release of acetylcholine, causing increased muscle tone leading to muscle spasms and rigidity.

Clinical Presentation

- Gradual onset over 1 to 7 days.
- Generalized tetanus (lockjaw): neurologic disease characterized by severe muscle spasms. Most common clinical presentation.
- Local tetanus: spasms proximal to infected wound site which usually progress to generalized tetanus.
- Neonatal tetanus: generalized tetanus in infants born to mothers lacking immunity.
- Cephalic tetanus: cranial nerve dysfunction secondary to infected head or neck wounds which may progress to generalized tetanus.

Diagnostic Evaluation

- Clinical diagnosis requiring exclusion of other causes of spasms.

Management

- Supportive care of spasms with minimal stimulation.
- Human tetanus immune globulin (TIG) 3,000 to 6,000 units intramuscularly in a single dose; optimal therapeutic dose not established.
- Intravenous immune globulin may be used as an alternative only in situations where TIG is unavailable.
- Antimicrobials used to decrease the number of vegetative forms.
  - Metronidazole or intravenous penicillin G.
- Primary vaccination with tetanus toxoid followed by regular boosters.
  - Follow CDC immunization recommendations.

Japanese Encephalitis

Background

- Present throughout eastern Asia, subcontinental India, and the western Pacific.

Definition

- Leading cause of vaccine-preventable encephalitis.
- Mosquito-transmitted viral illness.

Etiology/Types

- Japanese encephalitis virus (JEV) is transmitted to humans through bites from infected *Culex* mosquitoes; member of the family Flaviviridae.

- Humans generally do not attain high viral loads in the blood and are thus unlikely to infect mosquitoes.
- Transmission is most common among children during the summer and fall in some climate, but can be transmitted year-round in the tropics and subtropics.

Clinical Presentation

- Vast majority are asymptomatic.
- Clinical disease in <1% of patients presents after 5- to 15-day incubation period: acute encephalitis.
  - Headache, vomiting, fever.
  - Altered mental status, weakness, parkinsonism, seizures progressing to paralysis.
  - Mild leukocytosis, mild anemia, hyponatremia.
- 20% to 30% mortality with residual neurologic deficits or sequelae in about half of survivors.

Diagnostic Evaluation

- CSF analysis: normal glucose, elevated protein, leukocytosis with lymphocyte predominance.
- Serologic identification of anti-JEV IgM antibodies.

Management

- Supportive care only.
- Management of seizures, electrolyte disturbances, cerebral perfusion, and increased intracranial pressure.
- Inactivated vaccine, Ixiaro, approved for patients ≥17 years old.
- Inactivated vaccine for children (JE-Vax) no longer available in the United States.
  - Vaccination recommended for planned stays >1 month, or for travelers staying in rural areas during times of peak incidence.

Rabies

Background

- Primarily an animal infection transmitted to humans via saliva.

Definition

- Acute, highly fatal illness transmitted by animals, marked by neurologic changes.

Etiology/Types

- Rabies virus is an RNA virus in the Rhabdoviridae family.
- Wildlife such as bats, foxes, raccoons, and skunks are the most common source of infection of humans and domestic animals.

Pathophysiology

- Incubation period in humans is typically 1 to 3 months but may range from days to years.
  - Shorter incubation periods more common in settings of young age, immunocompromise, severe wounds, close proximity of wound to CNS, and high inoculum.
- Virus travels along nerves and replicates in tissues.

Clinical Presentation

- Prodromal period: 2- to 10-day period of viral invasion in CNS.
  - Fevers and behavioral changes with pain, paresthesia, or myoclonus at the site of infection.
- Rapid development of neurologic symptoms.
  - Anxiety, excitement, aggressiveness, fever, hydrophobia, hypersalivation, dysautonomia.
- Paralysis in 20% of patients.
- Coma.
- Highly fatal.

Diagnostic Evaluation

- Antemortem fluorescent microscopy of skin biopsy specimens, virus isolation from saliva, or antibody detection in previously unimmunized patients.
- Postmortem brain tissue analysis in humans and animals using immunofluorescence.

Management

- If available, suspected domestic animal sources should be confined and observed for 10 days for development of symptoms after a reported bite.
- Very few cases of human survival after development of symptoms.
- Postexposure prophylaxis against rabies with both vaccine and immunoglobulin is recommended for all patients presenting after a bite from a wild mammal or domestic animal suspected to be infected.
  - Rabies vaccine: 1 mL given intramuscularly on days 0 (first day of postexposure prophylaxis), 3, 7, and 14.
  - Rabies immune globulin: 20 IU/kg, injected to infiltrate the wound site as best as possible, with the remainder of the dose to be given intramuscularly.
  - In situations of delayed medical treatment, both vaccine and immune globulin should be administered regardless of the interval between exposure and treatment.

Common Diagnostic Testing

Jill C. Kuester

Blood Culture

Background/Definition

- Obtained to detect presence of bacteria in blood.

Procedure

- Preferably drawn prior to administering antibiotics.
- Drawn from at least two different sites.
  - Helps to determine contamination from skin bacteria.
  - Should not be drawn from IV catheter unless suspected catheter sepsis.
- Cultures must be transported to the laboratory immediately or at least within 30 minutes.

Testing

- Most organisms require at least 24 hours to grow.
- Often 48 to 72 hours are required for growth and identification of the organism.
- Anaerobic organisms may take longer to grow.

Clinical Considerations

- Obtain when a patient presents with fever and chills (signs of bacteremia) or other signs of infection.

Urine Culture and Sensitivity

Background/Definition

- Obtained to detect pathogenic bacteria in a patient with suspected UTI.
  - Can be obtained clean catch, urinary catheterization, or via indwelling urinary catheter; rarely via suprapubic tap.
- Negative result.
  - <10,000 bacteria per milliliter of urine.
- Positive result.
  - >100,000 bacteria per milliliter of urine; or >50,000 bacteria per milliliter of urine in catheter specimen.
- Indeterminate.
  - Between 10,000 and 100,000 bacteria per milliliter of urine.

Procedure

- Preferably obtained prior to administering antibiotics.
- Clean catch sample.
  - Midstream urine collection after cleaning urinary meatus.
- Catheterized sample.
  - Needed for patients who are unable to void or young infants.
  - Sterile technique.
- Indwelling catheterized sample.
  - Collected using aseptic technique with a needle at a point distal to the sleeve leading to the balloon.

Testing

- Most organisms require at least 24 hours to grow.
- Often 48 to 72 hours are required for growth and identification of the organism.
- Anaerobic organisms may take longer to grow.
  - Important to assess the sensitivity of bacteria to antibiotics.
  - Treatment tailored to safest, least expensive, and most effective antibiotic regimen.
- Cultures can be repeated after treatment to ensure resolution of infection.

Clinical Considerations

- Some institutions send UA prior to culture to save costs; culture is then sent if UA is suspicious for infection.

Cerebrospinal Fluid Culture and Sensitivity Analysis

Background/Definition

- Evaluation for presence of bacteria, blood, quantification of glucose and protein in CSF.

- CSF analysis; normal findings.
  - Culture: no organisms present.
  - Color: clear and colorless.
  - Blood: none.
  - Protein: 15 to 45 mg/dL CSF.
  - Glucose: 50 to 75 mg/dL CSF.
  - Cells:
    - Red blood cells (RBCs): 0 cells.
    - WBCs: total.
      - Neonate: 0 to 30 cells/μL.
      - 1 to 5 years: 0 to 20 cells/μL.
      - 6 to 18 years: 0 to 10 cells/μL.
      - Adult: 0 to 5 cells/μL.
      - Differential.
        - Neutrophils: 0% to 6%.
        - Lymphocytes: 40% to 60%.
        - Monocytes: 15% to 45%.

Procedure

- Lumbar puncture: temporary placement of a needle in the subarachnoid space of spinal column to obtain CSF.

Evaluation of CSF

- Color.
  - Normally clear/colorless.
  - Abnormal.
    - Cloudy appearance may indicate increased WBC count or protein.
    - Red tinge indicates presence of blood.
- Cells.
  - RBCs.
    - Number indicates amount of blood present in CSF.
    - Can be present as a result of "traumatic tap"; >1 WBC per 500 RBCs is considered pathogenic.
  - WBCs.
    - Neutrophils: indicative of bacterial meningitis/cerebral abscess.
    - Mononuclear lymphocytes: viral meningitis or encephalitis suspected.
- Protein.
  - Normally very little found in CSF; protein is a large molecule that does not cross blood–brain barrier.
  - Meningitis, encephalitis, and myelitis alter permeability of blood–brain barrier and allow protein to leak into CSF.
- Glucose.
  - Decreased when bacteria, inflammatory, or tumor cells present.
  - Assess blood glucose level simultaneously, and if the level in CSF is less than 60% of that in blood, it may indicate neoplasm or meningitis.
- Culture.
  - Should be drawn prior to start antibiotics; though initiation of antibiotics should not be delayed in cases when CSF sample cannot be obtained promptly.
  - Results and identification of organism within 24 to 72 hours.

- Gram stain will give preliminary information about organism.
- Antibiotics should be started right away, do no wait for identification of organism.

Testing Considerations

- Contraindications.
  - Increased intracranial pressure (can induce herniation).
  - Patients who are receiving anticoagulation; risk of epidural hematoma.
  - Patients with infection near the lumbar puncture site.

C-Reactive Protein

Background/Definition

- Nonspecific, acute-phase reactant used to diagnose inflammatory disorders or bacterial infectious disease.
- Normal findings <1.0 mg/dL or <10.0 mg/L.

Pathophysiology

- Abnormal serum glycoprotein liver produces during acute inflammatory process.
- Positive test indicates presence of disease (does not indicate cause).
- Shows earlier and more intense rise than ESR.
- Disappears when the inflammatory process is suppressed by salicylates or steroids.

Clinical Considerations

- Detectable 6 to 10 hours after inflammatory response.
- Disappears rapidly when inflammation subsides.

Testing Considerations

- Interfering factors.
  - Elevated test results occur with other entities, including medications such as estrogen and progesterone; not always indicative of inflammation or infection.

Erythrocyte Sedimentation Rate

Background/Definition

- Measurement of rate with which RBCs settle in saline or plasma over specified time period.
- Normal findings (Westergren method).
  - Male: up to 15 mm/hour.
  - Female: up to 20 mm/hour.
  - Child: up to 10 mm/hour.
  - Newborn: up to 0 to 2 mm/hour.
- Nonspecific (not diagnostic for specific disease or injury).

Procedure

- Specimen must be immediately transported to laboratory.

Testing

- Acute and chronic infections, inflammation, advanced neoplasm, and tissue necrosis increase protein content of plasma, causing RBCs to stack up on one another, increasing their weight and causing faster descent.

Clinical Considerations

- Can be used to detect occult disease in patients with vague symptoms.
- Fairly reliable indicator of course of disease.
  - Can be used to monitor disease therapy (especially autoimmune diseases).

Diagnostic Considerations

- Interfering factors.
  - Menstruation can cause elevated levels, and polycythemia is associated with decreased levels.
  - Some medications that affect ESR levels can impact results.
    - Increased ESR levels.
      - Dextran, methyldopa, oral contraceptives, penicillamine, procainamide, theophylline, and vitamin A.
    - Decreased ESR levels.
      - Aspirin, cortisone, and quinine.

D-Test for Macrolide-Inducible Resistance to Clindamycin

Background/Definition

- Test evaluates for the presence of macrolide-inducible resistance to clindamycin produced by an inducible methylase that alters the binding location for macrolides and clindamycin.

Procedure

- Small paper disk with antimicrobial amount applied to agar surface which has been inoculated with standardized inoculum of isolated organism.
- Antibiotic diffuses into agar medium.
  - Lack of zone inhibition around the disk indicates bacterial resistance to macrolide antibiotics.

Testing Considerations

- Organisms testing positive for D-test may still be sensitive to clindamycin; however, they are presumed to be resistant since resistance can be induced.
- In serious infections, bacterial isolates testing positive for D-test should lead to the avoidance of clindamycin (Figure 11.10).

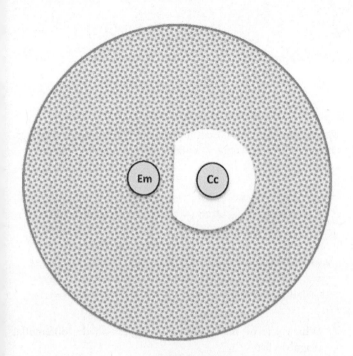

FIGURE 11.10 • **Positive D-Test.** Scheme illustrating a positive D-test for detecting inducible MLSB resistance in staphylococci. Erythromycin- and clindamycin-containing disks are placed onto an agar plate on which a staphylococcal strain was spread and grown overnight. Lack of an inhibition zone around the erythromycin disk indicates erythromycin resistance of the isolate. In case of clindamycin susceptibility, an O-shaped inhibition zone would be present around the clindamycin disk. However, the zone is blunted on the side facing the erythromycin disk where the diffusion zones of the two antibiotics meet. The typical D-shaped inhibition zone is due to the induction of clindamycin resistance by erythromycin in the colonies growing in this region.

Rapid Studies (Polymerase Chain Reaction)

Background/Definition

- Most useful for detecting/identifying pathogens for which cultures/serologic tests are slow or difficult to obtain, with high sensitivity and specificity.
- Greatest impact is in clinical virology and mycobacteriology (conventional methods are slow and insensitive).

Types

- Number of specimens that can be identified is rapidly increasing.
  - Examples include HIV, hepatitis B and C, cytomegalovirus, *M. tuberculosis*, *C. trachomatis*, and common respiratory viral pathogens in children.

Procedure

- Specimens can be sent from blood, nasopharyngeal swabs, CSF.
  - Should be sent in sterile containers/rapidly transported.
  - Turnaround time can be hours to days.

CASE STUDY: NEXT 2 QUESTIONS
A 10-year-old girl with a history of Acute Lmphoblastic Leuke-mia (ALL) has just completed her last round of chemotherapy 1 week ago. She has an oral temperature of 38.5°C and com-plains of abdominal pain and fever. The most recent ANC is 480 cells/μL. On physical examination, she has a central line and rebound abdominal tenderness.

1. What is the first priority/management for this child?
   a. Blood cultures, administration of Zosyn and Flagyl, admission to the floor.
   b. Abdominal ultrasound.
   c. Administration of Augmentin and observation for 24 hours.
   d. Admission to the floor, blood cultures, administration of Zosyn.

Answer: **A**

The priority in patient management is obtaining blood cultures from the central line while ordering antibiotics. The antibiotics should be administered within 1 hour and the patient should be admitted to the floor for at least 24 hours to monitor for effective-ness and vital sign stability. An abdominal ultrasound or an abdomi-nal CT may be useful in this child; however, imaging studies are not the first priority. This patient meets high-risk criteria secondary to her comorbidity and likely low ANC for >7 days, and Augmen-tin and observation are not adequate therapy in this scenario. The patient's disposition is not yet known; the child will require admis-sion; however, may require admission to a PICU. Transferring to an inpatient service should not happen until the initial management strategies are instituted and response to therapy is determined in order to determine the best disposition for this child.

2. Eight days later, the patient showed no improvement and contin-ued to be febrile with a temperature of 38.5°C PO and a cough that was new over the past 24 hours. A chest radiograph demon-strates a left lower lobe opacity. What is the next intervention?
   a. Resend blood cultures, CBC with differential, and obtain another chest radiograph.
   b. Start vancomycin in addition to the Zosyn, resend blood cultures, and obtain a chest radiograph in 24 hours.
   c. Discontinue Flagyl and consider an antifungal medication.
   d. Observe for 24 additional hours and obtain another chest radiograph if cough persists.

Answer: **B**

The addition of vancomycin is indicated to cover for pneumonia with demonstration of a new opacity in the left lower lobe and persistent fever for >4 to 7 days. Additional blood cultures assist in monitoring for improvement. Flagyl may be discontinued if the abdominal studies are negative; however, this is not a priority

with the new clinical examination and radiographic findings. Observation alone is not acceptable in this high-risk patient.

CASE STUDY
A 3-month-old presents to the emergency department (ED) with a 2-day history of poor feeding, decreased urine output, and lethargy, and is noted to have a bulging fontanelle. The child was born via vaginal delivery and was discharged home with mother. He has been febrile for the past 48 hours, unre-sponsive to acetaminophen.

3. Which one of the following is highest on the differential diagnosis list?
   a. Cardiac abnormality.
   b. Group B streptococcal meningitis.
   c. RSV pneumonia.
   d. *Bartonella henselae* infection.

Answer: **B**

The history of fever, lethargy, bulging fontanelle, and a known group B streptococcus (GBS) status in the mother at the time of birth places GBS high on the differential diagnosis. Although GBS usually occurs in infants <3 months of age, late-onset GBS can be deadly if not detected. A cardiac abnormality cannot be excluded in an infant with poor feeding; however, when accompanied by fever or other clinical symptoms, it is less likely. RSV is common in this age group and is as-sociated with fever and decreased PO intake; however, a bulging fon-tanelle is not noted in children with RSV infection. *Bartonella henselae* infection (cat scratch disease) is associated with fever and enlarged lymph nodes; however, it is not associated with a bulging fontanelle.

4. In the above scenario, the child is admitted to the hospital and cultures are obtained. Which one of the following results is most likely to determine the diagnosis?
   a. WBC of 20,000 on CBC, CSF culture with 0 RBC, WBC of <100 cells/μL, glucose of 67 mg/dL, and protein of 58 mg/dL.
   b. Urine culture with positive ketones.
   c. Blood culture with no growth to date.
   d. A CSF result with 3 red cells, WBC >1,000 cells/μL, glu-cose 38 mg/dL, protein 200 mg/dL, immature neutrophils.

Answer: **D**

CSF evaluation in bacterial meningitis is typically associated with a WBC count >1,000 cells/μL, low glucose, and high protein. It is also not uncommon to have a few RBCs in the sample, especially if the tap was traumatic. An elevated WBC count on a CBC sup-ports the diagnosis; however, it is not a specific finding of menin-gitis. Ketonuria is abnormal, though, it does assist in determining a diagnosis in this case. No growth on a blood culture is not useful in determining a diagnosis in this child.

5. A 16-year-old boy with acute myelogenous leukemia is admitted for 3 days of fever. He has been experiencing sinus pain and discharge over the past 2 weeks, and on examination, a dark spot is noted in his nares. Which one of the following is the appropriate next step(s)?
   a. Order a radiography of the sinuses.
   b. Obtain an induced sputum sample for culture.
   c. Obtain a CT of the sinuses, and consult a pediatric otolaryngologist for a biopsy.
   d. Start empiric therapy with amphotericin B.

Answer: **C**

Mucor often appears in the sinuses, and can be noted as a dark discoloration of the nasal tissue. *Mucor* is a medical emergency, as it is a highly aggressive fungus associated with high mortality if not aggressive treated. A radiograph may demonstrate sinusitis; however, it would not evaluate for *Mucor*. Sputum cultures will likely be obtained, but are secondary to CT and biopsy, which are diagnostic. Initiating empiric therapy is indicated; however, obtaining a biopsy sample first is recommended.

6. A 10-year-old girl is now 100 days out from a living donor liver transplant, and presents with new dysuria and fever for 2 days. A urine culture begins to grow *Aspergillus*. In choosing an antifungal agent, which one of the following treatment options is reasonable?
   a. Oral fluconazole.
   b. IV amphotericin B.
   c. IV voriconazole.
   d. No treatment as the fungus has only been isolated from her urine.

Answer: **B**

Oral formulations for invasive fungal disease are seldom appropriate because of the difficulty in achieving therapeutic levels in the blood. Fluconazole also has no activity against *Aspergillus*. IV voriconazole is a reasonable choice, but would be a difficult choice in light of its interactions with many immunosuppressive medications, which this patient is likely on. Urine isolates of invasive fungal species are real and should be treated as such.

7. A teenage patient with confirmed HIV infection presents to the ED with persistent nonproductive cough for 3 weeks. He has been mostly compliant with antiviral therapy, but sometimes forgets to take his medications. Heart rate (HR) and BP are normal, but respiratory rate (RR) is 32 breaths per minute and pulse oximeter reading is 88%. His lung examination is normal. A chest X-ray obtained shows "diffuse haziness in both lung fields but no focal consolidation." Which infection is most likely?
   a. Bacterial pneumonia, like *Strep. pneumoniae*.
   b. Viral infection.
   c. *Pneumocystis jirovecii* pneumonia (aka PCP).
   d. Tuberculosis.

Answer: **C**

Bacterial pneumonia, while overall much more common than PCP, usually has a focal finding on chest X-ray and the patients often have fever associated with it. Viral infections are usually associated with other symptoms such as rhinorrhea and fever. Tuberculosis is a very reasonable thought in the context of this patient, but does not usually cause persistent tachypnea or oxygen desaturations. Hilar adenopathy on chest X-ray would make the diagnosis more likely.

8. A 14-month-old boy presents to the ED with acute onset of fever, lethargy, and refusal to walk. A purplish rash is developing on his lower extremities that the parents tell you was not there just an hour ago. Vital signs include temperature of 39.5°C, HR of 180 beats per minute, RR of 46 breaths per minute, and BP of 74/42 mmHg. What is the most important next step in management?
   a. Administer 20 mL/kg isotonic fluid.
   b. Administer IV ceftriaxone.
   c. Start dopamine at 5 µg/kg/minute.
   d. Intubate the patient.

Answer: **B**

Antibiotic therapy is the most important step in treating a patient with meningococcemia. It is the only treatment that will ultimately cure the patient. Addressing emergency issues may also be required to stabilize the patient; however, administration of ceftriaxone is the most important initial endeavor. In clinical practice most of these steps will be done simultaneously.

9. A 19-month-old girl is admitted to the PICU with a diagnosis of meningococcemia. The patient is in severe septic shock, requiring inotropic support and mechanical ventilation. Which of the following populations would require prophylactic antibiotic treatment?
   a. Nurses working on the unit where the patient is admitted.
   b. The classmates of the patient's sibling.
   c. Patient's neighbor who played at the park with the patient last week.
   d. Physician who intubated the patient in the ED.

Answer: **D**

Anyone with close contact such as those living in the same household, those at the same childcare in the last 7 days, those with direct exposure to the patient's secretions, including those who were involved in the intubation or suctioning of secretions without protection, are at high risk and require chemoprophylaxis.

10. Which bacterial serotypes are covered with the meningococcal conjugate vaccine?
    a. A, C, Y, and W-135.
    b. A, B, C, Y, and W-135.
    c. C, Y, and W-135.
    d. A, B, and C.

Answer: **A**

The meningococcal vaccine covers four clinically significant serotypes of the bacteria which are A, C, Y, and W-13.

(continues on page 332)

11. In reviewing the charts of 10 patients diagnosed with meningococcus who had varying degrees of severity of illness, findings indicate the clinical courses included positive blood cultures with minimal symptoms to the extent of patients with severe sepsis and death. What is the most likely reason for this wide range in disease severity?
    a. Differing immune status of the patients.
    b. Amount of endotoxin in the patient's circulation.
    c. Documentation is likely wrong; all patients should have the same symptoms.
    d. The patients with less severe symptoms were immunized.

Answer: **B**

The amount of endotoxin circulating in the patient relates to the disease severity. The more endotoxin in the system, the more severe the symptoms are. Patients with complement deficiencies or asplenia are more likely to acquire meningococcus. However, this will not necessarily affect the severity of the disease. It is well known that the patients can have varying degrees of illness from just bacteremia, to meningitis, to severe sepsis, and death. The immunization status of the patient will merely protect them from contracting the disease.

CASE STUDY: NEXT 2 QUESTIONS

A previously healthy, 14-year-old girl presents to the ED with a 12-hour history of vomiting, muscle aches, and fever. She and her family recently returned from a camping trip in Colorado. The family prepared all their own meals, and the patient and her siblings swam in a small lake several times. On examination, she is ill-appearing and somnolent, but able to answer questions, and it is noted that she has redness of the conjunctivae and mouth. Temperature is 102.2°F, HR 140/minute, RR 30/minute, pulse oximetry of 97% on room air, BP 80/40 mmHg. Cardiac examination reveals tachycardia with regular rhythm and no murmurs. Lungs are clear to auscultation bilaterally. Extremities are warm with brisk capillary refill and bounding pulses. The skin is warm with an erythematous rash on the trunk, extending to the thighs.

12. Which of the following findings in the history would be suggestive of staphylococcal TSS?
    a. Siblings presenting with similar symptoms.
    b. Removal of a tick from the patient during the camping trip.
    c. History of similar symptoms requiring hospital admission 1 year previously.
    d. Recent antibiotic treatment for pharyngitis.

Answer: **C**

SIRS has a wide variety of causes. Staphylococcal TSS was historically reported in menstruating women using tampons. The overall incidence has declined, but 50% of staphylococcal TSS cases are still associated with menstruation and tampon use. Women who suffer menstrual TSS are at risk for recurrence. TSS is usually sporadic and it would be unusual for siblings to present simultaneously. A tick bite would suggest a vector-borne illness like RMSF.

Bacterial pharyngitis is typically caused by GAS, but pharyngitis is only rarely associated with streptococcal TSS. Family history is not known to play a role in the development of TSS.

13. What is the benefit of adding clindamycin to therapy with ceftriaxone and vancomycin to the treatment of TSS?
    a. Covers MRSA, which commonly causes TSS.
    b. Inhibits cell wall synthesis, resulting in bacterial death.
    c. Exerts anti-inflammatory effects on the host immune system.
    d. Inhibits bacterial toxin production.

Answer: **D**

Clindamycin binds to the 50S subunit of bacterial ribosomes and suppresses protein synthesis, including production of toxins causing TSS. Clindamycin is effective against streptococci and methicillin-sensitive strains of *Staph. aureus*. Clindamycin is effective against some strains of MRSA, but MRSA is rarely associated with TSS. β-Lactam antibiotics, such as penicillin and cephalosporins, inhibit bacterial cell wall synthesis. Several antibiotics are thought to have anti-inflammatory effects apart from their antibacterial activity, but this is not considered the major effect of clindamycin in TSS.

14. What is the role of superantigens in TSS?
    a. Bind simultaneously to antigen-presenting cells and helper T cells of the host immune system, triggering a massive inflammatory response.
    b. Are metabolized to proinflammatory cytokines in the host liver.
    c. Bind directly to the vascular endothelium, causing vasodilatation and capillary leak.
    d. Confer antibiotic resistance properties to the bacteria.

Answer: **A**

Superantigens are bacterial proteins that bypass the normal processing and presentation of antigens to helper T cells of the immune system. This triggers massive release of proinflammatory cytokines, resulting in fever, rash, and hypotension characteristic of the syndrome. A typical antigen activates less than 1% of host T cells, while superantigens may activate 20% to 30% of T cells.

15. A 3-year-old boy is admitted to the pediatric unit with refusal to walk and fever. He was started on empiric ceftriaxone and scheduled for an MRI in the morning to evaluate for osteomyelitis. There is concern in regard to his status, and he is noted to be in significant distress. Temperature is 103°F, HR 170/minute, RR 50/minute, BP 70/40 mmHg, and pulse oximetry of 98% on room air. He moans in response to voice and tactile stimulus, but does not open his eyes. There is an erythematous rash on his trunk. Lungs are clear to auscultation bilaterally, but the patient has moderate retractions and tracheal tugging. Abdomen is soft, nontender, and nondistended with active bowel sounds. Extremities are warm and well perfused with brisk cap refill and bounding pulses with the exception of the right leg. The right calf appears swollen and discolored. The child screams on palpation of the calf. In

addition to providing fluid resuscitation and broadening anti-biotic coverage, what is the most important consultation in the patient's management?

a. Cardiology for possible echocardiogram.

b. Pediatric surgery or orthopedics for evaluation of the right leg.

c. Infectious disease for antibiotic recommendations.

d. Radiology for an emergent MRI of the right leg.

Answer: **B**

Symptom and presentation indicate signs of the SIRS with shock. Hypotension, rash, and focal site of inflammation (right calf swelling and pain) should raise the suspicion of streptococcal TSS with necrotizing fasciitis. This requires immediate evaluation and possible debridement by surgery to prevent the spread of infection. The patient will require ICU care and infectious disease consultation may be desired, but the surgical evaluation is emergent. IVIG administration for toxin neutralization can be considered if the patient has refractory shock despite aggressive resuscitation. MRI may give useful information, but is time consuming and should not delay the surgical evaluation and management of the patient.

16. A 5-year-old febrile patient has had a CSF cell analysis and culture sent. The cell analysis shows protein 80 mg/dL, glucose 65 mg/dL, RBC 1,500 cells/mm^3, WBC 3 cells/mm^3. What is the most likely interpretation of these results?

a. Bacterial meningitis.

b. "Traumatic tap," contaminated with blood.

c. Viral meningitis.

d. Normal CSF findings.

Answer: **B**

Although it is important to consider herpes virus in any child who has RBCs present in the CSF, typically RBCs seen in the CSF without WBCs indicates a traumatic spinal tap. In this specimen, protein is elevated due to blood contamination from spinal blood vessel. The presence of WBC is due to the blood contamination. The WBC-to-RBC ratio is not greater than 1:500; therefore is not likely due to infection. Glucose would be decreased in the setting of bacterial infection.

17. Two sets of blood cultures from separate peripheral sites have been sent of a 5-year-old patient with likely bacteremia. One of the blood cultures has grown coagulase-negative *Staph. aureus*. The second has had no growth for 72 hours. What is the interpretation?

a. Pathologic organism which requires antibiotic treatment for 14 days.

b. Likely a contaminant; blood cultures can be repeated.

c. Likely a contaminant; treatment should still be continued for 14 days.

d. This is a pathologic organism which requires antibiotic treatment for 7 days.

Answer: **B**

Coagulase-negative *Staph. aureus* is a common contaminant and rarely pathogenic. Blood cultures can be repeated; however, treatment for this organism is not indicated.

18. A 16-year-old girl presents with a 1-week history of fever, chills, and cough. She is quite lethargic, dehydrated, and there is difficulty obtaining blood draw. Which of the following is most important to obtain?

a. CRP.

b. Lipase.

c. Blood culture.

d. ESR.

Answer: **C**

The patient is presenting with signs of bacteremia. Blood culture would be the most important to evaluate. CRP and ESR are non-specific findings and not diagnostic for specific disease or organism. Lipase is helpful in evaluating for pancreatitis, though is not indicated as a first line test for this adolescent.

19. A PICU patient with a diagnosis of sepsis has blood tests, including inflammatory markers monitored serially, and she is now clinically recovering. Which one of these nonspecific inflammatory markers will peak the highest at the beginning of disease and resolve more quickly than the others as the patient recovers?

a. ESR.

b. Albumin.

c. Platelet count.

d. CRP.

Answer: **D**

CRP is more sensitive and rapidly responsive, showing a more intense and earlier rise. It also predictably resolves more quickly than ESR. Albumin is a negative acute-phase reactant, which decreases with inflammation and infection. Platelet count can be an acute-phase reactant but the level can change for many reasons, not always a resolution of infection.

20. A patient presents with symptoms suspicious for meningitis. What CSF findings would be expected in the cell analysis, protein and glucose counts if it is bacterial meningitis?

a. Protein elevated, glucose elevated, neutrophils present.

b. Protein decreased, glucose elevated, no neutrophils present.

c. Protein elevated, glucose decreased, neutrophils present.

d. Protein decreased, glucose decreased, no neutrophils present.

Answer: **C**

Glucose in the CSF is decreased with bacterial infection and neutrophils are present in this setting as well. Protein is elevated in the CSF with bacterial infection because inflammation alters the permeability of the blood–brain barrier allowing protein to leak into the CSF.

21. A patient presents with urgency and frequency of urination. A catheterized urine culture reveals greater than 100,000 colony-forming units (CFU) of *E. coli* per milliliter of urine. The patient has been treated with appropriate antibiotic regimen,

(continues on page 334)

but continues to have symptoms. What culture results would be expected if the infection has been treated completely?
a. 50,000 CFU of *E. coli*.
b. Greater than 100,000 CFU of *E. coli*.
c. 1,000 CFU of *E. coli*.
d. 10,000 CFU of *E. coli*.

Answer: **C**

The infection has been treated if the clean catch specimen has less than 10,000 bacteria per milliliter of urine and is considered a negative result. If greater than 100,000, it is considered to be infection.

22. Which one of the following remedies should be recommended for symptomatic management of dengue fever?
a. Aspirin.
b. Ibuprofen.
c. Acetaminophen.
d. Naproxen.

Correct *Answer:* **C**

NSAIDs and salicylates should not be administered for pain management in patients with dengue fever to avoid contributing to blood dyscrasias.

23. A 13-year-old patient presents with a history of recent travel to subcontinental India complaining of fever, with noticeable mosquito bites upon examination. Which of the following findings on the CBC would increase your suspicion for malaria?
a. Elevated hematocrit.
b. Hemolytic anemia.
c. Leukocytosis.
d. Elevated mean corpuscular volume.

Answer: **B**

Malaria with high levels of parasitemia commonly causes normocytic hemolytic anemia, where a normal mean corpuscular volume would be expected. Dengue fever, another mosquito-borne illness, is associated with elevated hematocrit, while JEV can cause leukocytosis.

24. When a patient complaining of general malaise with symptoms of fever, chills, and myalgia mentions that he was recently cleaning out his flooded basement, which should be high on the differential diagnosis list?
a. Leptospirosis.
b. Dengue.
c. JEV.
d. Malaria.

Answer: **A**

While all possible answers may present with fever, chills, and myalgia, leptospirosis can commonly be contracted from contaminated water including the setting of a flood.

25. Ideally, children who are less than 17 years of age and are traveling to countries endemic for this disease should receive prophylaxis for which infectious process?

a. Malaria.
b. JEV.
c. Smallpox.
d. Hepatitis A.

Answer: **D**

Antimicrobial prophylaxis against malaria is recommended for children traveling to countries that are endemic for malaria, as it can cause a severe, critical illness. Currently, no vaccine exists for prevention of malaria.

26. Of the options listed below, what is the longest allowable time frame between suspected rabies exposure and when rabies vaccine and immune globulin should be offered?
a. 12 hours.
b. 3 days.
c. 1 month.
d. 3 months.

Answer: **D**

The Centers for Disease Control and Prevention recommend rabies immune globulin and vaccine for exposures, regardless of the time interval between exposure and initiation of postexposure prophylaxis. Thus, for this question, the longest time interval will always be the correct answer.

27. An 8-year-old girl presents to the ED with complaints of worsening headache, generalized muscle aches, and low-grade fever for 2 days. Upon physical examination, a light pink macular rash on her bilateral palms, wrists, and ankles is noted. She recently returned from a camping trip and has had multiple "close" exposures to wildlife. Empiric treatment with which antibiotic should be initiated before confirmatory laboratory testing is available?
a. Amoxicillin.
b. Vancomycin.
c. Doxycycline.
d. Ceftriaxone.

Answer: **C**

The patient's clinical symptoms of headache, myalgias, fever, and macular rash on her palms, wrists, and ankles are consistent with a diagnosis of RMSF. Serologic antibody testing may not be positive for RMSF until 7 to 10 days after onset of illness. Due to the potentially fatal nature of RMSF, antibiotic therapy with doxycycline should be initiated based on clinical suspicion of RMSF and should not be delayed for confirmatory testing.

28. A 6-month-old infant with no medical history and a diagnosis of RSV bronchiolitis is intubated and ventilated. The patient is currently on day 8 of illness and has demonstrated overall improvement in hypoxia and decreased ventilator needs. Two days ago, the patient developed copious thick yellow sputum and an increased oxygen requirement which has persisted. Vital signs are as follows: temperature 35.2°C, HR 175 beats per minute, RR 35 breaths per minute, BP 76/45 mmHg, Spo$_2$ 94% on Fio$_2$ 0.8. The chest radiograph demonstrates a

progressive right middle lobe infiltrate. Based on clinical suspicion, which diagnosis is highest on the differential list?

a. Pneumothorax.

b. Sepsis.

c. Secondary respiratory viral infection.

d. Ventilator-associated pneumonia.

Answer: **D**

Rationale: Hospital-acquired pneumonia is one of the most common hospital-acquired infections in both adults and children. This patient's clinical and diagnostic findings of a progressive infiltrate on chest X-ray with worsening gas exchange, temperature instability, new onset of purulent sputum, and tachycardia are most likely associated with a ventilator-associated pneumonia.

29. A 12-day-old term infant is admitted to the intermediate care unit with a 1-day history of lethargy, poor feeding, and recent fever of 38.5°C. The patient was born at 40 weeks gestation via spontaneous vaginal delivery to a G2 P2 mother who had an uncomplicated pregnancy with no known prenatal infections. The patient is lethargic, with mild jaundice, and bilateral upper extremity tremors. A sepsis evaluation was initiated and CSF analysis reveals a WBC count of 15 cells/mm^3, a RBC count of 8,000 cells/mm^3, protein level of 175 mg/dL, and a glucose level of 35 mg/dL. The white blood count differential is 2% neutrophils, 82% lymphocytes, and 16% mononuclear cells. Antibiotic therapy should include which of the following?

a. Valacyclovir.

b. Vancomycin.

c. Ceftriaxone.

d. Acyclovir.

Answer: **D**

Neonatal HSV can manifest as a life-threatening multisystemic disseminated disease, a localized CNS infection, or as a localized infection of the skin, eyes, and/or mouth. CSF analysis in individuals with HSV meningitis or encephalitis is significant for an elevated protein level, increased number of erythrocytes, and lymphocytic pleocytosis. Treatment with parenteral acyclovir should be administered to all neonates with a clinical suspicion of HSV regardless of disease manifestation due to the high morbidity and mortality risk of neonatal HSV infection.

30. A 1-year-old female infant presents to the ED with generalized weakness, diarrhea, and fever for 2 days. Temperature is 39.0°C, HR 102/minute, RR 20/minute, BP 80/39 mmHg, and SpO$_2$ 95% on room air. Physical examination is notable for a pale, tired-appearing female, with a diffuse maculopapular rash on her abdomen, trunk, and bilateral upper extremities with palmar involvement. Laboratory results are listed below:

Sodium	136 mEq/L	WBC count	6.8×10^3/μL
Potassium	3.5 mEq/L	Hemoglobin	10.5 g/dL
Chloride	100 mEq/L	Hematocrit	28.3%
Bicarbonate	21 mEq/L	Platelets	90×10^3/μL

Blood urea nitrogen	22 mEq/L
Creatinine	2.1 mEq/L
Glucose	92 mEq/L
Calcium	8.1 mEq/L
Magnesium	2.4 mEq/L
Phosphorus	4.9 mEq/L

Antibiotics should be selected to cover for which of the following organisms?

a. *Staph. aureus* and *Strep. pyogenes.*

b. Methicillin-resistant *Staph. aureus* and *E. coli.*

c. *Strep. pyogenes* and *E. coli.*

d. *Strep. pneumoniae* and *Staph. epidermidis.*

Answer: **A**

The patient's clinical presentation of fever, rash, hypotension, myalgias, and diarrhea in conjunction with laboratory findings depicting renal dysfunction and thrombocytopenia are consistent with a diagnosis of TSS as defined by the Centers for Disease Control and Prevention. The pathogenic mechanism of TSS includes multisystem organ involvement and shock due to exotoxin release from *Staph. aureus* and *Strep. pyogenes.*

31. A 5-year-old boy who recently received induction chemotherapy for acute myelocytic leukemia is admitted to the PICU with concern for sepsis with fever, lethargy, neutropenia, tachycardia, hypotension, and decreased peripheral perfusion. Using goal-directed therapy for the management of pediatric shock, the appropriate initial interventions should include which of the following steps in sequential order?

a. Administer oxygen, obtain blood and urine cultures, establish central venous access, administer antibiotics.

b. Administer oxygen, establish central venous access, administer antibiotics, rapid administration of up to and over 60 mL/kg of isotonic saline or colloid.

c. Administer oxygen, establish IV access, rapid administration of up to and over 60 mL/kg of isotonic saline or colloid, administer antibiotics.

d. Establish central venous and arterial access, administration of up to and over 60 mL/kg of isotonic saline or colloid, initiate vasopressor support.

Answer: **C**

According to the 2012 Surviving Sepsis Campaign, the sequential components of early goal-directed therapy include prompt recognition of decreased mental status and perfusion with early administration of oxygen, establishment of IV access, fluid administration, and antibiotic administration. Early and immediate vascular access can be established with two peripheral venous catheters.

32. A 10-year-old patient presents with abrupt fever, malaise, weakness, headache, and a maculopapular rash. Which of

(continues on page 336)

following tests should be used to confirm a diagnosis of West Nile virus?

a. Blood culture.

b. Sputum culture.

c. Serum West Nile virus IgM.

d. West Nile virus PCR, nasopharyngeal swab.

Answer: **C**

Rationale: Blood and sputum cultures will test for presence of bacteria, not virus. There is no nasopharyngeal swab PCR for West Nile virus; there is a PCR for CSF. Serum IgM for West Nile virus will confirm diagnosis.

33. Which of the following best describes the treatment plan for a child with West Nile virus?

a. Symptomatic and supportive care.

b. Doxycycline 100 mg 3 times per day for 14 days.

c. Referral to a neurologist.

d. Doxycycline 100 mg 3 times per day for 21 days.

Answer: **A**

Antibiotics treat bacterial infections and therefore will not treat West Nile virus. A neurologist may be involved if the patient has progression to neuroinvasive disease. With the patient's current symptoms, supportive care is the only treatment available.

34. A 6-year-old presents with an annular erythematous skin lesion and facial nerve palsy. What is the test of choice to confirm a diagnosis of Lyme disease?

a. Serologic assay.

b. Screening assays with confirmation by Western blot.

c. Blood cultures from two separate sites.

d. DFA.

Answer: **B**

Serologic assays are not sensitive within the first month of infection; therefore, confirmation with Western blot is the test of choice. Blood cultures will not reveal Lyme disease and DFA is the test of choice for tularemia.

35. A 10-year-old presents with fever, myalgia, decreased appetite, and emesis for 3 days and has been diagnosed with viral gastroenteritis. After questioning, parents do report a bug bite approximately 10 days ago after playing hide-and-seek in the backyard. What symptom below would place RMSF high on the differential diagnosis list?

a. Maculopapular lesion at tick bite site.

b. Rash on wrists, ankles, palms, and soles.

c. Erythema migrans rash at tick bite site.

d. Painful, swollen lymph nodes.

Answer: **B**

Rash on wrists, ankles, palms, and soles is supportive of a diagnosis of RMSF. In RMSF, the rash begins on wrists, ankles, palms, and soles but can rapidly spread to the trunk. Erythema migrans, also known as "target lesion," is a hallmark of Lyme disease. Maculopapular lesion at the tick bite is usually seen in tularemia. Painful, swollen lymph nodes can be seen in tularemia and bubonic plague.

Recommended Readings

Agarwal, A., McMorrow, M., & Arguin, P. M. (2012). Plasmodium species (malaria). In S. S. Long, L. K. Pickering, & C. G. Prober (Eds.), *Principles and practice of pediatric infectious diseases* (4th ed., pp. 1298–1306). Philadelphia, PA: Elsevier.

American Academy of Pediatrics. (2012). Group A streptococcal infections. In L. K. Pickering, C. J. Baker, D. W. Kimberlin & S. S. Long (Eds.), *Red book: 2012 Report of the committee on infectious diseases* (29th ed., pp. 668-680). Elk Grove Village, IL: Author.

American Academy of Pediatrics. (2012). Staphylococcal infections. In L. K. Pickering, C. J. Baker, D. W. Kimberlin, & S. S. Long (Eds.), *Red book: 2012 Report of the committee on infectious diseases* (29th ed.). Elk Grove Village, IL: Author.

Blessing, K., Toepfner, N., Kinzer, S., Möllmann, C., Geiger, J., Serr, A., . . . Berner, R. (2013). Lemierre syndrome associated with 12th cranial nerve palsy—a case report and review. *International Journal of Pediatric Otorhinolaryngology, 77*, 1585–1588.

Blyth, C. C., Palasanthiran, P., & O'Brien, T. A. (2007). Antifungal therapy in children with invasive fungal infections: A systematic review. *Pediatrics, 119*(4), 772–784.

Brook, I. (2012). Clostridium tetani (tetanus). In S. S. Long, L. K. Pickering, & C. G. Prober (Eds.), *Principles and practice of pediatric infectious diseases* (4th ed., pp. 966–970). Philadelphia, PA: Elsevier.

Castillo, S., Rake, A., & Farrington, E. (2012). Systemic inflammatory response syndrome and septic shock. In K. Reuter-Rice & B. Bolick (Eds.), *Pediatric acute care: A guide for interprofessional practice* (pp. 751–760). Burlington, MA: Jones & Bartlett Learning.

Centers for Disease Control and Prevention (CDC). (2007). *Summary of a review of the literature: Programs to promote chlamydia screening.* Infertility Prevention Social Marketing Campaign. Retrieved from http://www.cdc.gov/std/HealthComm/ChlamydiaLitReview2008.pdf

Centers for Disease Control and Prevention (CDC). (2010). Sexually transmitted diseases treatment guidelines, 2010. *Morbidity and Mortality Weekly Report (MMWR), 59*(RR-12), 1–116.

Centers for Disease Control and Prevention. (2010). Use of a reduced (4-dose) vaccine schedule or postexposure prophylaxis to prevent human rabies: Recommendations of the advisory committee on immunization practices. *Morbidity and Mortality Weekly Report (MMWR), 59*(RR-2), 5–6.

Centers for Disease Control and Prevention (CDC). (2012). Update to CDC's sexually transmitted diseases treatment guidelines, 2010: Oral cephalosporins no longer a recommended treatment for gonococcal infections. *Morbidity and Mortality Weekly Report (MMWR), 61*(31), 590–594.

Centers for Disease Control and Prevention (CDC). (2012). *2012 Case definitions: Nationally notifiable conditions infectious and non-infectious case.* Atlanta, GA: Author. Retrieved from http://www.cdc.gov/nndss/document/2012_Case%20Definitions.pdf

Centers for Disease Control and Prevention (CDC). (2013). *CDC/NHSN surveillance definition of healthcare-associated infection and criteria for specific types of infections in the acute care setting.* Retrieved from http://www.cdc.gov/nhsn/PDFs/pscManual/17pscNosInfDef_current.pdf

Centers for Disease Control and Prevention (CDC). (2013, July). *CDC/NHSN protocol clarifications.* Retrieved from http://www.cdc.gov/nhsn/PDFs/pscManual/10-VAE_FINAL.pdf

Dellinger, R., Levy, M., Rhodes, A., Annane, D., Gerlach, H., Opal, S., . . . The Surviving Sepsis Campaign Guidelines Committee Including the Pediatric Subgroup. (2013). Surviving sepsis campaign: International guidelines for management of severe sepsis and septic shock: 2012. *Critical Care Medicine, 41*(2), 580–637.

Ebert, V. (2012). Fever. In K. Reuter-Rice & B. Bolick (Eds.), *Pediatric acute care: A guide for interprofessional practice* (pp. 715–724). Burlington, MA: Jones & Bartlett Learning.

Egging, D. (2012). Sexually transmitted infections. In K. Reuter-Rice & B. Bolick (Eds.), *Pediatric acute care: A guide for interprofessional practice* (pp. 744–751). Burlington, MA: Jones & Bartlett Learning.

Gerber, M. A. (2011). Group A streptococcus. In R. M. Kliegman, B. F. Stanton, J. W. St. Geme, N. F. Schor, & R. E. Behrman (Eds.), *Nelson textbook of pediatrics* (19th ed., pp. 914–925). Philadelphia, PA: Elsevier Saunders.

Gilbert, D. N., Moellering, R. C., Eliopoulos, G. M., Chambers, H. F., & Saag, M. S. (Eds.). (2013). *The Sanford guide to antimicrobial therapy* (43rd ed.). Sperryville, VA: Antimicrobial Therapy.

Ginocchio, C., & McAdam, A. (2011). Current best practices for respiratory virus testing. *Journal of Clinical Microbiology, 49*(9 Suppl.), S44–S48.

Hayes, E. B., & Fischer, M. (2012). Flaviviruses. In S. S. Long, L. K. Pickering, & C. G. Prober (Eds.), *Principles and practice of pediatric infectious diseases* (4th ed., pp. 1099–1102). Philadelphia, PA: Elsevier.

Hile, L., Givvons, M., & Hile, D. (2009). Lemierre syndrome complicating otitis externa: Case report and literature review. *Journal of Emergency Medicine, 42*(4), e77–e80.

Horan, T., Andrus, M., & Dudeck, M. A. (2008). CDC/NHSN surveillance definition of health care-associated infection and criteria for specific types of infections in the acute care setting. *American Journal of Infection Control, 36,* 309–332.

Jordan, M. B., Allen, C. E., Weitzman, S., Filipovich, A. H., & McClain, K. L. (2011). How I treat hemophagocytic lymphohistiocytosis. *Blood, 118*(15), 4041–4052.

Karkos, P., Asrani, S., Karkos, C. D., Leong, S. C., Theochari, E. G., Alexopoulou, T. D., & Assimakopoulos, A. D. (2009). Lemierre's syndrome: a systematic review. *Laryngoscope, 119*(8), 1552–1559.

Leach, C., & Sumaya, C. (2009). Epstein-Barr virus. In R. Feigin, J. Cherry, G. Demmler-Harrison, & S. Kaplan (Eds.), *Feigin and Cherry's textbook of pediatric infectious diseases* (6th ed., pp. 2043-2070). Philadelphia, PA: Saunders Elsevier.

Leake, J. (2012). Infectious disorders: Travel organisms and parasites; vector-borne infections. In K. Reuter-Rice & B. Bolick (Eds.), *Pediatric acute care: A guide for interprofessional practice* (pp. 760–771). Burlington, MA: Jones & Bartlett Learning.

Leake, J. (2012). Vector-borne infections. In K. Reuter-Rice & B. Bolick (Eds.), *Pediatric acute care: A guide for interprofessional practice* (pp. 766–771). Burlington, MA: Jones & Bartlett Learning.

Mangram, A., Horan, T., Pearson, M., Silver, L., & Jarvis, W. (1999). Guideline for prevention of surgical site infection, 1999. The Hospital Infection Control Practices Advisory Committee, Center for Disease Control and Prevention. *Infection Control and Hospital Epidemiology, 20*(4), 247–278.

McGrath, N., Anderson, N., Croxson, M., & Powell, K. (1997). Herpes simplex encephalitis treated with acyclovir: Diagnosis and long term outcome. *Journal of Neurology, Neurosurgery & Psychiatry, 63,* 321–326.

Nadkarni, M. D., Verchick, J., & O'Neill, J. C. (2005). Lemierre syndrome. *Journal of Emergency Medicine, 28,* 297–299.

Nathalang, D. (2012). Viral infections. In K. Reuter-Rice & B. Bolick (Eds.), *Pediatric acute care: A guide for interprofessional practice* (pp. 771–789). Burlington, MA: Jones & Bartlett Learning.

National Network for Immunization Information (NNII). (2010, March 31). *Human papilloma virus: Understanding the disease.* Retrieved from http://www.immunizationinfo.org/vaccines/human-papillomavirus-hpv

O'Grady, N., Alexander, M., Burns, L., Dellinger, E., Garland, J., Heard, S., . . . Healthcare Infection Control Practices Advisory Committee (HICPAC). (2011). *Guidelines for the prevention of intravascular catheter-related infections.* Atlanta, GA: Centers for Disease Control and Prevention (CDC).

O'Keefe, C. (2012). Health care-associated infections. In K. Reuter-Rice & B. Bolick (Eds.), *Pediatric acute care: A guide for interprofessional practice* (pp. 724–728). Burlington, MA: Jones & Bartlett Learning.

Pong, A. (2012). Resistant organisms. In K. Reuter-Rice & B. Bolick (Eds.), *Pediatric acute care: A guide for interprofessional practice* (pp. 740–744). Burlington, MA: Jones & Bartlett Learning.

Reller, M. E. (2012). *Salmonella* species. In S. S. Long, L. K. Pickering, & C. G. Prober (Eds.), *Principles and practice of pediatric infectious diseases* (4th ed., pp. 814–819). Philadelphia, PA: Elsevier.

Root, R., & Abramo, T. (2013). Case report: A 10 month old with Lemierre syndrome complicated by purulent pericarditis. *American Journal of Emergency Medicine, 31*(274), e5–e7.

Sansalone, L. (2012). Meningococcemia. In K. Reuter-Rice & B. Bolick (Eds.), *Pediatric acute care: A guide for interprofessional practice* (pp. 724–728). Burlington, MA: Jones & Bartlett Learning.

Shah, S. S., Hall, M., Srivastava, R., Subramony, A., & Levin, J. E. (2009). Intravenous immunoglobulin in children with streptococcal toxic shock syndrome. *Clinical Infectious Diseases, 49,* 1369–1376.

Shapiro, E. D. (2012). *Leptospira* species (leptospirosis). In S. S. Long, L. K. Pickering, & C. G. Prober (Eds.), *Principles and practice of pediatric infectious diseases* (4th ed., pp. 942–952). Philadelphia, PA: Elsevier.

Siegel, J., & Grossman, L. (2008). Pediatric infection prevention and control. In S. Long, L. Pickering & C. Prober (Eds.), *Principles and practice of pediatric infectious diseases* (3rd ed., pp. 9–23). Philadelphia, PA: Elsevier.

Tilford, B. D. (2012). Toxic shock syndrome. In K. Reuter-Rice & B. Bolick (Eds.), *Pediatric acute care: A guide for interprofessional practice* (pp. 798–801). Burlington, MA: Jones & Bartlett Learning.

Todd, J. K. (2011). Staphylococcus. In R. M. Kliegman, B. F. Stanton, J. W. St. Geme, N. F. Schor, & R. E. Behrman (Eds.), *Nelson textbook of pediatrics* (19th ed., pp. 903–910). Philadelphia, PA: Elsevier Saunders.

Tristram, S., Jacobs, M., & Appelbaum, P. (2007). Antimicrobial resistance in *Haemophilus influenza. Clinical Microbiology Reviews, 20*(2), 368–389.

Tschudy, M. M., & Arcara, K. M. (2012). *The Harriet Lane handbook* (19th ed.). Philadelphia, PA: Mosby.

Wasilewska, E., Morris, A., & Yee, E. (2012). Case of the season: Lemierre syndrome. *Seminars in Roentgenology, 47,* 103–105.

Willoughby, R. E. (2012). Rabies virus. In S. S. Long, L. K. Pickering, & C. G. Prober (Eds.), *Principles and practice of pediatric infectious diseases* (4th ed., pp. 1145–1149). Philadelphia, PA: Elsevier.

Trauma

Trauma Systems

Marcella D. Bono

Background/Definition

- A trauma system is a defined group of health care providers and entities from prehospital through rehabilitation within a specific geographic location designed to optimize the care of injured patients.
- State level.
  - Policies and guidelines are in place for trauma center designation.
  - Field triage guidelines for emergency medical system providers.
  - Trauma center levels of care with identified resources.
- The American College of Surgeons (ACS) Committee on Trauma verifies trauma centers and provides guidelines for trauma care.
  - ACS guidelines are often more stringent than state requirements.
- Trauma centers within trauma systems submit data to the state through the trauma registry.
- In addition to establishing guidelines for the care of injured patients, trauma system members work together to develop and provide injury prevention resources for the community.
- Injury prevention in children often focuses on motor vehicle safety such as the appropriate use of car seats and seat belts, pedestrian safety, home safety, burn prevention, and firearm safety.

Trauma Survey

Marcella D. Bono

Background

- Unintentional injuries are the number one killer of children 1 to 19 years of age.

Definition

- Trauma survey: a systematic approach to the assessment of an injured patient used to quickly identify and evaluate injuries.
- Types.
  - Primary survey.
    - Airway and cervical spine protection.
      - Assess patency.
      - Protect cervical spine.
    - Breathing and ventilation.
      - Inspect for chest wall excursion.
      - Auscultate breath sounds.
      - Identify flail chest, closed or open pneumothorax.
    - Circulation.
      - Level of consciousness.
      - Skin color.
      - Pulse.
      - Hemorrhage control.
    - Disability.
      - Level of consciousness.
      - Pupil size.
      - Spinal cord injury (SCI) level if applicable.
      - Glasgow Coma Scale.
    - Exposure.
      - Completely undress patient.
  - Secondary survey.
    - Vital signs.
    - History.
      - AMPLE.
        - Allergies.
        - Medications.
        - Past illness/pregnancy.
        - Last meal, last menstrual period.
        - Events/Environment related to injury.
    - Head to toe physical examination.

Abdominal Trauma
Kristen Hittle

Abdominal Trauma: Liver Laceration, Pancreas Laceration, and Splenic Laceration

Background
- Abdominal trauma is the primary cause of morbidity and mortality.
- The spleen is the most commonly injured organ; however, the liver is also at high risk due to its large size and anatomical location.
- Pancreatic injuries are challenging to diagnose with initial imaging, and symptoms often present hours after the original trauma.

Definition
- Injury to a solid organ(s) in the abdomen that are graded on an injury scale that delineates severity.

Etiology/Types
- Blunt injury: motor vehicle collisions, falls, bicycle accidents, all-terrain vehicle accidents, sports injuries, nonaccidental trauma.
- Penetrating injury: firearms, stabbings, impalement.

Clinical Presentation
- Abdominal pain, distension, tenderness, guarding, ecchymosis (e.g., "seat belt sign" or handlebar marking), abrasions, referred pain (Kehr sign), signs of a penetrating wound, hypotension, and tachycardia.

Diagnostic Evaluation
- Abdominal computed tomography (CT) with and without contrast.
- Abdominal ultrasound (focused assessment with sonography for trauma).
- Diagnostic peritoneal lavage.
- Magnetic resonance cholangiopancreatography or endoscopic retrograde cholangiopancreatography for pancreatic injuries.

Management
- Based on grade of injury and hemodynamic status.
- Nonoperative.
  - Liver and Spleen: bed rest, serial abdominal examinations, hemodynamic monitoring, nothing by mouth (NPO), maintenance IV fluids, frequent hemoglobin and hematocrit monitoring, transfusions as indicated.
  - Pancreas: bed rest, serial abdominal examinations, hemodynamic monitoring, NPO, Salem sump placement for gastric decompression, parenteral nutrition, elemental enteral nutrition, octreotide infusion.
- Operative.
  - Liver: hepatic artery embolization, exploratory laparotomy.
  - Spleen: repair, partial splenectomy, total splenectomy.
  - Pancreas: endoscopic stent placement, laparotomy with pancreatectomy, Whipple procedure (pancreaticoduodenectomy).

Pediatric Burns
Elizabeth Leachman

Background
- Leading cause of injury-related death in children of all ages.
- Flame, scald, contact, cold, and radiation burns are the most common types of burns in childhood.
- Scald burns are the most common cause of burns in infants, toddlers, and preschoolers.
- Contact burns are most common in toddlers.
- Curiosity and naivety lead to most burn injuries in school-age and teenage children.
- Burns are dynamic injuries and often evolve into deeper injuries over time.
- Most burns have a combination of depths. The center of the burn usually demonstrates a higher degree of burn than the periphery.
- The depth of the burn is directly related to the etiology of the burn and the amount of time the skin is in contact with the source.
- Special characteristics of children.
  - Thinner skin and the less resistance to heat.
  - Slower reflexes.
  - Greater body surface area and percentage of water in relation to weight.
  - Lower tolerance of hypothermia.
  - Accentuated metabolism which can lead to metabolic acidosis.

Definition
- Damage to varying layers of the skin caused by heat, cold, electricity, chemicals, or friction.

Etiology
- Scald burn: caused when skin comes in contact with hot fluid such as coffee, tea, or soup.
- Contact burn: caused when skin touches a hot object such as a stove, iron, grill, or muffler.
- Mechanical burn: friction with a surface such as a treadmill, rope, or pavement.
- Flame burn: contact with fire.
- Electrical burn: occurs when electrical current travels from the contact site into the body. In children, these burns most often occur when the child inserts a metal object, such as a hair pin, into a household electrical socket. There is usually an entrance and exit wound.
- Chemical burn: occurs when skin comes in contact with strong acids (e.g., drain and toilet cleaners) or strong alkalis (e.g., fertilizers, detergents, oven cleaners).

- Inhalation burn: Hot gases or smoke results in burns in the oropharynx.

Pathophysiology

- The skin is the largest organ in the body offering protection from infection, fluid loss, and heat loss. The epidermis prevents infection and fluid loss. The dermis prevents heat loss and consists of hair follicles, sweat glands, nerve fibers, and connective tissue.
- Burns cause an increase in capillary permeability, which leads to loss of fluid and proteins, including immune globulins, increasing the risk of infection and dehydration.
- Loss of the protective skin barrier in children increases the risk of hypothermia and metabolic acidosis.

Clinical Presentation

- Superficial burn: involves the outer layer epidermis which results in pain and erythema. The tissue remains intact and the burn usually heals without scarring in 4 to 5 days.
- Superficial partial-thickness burn: involves the epidermis and superficial layer of the dermis, causing blistering, erythema, blanching, and pain. Typically heals in 7 to 10 days. Scarring is minimal.
- Deep partial-thickness burn: involves the epidermis and more than 50% of the dermis, which causes destruction of nerve endings and is erythematous, moist, nonblanching, and less painful. Typically heals in 2 to 3 weeks and causes scarring.
- Full-thickness burn: involves the entire epidermis and dermis which appears white, waxy, nonblanching, and is insensate due to the complete destruction of nerve fibers. Typically takes over a month to heal with significant scarring.

Evaluation

- Initial evaluation: airway, breathing, and circulation, followed by disability and evaluation of the burn (depth and total body surface area [TBSA]).
- During evaluation, address thermoregulation with heat lamps or warmed fluids. A sheet or blanket will also limit burn exposure to the environment and decrease pain.
- TBSA in children is calculated using the Lund and Browder chart or palmar surface. The child's palm, including fingers, is approximately 0.8% to 1% of the TBSA.

Management

- Superficial burns: thin layer of moisturizer every 6 to 8 hours.
- Superficial partial-thickness burns: Xeroform, Mepilex AG.
  - Xeroform: petrolatum gauze infused with 3% bismuth tribromophenate.
  - Mepilex AG: silver-impregnated antimicrobial dressing, lasts 5 to 7 days.
- Deep partial-thickness burns: Mepitel and Acticoat.
  - Acticoat: silver-impregnated rayon/polyester/polyethylene mesh. Active release of antimicrobial silver ions into burn wound when moistened; lasts 3 to 7 days. Antimicrobial activity up to 96 hours.
- Full-thickness burns: silver sulfadiazine, skin grafting.

- Silver sulfadiazine 1% cream: absorbed into epidermis and dermis. Bactericidal against gram-positive and gram-negative organisms, fungi, and some viruses.
- Tetanus: booster injection if >5 years since the last tetanus vaccine.
  - <7 years: DTaP.
  - >7 years: Tdap or Td if child has already received one Tdap. Latest recommendations can be found on the CDC website at: http://www.cdc.gov/vaccines/
  - If contraindication to pertussis vaccine: Td.
  - Not previously immunized: Tetanus IG plus appropriate tetanus vaccine.
- Partial-thickness burns <10% of TBSA and full-thickness burns <2% TBSA can usually be managed in the outpatient setting.
- Partial-thickness burns 10% to 20% and full-thickness burns >5% should be admitted to the hospital.
- Burns >10% TBSA require intravenous crystalloid fluid resuscitation.
- Patients with burns greater than 15% should be resuscitated using the Parkland formula.
  - Parkland formula: 4 mL × TBSA (% burned) × Body weight (kg).
  - Administer half of the volume in the first 8 hours.
  - Administer second half of the formula in the remaining 16 hours.
  - Titrate fluid resuscitation to achieve urine output of 1 mL/kg/hour.
  - Maintenance fluid (normal saline, lactated Ringer) added for children <5 years of age. Normal saline or lactated Ringer plus 5% dextrose added for children <20 kg.
- Consulting services: physical therapy for mobility, occupational therapy for splint fabrication, nutrition, case management, social work, child life, plastic surgery.

PEARLS
- *Prevention of burns is the most important concept for children, which includes information about water heater temperatures, keeping hot and caustic substances, and household objects like electrical cords away from young children.*
- *Installing smoke detectors and teaching children to "Stop, drop, and roll" when clothing is burning and what to do in a suspected fire situation are other important teaching points.*

Drowning/Submersion Injuries
Alexandra K. Yockey

Background

- Approximately 3,500 fatal unintentional drownings annually; approximately 10 deaths per day. The number of unreported or nonfatal submersions may be several hundred times higher.

- Children at the greatest risk of submersion injuries are <5 years of age; another peak in incidence is between 16 and 24 years of age; males predominate in all age groups, and minority children are at higher risk than whites.
- Factors impacting submersion injury: alcohol or drug consumption, lack of supervision, lack of protective barriers, trauma, and lack of ability to swim.
- Only a few inches of water are required for a child to drown, making bathtubs and other small reservoirs of water (e.g., toilets or buckets) just as deadly as large bodies of water.

Definition

- A process resulting in primary respiratory injury from submersion/immersion in a liquid medium.
- Terms such as *near-drowning*, *secondary drowning*, and *wet* versus *dry drowning* should not be used as they can be ambiguous or confusing.

Pathophysiology

- Drowning is typically preceded by panic, breath holding, and struggling to stay above the surface. Involuntary laryngospasm occurs as water comes into contact with the airway after submersion, causing a conscious person to cough and inhale more water. Aspiration of water and vomitus causes further laryngospasm, leading to hypoxemia and loss of consciousness. Hypoxemia stimulates a shift in the acid–base balance, resulting in arrhythmias, myocardial and cardiac arrest due to metabolic or respiratory acidosis.
- Water entering the airway triggers an inflammatory cascade, causing pulmonary vasoconstriction and pulmonary edema. Surfactant is denatured and the lungs become noncompliant and difficult to ventilate with increased atelectasis. Intrapulmonary shunting with ventilation/perfusion mismatching can occur in this setting.
- Cerebral ischemia results from inadequate blood flow to the brain, and if deprived of oxygen for an extended amount of time, the brain tissue begins to die, causing cerebral infarcts. The injured brain then begins to swell, resulting in cerebral edema and increased intracranial pressure (ICP), further injuring the nervous system.
- Submersion injuries do not directly cause cardiovascular injury; it is the resultant hypoxia and pulmonary injury that affect the myocardium.
- Hypothermia and electrolyte disturbances result in arrhythmias. The cardiovascular system is able to recover from hypoxia if oxygenation and acid–base balance are restored.

Clinical Presentation

- Varies based on length of submersion, temperature, and degree of hypoxia, along with possible causes of drowning (e.g., seizure, trauma, or arrhythmia).
- Children may present to the emergency department (ED) asymptomatic. A thorough evaluation is still required as even mild hypoxia can increase permeability of pulmonary capillaries, with alveolar fluid leak and surfactant damage.

- Respiratory dysfunction may take hours to manifest, making it crucial for children to be observed for a prolonged time frame after submersion incident. Pulse oximetry should be monitored; if abnormal or in the presence of respiratory distress, arterial blood gas (ABG) values and chest radiograph should be obtained.
- Symptomatic patients present anywhere on a continuum of symptoms: anxiety, vomiting, cough, wheezing, hypothermia, altered mental status, metabolic acidosis, respiratory failure, and finally respiratory/cardiac arrest.

Evaluation

- ABCs (airway, breathing, and circulation) algorithm for pediatric advanced life support. ABG values are helpful in evaluating the degree of hypoxemia in children who have been submerged; should be obtained on all symptomatic children and those with a prolonged event who are asymptomatic.
- Vital signs: heart rate, respiratory rate, blood pressure, temperature, and pulse oximetry on every submersion victim.
- Chest radiograph: evaluation for atelectasis, pulmonary edema, and aspiration.
- Further imaging and testing will depend on the degree of deterioration and other coinciding injuries related to the incident.

Management Occurs in Three Phases

- Prehospital: Rescue victim from the source of submersion. Immediate resuscitation by witnesses is proven to increase survival rates. Unlike standard basic life support, which is very compression driven, opening and maintaining the airway is priority.
  - Routine cervical spine immobilization is not indicated unless there is obvious trauma.
  - The basic life support algorithm should be initiated if the child is not breathing and/or pulseless. Supplemental oxygen should be administered to all submersion victims. All submersion victims should be taken to the hospital for evaluation regardless of severity of injury.
- ED: First priority is establishing an airway. Indications for intubation include unconscious child, peripheral arterial carbon dioxide ($Paco_2$) levels >50 mmHg, inability to maintain peripheral arterial oxygen (Pao_2) >90% with supplemental oxygen. Positive end-expiratory pressure should be used to prevent atelectasis and overcome intrapulmonary shunting.
  - Noninvasive ventilation with either continuous positive airway pressure or bilevel positive airway pressure may be indicated in alert patients with ongoing respiratory symptoms despite supplemental oxygen.
  - Chest radiograph is indicated on all submersion victims.
  - Gastric decompression via orogastric or nasogastric tubes should be placed to minimize aspiration risk in patients with altered level of consciousness.
  - Hypothermia can be both protective and harmful. Remove all wet clothing and cover patient. Evaluate for hypothermia, hypoglycemia, and electrolyte abnormalities; common in submersion injuries.

- Inpatient: focus of hospitalization is supportive; primary goal is preventing secondary cerebral injury. The initial cerebral ischemic injury occurs during the time a victim is submerged. Secondary cerebral injury occurs later from prolonged hypoxemia, cerebral edema, acidosis, hypovolemia, seizures, and electrolyte imbalances.
  - Respiratory treatments and interventions should be tailored by clinical condition and ABG values once in a controlled environment.
  - Hypercapnia should be avoided; increased cerebral hypertension further compounds cerebral edema.
  - Aspiration pneumonitis can further complicate pulmonary status; antibiotic therapy for aspiration is controversial.
  - Normalize blood pressure; vasoactive agents may be required. Hypotension decreases blood flow to the brain, further compromising oxygenation, potentially resulting in poor neurologic outcomes. poor neurologic outcomes.
  - Hypervolemia can exacerbate pulmonary edema and should be avoided. The use of diuretics and fluid restriction may be indicated in some cases.
  - Hypermetabolic states (e.g., seizure and fever) should be treated aggressively to avoid secondary brain insults/injury.
  - Electroencephalography (EEG) should be used to detect subclinical seizures, especially in patients requiring neuromuscular blocking agents.

PEARL

- *The best treatment and management for submersion injuries is prevention. Community awareness of risks, CPR training, and education of first responders will help save lives.*

Pneumothorax Resulting from Trauma

Anne Vasiliadis

Background

- Air leak syndromes include any pathology in which air enters a normally closed space within the thorax.

Definition

- A pneumothorax is an abnormal collection of air between the visceral and parietal pleura in the thoracic cage. In the case of trauma, pneumothorax can be a result of blunt, crushing, or penetrating injury directly to the chest.
- A *tension* pneumothorax can occur as a result of lung laceration or injury to a major airway and can cause sudden or acute symptoms.

Incidence

- Chest trauma is infrequent in children; responsible for 4% to 8% of all pediatric traumas. Blunt injuries are responsible for 85% of chest injuries.

- May occur as a result of increased intrathoracic pressure (e.g., mechanical ventilation).

Pathophysiology

- Acute increase in transpulmonary pressure; causes alveolar overdistention and rupture.

Clinical Presentation

- History of blunt trauma, fall, or other trauma event.
- Review of symptoms: typically pleuritic chest pain (e.g., sharp and worse with inspiration), dyspnea, or may be asymptomatic. The chest pain usually resolves or changes to a dull pain within 1 to 3 days despite the persistence of the pneumothorax.

Physical Examination

- Ipsilateral hyperresonance to percussion.
- Ipsilateral decreased air entry.
- Ipsilateral decreased vocal fremitus.

Clinical Findings

- Hypoxia.
- Tachycardia.
- Increased peak inspiratory pressures or decreased expired tidal volumes (if on mechanical ventilation).
- Tension pneumothorax: tracheal deviation, asphyxia, and decreased cardiac output leading to hypotension, tachycardia, and hypoxemia. A *medical emergency* requiring immediate intervention.

Diagnostic Evaluation

- Radiography: Diagnosis is typically confirmed with a posterioanterior chest radiograph. A lateral decubitus radiograph may be needed if suspicion is high with normal posterioanterior radiograph. CT is not necessary to diagnose pneumothorax, but may help identify underlying blebs/bullae or very small pneumothoraces not detected by radiography (Figure 12.1).
- Estimation of size: Clinical history is not a reliable indicator of size. There are multiple equations for calculating size of pneumothorax in adults, but these methods are not accurate in the pediatric population.
- Laboratory findings: ABG analysis may reveal decreased Pao_2.

Management

- Treatment is dictated by the type and size of pneumothorax and clinical condition of the patient.
- Observation: Clinically stable patients may only require observation with pulse oximetry and cardiorespiratory monitoring. During observation, patient should receive 100% oxygen delivered via face mask to wash out nitrogen from pleural space.
- Needle aspiration: Air is aspirated via a temporary needle inserted at the second intercostal space, midclavicular line.
- Thoracostomy tube: Catheter is placed in the pleural space at fourth, fifth, or sixth intercostal space at the midaxillary line and connected to water seal or suction.

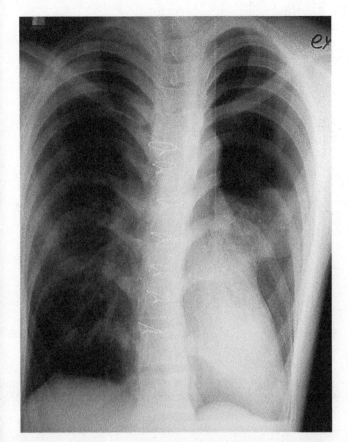

FIGURE 12.1 • **Pneumothorax Chest Radiograph.** Large left pneumothorax in otherwise healthy 16-year-old boy.

Pulmonary Contusions

Catherine Walsh

Definition

- Injury to lung parenchyma with edema and hemorrhage without associated pulmonary laceration.

Background

- Most common traumatic chest injury in children.
- Early diagnosis and intervention may improve outcomes.
- Fewer short- and long-term complications in pediatric populations than in adults.

Etiology

- Pulmonary contusions are the most common pediatric thoracic trauma injury.
- Children are more likely to have pulmonary contusions without other chest wall injury (e.g., rib fractures) due to high chest wall compliance.
- Child thorax offers less protection to lung tissue than adult.
- Flail chest and scapular fractures are rare in children, but are almost always associated with pulmonary contusions.
- Most commonly seen in children struck by vehicles.
- Associated with blunt chest wall trauma.
- Suspect in patients who have sustained falls, rapid deceleration, or blast injuries. Due to severe mechanism of injury (MOI), patients frequently sustain damage to other body systems.

Pathophysiology

- Lung tissue injury due to hemorrhage, edema, and alveolar collapse. Results in poor gas exchange, increased pulmonary vascular resistance, and inflammatory reaction.
- Deceleration at different rates results in shearing of alveolar tissue and hemorrhage.
- Alveolar membrane is disrupted, resulting in increased cell membrane permeability and fluid extravasation.
- Parenchymal damage is caused by overexpansion of intrapulmonary air.
- Pathophysiologic changes peak 24 to 48 hours after injury and typically resolve within 7 days.
- Subsequent respiratory impairment may be due to local inflammatory response from sequestered blood, systemic response from associated injuries, and possible nosocomial pneumonia.
- Posttraumatic empyema is rare, but has potentially severe sequelae.

Clinical Presentation

- Initial presentation may be subtle. Symptoms may include tachypnea, hypoxemia, hypercarbia, hemoptysis, and respiratory distress.
- May be associated sign of chest wall injury.
- ABG may be normal or demonstrate hypoxemia.
- Delayed presentation may occur as *symptoms peak 24 to 48 hours after injury.*

Diagnostic Evaluation

- Goal of primary evaluation is to identify potential life-threatening conditions.
- High suspicion determined by mechanism and type of injury.
- Radiographic findings of consolidation: Chest radiography and CT are the primary forms of testing. Bedside ultrasound can be used for unstable patients.
- Chest radiography:
  - Irregular opacification in area of chest wall injury/impact.
  - Chest radiograph changes may not be noted until 4 to 6 hours after injury, and changes may not appropriately reflect extent of injury.

- Enlargement of contusion in the first 24 hours after injury is likely indicative of increased morbidity.
- May underestimate severity of ventilation/perfusion mismatch.
- May be difficult to separate degree of contusion from other conditions including aspiration, pneumonia, and fluid overload (Figure 12.2).
- CT.
  - Highly sensitive, but may detect mild and asymptomatic contusions.
  - More accurate in differentiating other causes of consolidation. Subpleural sparing is seen in pulmonary contusions but unlikely with atelectasis or pneumonia.
  - Better able to calculate extent of injury and predict need for respiratory support.

Management

- PRIMARY management is supportive. Most children with pulmonary contusions require no intervention.
- Address life-threatening injuries and ensure oxygenation, ventilation, cardiovascular support.
- Close monitoring; injury evolves over first 24 to 48 hours after injury.

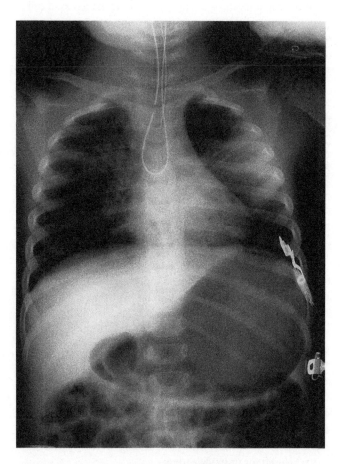

FIGURE 12.2 • **Pulmonary Contusion Chest Radiograph.** This 3-year-old child was struck by a car. The radiograph shows the pulmonary contusion, looking much like pneumonia. Note the malpositioned nasogastric tube and the resultant distended abdomen.

- Supplemental oxygen for hypoxia.
- Pulmonary toilet, fluid management, and pain control are essential.
- Fluids:
  - Judicious fluid administration. Avoid underresuscitation, which may result in hypovolemia and hypoxemia; overresuscitation may result in pulmonary edema.
- No benefit of prophylactic antibiotics or corticosteroids.
- Intubation:
  - Most commonly used for patients with extra-thoracic injuries.
  - For patients requiring respiratory support, the goal is to maximize oxygenation and minimize secondary lung injury.
  - Use of positive pressure improves alveolar recruitment.
  - Single lung ventilation for unilateral injuries may improve oxygenation and ventilation/perfusion mismatch.
- Pain may contribute to hypoventilation, atelectasis, and respiratory deterioration.
  - Patients with boney chest wall injury may benefit from regional analgesia.
- Positioning.
  - Frequently change patient position.
  - Prone position and injured lung in dependent position may improve perfusion.
- Complications include pneumonia and acute respiratory distress syndrome.
  - Risk for pneumonia due to blood in alveolar space and decreased pulmonary toilet. Appropriate antibiotic coverage for patients with fever with worsening respiratory function.
- Long-term consequences rarely seen in children.

PEARLS

- *Pulmonary contusions are frequently seen with injury to other organ systems.*
- *Primary goal is to identify other life-threatening injuries. Management is primarily supportive.*
- *Injury may evolve over 24 to 48 hours.*
- *Severe pulmonary hemorrhage may be associated with diffuse hemorrhage, related liver damage, massive hilar contusions.*

Limb Trauma: Fractures and Sprains

Cathy Haut

Background

- Unintentional or accidental limb injuries occur as a result of sports injuries, motor vehicle accidents (MVAs), and falls.
- More than 3.5 million children <14 years of age are injured each year playing sports or involved in recreational activities.
- When evaluating limb trauma, it is important to note the MOI, which represents the effect that energy has on human tissue, thus the expected severity of the injury.

- Fractures are extremely common injuries sustained by children as a result of trauma, with lifetime risk of sustaining a fracture, 42% to 60% of boys and 27% to 40% of girls sustaining fractures during childhood.

Fractures

Background/Definition

- A fracture is a break or disruption in the continuity of bone. Fractures in children can involve the epiphysis or metaphysis; disrupting the epiphyseal plate may interfere with bone growth.
- Most fractures in children are a result of low-velocity trauma. Fractures in children <2 years of age: highly suspicious for child maltreatment.

Etiology/Types

- Epiphyseal injuries occur most frequently with distal radius and ulnar fractures, excluding phalangeal fractures. The MOI is usually a fall on an arm or hand; ages 11 to 15 years are the most common group affected with injury to the radius and ulna.
- Forearm and wrists are the most common fracture sites in children >5 years of age, and categories include fracture dislocations, midshaft, and distal fractures.
- Clavicle fractures occur frequently in children resulting from a fall landing on the shoulder.
- Humerus fractures include the supracondylar site and can be associated with an acute vascular injury. Injury to the shaft of the humerus results from twisting mechanism. Distal humeral fractures occur more often in the lateral epicondyle.
- Young children and adolescents sustain femur fractures which are often associated with a MVA involving high-energy force.
- Tibial fractures are diaphyseal in school-age children and nondisplaced often from MVAs and sports injuries.
- Ankle fractures, often the result of direct trauma, are more likely to involve the tibia and fibula than the talus.
- Foot fractures involve the metatarsals and phalanges and are usually not displaced.
- Pelvic fractures, uncommon in children, are usually the result of a crush-type injury or high-energy force. Abdominal hemorrhage and damage to other soft tissue in the abdominal area should be suspected with pelvic fracture.
- Hip fractures can result in avascular necrosis of the femoral head, damage to the physis with growth arrest, malunion, and nonunion. Hip fractures are uncommon except for pelvic avulsion fractures occurring in adolescent boys.
- Spinal fractures, rare in children, most often involve the cervical spine, from significant direct trauma in MVA, fall, or pedestrian-struck MVA.

Classification of Fractures

- Either open or closed.
  - Open: Wound communicates with fracture.
    - Result of high-energy trauma or penetrating wound.
  - Closed: Skin is intact.

Explanation of Classification or Type of Fractures

- Plastic deformation: a bending of the bone which causes a small fracture that does not cross the bone. Most common in the ulna.
- Buckle (torus) fractures: fracture on the tension side of the bone near the softer metaphyseal bone; crosses the bone and buckles the harder bone on the opposite side, causing a bulge.
- Greenstick fracture: Bone is bent with an initial fracture which does not go through bone.
- Complete fracture: involves total width of bone.
- Spiral: occurs from a rotational or twisting force.
- Oblique: viewed diagonally across the diaphysis.
- Transverse is usually diaphyseal.
- Epiphyseal: through the physis or growth plate.

Pathophysiology

- Limb injury results in a break in the continuity of the bone, followed by a staged healing process which involves coagulation of blood between bone fragments, formation of bone matrix, and mineralization of the matrix.

Clinical Presentation

- History of injury or trauma.
- Inability to stand, walk, or use injured part, with substantial pain or point tenderness.
- Visible or palpable limb deformity and ecchymosis, crepitus, or grating.
- Spontaneous onset of pain (usually seen with pathologic fractures).
- Local swelling and marked tenderness, possible movement between bone fragments, muscle spasm.

Diagnostic Evaluation

- Radiographs of suspected limb fractures should include the joint above and below the injury.
- Comparison views of the opposite extremity are often obtained to help distinguish the fracture line from the growth plate.
- In some situations, oblique radiographs are warranted in order to identify a fracture that is difficult to detect.
- Further radiologic studies may be indicated in certain instances to evaluate a fracture: ultrasound, tomography, CT, magnetic resonance imaging (MRI), bone scan, fluoroscopy.
- Vascular assessment may include the use of Doppler studies, compartment pressure monitoring, and/or angiography.

Management

- Dependent on the type of fracture, location, and the age of the child.
- Treatment may consist of immobilization by cast, splint, or brace, closed reduction followed by a period of immobilization in a cast or splint, or open reduction with or without internal fixation, and usually followed by a period of immobilization in a cast or splint. Closed reduction and percutaneous pinning followed by a period of immobilization. Closed or open reduction and application of an external fixator.

- Traction (i.e., skin, skeletal) followed by a period of immobilization.
- Immobilization for most fractures ≤12 weeks.
- Simple fractures that are closed and nondisplaced can heal enough to be free from immobilization within 3 weeks.

Potential Complications from Fractures or Treatment of Fractures

- Infection, avascular necrosis, vascular injuries, delayed union, nonunion, malunion, epiphyseal arrest, nerve and visceral injuries, tendon and joint injuries, fat embolism, compartment syndrome (see Musculoskeletal section), osteoarthritis, reflex sympathetic dystrophy.

Sprains

Definition

- Injury to a ligament resulting from excessive stretching force.

Etiology

- Typical causes are falls or sports-related injury, mostly in basketball, running, and soccer, grades I to III. Ankle sprains constitute approximately 25% of all sports-related injuries; 75% of sprains involve the ankle.
  - Grade I: minimal discomfort, minimal or no loss of function.
  - Grade II: ligaments are partially torn with tenderness, swelling, and ecchymosis with mild-to-moderate loss of function.
  - Grade III: completely torn ligament with unstable joint, significant tenderness, swelling, and ecchymosis with loss of function.

Pathophysiology

- An injury to the articular ligament, which is a connective tissue connecting the bone to another bone.

Clinical Presentation

- History of feeling a tear or hearing a pop with activity, swelling, and pain, typically in the wrist or ankle.
- Pain and swelling in shoulder, knee, or elbow can also indicate sprain, but these areas are much less common.

Diagnostic Studies

- Imaging is not usually indicated for a sprain.
- Ottawa ankle rules provide guidelines for deciding about radiography: Radiographies are ordered only if there is point tenderness on the lateral or medial malleolus and the distal 6 cm of the posterior edge of the tibia or fibula or if inability to bear weight or take four unassisted steps in the examination room.

Management

- Provide relief of discomfort with ice, rest, and nonsteroidal anti-inflammatory drugs or acetaminophen, maintain joint stability with Ace wrap or splint, and minimize swelling.
- RICE: rest, ice, compression, elevation.
- Complete healing should occur between 4 and 6 weeks.

PEARL
- *Prevention of fractures and sprains is the most important management through the use of supervision of young children, protective gear, well-fitting shoes, and warming up/stretching prior to exercise.*

Ophthalmic and Facial Trauma
Cathy Haut

Background

- Young children are more susceptible to facial trauma due to their greater cranial mass to body ratio.
- MOI is important to assist in determining the severity of injuries.

Definition

- Physical trauma to the face involving soft tissue injuries, fractures to the nose or orbits, and eye injuries.

Types

- Eye and orbital injuries.
- Midface, nose, and jaw injuries.
- Malocclusion of the jaw with mandibular fracture.

Pathophysiology

- Facial trauma may be blunt or penetrating and occurs within three functional divisions of the face: upper third, midface, and lower third. Trauma can affect muscle movement, cranial nerve innervation, and function.

Clinical Presentation

- History of injury: fall, sports-related, or MVA.
- Pain, bleeding, bruising.

Diagnostic Studies

- Orbital assessment includes evaluation of visual acuity, pupillary size and response, visual fields, diplopia, and extraocular muscle function.
- Subconjunctival hemorrhage or hyphema requires urgent ophthalmologic consultation.
- Compare preinjury photo with current status.
- Radiographies of facial bones and orbits.
- CT of head and orbits may be necessary to detail cranium, midfacial structures, and mandibular condyle.

Management

- ABCs are most important.
- Airway compromise from inflammation is possible.
- Soft tissue laceration repair, irrigation of mouth and/or lip lacerations.
- Fracture reduction and fixation.
- Dental repair.

Additional Ophthalmic Injuries
Cathy Haut

Corneal Abrasion

Presentation

- Pain, redness, tearing, photosensitivity, blurred vision, and foreign body sensation.
- *Most corneal abrasions will resolve without therapy.*

Evaluation

- Fluorescein dye under blue light can be used to determine an accurate diagnosis.

Management

- Urgent consultation is needed for suspected corneal ulcerations (microbial keratitis).
- Ophthalmologic consultation is indicated if symptoms do not resolve within 1 week or for more involved damage.
- Patching and/or antibiotic topical treatments are not warranted unless indicated by ophthalmology or to treat abrasions in children who wear contact lenses.

Corneal and Conjunctival Foreign Body

Presentation

- Pain, conjunctival injection, tearing, photosensitivity, blurred vision, and foreign body sensation.

Evaluation and Management

- Removal of obvious foreign body.
- May require removal under anesthesia.
- If global penetration is suspected, CT is indicated.
- Fourth-generation fluoroquinolone or ciprofloxacin drops should be used 4 times a day until the eye is healed.
- *Steroid-containing eye drops should never be used.*

Spinal Cord Injury
Kimberly L. DiMaria & Cheryl N. Bartke

Background

- Pediatric SCI is relatively rare, representing about 5% of all spinal cord injuries. Younger children are more likely to sustain cervical spine injuries, specifically C1-C2, while older children typically sustain lower cervical injuries. Mortality rates in pediatric patients are higher than in adults.

Definitions

- SCI is defined as damage to the spinal cord resulting in motor, sensory, or autonomic dysfunction.
- The impairment can be either temporary or permanent.

- Tetraplegia, formerly referred to as quadriplegia, refers to paresis of all four extremities as a result of an injury to the cervical area of the spinal cord.
- Paraplegia is used to describe an injury to the spinal cord in the thoracic, lumbar, or sacral regions, causing paresis of the lower extremities.

Etiology

- Common causes of pediatric SCI include falls, MVAs, sports-related injuries, gunshot wounds, birth trauma, malignancies, and nonaccidental trauma.

Types

- SCIs have been categorized into two types: incomplete and complete.
- An incomplete SCI refers to an injury in which some degree of sensory and/or motor function is preserved up to three vertebrae below the level of injury.
- Complete SCIs are defined as absolute loss of motor, sensory, and reflex functions at three neurologic levels below the level of injury.
- SCI without radiographic abnormality (SCIWORA) is the presence of an SCI in the absence of evidence on an imaging study such as radiography or CT. Recent advances in MRI technology have improved the sensitivity of identification of SCI, making the diagnosis of SCIWORA less common.

Pathophysiology

- Divided into primary and secondary injury phenomena.
- The primary injury process occurs at the moment of injury or in the minutes following and includes immediate cell death, axonal damage, and vascular injury.
- Secondary injury develops minutes to weeks after injury and is a result of edema, and other sequelae of inflammation. During secondary injury, neurons die either by necrosis or apoptosis, both of which lead to demyelination and axonal degeneration near the level of injury. Following neuronal death, glial scar formation occurs which ultimately results in an axon's inability to regenerate.
- Patients who sustain an SCI experience one or more of the following complications:
  - Spinal shock: temporary loss of sensory, motor, autonomic, and reflex function below the level of injury. Resultant flaccid paralysis results in venous pooling and, subsequently, relative hypovolemia.
  - Neurogenic shock: potentially life-threatening complication leading to hypotension, bradycardia, and hypothermia. The sympathetic nervous system response below the level of injury can be inadequate to oppose the parasympathetic response.
  - Autonomic dysreflexia: inappropriately strong sympathetic response to triggers that occur below the level of injury. Patients develop vasoconstriction, hypertension, and reflexive bradycardia. Triggers may include bladder and bowel distention.

Clinical Presentation

- Depends on the level and type of injury.
- Presentation can range from slight tingling and numbness to total lack of sensation and movement.

Diagnostic Evaluation

- Radiographies.
  - Identify injury to vertebrae that surround the spinal cord, but not the spinal cord itself. Bony injury typically accompanies traumatic SCI. Cervical radiographies should include anterioposterior, lateral, and odontoid views. Flexion–extension views should be performed only by experienced professionals and in patients who are able to follow commands and answer questions appropriately.
- CT.
  - Useful if radiographs are inconclusive or abnormal. A spinal CT is more sensitive at detecting fractures than a radiograph, but cannot be used to evaluate the spinal cord itself. Hematomas are visible on CT.
- MRI.
  - The most sensitive test to evaluate injury to the spinal cord, surrounding ligaments, and soft tissue. It is also useful in identifying the extent and severity of SCI and can evaluate for hematomas and herniated disks.

Management

- Stabilization of the spine is the most important initial management strategy for any patient with a known or suspected SCI.
  - Application of a C-collar and logrolling the patient during position changes are critical.
- Evaluate and manage the patient's ABCs.
  - Intubation of a patient with an SCI can be challenging because of the concurrent cervical spine immobilization.
- Treat shock with isotonic fluid resuscitation. Evaluate for hemorrhagic and neurogenic shock. Vasopressors are often required for patients with neurogenic shock. Hypotension can cause secondary injury to the spine.
- Obtain a thorough history of the event, including MOI.
- Obtain appropriate imaging studies to diagnose SCI.
- Consult a neurosurgeon and orthopedic surgeon for possible spine stabilization or decompression.
- Serial neurologic examinations are essential to evaluate for secondary injury caused from spinal cord swelling.
- Corticosteroid administration is controversial and may be considered in SCI. If steroids are part of the treatment plan, they should be administered within 8 hours from the time of injury.
- It is common for patients who sustain an SCI to develop an ileus. Therefore, gastric decompression is recommended to prevent emesis and subsequent aspiration.
- Autonomic dysreflexia is commonly triggered by bladder or bowel distention. Efforts such as urinary catheterization and a bowel regimen should be taken to prevent and minimize these triggers.

PEARLS

- *Hypotension and hypoxia perpetuate secondary SCI. Therefore, adequate management of blood pressure and oxygenation are essential.*
- *Spinal cord injuries are described by location and type of injury.*
- *Patients who sustain a complete SCI typically regain one more level of function beyond the level of deficit that was observed upon initial evaluation of injury.*
- *The first 24 hours after injury are crucial for therapeutic interventions.*

Suicide

Alexandra K. Yockey

Background

- Suicide is the third leading cause of death in children and adolescents in the United States, with higher incidence of suicide completion among males.
- More than half of male suicide occurrences involve a firearm; most female suicides are caused by poisoning.

Definitions

- Suicide: the act or an instance of taking one's own life voluntarily and intentionally.
- Suicide attempt: a nonfatal self-directed potentially injurious behavior with any intent to die as a result of the behavior. This attempt may or may not result in injury.
- Suicidal ideation: thinking about, considering, or planning for suicide.
- Suicide affects not only the person committing the act, but the community around them. Attempted suicides and the sequelae which follow are frequently costly to the individual and the community.

Etiology

- Suicide is the result of both environmental and psychological factors which include:
  - Mental illness.
  - Alcohol or drug abuse.
  - Family history or previous attempts.
  - Physical or sexual abuse.
  - Social stresses.
  - Sexual orientation.
  - Impulsive or aggressive propensities.
  - Physical illness or pain.
  - Access to means.
- It is possible for someone to have these elements and not be suicidal. Individuals can have protective elements such as connectedness, problem solving skills, and access to mental health care which ameliorate the risk factors.
- Methods for suicide in children and adolescents:

- Firearms.
- Poisoning.
- Suffocation.
- Falls.
- Males are more likely to die from suicide; females are more likely to attempt suicide. This may be due to males using more lethal mechanism. Those who survive a suicide attempt may have long-term physical disabilities and medical needs. Individuals may suffer from brain injury or organ failure.

Evaluation

- Past suicide attempts and past/current thoughts about suicide, and the circumstances surrounding them.
- Depression is a chief catalyst for suicide and suicidal thoughts. Suicides are not always thought out in advance. Often, attempts are impulsive, spurred by a sudden stressor (e.g., a breakup or fight).
- The American Association of Suicidology developed a mnemonic for evaluating warning signs of a person at risk: IS PATH WARM.
  - I—Ideation
  - S—Substance abuse
  - P—Purposelessness
  - A—Anxiety
  - T—Trapped
  - H—Hopelessness
  - W—Withdrawal
  - A—Anger
  - R—Recklessness
  - M—Mood changes
- The Suicide Prevention Resource Center categorizes people as high, moderate, or low risk for suicide.
  - High risk.
    - History of serious or nearly lethal attempts or planning.
    - Recently institutionalized for a psychiatric disorder or recent psychiatric disorder.
    - Persistent suicidal ideation, psychosis, or history of aggression and impulsive acts.
  - Moderate risk.
    - Under medical care of a psychiatric specialist.
    - Suicidal ideation without plans or attempts.
    - No other identified signs.
  - Low risk.
    - Mild suicidal ideation, but without attempt.
    - Social support.
    - No previous attempts.

Management

- Stabilization and management of acute injury.
- Patient should not be left alone; doors should be monitored to avoid elopement.
- All harmful items or possible weapons must be removed from their vicinity.
- Continued care of the child who has attempted suicide is based on risk criteria for hospitalization based on psychiatric evaluation.
- The treatment path should be tailored to the individual's needs and level of suicide risk.

Traumatic Brain Injury: Moderate or Severe

Myra L. Popernack

Background

- Pediatric traumatic brain injury (TBI) is a leading cause of injury-related deaths and disability for age groups newborn to 4 years old and 15 to 19 years old, with males more likely to experience a TBI.
- Injured patients often have associated preexisting comorbidities such as learning disabilities, risk-taking behaviors, attention deficit hyperactivity, or psychiatric disorders.
- Survivors of TBI account for a significant number of admissions to pediatric rehabilitation to address cognitive, mobility, and functional deficits.

Definition

- An acquired brain injury from a blow to the head or a penetrating head injury that disrupts the normal function of the brain.

Etiology/Types

- Diffuse or focal injuries from trauma, postembolic events, postinfection, and postsurgical sequelae.
- MOI includes falls, struck-by/struck-against injuries, assault, and motor vehicle crashes.
- Severity is classified as mild, moderate, or severe.

Pathophysiology

- TBI results in primary and secondary brain injury. The primary event results in direct injury or disruption to the brain parenchyma; however, the secondary injury occurs as the result of a cascade of biochemical, cellular, and metabolic responses influenced by associated hypoxia and hypotension, affecting long-term outcomes.
- Diffuse axonal injury occurs when rapid acceleration, deceleration, or rotational forces results in axonal shearing at the interface of gray and white matter. This leads to cell edema, damage, or death. No surgical intervention is available; therefore, supportive treatment is maximized.

Clinical Presentation

- Altered level of consciousness; respiratory distress or respiratory failure; hemodynamic instability with shock; signs associated with increased ICP; abnormal brain imaging including extra-axial hemorrhages, skull/cervical spine fractures, or cerebral edema; seizures; vomiting; visual disturbances; motor or sensory impairments.

Diagnostic Evaluation

- Head CT, head MRI, diffusion tensor imaging (if available).

Management

- Intensive observation and monitoring with management of cerebral edema and increased ICP via external ventricular drainage to keep ICP <20 mmHg and optimal cerebral perfusion pressure for age; mild hyperventilation; hyperosmolar therapy; hypothermia.

- Surgical intervention for extra-axial hemorrhage/cerebral edema when indicated, such as evacuation or decompressive craniectomy.
- Maintain hemodynamic stability with optimal oxygenation/ventilation.
- Control seizures; provide pain control, sedation, and neuromuscular blockade as indicated.
- Optimize nutritional status with parental nutrition and introduction of enteral feedings when appropriate.
- Provide deep vein thrombosis prophylaxis when appropriate.
- Institute speech–language pathology program and occupational and physical therapies as soon as clinically appropriate.
- Manage comorbidities such as obstructive hydrocephalus and solid organ or skeletal injuries.

PEARLS

- *The location and extent of the brain injury, the MOI, and the initial modalities applied to minimize secondary brain injury significantly impact neurocognitive and motor/sensory recovery.*
- *There are two theories of the mechanism of recovery from pediatric TBI associated with rehabilitation. The first phase is restitution which results from the natural process of healing with reactivation of neural pathways and restoration of function. The second phase involves substitution which results from transfer of functions from injured brain areas to uninjured areas which compensate for deficits. Early in the acute stage of recovery, these two phases overlap; however, substitution is theorized to be the underlying mechanism after the first 6 months.*
- *Rehabilitation utilizes strategies to optimize functional independence and neurocognitive recovery throughout recovery. Evidence demonstrates that the natural recovery process continues beyond the initial 6 months after injury.*
- *The Rancho Los Amigos Scale is a 10-level behavior/response scale used to evaluate the state of consciousness through interaction of the patient with the environment or response to stimuli. This assessment reflects the level of brain damage. In the acute care setting, the first 8 levels are most applicable and may indicate prognosis for outcome.*

Concussion

Andrea M. Kline-Tilford

Background

- A clinical syndrome of altered brain function as a result of biomechanical injury. Typically results in disturbance in memory and orientation; may be associated with loss of consciousness. Football is associated with the highest risk for concussion. Some athletes may be at a higher risk due to age, gender, sport, and equipment.

Etiology

- Traumatic blow to the head.
- Can be related to any form of trauma; however, frequently related to sports injuries in children and adolescents.

Pathophysiology

- Primarily due to acceleration/deceleration and rotational forces to the head.
- Neuronal membrane disrupted resulting in potassium efflux and release of an excitatory amino acid, glutamate.
- Ultimately, reduced neuronal activity, increased lactate levels, reduced cerebral blood flow, and cell death.

Presentation

- Signs.
  - Dazed or stunned immediately after injury, clumsy movements.
  - Confused about position/assignment.
  - Forgets instructions, delay in answering questions.
  - Unsure of score of opponent.
  - Loss of consciousness; though, not required.
  - Personality, mood, or behavior changes.
  - Retrograde and/or antegrade amnesia.
- Symptoms.
  - Headache.
  - Nausea/Vomiting.
  - Dizziness; difficulty with balance, feeling groggy, confusion.
  - Visual disturbances (e.g., blurred vision), sensitivity to light and/or sounds.
  - Memory or concentration difficulties.
  - Changes in sleep (e.g., difficulty falling asleep; more sleep than usual; loss of sleep).

Evaluation

- Standardized Symptom Scale or Graded Symptom Checklist.
  - Post-Concussion Symptom Scale (PCSS) and Graded Symptom Checklist.
    - Administered by trained professional or self-report.
    - Accurately identifies in athletes with 64% to 89% sensitivity and 91% to 100% specificity.
    - Incorporates questions on headache, nausea, sleep disturbances, light sensitivity, dizziness.
    - Performed on the sideline after injury by licensed health care profession; information provided to the health care professional who will be evaluating the injured athlete.
- Additional tools are available (e.g., neuropsychologic testing, balance error scoring, sensory organization test); though, lower sensitivity and specificity.
- Best evaluation may incorporate using a combination of diagnostic measures.

Management

- ABCs, stabilization of cervical spine.

- Assume cervical spine instability in any athlete or trauma victim with loss of consciousness.
- Neurologic examination and inquiry of symptoms.
- Any child suspected of suffering a concussion should be immediately removed from the game in order to prevent further injury.
- Regular monitoring over next few hours.
- Imaging.
  - CT.
    - Typically, normal in concussion.
    - Indicated in children with loss of consciousness, posttraumatic amnesia, persistent altered mental status (Glasgow Coma Scale <15), focal neurologic deficit, skull fracture, or deteriorating clinical condition.
    - Used to evaluate more serious TBI (e.g., intracranial hemorrhage) rather than to diagnose concussion.
    - Imaging study of choice to diagnosis intracranial hemorrhage in the first 24 to 48 hours after injury.
  - MRI.
    - May be more appropriate radiographic testing modality if >48 to 72 hours after injury.
    - Superior to CT in identifying cerebral contusion, petechial hemorrhage, and white matter changes.
- Prohibited to return to play until formal evaluation by a licensed health care professional trained in the evaluation and management of concussion.
  - Able to return to play after resolution of concussion symptoms; gradual.
  - Progression through systematic tasks; must be asymptomatic during progress to be able to return to play.
    - Rest until asymptomatic.
    - Light aerobic exercise.
    - Sport-specific training.
    - Noncontact drills.
    - Full-contact drills.
    - Game play.
- Cognitive rest (e.g., temporary leave of absence from school, reduction in workload, increased time to complete assignments or take tests).
- If repeated concussions or persistent concussive symptoms, recommend retiring from sport.

PEARLS

- *History of concussion may be associated with more severe and longer duration of deficits and symptoms.*
- *Repeated concussions risk longer-term neurobehavioral or cognitive impairments.*
- *Mild brain injury can occur with or without loss of consciousness.*

Child Maltreatment

Definition/Background

- Any act on the part of the caretaker which results in serious physical or emotional harm, sexual abuse or exploitation, or death.

- Inclusive of neglect, physical abuse, sexual abuse, emotional abuse, and threat of harm.
- Over 3 million reports of child maltreatment are investigated every year in the United States.
- Youngest children have the highest rate of victimization.
- Child neglect is the most common type of child maltreatment.

Emotional Maltreatment

Background/Definition

- Described as psychological abuse.
- Fails to adequately provide children with love, affection, or nurturance.
- The child may be humiliated, terrorized, isolated, rejected, exposed to violence, or deprived of basic needs.
- May impair child's ability to experience normal emotions, attachments, or intellectual curiosity.
- Difficult to measure.
- Often goes unreported.
- May result from physical or sexual abuse, or a separate indication.
- Contributory factors to emotional abuse include:
  - Mental illness, substance abuse, or developmental delay of caregivers.
  - High stress levels, including economic stressors.
  - Caregivers had poor parenting; lack of role models.
  - Chronic illness in child.

Clinical Presentation

- Pediatric providers in pivotal position to recognize presenting symptoms:
  - Poor adherance with preventive visits and immunizations.
  - Caregiver's attitude revealing frustration, depression, and negative attitude toward the child.
  - Caregiver may be socially isolated, emotionally detached, hostile, and unable to identify any positives about the child.
  - Child may present with behavioral problems, school issues, appearing withdrawn, acting out; infant may be increasingly demanding, causing the caregiver to withdraw further.
  - Physical symptoms include a poor growth pattern, failure to thrive, poor hygiene, untreated medical conditions, inappropriate clothing, flattened occiput from being left in one position.

Diagnostic Evaluation

- Thorough psychosocial assessment of child and family.
- Home assessment by a community agency may provide the complete picture.
- Documented pattern over time also provides insight.
- Thorough physical examination including a careful skin/mobility assessment to evaluate for possible associated physical abuse.
- Detailed objective documentation.

- Minimal diagnostic studies; however, consider complete blood count (CBC), electrolytes, lead level, tuberculosis, and human immunodeficiency virus (HIV) testing to determine extent of medical issues or failure to thrive.
- Evaluation for other children in home.

Management

- Mental health consults for caregivers and child.
- Child protective services (CPS) referral, if indicated.
- Close follow-up for the child and family; in person and via telephone.
- Treatment of underlying conditions, as appropriate.
- Safe disposition for the child is essential.

Fabricated Illness/Munchausen Syndrome by Proxy

Background/Definition

- An atypical form of child maltreatment that involves the methodical fabrication of an illness in a child by the caregiver.
- A complex diagnosis that involves many challenges and possibly legal issues.
- The symptoms may be credible and consistent with some illnesses.
- If not identified, a healthy child may experience trauma/death.

Etiology/Types

- Estimated 600 new cases in the United States every year.
- Perpetrator is usually a mother.
- Perpetrator often has some medical/health care background or knowledge.
- Caregiver falsifies the history/symptoms to meet own emotional needs.
- Most common causes of death are suffocation and poisoning.
- Child is victimized by multiple office visits, hospitalizations, tests, procedures, treatments.

Clinical Presentation

- Wide range of presenting symptoms/laboratory findings.
- Most common presentation is apnea.
- Other frequent symptoms include seizures, bleeding, vomiting, diarrhea, fever, rash.

Evaluation

- Differential diagnosis; expansive.
- Meticulous physical examinations/comprehensive psychosocial history of child/caregiver.
- Examine patterns of illness.
- Consider Munchausen syndrome by proxy (MSBP) with elusive diagnosis despite testing.
- Testing may include:
  - Routine/extensive blood work.
  - Toxicology studies.
  - Video monitoring; may need collaboration with hospital counsel.
  - Careful and close observation.

- Extensive records review, including admissions to other hospitals/health systems.
- Interdisciplinary team.

Management

- Detailed documentation of physical examination, comprehensive history, patterns.
- Medical testing/procedures/treatments as indicated.
- Team collaboration including health care providers, child abuse experts, CPS, legal, family members.
- Safe disposition of child: may include removal from suspected caregiver to evaluate when child is in alternative environment.

Child Neglect

Background/Definition

- Most common form of child maltreatment.
- Defined as the parental/caregiver omission in care that may result in the actual/potential harm to the child.
- Estimated to account for 78% of all cases of child maltreatment (USDHHS, 2011).
- May range from subtle to severe, intentional, or an inability to meet needs secondary to poverty, caregiver inability, or mental illness.
- Perpetrator most often the mother.
- Risk factors include:
  - Poverty.
  - Single parenting.
  - Young maternal age.
  - Limited family support.
  - Poor economic community resources.
- Common types of neglect:
  - Lack of supervision.
  - Lack of health care.
  - Inconsistent education.
  - Environmental hazards.
  - Lack of clothing, food, heat.
  - Lack of nurturance and emotional support.

Clinical Presentation

- Poor hygiene.
- Inappropriate clothing.
- Lack of medical/dental care; immunizations.
- Hunger or fatigue.
- Excessive school absence.
- Environmental hazards, including lack of heat and food, fire hazards, unsanitary conditions.
- Multiple illness/injuries secondary to poor supervision.
- Poor growth patterns or obesity.

Evaluation

- Neglect—purposeful or secondary to inability to care for child.

Management

- Multifaceted issue that requires an interprofessional team approach with health care providers, community agencies.

- Consider child protective service team evaluation; CPS if indicated.
- Careful physical examination and comprehensive psychosocial evaluation with careful documentation.
- Medical tests/procedures/treatments as indicated.
- Safe disposition of child; may require removal from home if situation is unsafe.

Sexual Abuse

Definition

- Defined as engaging a child in sexual activity that the child cannot understand, for which the child is developmentally unprepared, and cannot give informed consent, or that violates societal taboos.
- Involves both touching and nontouching behaviors.

Etiology/Types

- Often occurs with other types of child maltreatment (e.g., emotional abuse, physical abuse, neglect).
- Characteristics placing children at increased risk.
  - Female gender—2.5 to 3 times more common than males.
  - Increased age—35% of sexually abused children are 12 to 15 years of age; 23.7% 8 to 11 years of age; 22.4% 4 to 7 years of age; and 6.5% <4 years of age.
  - Developmental or physical disability.

Clinical Presentation

- Sexual abuse as chief complaint (current disclosure of abuse).
- Sexually transmitted infection (STI) (no current disclosure of abuse).
- Pregnancy (no current disclosure of abuse).
- Symptoms of sequelae without disclosure of abuse.
  - Sexualized behaviors.
  - Attention deficit hyperactivity disorder symptoms.
  - Posttraumatic stress disorder.
  - Depression.
  - Suicide.
  - Substance abuse.
  - Borderline personality disorder.
  - Eating disorders.

Evaluation and Management

- Acute presentation (within 72 hours of latest incident of sexual abuse).
  - Consider forensic evidence collection.
  - Consider HIV prophylaxis.
    - HIV prophylaxis should be considered whenever a child presents with an acute history of sexual abuse which includes anal–genital or genital–genital contact.
    - Risk of transmission increases if there is anogenital injury noted on examination or if perpetrator is known to be at high risk for having HIV (e.g., intravenous [IV] drug user, male or has sex with males, prison inmate), or if perpetrator is unknown to victim and therefore risk cannot be determined.
  - Adolescent female: Consider pregnancy prophylaxis.

- Adolescent male/female: Consider STI prophylaxis for *Chlamydia*, *Gonorrhea*, and trichomoniasis.
  - Consider referral to ED/child protective service team for acute expert care.
- Chronic presentation (>72 hours from latest incident of sexual abuse).
  - Consider referral to child protective service team for expert care.
- Psychosocial history.
- Medical history.
- Forensic interview.
- Complete physical examination including anogenital examination.
  - Ability to recognize normal anogenital anatomy is needed in order to perform a competent anogenital examination.
  - Less than 5% of children who are sexually abused will have an abnormal finding on anogenital examination.
  - A child can have a normal anogenital examination following sexual abuse including penile penetration of the vagina.
  - The lack of physical trauma upon anogenital examination of child sexual abuse victims can be explained by:
    - Elasticity of the genital structures and anus.
    - Nature of the sexual abuse behavior (nontouching; fondling).
    - Sensitivity of the prepubertal hymen to touch.
- Consider STI testing.
  - A positive genital chlamydia culture in a child older than 3 years is diagnostic of sexual abuse and must be reported to CPS.
- Report concerns of suspected sexual abuse to CPS.
- Referral for mental health counseling.

Physical Abuse

Background

- Physical abuse accounts for 16.1% of the approximately 772,000 substantiated cases of child maltreatment occurring in the United States annually.

Definition

- Physical abuse is any action that inflicts injury on a child.
- Physical abuse may take the form of skin injuries, musculoskeletal injuries, visceral injuries, or head injuries.

Etiology/Types

- Risk factors.
  - Parental/Caregiver.
    - Substance use.
    - Mental illness.
    - Domestic violence.
    - Single parenting.
    - Nonrelated adult living in the home.
  - Child.
    - Younger age.
    - Prematurity.
    - Low birth weight.
    - Developmental or physical disability.

- Societal.
  - Poverty.
  - Increased family size.
  - Social isolation.
- Types.
  - Cutaneous.
    - Most common findings in physical abuse.
    - Accidental skin injuries are common in ambulatory children and typically present over boney prominences such as the forehead, knees, shins, and elbows.
    - Bruises over protected areas of the body such as abdomen, genitals, behind the ears, or bruises in nonambulatory children raise suspicion for physical abuse.
    - Patterned injuries raise concern for abuse.
    - Most pediatric burns in the United States are accidental scald burns involving hot liquids in the kitchen.
    - Immersion burns are an inflicted scald burn that occurs when a child is forcefully held in hot liquid. The pattern is characteristic: The burns tend to be circumferential, demonstrate uniform thickness, and leave a clear line of demarcation between injured and uninvolved skin.
    - Contact burns with a clear outline of an implement located on a protected area of the body, or on multiple surfaces of the body raise concern for inflicted injury.
  - Skeletal injuries.
    - Short vertical falls rarely result in significant injury; however, falls from somewhat greater heights may result in a simple linear skull fracture.
    - Injuries concerning for physical abuse include:
      - Posterior rib fractures.
      - Fracture in a child <1 year of age.
      - Classic metaphyseal lesions.
  - Abusive head trauma (AHT).
    - Can result from blunt trauma, shaking, or rotational forces.
    - Retinal hemorrhages are found in 65% to 80% of patients with AHT.
    - Retinal hemorrhages, rib fractures, and classic metaphyseal lesions are other injuries associated with AHT.
    - Subdural hemorrhage is the most common form of intracerebral bleed in AHT.
  - Visceral injury.
    - Any organ in the body may be impacted.
    - Bruising *absent* in up to 80% of abdominal injuries.
    - Intrathoracic injuries more common in children <5 years of age.
    - Abusive abdominal injuries more common in younger children (e.g., infants and toddlers), and accidental abdominal trauma more common in older school-age children (e.g., >7 years of age).
    - Duodenal injuries more common in abusive injuries when compared with accidental injuries.

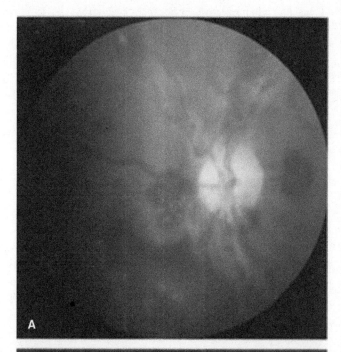
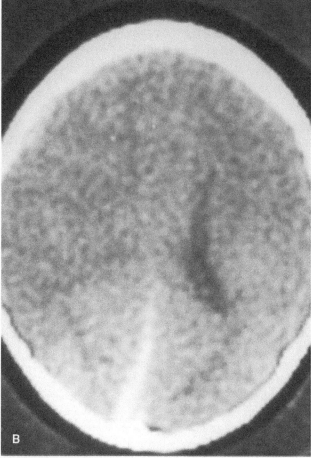

FIGURE 12.3 • **Retinal Hemorrhages and Subdural Bleed.** Manifestations of abusive head trauma. **A:** Retinal hemorrhages as seen on fundoscopic examination. **B:** CT showing intrahemispheric subdural bleeding and right cortical brain swelling.

Clinical Presentation

- Historical indicators of abusive injury.
  - No history of trauma despite signs of trauma on presentation.
  - History of minor trauma out of proportion to injury severity.
  - Multiple histories of injury.
  - Inconsistent history from same caregiver or between caregivers.
  - Evolving history over time.
  - History inconsistent with the developmental level of the pediatric patient.
  - Injury attributed to a sibling or pet.
  - Delay in seeking medical care.

Diagnostic Evaluation

- Obtain a comprehensive history.
  - MOI.
  - Caregivers.
  - Birth history.
  - Medical history.
  - Family history.
  - Developmental history.
  - Nutritional history.
  - Social history.
- Evaluation (modified based on infant/child presentation).
  - CBC with platelets.
- Prothrombin time (PT)/Partial thromboplastin time (PTT).
  - An underlying bleeding disorder can cause bruising disproportionate to the force of injury.
  - PT/PTT/CBC with platelets is completed to rule out an underlying bleeding disorder.
- Creatine kinase.
- Liver function tests, amylase, lipase.
  - Evaluates for abdominal trauma/injury.
- Urinalysis.
  - Evaluates for kidney trauma.
- Skeletal survey.
  - If <2 years of age, a skeletal survey should be completed on presentation and repeated in 2 weeks because skeletal injuries specific to abuse can be difficult to see in radiographs obtained shortly after the incident.
- Cranial imaging (CT).
  - Evaluates for intracranial hemorrhage or cerebral edema.
- Ophthalmologic examination.
  - Evaluation for retinal hemorrhages (AHT) (Figure 12.3).
- Additional tests as needed to evaluation for underlying medical conditions not related to abuse.

Management

- Obtain a comprehensive history.
- Thoroughly document (written and photo) all injuries.
- Rule out underlying potential medical explanation for the injuries.
- Report concerns of suspected physical abuse to CPS.

A 7-year-old boy with a history of attention deficit hyperactivity disorder was struck by a motor vehicle traveling at 50 mph. He was hit on his left side and thrown 30 feet onto the pavement. He presented to the ICU intubated for respiratory failure, with a Glasgow Coma Score (GCS) of 3 and a left femur fracture. After aggressive resuscitation efforts and emergent left frontoparietal craniectomy with evacuation of a left subdural hematoma, he stabilized and was extubated. He remained minimally responsive to painful stimuli upon presentation to the pediatric rehabilitation unit for ongoing treatment.

1. Based on the GCS, what is the severity classification of the TBI?
   a. Mild.
   b. Moderate.
   c. Severe.
   d. Comatose.

Answer: **C**

GCS is a standardized 15-point test using three measures: eye opening, best verbal response, and best motor response. Although there are several severity rating scales, GCS is most commonly used to initially grade the severity of TBI. TBI is graded as mild (GCS 13–15), moderate (GCS 9–12), and severe (GCS 3–8). This child's GCS was 3, indicating a severe TBI.

2. Based on the mechanism and location of this child's brain injury, what areas of impaired motor function are anticipated interfering with functional independence?
   a. Left upper extremity paresis.
   b. Left lower extremity flaccidity.
   c. No spontaneous eye opening.
   d. Right hemiplegia.

Answer: **D**

The brain has two cerebral hemispheres with contralateral effects; hence, the left controls the right-sided movements. The child sustained a left subdural hematoma in the frontoparietal region where the motor sensory strip resides; therefore, right hemiparesis would be anticipated. The child had a posttraumatic generalized seizure in the ED upon arrival, followed by a single focal seizure 12 hours later. IV phenytoin was administered in a loading dose with continued maintenance therapy. No further seizures were clinically evident.

3. What is the most appropriate ongoing management for a single posttraumatic seizure within the first 7 days after injury?
   a. Continue phenytoin IV for 3 weeks via central access.

b. Begin phenobarbital in addition to continuing phenytoin.
   c. Discontinue antiepileptic medication after 7 days.
   d. Perform continuous EEG for 48 hours.

Answer: **C**

In severe TBI and the very young infant/child, there is an increased risk of early posttraumatic seizures which includes seizures up to 7 days after injury. However, there is no data to support the use of prophylactic antiepileptic medications for the prevention of late posttraumatic seizures (e.g., >7 days). There are potential complications and cognitive effects associated with the use of some antiepileptics; therefore, medications should be used only when clinically appropriate. There are data to support the use of levetiracetam versus phenytoin for treatment of seizures if ongoing anticonvulsant prophylaxis is indicated.

On admission to the rehabilitation facility, the boy is intermittently responsive to noxious stimuli with slight movement of his left arm and increased tone on the left side. Right hemiparesis remained. Overall, his response is described as generalized and nonpurposeful. Intensive speech-language pathology program and occupational and physical therapies to address all deficits were initiated to address neurocognitive stimulation, neuromuscular reeducation, and strengthening.

4. Using the criteria of the Rancho Los Amigos Scale of Cognitive Levels to describe the level of behavioral response, which is the appropriate rating?
   a. Rancho Los Amigos Level VII.
   b. Rancho Los Amigos Level II.
   c. Rancho Los Amigos Level III.
   d. Rancho Los Amigos Level I.

Answer: **B**

The criterion to meet Rancho Los Amigos Level II is a generalized response with inconsistent and nonpurposeful reaction to stimuli in a nonspecific manner. Responses may be delayed and include physiologic changes, gross body movements, and/or vocalizations. A patient at Level I exhibits no response to stimuli. Progression to Level III occurs when the response to stimuli is more localized, such as withdrawal from painful stimuli or inconsistent following of simple, one-step commands. Level VII exhibits automatic but appropriate responses although "robotic-like" and demonstrates decreased safety awareness and impaired judgment.

At the time of injury, an emergent left frontal decompressive craniectomy was done for management of acute cerebral edema and the bone segment was stored for future replacement. On admission to the rehabilitation facility, the left bone flap was absent and the area was full and soft. He was positioned with the head of the bed elevated at 30 to 40 degrees at all times. Initially the site fluctuated in fullness; however, within 2 weeks, it showed increasing depression of the area.

When rounding in the morning, it is noted that the area of absent bone flap was full and tense. He was slightly more difficult to arouse to painful stimuli. His pupils were reacting sluggishly to light but were equal. His nurse reported his vital signs were stable, including being afebrile; however, he had a single small emesis during turning overnight.

5. Which one of the following diagnoses is highest on the differential list?
    a. Aspiration pneumonia.
    b. Hydrocephalus.
    c. Viral infection.
    d. Uncal herniation.

Answer: **B**

Obstructive hydrocephalus is a common complication following an acquired TBI, meningitis, or cerebral hemorrhage. Early detection of subtle signs of increased ICP, especially in the presence of an absent bone flap, requires immediate evaluation by a neurosurgeon. Imaging studies such as an MRI or CT to evaluate for hemorrhage or obstructed cerebral spinal fluid flow with dilated ventricles should be completed without delay to prevent brain herniation or death.

Imaging studies verified the presence of obstructive hydrocephalus, and a ventriculoperitoneal shunt was surgically inserted. The child transitioned to Rancho Los Amigos Level III with increased physical responsiveness, visual tracking of persons or objects of interest, and inconsistent but purposeful withdrawal of his left side to painful stimuli. He remained aphasic without vocalizations.

6. Which area of the brain is responsible for production of speech?
    a. Amygdala.
    b. Basal ganglia.
    c. Wernicke area.
    d. Broca area.

Answer: **D**

Injury to the left frontotemporal, where Broca area is located, may result in a motor aphasia or dysarthria. Although the patient will understand, he may have difficulty expressing thoughts. The Wernicke area is located in the parietal-temporal area and is responsible for language comprehension and receptive speech. Injury in this area may result in fluent aphasia in which the patient may express thoughts fluently with a nonsensical speech pattern.

7. During which survey are life-threatening conditions identified and treated?
    a. Primary.
    b. Secondary.
    c. Initial.
    d. Tertiary.

Answer: **A**

It is important to identify and treat life-threatening conditions as quickly as possible through the orderly evaluation of the airway, breathing, circulation, disability, and exposure which occurs during the primary survey. This step must be completed before moving on to a more extensive multisystem assessment.

8. When child maltreatment is suspected, the provider should obtain a detailed history during which portion of the survey?
    a. Primary: It is important to obtain the information as soon as the patient arrives in order to direct care.
    b. Secondary: The information will be obtained in the appropriate sequence after life-threatening injuries have been identified and treated.
    c. Tertiary: The information should be obtained after the patient has been evaluated and treated as long as it is within 24 hours of admission.
    d. Definitive: The information should be obtained when the patient reaches the location where definitive care will be provided as they have more experience with these evaluations.

Answer: **B**

The trauma survey should be completed in a consistent, orderly fashion beginning with the primary survey in which life-threatening injuries are identified and treated. The history is obtained during the secondary survey. Abuse is suspected when identified injuries are not in proportion to the history or when there are discrepancies in the history over time or among the child's caregivers.

9. A 16-year-old presents to the ED for a respiratory infection. She is noted to have lacerations to her bilateral wrists in advanced stages of healing and has an overall flat affect. What is the most important next step?
    a. Evaluate and treat the upper respiratory tract infection and inform her PCP of the encounter.
    b. Ask additional questions about her family and school to engage her.
    c. Inquire if she has thought of committing suicide or currently has plans to end her life.
    d. Consult the social worker to complete a formal evaluation.

Answer: **C**

Although delving into the personal life of an adolescent is important, matter-of-fact, direct questions will provide a better assessment of the patient's immediate intent and risk level. These are difficult topics for patients and health care providers, so the approach should include nonjudgmental language and questions.

10. A 3-year-old has been submerged in his backyard pool for approximately 10 minutes. Bystander cardiopulmonary resuscitation was initiated and bag mask ventilation has begun. He now has a thready pulse but remains unresponsive. The next step in management is to:
    a. Obtain a chest radiograph.
    b. Place an endotracheal tube.
    c. Obtain an ABG values.
    d. Administer a fluid bolus.

Answer: **B**

(continues on page 358)

The first step in management for any patient is to assess and treat airway, breathing, and circulation issues. Placing an endotracheal tube will support ventilation. Establishing and maintaining an airway is the first priority in submersion victims.

11. What is the primary catalyst for secondary injury in a drowning victim?
    a. Hypotension.
    b. Hypoxemia.
    c. Hyperglycemia.
    d. Hypovolemia.

Answer: **B**

The initial assault to the body is caused during submersion, which cannot be reversed. Although all the above answers can lead to secondary injury, hypoxemia is attributed to worse mortality and morbidity.

12. Which of the following is an example of an incomplete SCI?
    a. Tetraplegia.
    b. Spinal shock.
    c. Sacral sparing.
    d. Autonomic dysreflexia.

Answer: **C**

Sacral sparing is an example of an incomplete SCI in which some degree of sensory and/or motor function is preserved up to three vertebrae below the level of injury. Tetraplegia is an example of complete SCI and refers to paresis of all four extremities as a result of an injury to the cervical area of the spinal cord. Spinal shock and autonomic dysreflexia are complications that can occur in conjunction with an SCI.

13. What measure can be used to prevent the most common cause of SCI in children?
    a. Avoiding placing an infant in a car seat on a table.
    b. Using a helmet during football season.
    c. Utilizing a gun safe in homes with guns.
    d. Using a seat belt with shoulder harness in vehicles.

Answer: **D**

The most common cause of SCI in children is motor vehicle collision. Falls, acts of violence, and sports are also common causes of injury in children. Using a seat belt with a shoulder harness will help to prevent these injuries.

14. What is the most effective diagnostic test for evaluating suspected SCI?
    a. Plain radiographies.
    b. Spinal CT.
    c. MRI.
    d. PET scan.

Answer: **C**

An MRI is the most sensitive diagnostic test to evaluate spinal cord, ligamentous, and soft tissue injuries. Radiographies are not practical for a full spinal evaluation and are not adequate for evaluating the spinal cord. A spinal CT is very sensitive for identifying fractures, but not the spinal cord itself.

15. A 6-year-old, after trauma resulting from a fall from a second story roof, is exhibiting complete paralysis below C6. The radiographies and CT are negative for a fracture. What is the most likely etiology of the paralysis?
    a. Neurogenic shock.
    b. Autonomic dysreflexia.
    c. Refusal to cooperate.
    d. SCIWORA.

Answer: **D**

Rationale: SCIWORA is an injury that occurs only in children, most commonly younger than 9 years of age. The spinal processes remain partially cartilaginous and may not demonstrate fractures. However, the impact of the injury can cause partial or complete spinal cord transection.

The next two questions refer to the case below:
An 18-month-old male toddler presents to the ED with burns to his face, anterior chest, and left shoulder. The toddler had grabbed a coffee mug from the table, resulting in spilling hot liquid on himself. There are large fluid-filled bullae on the baby's chest and shoulders and some skin is beginning to slough. The post-debridement tissue is pink, moist, and blanching.

16. Considering the description of the injury and skin, how would the burns be classified?
    a. Superficial.
    b. Superficial partial-thickness.
    c. Deep partial-thickness.
    d. Superficial partial and deep partial-thickness.

Answer: **B**

Superficial, partial-thickness burns involve the first layer and some of the second layer of skin, known as the dermis and epidermis.

17. What is the best recommendation for treatment of this type of burns?
    a. Moisturizer to the face, silver dressing to the chest and shoulder.
    b. Silver sulfadiazine cream to all burned areas.
    c. Moisturizer to the face, silver sulfadiazine to the chest and shoulder.
    d. Silver dressing to all burned areas.

Answer: **A**

Silver dressings provide antimicrobial activity and conform easily to body surface areas, making them an important part of burn therapy. Silver dressings should not be applied to the face, so moisturizers without alcohol are sufficient. Silver sulfadiazine (Silvadene) cream has not shown increased healing times for burns and does not provide a topical protective dressing as does silver dressings.

18. An 18-month-old has had a 2-day history of emesis and increased fussiness. Examination reveals ecchymosis on his abdomen and mild right upper quadrant edema. What diagnostic testing is indicated to evaluate these physical findings?
    a. Abdominal CT with and without contrast.
    b. Abdominal CT without contrast.
    c. Abdominal ultrasound.
    d. Skeletal survey.

Answer: **A**

CTs with and without IV contrast are the primary diagnostic tool for abdominal injuries when blunt trauma is suspected.

19. A 13-year-old boy is admitted to the hospital for observation after sustaining a grade III liver laceration while at football practice. Based on current guidelines, how long does he need to maintain strict bed rest?
    a. Bed rest is not indicated.
    b. Two nights.
    c. Four nights.
    d. Until the hemoglobin levels are stable.

Answer: **B**

The Trauma Committee of the American Pediatric Trauma Society published guidelines in 1999 that recommended that strict bed rest should be maintained for the length of time related to the degree of injury, 1 day for each grade of injury plus 1 additional day. Recent research has indicated that it is safe to use an abbreviated period of bed rest, 1 day for grades I and II injuries and 2 days for grades III and IV injuries. In addition to being safe, there is also a reduction in length of hospitalization.

20. An 8-year-old was involved in a motor vehicle collision while she was only wearing a lap belt. A lumbar spine fracture was identified, but no solid organ injury was noted on an abdominal CT. There is concern that she may have sustained abdominal injury despite the CT findings. Which one of the following methods would provide the first indication of an intra-abdominal injury?
    a. Abdominal pain that is only transiently relieved with pain medications.
    b. Increasing serum amylase and lipase levels.
    c. Physical examination findings of increased abdominal rigidity and a palpable mass.
    d. A repeat CT.

Answer: **C**

Pancreatic injuries are frequently not detected on initial imaging; however, physical examination findings should be the first sign to alert a provider to a change in status and the need for additional testing. Amylase levels are not a reliable indicator of the severity of an injury and can be misleading, resulting in an increased frequency of unnecessary CTs.

21. A 13-year-old involved in a motor vehicle collision presents with an open skull fracture and has a GCS of 5. This patient should be transported to the nearest level I or II pediatric trauma center primarily because this institution:
    a. Provides the closest opportunity for intensive care.
    b. Has the specialized resources needed for the care of the patient.
    c. Will offer pediatric surgery with pediatric anesthesiology.
    d. Can provide social support and rehabilitation for the child and family.

Answer: **B**

The hospital has the specialized resources needed for the care of the patient. Pediatric trauma centers have pediatric specific requirements for the care of injured patients in addition to requirements associated with adult trauma centers. This not only includes access to pediatric-specific medical specialties, but also pediatric-specific nursing care and rehabilitative services.

22. A 9-year-old, weighing 38 kg, has been brought to the ED after being struck by a car. Injuries include left pulmonary contusions with overlying rib fractures on chest radiograph. Vital signs include heart rate of 100 beats per minute, respiratory rate 20 breaths per minute, and oxygen saturation 96% on room air. IV fluids should be ordered at what rate?
    a. 58 cc/hour.
    b. 78 cc/hour.
    c. 95 cc/hour.
    d. 100 cc/hour.

Answer: **B**

This patient presents as hemodynamically stable, and goal therapy should be to provide adequate tissue perfusion and avoid overresuscitation. Therefore, patient should be placed on a weight-based maintenance rate. Ongoing evaluation for signs of fluid deficit can be treated with fluid boluses as indicated by vital signs and physical examination.

23. When diagnosing and managing a pulmonary contusion, it is important to acknowledge that this injury:
    a. Is always symptomatic on initial presentation.
    b. Requires chest CT for diagnosis.
    c. Peaks at 24 to 48 hours after the injury.
    d. Requires prophylactic antibiotic therapy.

Answer: **C**

A child with a pulmonary contusion may or may not be symptomatic on presentation. Although CTs are much more sensitive and may be useful in predicting the clinical severity, pulmonary contusions can be diagnosed with chest radiography and not all patients require CT. Pulmonary contusions peak at 24 to 48 hours after the injury and typically resolve within 1 week of injury. Antibiotic therapy is not recommended for prophylaxis, but may be required for patients who develop pneumonia.

24. An adolescent who is a long-distance runner complains of pain and swelling of his right ankle. He remembers tripping

(continues on page 360)

on a trail run a week ago. He is able to bear full weight and walk without limping. The ankle is mildly swollen and pain is noted with weight bearing. The best guidance includes:

a. This is most likely a sprain and using the RICE (rest, ice compression, and elevation) protocol is the best management.

b. A radiograph of the ankle should be obtained to evaluate for a fracture.

c. The child should be seen by an orthopedist as soon as possible.

d. This is most likely an ankle strain and the child should avoid exercise for 2 weeks.

Answer: **A**

The Ottawa ankle rules indicate that imaging is not usually indicated for a sprain. Radiographs are only ordered if there is point tenderness or if inability to bear weight or take four unassisted steps in the examination room. The RICE protocol is the best initial management.

25. An 11-year-old with multiple injuries as a result of being struck by a car while riding his bike has been admitted to the PICU. The child had a normal chest radiograph in the ED. The next morning he developed shortness of breath and an acute decrease in his oxygen saturation. What is the most likely diagnosis?

a. Pulmonary contusion.

b. Hemothorax.

c. Pneumonia.

d. Flail chest.

Answer: **A**

Pulmonary contusions are the most common chest injury in children resulting typically from high-energy impact injuries such as pedestrian-struck crash. Pulmonary contusion often has subtle symptoms and no other obvious injury to the chest or chest wall. Symptoms of respiratory distress can occur within 24 to 48 hours after the injury.

26. An adolescent football player sustains a head injury on the playing field and develops memory loss, photophobia, and headache within 4 hours of the injury. What is the best plan for this child?

a. Refrain from playing sports until evaluation by a health professional and a head CT.

b. Rest overnight and if symptoms are not present, child may resume play.

c. Refrain from playing any sports until seen in the ED and evaluated by a neurologist.

d. Obtain a head CT and rest for 2 to 3 days, returning to practice under the guidance of the coach.

Answer: **A**

A child with symptoms of a concussion should be evaluated by a health care professional with the use of a formal screening tool and if indicated imaging studies. Return to play is determined by the extent of symptoms and by a health care professional.

27. According to the AO Muller rating table, a Salter–Harris III fracture is considered a fracture involving what area of the bone?

a. Paraphyseal.

b. Diaphyseal.

c. Metaphyseal.

d. Epiphyseal.

Answer: **D**

Salter–Harris fractures are those that result in injury to the growth plate of the long bone. These types of fractures are very common in children and a type III fracture goes through the growth plate and epiphysis, sparing the metaphysis.

28. A 2-year-old fell into the pool of a neighbor and was found shortly after. Emergency medical service was called, and on their arrival, the child was awake, but lethargic with a pulse oximetry reading of 99%. The parents did not want the child taken to the ED at this point. What is the most appropriate management?

a. Allow the parents to monitor the child's status over the next 24 hours.

b. Make an appointment with the PCP to examine the child the next day.

c. Transport the child to the ED for evaluation and longer-term monitoring.

d. Have the parents transport the child to the ED, evaluate for a short time, and if stable, discharge home.

Answer: **C**

Children who have suffered submersion injuries experience a variety of symptoms and can become worse despite initial presentation. Pulse oximetry should be monitored, and if abnormal or if respiratory distress develops, ABG values and chest X-ray should be obtained. Respiratory dysfunction may take hours to manifest, making it crucial children be observed for several hours after a submersion incident.

29. Which of the following best describes typical diagnostic findings in a child presenting without loss of consciousness after suffering a concussion?

a. MRI demonstrates gray matter change.

b. Skull radiograph demonstrates discrete fractures.

c. Electroencephalograph demonstrates focal spike waves.

d. CT demonstrates no intracranial abnormality.

Answer: **D**

Most children suffering a concussion without loss of consciousness will have a normal head CT. MRI is generally not needed in children presenting after concussion without a loss of consciousness. MRI is superior to CT in identifying cerebral contusion, petechial hemorrhage, and white matter changes. Skull radiographs are not typically indicated in children with concussive injuries. EEG monitoring is not needed in patients suffering from a concussion unless there is concern for seizure activity.

30. When counseling a child and his family after sustaining a concussion while playing football, development of which of the following conditions has been associated with repeated concussive injuries?

a. Seizure disorder.

b. Intracranial malignancy.

c. Cognitive impairments.

d. Schizophrenia.

Answer: **C**

Long-term neurobehavioral and cognitive impairments have been demonstrated in individuals sustaining repeated concussion injuries. This information should be shared with families of children after sustaining a concussion. The other conditions listed are not associated with repeated concussions.

31. The most common presentation of MSBP is:

a. Head trauma.

b. Vomiting.

c. Apnea.

d. Cutaneous injuries.

Answer: **C**

Rationale: Apnea is the most common presenting symptom of a fabricated illness. It is easy to invoke medical interest as apnea may be an acute life-threatening event.

Recommended Readings

Abend, N., Huh, J., Helfaer, M., & Dlugos, D. (2008). Anticonvulsant medications in the pediatric emergency room and intensive care unit. *Pediatric Emergency Care, 24*(10), 705–718.

American Association of Suicidology (AAS). (2012). *Know the warning signs.* Retrieved from http://www.suicidology.org/stats-and-tools/suicide-warning-signs

American College of Surgeons Committee on Trauma. (2006). *Resources for optimal care of the injured patient 2006.* Chicago, IL: American College of Surgeons.

American College of Surgeons Committee on Trauma. (2012). *Advanced trauma life support for doctors (ATLS) student manual* (9th ed.). Chicago, IL: American College of Surgeons.

American Heart Association. (2008, March 31). *Hands-only CPR simplifies saving lives for bystanders. Statements and guidelines.* Retrieved from http://newsroom.heart.org/pr/aha/hands only-cpr-simplifies-saving-228211.aspx

Asarnow, J., Berk, M., Hughes, J. L., & Anderson, N. L. (2014). The SAFETY Program: A treatment-development trial of cognitive-behavioral family treatment for adolescent suicide attempters. *Journal of Clinical Child and Adolescent Psychology, 25,* 1–10.

Avdimiretz, N., Phillips, L., & Bratu, I. (2012). Focus on pediatric intentional trauma. *Journal of Trauma Acute Care Surgery, 72*(4), 1031–1034.

Biagas, K. (2008). Drowning and near drowning: Submersion injuries. In D. G. Nichols (Eds.), *Rogers' textbook of pediatric intensive care* (4th ed., pp. 408–413). Philadelphia, PA: Lippincott Williams & Wilkins.

Catroppa, C., & Anderson, V. (2006). Planning, problem-solving and organizational abilities in children following traumatic brain injury: Intervention strategies. *Pediatric Rehabilitation, 9*(2), 89–97.

Centers for Disease Control and Prevention (CDC). (2012). *Unintentional drowning: Get the facts.* Retrieved from http://www.cdc.gov/HomeandRecreationalSafety/WateSafety/waterinjuriesfactsheet.html

Centers for Disease Control and Prevention. Web-based Injury Statistics Query and Reporting System (WISQARS). (2012, March 9). *Fatal injury reports.* National Center for Injury Prevention and Control. Retrieved from http://www.cdc.gov/injury/wisqars/index.html

Centers for Disease Control and Prevention (CDC). (2012, April 20). Vital signs: Unintentional injury deaths among persons aged 0–19 years—United States, 2000–2009. *Morbidity and Mortality Weekly Report (MMWR), 61*(15), 270–276.

Centers for Disease Control and Prevention (CDC). (n.d.). *Injury prevention and control: Traumatic brain injury.* Retrieved from www.cdc.gov/traumaticbraininjury/statistics

Cheng, A. (2008). Drowning and submersion injuries. In A. Cheng, A. Mikrogianakis, & R. Valani (Eds.), *The hospital for sick children manual of pediatric trauma* (pp. 219–224). Philadelphia, PA: Lippincott Williams & Wilkins.

Cohn, S. M., & Dubose, J. J. (2010). Pulmonary contusion: An update on recent advances in clinical management. *World Journal of Surgery, 34*(8), 1959–1970. doi:10.1007/s00268-010-0599-9

Committee on Pediatric Emergency Medicine. (2011). Pediatric and adolescent mental health emergencies in the emergency medical services system. *Pediatrics, 127,* e1356–e1366.

Cooper, A., Barlow, B., DiScala, C., & String, D. (1994). Mortality and truncal injury: The pediatric perspective. *Journal of Pediatric Surgery, 29*(1), 33–38.

Dean, N. L. (Ed.). (2009). Drowning. *The Merck manual online.* Retrieved from http://www.merckmanuals.com/professional/injuries_poisoning/drowning/drowning.html#v111276

Donnino, M., Gabrielli, A., Jeejeebhoy, F. M., Lavonas, E. J., Morrison, L. J., Shuster, M., . . . Vanden, T. L. (2010, November 2). 2010 American Heart Association guidelines for cardiopulmonary resuscitation and emergency cardiovascular care. Part 12: Cardiac arrest in special situations. *Circulation, 122,* S829–S861. doi:10.1161/CIRCULATIONAHA.110.971069.

Giunta, Y. P., Rocker, J. A., & Adam, H. M. (2008). Sprains. *Pediatrics in Review, 29*(5), 176–178.

Giza, C. C., Kutcher, J. S., Ashwal, S., Barth, J., & Zafonte, R. (2013). Summary of evidence based guideline update: Evaluation and management of concussion in sports. *American Academy of Neurology, 80*(24), 2250–2257.

Halstead, M. E., Walter, K. D., & Council on Sports Medicine and Fitness. (2010). Clinical report—Sport-related concussion in children and adolescents. *Pediatrics, 126,* 597–615.

Hamrick, M. C., Duhn, R. D., Carney, D. E., Boswell, W. C., & Ochsner, M. G. (2010). Pulmonary contusion in the pediatric population. *American Journal of Surgery, 76*(7), 721–724.

Herman, R., Guire, K. E., Burd, R. S., Mooney, D. P., & Ehlrich, P. F. (2011). Utility of amylase and lipase as predictors of grade of injury or outcomes in pediatric patients with pancreatic trauma. *Journal of Pediatric Surgery, 46,* 923–926.

Holmes, J. F., Sokolove, P. E., Brant, W. E., & Kuppermann, N. (2002). A clinical decision rule for identifying children with thoracic injuries after blunt torso trauma. *Annals of Emergency Medicine, 39*(5), 492–499.

Gilbride, J. (2005). Not just skin deep: A history of pediatric burn trauma. *Pediatric Nursing, 31*(5), 421–413.

Gupta, R., Bathen, M. E., Smith, J. S., Levi, A. D., Bhatia, N. N., & Steward, O. (2010). Advances in the management of spinal cord injury. *Journal of the American Academy of Orthopaedic Surgeons, 18,* 210–222.

Idris, A. H., Berg, R. A., Bierens, J., Bossaert, L., Branche, C. M., Gabrielli, A., . . . American Heart Association. (2003). Recommended guidelines for uniform reporting of data from drowning: The "Utstein style". *Circulation, 108*(20), 2565–2574.

Landry, G. L. (2011). Head and neck injuries. In R. M. Kliegman, B. F. Stanton, J. W. St Geme, N. F. Schor, & R. E. Behrman (Eds.), *Kliegman: Nelson textbook of pediatrics* (pp. 2418–2420). Philadelphia, PA: Elsevier.

Lane, W. G., Lotwin, I., Dubowitz, H., Langenberg, P., & Dischinger, P. (2011). Outcomes for children hospitalized with abusive versus noninflicted abdominal trauma. *Pediatrics, 127*(6), e1400–e1405.

Leetch, A. N., & Woolridge, D. (2013). Emergency department evaluation of child abuse. *Emergency Medicine Clinics of North America, 31*(3), 853–873.

Maguire, S. A., Upadhyaya, M., Evans, A., Mann, M. K., Haroon, M. M., Tempest, V., . . . Kemp, A. M. (2013). A systematic review of abusive visceral injuries in childhood—their range and recognition. *Child Abuse and Neglect, 37*(7), 430–435.

Mathison, D. J., & Agrawal, D. (2010). Update on the epidemiology of pediatric fractures. *Pediatric emergency care, 26*(8), 594–603.

Narang, S., & Clarke, J. (2014). Abusive head trauma: Past, present, and future. *Journal of Child Neurology, 29*(12), 1747–1756.

NSW Health. (2004, September 1). *Suicide risk assessment and management protocols: General hospital ward.* Retrieved from http://www.health.nsw.gov.au/pubs/2004/general_hosp_ward.html

Ochfeld, E., Newhart, M., Molitoris, J., Leigh, R., Cloutman, L., Davis, C., . . . Hillis, A. E. (2010). Ischemia in broca area is associated with broca aphasia more reliably in acute than in chronic stroke. *Stroke, 41*(2), 325–330.

Parent, S., Dimar, J., Dekutoski, M., & Roy-Beaudry, M. (2010). Unique features of pediatric spinal cord injury. *Spine (Phila Pa 1976), 35* (21 Suppl.) S202–S208.

Parent, S., Mac-Thiong, J. M., Roy-Beaudry, M., Sosa, J. F., & Labelle, H. (2011). Spinal cord injury in the pediatric population: A systematic review of the literature. *Journal of Neurotrauma, 28*, 1515–1524.

Proctor, M. R. (2002). Spinal cord injury. *Critical Care Medicine, 30* (11 Suppl.) S489–S499.

Quan, L., Mack, C. D., & Schiff, M. A. (2014). Association of water temperature and submersion duration and drowning outcome. *Resuscitation, 85*(6), 790–794.

Reed, J., & Pomerantz, W. (2005). Emergency management of pediatric burns. *Pediatric Emergency Care, 21*(2), 118–129.

Semple-Hess, J., & Campwala, R. (2014). Pediatric submersion injuries: Emergency care and resuscitation. *Pediatric Emergency Medicine Practice, 11*(6), 1–21.

Simon, B., Ebert, J., Bokhari, F., Capella, J., Emhoff, T., Hayward, T., 3rd, . . . Eastern Association for the Surgery of Trauma. (2012). Management of pulmonary contusion and flail chest: An eastern association for the surgery of trauma practice management guideline. *Journal of Trauma and Acute Care Surgery, 73*(5, Suppl. 4), S351–S361. doi:10.1097/TA.0b013e31827019fd

St. Peter, S. D., Sharp, S. W., Snyder, C. L., Sharp, R. J., Andrews, W. S., Murphy, J. P., & Ostlie, D. J. (2011). Prospective validation of an abbreviated bedrest protocol in the management of blunt spleen and liver injury in children. *Journal of Pediatric Surgery, 46*, 173–177.

Suicide Prevention Resource Center (SPRC). (2008). *Suicide risk: A guide for evaluation and triage.* Retrieved from http://www.sprc.org/library_resources/items/suicide-risk-guide evaluation-and-triage

Swoboda, S. L., & Feldman, K. W. (2013). Skeletal trauma in child abuse. *Pediatric Annals, 42*(11), 236–243.

Thorpe, E. L., Zuckerbraun, N. S., Wolford, J. E., & Berger, R. P. (2014). Missed opportunities to diagnose child physical abuse. *Pediatric Emergency Care, 30*(11), 771–776.

United States Consumer Product Safety Commission. (2012). *Recalls and safety news.* Retrieved from http://www.cpsc.gov/cpscpub/prerel/prhtml12/12186.html

Wanek, S., & Mayberry, J. C. (2004). Blunt thoracic trauma: Flail chest, pulmonary contusion, and blast injury. *Critical Care Clinics, 20*(1), 71–81.

Warner, D., & Knape, J. (2006). Brain resuscitation in the drowning victim: Task force on brain resuscitation. In J. J. L. M. Bierens *Handbook on drowning: Prevention, rescue, treatment* (pp. 433–478). Berlin, Germany: Springer-Verlag.

World Health Organization. (2012). *Mental health suicide prevention.* Retrieved from http://www.who.int/mental_health/prevention/suicide/suicideprevent/en/

Williams, C. (2011). Assessment and management of paediatric burn injuries. *Art & Science, 25*(25), 60–64.

Toxicology

Overview

Poisonings

- Event resulting from the ingestion of, or contact with, a harmful substance.
- May be the result of an overdose or incorrect use of a medication.
- Children <3 years of age account for approximately 46% of poisonings.
- Male predominance <13 years of age.
- Female predominance >13 years of age.
- More than 90% of poisonings occur inside the child's residence.

Poison Control Centers

- National poison control hotline.
  - 1-800-222-1222.
  - Consultation is free to health care professionals and the general public.
  - Most callers are *not* referred to a health care facility.
    - Results in significant health care cost savings.

Selected Poisonings

Acetaminophen

Shawna Mudd

Background

- Also known as *N*-acetyl-*p*-aminophenol and paracetamol.
- Commonly used and widely available analgesic and antipyretic.
- Dispensed as a single product, but also found in many combination preparations.
- Common in pediatric overdoses.

Etiology

- Commonly occurs through dosing errors.
- Unintentional ingestions are common in young children.
- Intentional ingestions occur more often in older children/adolescents.

Pathophysiology

- Rapidly absorbed from the gastrointestinal (GI) tract.
  - Primarily in the small intestine.
- Metabolized primarily by the liver.
  - When ingested in *normal* therapeutic levels, primarily metabolized by the liver.
    - Metabolized to sulfate and glucuronide conjugates.
    - A small amount is metabolized to *N*-acetyl-*p*-benzoquinone imine (NAPQI).
    - NAPQI is then rapidly conjugated with glutathione and is inactivated to nontoxic cysteine and mercapturic acid conjugates.
  - Toxic ingestions (as little as 4,000 mg in a single day).
    - Glutathione conjugation becomes insufficient to meet the metabolic demand.
    - Result in elevated NAPQI levels.
    - Subsequent hepatocellular necrosis and can lead to irreversible liver failure.

Clinical Presentation

- Initial symptoms, mild.
  - Vomiting.
  - Malaise.
- >24 hours, symptoms progress.
  - Increased alanine transaminase (ALT) and aspartate transaminase (AST).
- >72 hours, peak toxicity.
  - Coagulopathy.
  - Encephalopathy.
  - Liver failure.
  - Cerebral edema (some cases).
  - Possibly, death.

Diagnostic Evaluation

- Determine quantity and dosage form ingested.
- Determine time of ingestion.
- Refer to an emergency department (ED) for:

363

- Children <6 years of age.
  - >200 mg/kg in children <6 years of age in a 24-hour period.
  - >150 mg/kg per 24-hour period for the preceding 48 hours.
  - >100 mg/kg per 24-hour period for 72 hours or longer.
- Acetaminophen level.
  - Draw 4 hours after ingestion, or immediately on presentation if more than 4 hours has elapsed since ingestion.
  - If presenting <4 hours after ingestion, consider waiting to draw level until 4 hours has passed.
  - A 4-hour postingestion level is the first value plotted on the acetaminophen serum level nomogram.
  - Serum acetaminophen levels should be drawn, as well as liver function tests.
    - See Figure 13.1.
- If the ingestion occurred over time, obtain the level 4 hours after the first dose was taken or immediately on presentation if >4 hours have elapsed.
  - Example: Child began ingesting acetaminophen at 4 p.m. and continued taking additional medication until 7 p.m.; the 4-hour mark will be considered from the 4 p.m. time of first ingestion, and the first level should be obtained at 8 p.m. (or immediately if the child is presenting later than 4 hours after the ingestion).
- Acetaminophen serum level nomogram.
  - Used to assist in determining severity of toxicity and therapy.
    - Stratifies risk level of ingestion.
    - Based on serum level and time after ingestion.

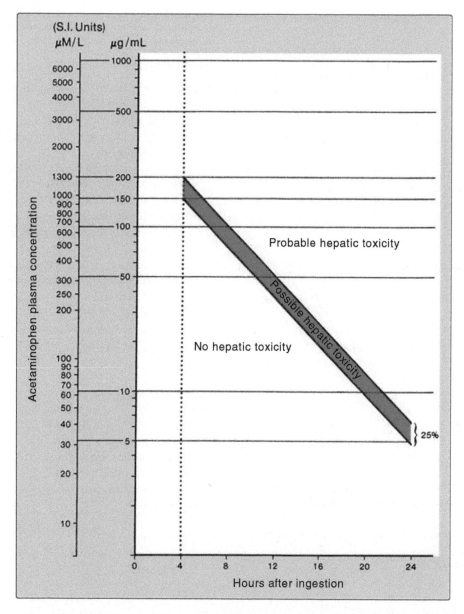

FIGURE 13.1 • **Rumack–Matthew Nomogram for Acetaminophen Poisoning.** Acetaminophen concentration plotted versus time after exposure to predict potential toxicity and antidote use.

- First level is 4 hours after ingestion.
- Limitations:
  - Levels obtained prior to 4 hours after ingestion are not interpretable on the nomogram.
  - Patients presenting late may no longer have a detectable level or may have a low level and may have ingested a lethal dose.
  - Less predictive in chronic ingestion (rather than acute ingestion).
  - Less predictive in extended-release formulations.

Management

- Antidote: *N*-acetylcysteine (NAC).
  - Available formulations.
    - Intravenous (IV) (Acetadote).
    - Oral (Mucomyst).
  - Mechanism of action.
    - Unclear; likely maintains or restores glutathione levels, allowing for metabolism of acetaminophen without development of hepatocellular necrosis, or may act as an alternative substrate for conjugation with acetaminophen toxic metabolites.
  - Administer within 8 hours of acetaminophen ingestion for greatest efficacy.
  - Administer in cases with any signs of hepatotoxicity, even if the acetaminophen level is low or undetectable.
  - Any child with an unknown amount of acetaminophen ingestion or questionable history should have an acetaminophen level drawn and consideration for NAC administration.
- Activated charcoal (AC).
  - Consider administration if child presents to medical attention immediately after ingestion (<2 hours postingestion; ideally <1 hour postingestion).
  - May also be beneficial in cases of multidrug ingestion.

Alcohols (Ethanol, Methanol, Ethylene Glycol)
Shawna Mudd

Background

- Toxic symptoms result from either intentional or accidental ingestion of alcohol-containing products.
- Many alcohol products exist that are intended for human consumption; however, some are not intended for human consumption.
- All can pose serious health risks for children.

Etiology/Types

- Ethyl alcohol (ethanol).
  - The alcohol most commonly recognized; produced by the fermentation of grains, "grain alcohol."
  - Alcoholic beverages and distilled spirits.

- Found in accessible household products—hand sanitizer, mouthwash, colognes, and others.
- Methyl alcohol (methanol).
  - Produced from the distillation of wood, "wood alcohol."
  - Found in industrial solvents, gasoline blends, plastic products, windshield wiper fluid, paint strippers, glass cleaners, hobby and craft adhesives, food warming cans used under chafing dishes (e.g., Sterno), and others.
- Ethylene glycol.
  - Used in various solvents.
  - Primary component of automobile antifreeze.
  - Found in herbicides/pesticides, liquid detergents, paints and paint products, among others.
  - *May have a sweet taste and attractive color which can pose a particular danger to children.*

Pathophysiology

- Ethanol, methanol, and ethylene glycol are rapidly absorbed from the GI tract and have inherent sedating central nervous system (CNS) properties.
- Methanol can result in mild toxicity through cutaneous absorption and inhalation, but this is not common.
- End products of methanol and ethylene glycol metabolism in the liver, primarily by alcohol dehydrogenase and aldehyde dehydrogenase, produce the significant toxicity associated with their consumption.

Clinical Presentation

- All present with generalized nonspecific CNS depression.
- Ethanol.
  - Symptoms similar to other sedatives.
  - Vomiting due to GI distress.
  - Slurred speech, ataxia, lethargy, and coma.
  - Respiratory depression.
  - Hypotension.
  - Bradycardia.
  - Facial flushing.
  - Profound hypoglycemia secondary to impaired gluconeogenesis can be problematic, and often is a delayed presentation.
  - An odor to the breath can sometimes be detected.
- Methanol.
  - Similar to ethanol intoxication in its initial presentation, but the initial inebriation period may diminish for periods ranging from 6 to 30 hours, during which the patient is fairly asymptomatic despite the fact that toxic metabolism is occurring.
  - Severe metabolic acidosis.
  - Visual complaints (e.g., blurred vision or seeing spots), headache, seizures.
  - Tachypnea or hyperpnea.
  - Pulmonary edema and renal failure.
  - Coma.
- Ethylene glycol.
  - Similar to ethanol intoxication in its initial presentation, except that no odor is generally present on the breath.

- CNS depression may worsen over time.
- Tachypnea and hyperpnea.
- Shock.
- Pulmonary edema.
- Acute renal failure.
- Acute respiratory failure.
- Cerebral edema.
- Ocular complaints are generally *not* present.

Diagnostic Evaluation

- Any symptomatic patient or any patient suspected of ingesting methanol or ethylene glycol should be managed in the ED/hospital setting.
- Patients require cardiorespiratory monitoring and supportive treatment as appropriate (e.g., airway, breathing, and circulation).
- Laboratory.
  - Serum ethanol (blood alcohol), ethylene glycol, and methanol levels.
  - In cases of suspected methanol or ethylene glycol ingestions, laboratory evaluation for metabolic acidosis is necessary.
  - Electrolytes with calcium and anion gap calculation.
  - Serum osmolality (a large serum osmolality gap should raise suspicion for ingestion of methanol or ethylene glycol).
  - Arterial or venous blood gas values.
  - Blood glucose level.
  - BUN and creatinine level.
  - Hepatic panel/Liver function tests.
  - Additional testing may include urinalysis and amylase, lipase, and creatine kinase levels.

Management

- Ethanol.
  - Conservative observation with cardiorespiratory monitoring.
  - Supportive treatment as appropriate.
    - Supplemental oxygen.
    - IV fluids.
    - Glucose (if hypoglycemia is present).
    - Electrolyte monitoring (particularly if frequent vomiting/diarrhea).
    - *Gastric decontamination or emptying is not recommended.*
- Methanol and ethylene glycol.
  - Supportive cardiovascular and respiratory care.
  - Prompt treatment of hypoglycemia.
  - Key to treatment of methanol and ethylene glycol toxicity is to interfere in the production of toxic metabolites through the IV administration of fomepizole or by the oral or IV administration of ethanol.
  - Dialysis effectively clears alcohols; however, it is infrequently needed unless the patient is deteriorating with the administration of fomepizole or ethanol.
    - May be needed in the cases of concomitant renal failure.

Metformin
Mark D. Weber

Background

- Overdose of oral hypoglycemic agents, such as metformin and sulfonylureas, is rare in children.
- Metformin overdose leads to lactic acidosis but rarely hypoglycemia.
- Sulfonylureas (e.g., glipizide, glyburide, glimepiride) can cause rapid decrease in glucose levels.

Etiology

- Inadvertent or accidental ingestion.
- Suicide attempt.

Pathophysiology

- Metformin is an oral antihyperglycemic agent which improves glucose tolerance in patients with type 2 diabetes.
- Increases glucose tolerance through reducing the basal and postprandial blood glucose level in patients with type 2 diabetes.
- Decreases hepatic glucose production and intestinal absorption of glucose.
- Increases peripheral glucose uptake and utilization, resulting in improved insulin sensitivity.
- The pharmacologic properties of metformin are unique and are unlike other classes of oral antihyperglycemic agents (e.g., sulfonylureas) which can result in acute hypoglycemia.
  - The exact mechanism of sulfonylureas' hypoglycemic effect is unknown.
  - Sulfonylureas bind to receptors that are associated with potassium channels sensitive to adenosine triphosphate in β-cell membrane.
  - The binding inhibits efflux of potassium ions from the cells, cascading and resulting in release of preformed insulin.

Clinical Presentation

- Nausea, abdominal pain, diarrhea.
- Dizziness.
- Hypoglycemia; rare in metformin overdose (common in other classes of oral antihyperglycemic agents).
- Lactic acidosis is primarily noted in adults with preexisting liver and renal insufficiencies.

Diagnostic Evaluation

- Baseline blood glucose level.
- Comprehensive metabolic panel.
- Hepatic function panel.
- Lactic acid level.

Management

- Gastric lavage with AC; depending on time of presentation related to ingestion.
- Glucose-level monitoring.
- Hemofiltration, in cases of severe lactic acidosis.

β-Blockers

Melanie Muller

Background

- Most ingestions are acute, accidental, occur in a residence and in children <6 years of age.

Definition

- Intentional or unintentional ingestion of toxic doses of β-blockers.

Pathophysiology

- β1-Receptors are found primarily in myocardial tissue and affect heart rate, contractility, and AV conduction.
- Blocking these receptors results in decreased myocardial contractility and decreased conduction through the AV node.
  - *Results in bradycardia and hypotension.*
- β2-Receptors are primarily found within the smooth muscles of peripheral vasculature and bronchioles.
- β-Blockers typically antagonize selective β-adrenergic receptors; however, some medications have both antagonistic and agonistic properties.
- β-Blocker medications may also have the following characteristics that affect clinical presentation after ingestion.
  - Membrane stabilizing activity (MSA)—inhibits myocardium fast sodium channels which could widen QRS and cause dysrhythmia (e.g., propranolol and acebutolol).
  - Lipophilicity—high lipid solubility, therefore crossing the blood–brain barrier, increasing the patient risk for CNS sequelae following a toxic ingestion (e.g., propranolol and metoprolol).
  - Intrinsic sympathomimetic activity—partial agonistic or activating effects on receptors, therefore potentially decreasing the risk of severe bradycardia and hypotension with toxic ingestion (e.g., labetalol and propranolol).

Clinical Presentation

- Widely variable depending on the amount ingested and the specific drug that was ingested.
- Ranges from asymptomatic to cardiac arrest.
- *Most patients become symptomatic within 2 hours after the ingestion, except in the case of extended-release medications in which symptomatology can be delayed for up to 24 hours.*
- Most common presentations include:
  - Bradycardia.
  - Hypotension.
- Ventricular dysrhythmias can be associated with the ingestion of β-blockers with MSA properties.
- Seizures and neurologic sequelae can occur if patient experiences severe hypotension or if medication ingested possesses lipophilicity.

Diagnostic Evaluation

- Accurate history.
  - Name of agent ingested.
- Approximation of number of pills ingested and concentration.
- Approximate time of ingestion.
- Possibility of co-ingestion.
- Any interventions performed prior to seeking assistance.

Evaluation

- EKG.
- Serum electrolytes.
- Urine and serum toxicology screen.
- Acetaminophen and salicylate levels to evaluate for co-ingestion.

Management

- Depends on the amount ingested and patient symptomatology.
- First, evaluate airway, breathing, and circulation.
- Consider AC (1 g/kg/dose) if within 1 hour of ingestion.
- Fluid bolus (normal saline 20 mL/kg) for hypotension.
- Atropine administered IV for bradycardia.
- Glucagon infusion for moderate to severe ingestions.
- Sodium bicarbonate if the β-blocker ingested possesses MSA properties.
  - Helps to prevent dysrhythmias.

PEARL

- *In general, individuals with a history of bronchoreactivity should not take β-blocking medications.*

Bath Salts/Spice

Mark D. Weber

Background

- Bath salts are compounds that originate from the khat plant (*Catha edulis*).
- Marketed as "bath salts" or "plant food."
- Labeled as "not to be used for human consumption" in order to avoid legislative regulation.
- Effects are similar to that of cocaine or amphetamines.

Definition

- A synthetically prepared or naturally derived drug from the khat plant that provides effects similar to cocaine or amphetamines.
- Common street names.
  - Plant food.
  - Bath salts.
  - Meow meow.
  - New cocaine.

Clinical Presentation

- Initial effects include:
  - Hypertension.
  - Tachycardia.
  - Euphoria.
  - Alertness.
  - Hyperactivity.

- Additional effects may include acute coronary vasospasm, myocardial infarction, esophagitis, gastritis, liver dysfunction, and increase of preexisting psychosis.

Diagnostic Evaluation

- Not detected by standard drug/toxicology screen analysis.
- Advanced detection can be performed by mass spectrometry.

Management

- Low-dose benzodiazepines to manage agitation.
- Benzodiazepines to treat seizures.
- Surface cooling and/or dantrolene to treat hyperthermia.
  - Prevention of rhabdomyolysis.
- Nitroglycerine, morphine, and antiplatelet drugs for coronary vasospasm.

Benzodiazepines

Dana L. Lerma

Background

- Class of medications that provide a sedative-hypnotic effect.
- Used in the treatment of anxiety, seizures, procedural sedation, withdrawal states, and as muscle relaxants.
- While benzodiazepine overdose is relatively common, they generally involve a co-ingested agent.
- Overall, patient outcomes are generally good when benzodiazepine ingestion occurs alone.

Pharmacology

- Benzodiazepines act on γ-aminobutyric acid A receptors, an inhibitory neurotransmitter in the CNS.

Clinical Presentation

- Mild to moderate toxicity:
  - CNS depression.
    - Drowsiness, fatigue, confusion, memory loss, ataxia, and slurred speech.
  - Paradoxical excitement is not uncommon in children.
  - Respiratory depression is uncommon, but may occur.
  - Tachycardia or bradycardia may be present; although with mild toxicity, vital signs are normally stable.
  - Nausea and vomiting.
- Severe toxicity.
  - More profound CNS depression.
  - Respiratory depression and/or arrest.
  - Hypothermia and hypotension are common.
  - Possible coma or death.

Diagnostic Evaluation

- Urine toxicity screen should be sent. However, not all benzodiazepines are detected on routine urine drug/toxicology tests, including midazolam, lorazepam, and clonazepam.

- Routine laboratory testing should be completed, including glucose to evaluate for hypoglycemia as cause of decreased mental status.
- Acetaminophen, salicylate, and ethanol are common co-ingestions.
  - Evaluation of these serum levels is indicated.

Management

- Primarily supportive.
- Flumazenil is a rapid benzodiazepine receptor antagonist; only indicated in iatrogenic oversedation or respiratory depression.
- Intubation may be required in patients with respiratory depression and loss of airway reflexes.
- Fluid resuscitation for hypotension.
- Rarely, vasopressors are required to maintain adequate blood pressure.
- AC is generally only beneficial when benzodiazepines are co-ingested with another toxic substance.

PEARL

- *A negative urine toxicology test does not exclude the possibility of benzodiazepine ingestion.*

Carbon Monoxide

Mark D. Weber

Background

- Inhalation of carbon monoxide (CO) from surrounding environment, leading to tissue hypoxia.

Definition

- Acute CO poisoning results from brief exposure to high levels.
- Chronic CO poisoning results from long-term exposure to low levels (e.g., tobacco smokers).
- Mild CO poisoning (CO <30%) may not be associated with any symptoms.
- Moderate CO poisoning (CO level 30%–40%).
- Severe CO poisoning (CO level >40%) may result in loss of consciousness.
  - Death has been associated with CO levels >60%.

Etiology

- Exposure to:
  - Smoke inhalation.
  - Space heaters; fuel burning.
  - Furnaces, charcoal grills, fireplaces, portable generators.
  - Water heaters.
  - Cooktop ranges.
  - Wood-burning stoves.
    - Typically, exposure to these is not of concern unless they are not kept in proper working order or if used in a close or partially closed space.
  - Car/truck exhaust.
    - Typically not a concern unless running a car/truck in a closed garage/space with inadequate ventilation.

Pathophysiology

- CO has a 200 times greater affinity for hemoglobin than does oxygen.
  - Large amounts of carboxyhemoglobin (COHb) hinder oxygen delivery to the body.
- The relative oxygen saturation of the hemoglobin molecule is then decreased leading to tissue hypoxia (Figure 13.2).

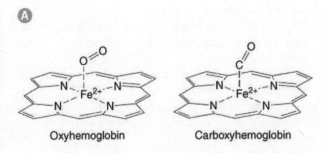

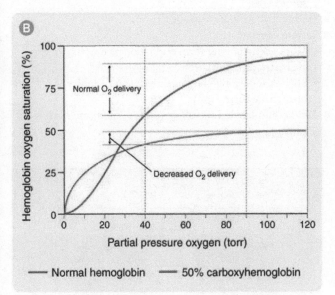

FIGURE 13.2 • Mechanism of Carbon Monoxide Poisoning.
A: The binding site of hemoglobin is a ferrous heme that can reversibly bind oxygen. CO prevents oxygen binding by forming a bond to ferrous heme that is significantly stronger than the heme–oxygen bond (shorter bold line). **B:** CO interferes strongly with oxygen transport because it both prevents oxygen binding and increases the affinity of heme for oxygen. Under normal conditions (blue line), hemoglobin is 85% saturated with oxygen in the alveoli (where the partial pressure of oxygen is approximately 90 torr). At tissue partial pressures (40 torr), normal hemoglobin is 60% saturated with O_2. Thus, under normal conditions, 25% of the hemoglobin sites deliver their oxygen to the tissues. When 50% of oxygen binding sites are occupied by CO (red line), hemoglobin oxygen saturation can be no more than 50% at a partial pressure of 90 torr. At tissue partial pressures (40 torr), the hemoglobin oxygen saturation is still over 35%, indicating that less than 15% of the heme sites can deliver their oxygen to the tissues.

Clinical Presentation

- Symptoms include headache, nausea, dizziness, vomiting, seizures, shortness of breath, hypotension, confusion, loss of consciousness (moderate to severe poisonings).
- May initially seem like a flu-like illness.
- Can lead to cardiopulmonary arrest, coma, and death.
- Cherry-red skin is a rare finding.

Diagnostic Evaluation

- Arterial or venous blood gas analysis to assess COHb percentage—normal <2%.
- Traditional pulse oximetry may be unable to detect CO binding to hemoglobin, resulting in falsely elevated oxygen saturation reading.
  - Hemoglobin is saturated, however, with a mixture of oxygen and CO.
  - Pulse oximeters are unable to discern what substance is bound to the hemoglobin and report a total percentage of saturation; in cases of CO toxicity, the combination of oxygen and CO bound to hemoglobin.

Management

- Supplemental oxygen.
  - Preferably, non-rebreather to maximize oxygen concentration.
- Intubation if level of consciousness and respiratory rate indicate.
- Hyperbaric oxygen therapy.
  - Controversial, but may speed recovery and removal of CO.

PEARL

- *Tobacco smokers typically have an elevated baseline COHb level of approximately 5% to 8%.*

Caustic Agents

Andrea M. Kline-Tilford

Background/Definition

- Remains an important public health problem despite education and regulatory efforts to decrease its occurrence.
- Approximately 5,000 to 15,000 caustic ingestions in the United States annually.
- Bimodal pattern.
  - First peak is at 1 to 5 years of age.
    - Most are accidental.
  - Second peak is at 21 years and older.
    - Most are intentional/suicide attempts.
- Results in widespread injury.
  - Lips, oral cavity, pharynx, and upper airway.
- Most serious injuries are a result of involvement of the esophagus.
  - About 18% to 46% of caustic ingestions are associated with esophageal burns.

- Short-term complications:
  - Perforation.
  - Death.
- Long-term complications:
  - Strictures.
  - Lifelong risk of esophageal carcinoma.

Etiology

- Determined by the identity of the agent, amount consumed, concentration, and duration of exposure to the tissue.
- Tissue injury is caused by a chemical reaction.
- Greatest concern is acids with a pH <3 and alkalis with a pH >11 (Table 13.1).

Clinical Presentation

- Injuries often present hours to days after the ingestion.
  - Appearances may change after initial presentation; initial presentation may appear deceptively harmless.
- Injuries divided into three categories:
  - Airway/facial burns.
  - Esophageal/GI burns.
  - Splash burns.
- Burning sensation in the mouth, perioral edema.
- Esophageal/pharyngeal edema.
  - Esophageal injury is rapid.
  - Acute tissue penetration and deep tissue injury continues for hours.
  - Injury progresses for the first week after the ingestion.
    - Inflammation.
    - Vascular thrombosis.
    - Ulceration, fibrous crust formation, and granulation tissue develop in the first few days after the event.

- Dyspnea, dysphagia, drooling.
- Stridor.
- Recurrent emesis.
- Hematemesis.

Diagnostic Evaluation

- History and physical examination.
- Nothing by mouth.
  - Aggressive IV hydration.
- Chest and abdominal radiographs.
  - Evaluate for free air in mediastinum (esophageal perforation), air under diaphragm (gastric perforation) (see Figure 13.3).
  - Baseline chest radiograph in anticipation that aspiration pneumonia may develop.
- Laryngoscopy: often fiber-optic, to reduce the likelihood of bleeding or increased damage to area associated with procedure.
  - Surgical airway may be required (e.g., tracheostomy) in some cases.
- Endoscopy (airway, esophageal).
- Barium esophagram.
  - More useful in long-term evaluation of esophagus, especially stricture formation.
  - High false-negative rate in early stages of injury (e.g., prior to stricture formation).
- Technetium-labeled sucralfate (nuclear medicine study) (Figures 13.4A & B).

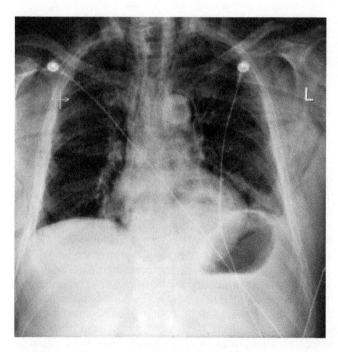

FIGURE 13.3 • Pneumomediastinum Due to Esophageal Perforation. Posteroanterior chest radiograph shows extensive air within the mediastinum, as well as lucencies around the aortic arch and along the tracheal air column and associated subcutaneous air.

TABLE 13.1	Commonly Ingested Caustic Agents
Type of Agent	**Examples of Agents**
Acid	Hydrochloric acid, nitric acid, sulfuric acid (e.g., swimming pool cleaners, rust removers, toilet bowl cleaners), acetic acid (e.g., descaling agents).
Alkali	Potassium hydroxide, sodium hydroxide (e.g., liquid drain cleaners, oven cleaners, disk batteries), ammonia (household cleaning agents), sodium metasilicate (e.g., dishwashing agents), lithium and calcium hydroxide (hair relaxers).
Other	Bleach/Hypochlorous acid. Peroxide (Mildew cleaners).

Adapted from Lupa, M., Magne, J., Guarisco, L., & Amedee, R. (2009). Update on the diagnosis and treatment of caustic ingestion. *The Ochsner Journal, 9*, 54–59.

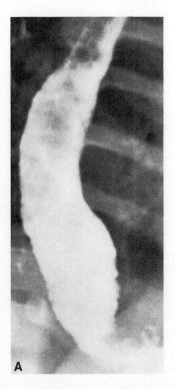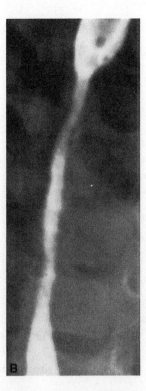

FIGURE 13.4 • **Corrosive Esophagitis Esophagram.**
A: Dilated, boggy esophagus with ulceration 8 days after the ingestion of a caustic agent. **B:** Stricture formation is evident on an esophagram obtained 3 months after the caustic injury.

Management

- Pain control.
- Nasogastric tube may be required as a stent for injured area and provide nutrition.
  - Placed under endoscopic guidance.
  - Generally left in place for 14 to 21 days.
- Strictures often require repeated balloon dilation via endoscopy.
- Antibiotics often used, though no evidence to support that they affect stricture formation or rates of infection.
- Steroids, controversial.
- Avoid induction of emesis; may lead to worse injury from additional exposure to corrosive agent.

PEARLS

- *Alkaline disk battery ingestion results in damage and leakage within 1 hour, and if lodged in the esophagus, perforation 8 to 12 hours after the ingestion.*
- *Evaluate for potential splash burns to skin and eyes.*
- *Most long-term sequelae occur in the esophagus.*
- *The presence or absence of burns on the lips, mouth, and oropharynx immediately after the event does not always correlate with the extent of injury in the esophagus or GI tract.*

Calcium Channel Blockers

Lara G. Smith & Mark D. Weber

Background/Definition

- Antihypertensive.
- Lethal prescription drug ingestion.
- Appealing to children because of candy-like appearance.
- Several formulations: short-acting, long-acting, ultra-long-acting.
- Relaxation of smooth muscle in the coronary vasculature and dilation of the coronary vessels.
- Metabolized in the liver into inactive metabolites.
- Half-life.
  - Dependent on agent ingested.
    - Example: Nifedipine has a half-life of 2 to 5 hours; amlodipine has a half-life of 30 to 50 hours.
  - It is vital to determine the agent ingested to anticipate patient course.

Pathophysiology

- Binds to L-type, slow calcium channels in cell membranes.
- Binding reduces the flow of calcium into the cell.
- Inhibition of depolarization in cardiac pacemaker cells.
- Metabolized primarily in the liver.

Clinical Presentation

- Cardiovascular.
  - Hypotension, bradycardia, bradyarrhythmias.
  - Conduction abnormalities of sinoatrial/atrioventricular
  - (SA/AV) node, idioventricular arrhythmias.
  - Shock.
  - Death.
- Other effects.
  - Altered mental status, seizures.
  - Respiratory depression.
  - Hyperglycemia.
  - Bowel ischemia.
- Verapamil and diltiazem can result in cardiac failure.

Management

- Monitoring.
  - Blood pressure.
  - EKG.
  - Blood glucose levels.
- Treatment.
  - Aggressive supportive care.
  - Fluid resuscitation for hypotension.
  - Atropine for symptomatic bradycardia.
  - Calcium, IV.
  - High-dose insulin may improve hypotension.
  - Glucagon may help improve cardiac contractility and conduction.
  - IV lipid administration may act as a "lipid sink" for absorbing lipophilic drugs

Clonidine
Lara G. Smith

Background/Definition

- α-Adrenergic agonist agent.
- Analgesic, nonnarcotic.
- Antihypertensive agent.
- Stimulates α2-adrenoreceptors in the brainstem, resulting in reduced sympathetic outflow.
- Results in decreased vasomotor tone and heart rate.
- Metabolism.
  - Hepatic metabolism to inactive metabolites.
  - Undergoes enterohepatic recirculation.
- Half-life.
  - In children, 8 to 12 hours.

Clinical Presentation

- Symptoms generally develop within 1 hour of ingestion.
- Hypotension.
- Bradycardia.
- Lethargy.
- Respiratory depression.

Management

- Monitoring.
  - Blood pressure.
  - EKG.
  - Respiratory status.
- Treatment.
  - Aggressive supportive care.
  - No antidote available.

Digoxin
Lara G. Smith

Definition/Background

- Antiarrhythmic agent.
- Increases the force of myocardial contraction.
- Inhibits ATPase.
- Decreases conduction through SA and AV nodes.
- Increases vagal tone.
- Metabolism.
  - Metabolized in the stomach and intestines.
  - Eliminated through the urine.
  - The metabolites can contribute to the therapeutic and toxic effects.

- Half-life.
  - In infants, 18 to 25 hours.
  - In children, 35 hours.

Clinical Presentation

- Arrhythmias.
  - Often tachyarrhythmias; possibly fatal.
- Impaired cardiac conduction.
- Nausea and vomiting (often the first sign).
- Dizziness, headache, mental disturbances.
- Shock.

Management

- Monitoring.
  - Electrolyte levels.
    - Especially serum potassium.
  - Continuous EKG.
  - Blood pressure.
- Treatment.
  - Aggressive supportive care.
  - Atropine can be used for bradycardia.
  - Antidote is Digoxin Immune Fab (Digibind).

Hydrocarbons
Lara G. Smith

Background/Definition

- Found in a wide variety of chemical substances available commercially, most commonly in lamp oil, kerosene, mineral spirits, glues, gasoline, solvents, paints.
- Recreational use of *inhaled* hydrocarbons is a significant health issue in pediatrics.
  - Inhalants are the second most widely used illicit drug class among adolescents.
  - Low cost, accessible.
  - Most pressurized aerosolized agents can be abused.
    - Propellants used in most aerosolized materials are hydrocarbons.
  - Performed through huffing, sniffing, or bagging.
  - Recognition and treatment remains challenging for caregivers and health care providers.

Clinical Presentation

- Liquid ingestion (most commonly an unintentional ingestion).
  - Most common injury is aspiration with resultant pneumonitis.
  - Lower viscosity agents causing greater injury because of their distribution.
  - Injury to the epithelial tissue of the respiratory tract results in:
    - Inflammation and bronchospasm.
    - Poor oxygen exchange.
    - Atelectasis.
    - Pneumonitis.

- Contact with alveolar membranes results in:
  - Hemorrhage.
  - Edema.
  - Surfactant inactivation.
  - Leukocyte invasion.
  - Vascular thrombosis.
- Some agents can be absorbed and result in transient CNS depression.
- Some agents can cause renal and bone marrow toxicity.
- Methemoglobinemia.
- Inhalants (primarily intentional).
  - Absorption across the pulmonary vascular bed.
  - Side effects noted 15 to 30 minutes after inhalation.
  - Two primary systems are impacted.
    - Cardiac.
      - Arrhythmias.
      - Increased oxygen demand.
      - Acute myocardial infarction.
    - CNS.
      - Impaired motor function.
      - Euphoria, hallucinations, confusion, disinhibition, slurred speech.
      - May follow with drowsiness, CNS depression, and sleep.
    - Other systems.
      - Renal tubular acidosis.
        - Hypokalemia.
        - Hyperchloremia.
      - Frostbite/Burns.
        - Face, trachea, esophagus.
      - Bone marrow damage/Aplastic anemia.
      - Leukemia.
      - Toxic hepatitis.
  - Highly lipid soluble; crosses the blood–brain barrier.
  - *Chronic use results in cerebral atrophy and neuropsychological changes.*

Management

- Monitoring.
  - Vital signs.
  - Respiratory status.
    - Can progress to respiratory failure quickly (aspiration of liquid hydrocarbons).
    - Chest radiograph findings often lag behind clinical symptoms.
  - Evaluation of serum electrolytes, renal function, hepatic function.
- Treatment.
  - ABCs.
  - Aggressive supportive care.
  - *Active removal of agent is contraindicated unless highly toxic hydrocarbon ingested.*
  - Avoid the use of catecholamines, inotropic agents, and bronchodilators due to myocardial sensitization of catecholamines.
    - Use amiodarone to treat arrhythmias (inhalants).
  - Correct electrolytes.

Iron

Lara G. Smith

Background/Definition

- Iron salt.
- Replenishes depleted stores in bone marrow.
- Pharmacokinetics:
  - 10% to 30% absorbed depending on stores.
  - Little is known about absorption rate, timing of peak level, or rate at which serum levels decline.

Clinical Presentation

- Nausea/vomiting.
- Diarrhea.
- Abdominal pain.
  - Typically develops 30 minutes to 6 hours after ingestion.
- Hematemesis.
- Bloody diarrhea.
- With more severe poisonings.
  - Hypotension.
  - Drowsiness.
  - Metabolic acidosis.
  - Hepatic necrosis.
  - Coma.

Diagnostic Evaluation

- Serum iron levels.
  - Mild <300 µg/dL.
  - Moderate 300 to 500 µg/dL.
  - Severe >500 µg/dL.
  - Serum levels often correlate with clinical severity.

Management

- Close clinical monitoring.
- Abdominal radiograph may demonstrate retained tablets.
- Whole-bowel irrigation may be of benefit.
  - Administration of a polyethylene glycol electrolyte solution orally or using a nasogastric tube.
  - Speeds passage of undissolved tablets.
  - Continue until abdominal radiograph is free of tablet fragments or until effluent is clear.
- Moderate to severe poisonings.
  - Deferoxamine administration.

- Iron-chelating agent of choice.
- Continuous IV infusion (most commonly) or intramuscular.
- Binds absorbed iron.
- Iron–deferoxamine complex is excreted through urine.
- No clear end point to therapy, though frequently:
  - Moderate toxicity: 6 to 12 hours.
  - Severe toxicity: 24 hours.
- Observe for recurrence of signs of toxicity after deferoxamine infusion has been stopped.
- Adverse events associated with administration are rare.
  - Pulmonary toxicity has been reported in administration >24 hours.
  - Monitor for rate-related hypotension.
- Results in vin rosé, reddish discoloration of the urine.
- Follow-up.
  - Gastric scarring.
  - Pyloric stenosis.
  - Intestinal strictures can develop 2 to 4 weeks later.

PEARL
- *Serum iron levels may not be available in a timely manner.*

3,4-methylenedioxy-methamphetamine (MDMA)/Ecstasy
Lara G. Smith

Background/Definition

- Psychoactive drug with stimulant and hallucinogenic properties.
- Increases the activity of serotonin, dopamine, and norepinephrine.
- Produces a feeling of euphoria and increased energy.
- Metabolized in the liver.
- Produces an active metabolite that is a more potent neurotoxin than the parent drug; destroys serotonin-producing neurons.
- Half-life.
  - Approximately 7 hours.

Clinical Presentation

- Euphoria, relaxation, double or blurred vision.
- Increased energy.
- Jaw clenching/bruxism.
- Sweating.
- Dry mouth.
- Increased doses can be associated with agitation, panic attacks, hallucinations.
- Rare cases: hyperthermia, rhabdomyolysis, cerebral edema, and death.

Management

- Monitoring.
  - Vital signs, especially heart rate and temperature.

- Electrolytes.
  - Particular attention to renal function.
- Bedside glucose testing.
  - Always indicated in cases of altered mental status.
- Liver function tests, coagulation panel.
- Creatine kinase.
  - Evaluates for rhabdomyolysis.
- Urine dipstick for myoglobin.
  - Evaluates for rhabdomyolysis.
- Urine toxicology screen.
  - Nonspecific; only tests for amphetamine.
  - Often only positive if a high amount has been ingested.
- 12-lead EKG and cardiac enzymes/troponin, if complaints of chest pain.
- Complete blood count, if fever, to evaluate for infection.
- Pregnancy test; females if postmenarchal.
- Supportive care.
- Short-acting benzodiazepine (e.g., lorazepam) if anxiety, extreme agitation, panic reactions.
- If hyperthermia, aggressive cooling and dantrolene administration.
- Follow-up.
  - Long-term use can result in impaired cognitive functioning, inattention, depersonalization related to damage to serotonin-producing neurons.
  - Counseling related to use of agent.

PEARLS
- *High incidence of co-ingestion.*
- *Drugs thought to be 3,4-methylenedioxy-methamphetamine (MDMA) often contain more than one substance and at times no MDMA at all.*

Opioids
Lara G. Smith

Background/Definition

- Analgesic.
- Narcotic.
- Binds to opiate receptors in the CNS, inhibiting ascending pain pathways.
- Alters the perception of and response to pain.
- Metabolized in the liver to active and/or inactive metabolites depending on the agent.
- Half-life.
  - Dependent on the agent utilized.
    - Short-acting.
    - Long-acting.
    - Immediate-release.
    - Extended-release.

Clinical Presentation

- Decreased pain perception and sensation.

- Respiratory depression in high levels of opioid ingestion.
- Cardiovascular instability.
- Chills.
- Ataxia.
- Lethargy.
- Coma.
- Urinary retention.
- Ileus.
- Histamine release.

Management

- Aggressive supportive care.
- May require respiratory and/or cardiovascular support.
- Identification of class of medication ingested to assist in determining the half-life.
- Naloxone (Narcan) is the reversal agent for narcotics.
  - Use judiciously if long-term opioid use, because of the risk of precipitating acute withdrawal.
  - Multiple doses or continuous infusion of naloxone may be necessary because of a shorter half-life than the agent ingested.

Organophosphates
Monika Chauhan

Background/Definition

- Commonly used as pesticides.
  - Malathion.
  - Parathion.
  - Diazinon.
- Nerve agents developed for chemical warfare can produce a similar toxidrome.

Pathophysiology

- Organophosphates are inhibitors of acetylcholinesterase.
- Exert their toxicity by excessive cholinergic stimulation of nicotinic and muscarinic receptors in autonomic and central nervous systems.
- Parasympathetic manifestations predominate the autonomic component of toxicity.

Clinical Presentation

- Muscarinic symptoms.
  - Can be remembered by the mnemonic DUMBBELS: Diarrhea, Urinary incontinence, Miosis, Bradycardia, Bronchorrhea, Emesis, Lacrimation, and Salivation.
- Nicotinic effects include fasciculations, weakness, paralysis, tachycardia, hypertension, and agitation.
- Central effects include lethargy, coma, agitation, and seizures.
- Pungent garlic breath/vomitus.
  - Sulfurated organophosphate ingestions.

Diagnostic Evaluation

- Based on history and evidence of accidental or intentional exposure to a pesticide or nerve agent.

Clinical Manifestations

- Consistent with cholinergic toxidrome features detailed earlier.

Management

- Acute airway management may be necessary for acute respiratory failure resulting from diaphragmatic paralysis or secondary to bronchorrhea and bronchospasm.
- Administration of three pharmacologic agents as antidotes:
  - *Atropine* is used to reverse muscarinic manifestations, though it has no effect on nicotinic manifestations.
  - *Pralidoxime* is used to reverse nicotinic effects, primarily muscular weakness.
    - It should be administered as soon as possible, i.e., before the organophosphate binds irreversibly to cholinesterase (a process referred to as *aging*).
  - *Benzodiazepines* are administered to treat seizures.

Salicylate
Monika Chauhan & Bradley D. Tilford

Background

- Aspirin or acetylsalicylic acid is the most common form of salicylate.
- Other examples include oil of wintergreen, bismuth subsalicylate, trolamine salicylate, and magnesium salicylate.

Pathophysiology

- Stimulate the respiratory center in the brainstem.
  - Results in hyperpnea and respiratory alkalosis, initially.
    - Sometimes children present later in salicylate poisonings and this stage is no longer noted.
- Interferes with Krebs cycle.
  - Adenosine triphosphate production is limited.
  - Uncouples oxidative phosphorylation.
    - Accumulation of lactic and pyruvic acids.
    - Heat generation: pyrexia.
    - Ketone production: result of fatty acid metabolism.
  - Wide anion gap metabolic acidosis.
    - Ultimately, may be replaced by a respiratory acidosis.
  - Abnormalities in glucose metabolism.

Presentation

- *Toxicity from salicylate overdose involves all body organ systems.*
- Nausea.
- Vomiting.
- Hematemesis.
- Gastric pain.
- Tinnitus.
- Mixed respiratory alkalosis and metabolic acidosis.
- Hypoglycemia.

- Hypokalemia.
- Hyperpyrexia.
- Severe and life-threatening manifestations include:
  - Coma, cerebral edema.
  - Pulmonary edema.
  - Rhabdomyolysis.
  - Arrhythmias, asystole.

Diagnosis

- Careful history may reveal acute or chronic salicylate ingestion.
- Serum salicylate levels.
  - Confirm the ingestion.
  - Assess severity.
  - Determine need for hemodialysis.
  - Serial salicylate level measurement is needed (e.g., every 2–3 hours) until a peak is determined.

Management

- Careful observation.
- Because of its potential to result in severe morbidity and mortality, consideration should be given to multiple modes of decontamination.
  - GI decontamination.
  - AC.
- Correction of fluid and electrolyte abnormalities.
  - Often dehydrated on presentation.
  - Restoration of fluid and electrolyte balance.
- Correction of hypoglycemia by providing:
  - Dextrose bolus.
- Alkalinization of the urine (enhances urinary excretion of salicylate)/treat wide anion gap.
  - Sodium bicarbonate infusion.
    - Typically, 5% dextrose solution with 150 mEq of sodium bicarbonate per liter.
      - Often infused at 1.5 to 2 times maintenance rate.
    - Goal urine production 1 to 2 mL/kg/hour.
    - Goal urine pH 7.5 to 8.
    - May discontinue alkalinization when salicylate levels <30 mg/dL.
- Consider chest radiography; evaluate for noncardiogenic pulmonary edema.
- Treat seizures.
  - Benzodiazepines.
- Emergent hemodialysis.
  - May be indicated for a serum salicylate level approaching 100 mg/dL in an acute ingestion.
  - Consider for severe manifestations.
    - Pulmonary edema.
    - Renal failure.
    - Cardiovascular instability/congestive heart failure.
    - Altered mental status.
    - Severe electrolyte or acid–base abnormalities.
    - Progressive deterioration in vital signs.

PEARLS

- *Chronic administration during a viral illness has been associated with Reye syndrome.*
  - *Symptoms include vomiting, hypoglycemia, hepatic dysfunction, and encephalopathy.*
- *Large ingestions of enterically coated salicylates may result in bezoars; slow dissolving.*

Tricyclic Antidepressants

Monika Chauhan & Bradley D. Tilford

Background/Definition

- Tricyclic antidepressants (TCAs) include amitriptyline, clomipramine, desipramine, doxepin, imipramine, and nortriptyline.
- Produce a variety of clinical effects.

Clinical Presentation

- TCA ingestion should be suspected in the presence of *anticholinergic toxidrome* features.
  - Agitation, delirium.
  - Mydriasis.
  - Dry mouth.
  - Tachycardia, hypertension.
  - Warm dry skin.
  - Fever.
  - Urinary retention.
  - Decreased bowel sounds.
- TCAs can cause profound hypotension by α-adrenergic blockade.
- Respiratory failure and coma can occur by CNS depressant effect.
- Cardiac conduction abnormalities.
  - Result of sodium channel blockage in the myocardium.
  - Widened QRS complex and prolonged QT interval on EKG.
  - Life-threatening dysrhythmias, including ventricular tachycardia or fibrillation, can occur.

Diagnostic Evaluation

- Can be detected on serum drug screen testing.
- *Diagnosis is typically made based on history of TCA use or presence in the home and the anticholinergic clinical manifestations.*

Management

- Acute airway management may be necessary because of respiratory failure from CNS depression.
- Seizures management.
  - Benzodiazepines.

- EKG abnormalities and dysrhythmias.
  - Sodium bicarbonate.
    - Goal of achieving an arterial pH of 7.45 to 7.55.
    - Sodium bicarbonate is thought to act in two ways.
      - Sodium loading may overcome TCA blockage of myocardial sodium channels.
      - Increasing pH may increase protein binding of TCA, resulting in a reduction of free drug in the serum.
- Hypotension.
  - Inotropic agents.
    - Norepinephrine often preferred.

PEARLS

- *Some medications are contraindicated in TCA overdose.*
  - *Physostigmine, a cholinesterase inhibitor, has been associated with seizures, asystole, and death in setting of TCA overdose.*
    - *It should not be used to treat anticholinergic manifestations of TCAs.*
  - *β-Blockers should not be used for tachycardia due to potential for hypotension.*
  - *Class 1A and 1C antiarrhythmics (e.g., quinine, procainamide, disopyramide, flecainide) may worsen cardiac conduction and should be avoided.*

Toxidromes

- A group of clinical symptoms that can be used to classify certain classes of ingestions.
- See Table 13.2 for the various toxidrome features.

Methods of Gastrointestinal Decontamination

General Considerations

- Consider in:
  - Children with a recent toxicologic exposure of a known or potentially toxic substance.
  - Children exhibiting signs and symptoms of a poisoning.
  - Children who have ingested a toxin that may result in a delay in symptoms.
- Carefully select patients who may benefit from gastric decontamination.

Syrup of Ipecac

- Emetic agent.
- *Not* recommended for *routine* administration in poisoned patients.
  - If present in the home, it should be disposed of properly.
- Should only be considered when it can be administered within 60 minutes of the ingestion.
- May delay the administration of or the effectiveness of orally administered anecdotes, AC, or whole-bowel irrigation.

- Potential complications.
  - Pulmonary aspiration.
  - Tissue injury.
    - If used in an ingestion of a caustic agent.
  - Prolonged vomiting.
- Availability is scarce.
  - Only manufacturer has stopped production.
- Dose.
  - For 6 to 12 months of age 5 to 10 mL, followed by 120 to 240 mL of water.
  - For 1 to 12 years of age 15 mL, followed by 120 mL to 240 mL of water.
  - Do not administer with milk or carbonated beverages.

Gastric Lavage

- Conditions for use.
  - Ingestion of a potentially life-threatening toxin.
  - Performed within 1 hour of ingestion.
  - At best, removes 40% of stomach contents.
- Potential complications.
  - Pulmonary aspiration.
  - Laryngospasm.
  - Tension pneumothorax.
  - Atrial and ventricular ectopy.
  - Hyper/hyponatremia.
  - Hypothermia.
- Contraindications.
  - Ingestion of caustic agents.
  - Hydrocarbon ingestion.
  - Hemodynamic instability.
  - GI bleed.
  - Unprotected airway.

Activated Charcoal

- Tasteless and odorless black powder.
- Specially treated charcoal that results in a very large surface area.
  - Allows for significant adsorption of a variety of toxins.
- Indication.
  - Ingestion of a toxin known to adsorb to AC.
  - Most effective when administered within 1 hour of ingestion.
  - Should *not* be administered to asymptomatic patients presenting several hours after an ingestion.
- Few agents *not* well adsorbed by AC include:
  - Alcohols.
  - Acids and alkalis.
  - Iron.
  - Potassium.
  - Magnesium.
  - Sodium.
  - Lithium salts.
  - Hydrocarbons.
- Administration.
  - Charcoal with sorbitol: oral dosing.
    - Infants <1 year of age.
      - Not recommended.

TABLE 13.2 Toxidromes

Toxidrome	Presentation	Vital Sign Changes	Causative Agents (Sampling)	Mnemonic
Anticholinergic	Agitation, delirium, flushed skin, mydriasis, dry mouth, urinary retention, decreased bowel sounds, memory loss, seizures, coma.	Tachycardia. Hyperthermia. Hypertension. Fever.	Antihistamines. Scopolamine. Jimson weed. Angel's trumpet. Mushrooms. Tricyclic antidepressants. Atropine. Oxybutynin.	Hot as a hare, dry as a bone, red as a beet, blind as a bat
Cholinergic, Muscarinic	Salivation, lacrimation, urination, defecation, GI cramps, emesis, diarrhea, urination, miosis, bronchorrhea, bradycardia, bronchoconstriction, emesis, lacrimation, and salivation.	Bradycardia. Hypothermia.	Organophosphates. Carbamates. Mushrooms (some). Physostigmine. Pilocarpine. Pyridostigmine.	SLUDGE. DUMBBELS.
Opiate/Narcotic	Altered mental status, unresponsiveness, miosis, shock.	Shallow respirations. Slow respiratory rate. Bradycardia. Hypothermia. Hypotension.	Opiates. Propoxyphene. Dextromethorphan.	
Sedative-Hypnotic	Coma, stupor, confusion, sedation, progressive deterioration of CNS function.	Apnea.	Barbiturates. Benzodiazepines. Ethanol. Anticonvulsants.	
Sympathomimetic	Delusions, paranoia, diaphoresis, piloerection, mydriasis, hyperreflexia, seizures, anxiety/agitation, pallor, cool skin.	Tachycardia. Bradycardia (if pure α-agonist). Hypertension.	Cocaine. Amphetamines. Methamphetamine. Phenylpropanolamine. Ephedrine. Pseudoephedrine. Albuterol. Ma huang. Caffeine. Ketamine, phencyclidine (PCP), terbutaline, theophylline.	

- 1 to 12 years of age.
  - 1 to 2 g/kg or 25 to 50 g.
- Adolescents/Adults.
  - 30 to 100 g.
- Sorbitol is a cathartic.
  - If repeated doses are needed, administer charcoal without sorbitol to minimize associated electrolyte disturbances.
- Charcoal without sorbitol.
  - May be administered as repeated dosing until signs of toxicity resolve or serum drug levels have returned to subtherapeutic range.

- Strategies for improving palatability.
  - Administer in an opaque cup with lid and straw.
  - Add a flavor.
    - Chocolate syrup.
    - Fruit syrup.
  - Avoid mixing with milk, sherbet, or marmalade.
    - Reduces the adsorption capacity of the charcoal.
- May require administration via nasogastric tube.
- Contraindications.
  - Unprotected airway.
  - Hydrocarbon ingestion.
  - Caustic ingestion.
  - Anatomically nonintact GI tract.

Cathartics

- Strong laxative agents.
- Decrease the transit time of ingested toxins.
- Most commonly used agents.
  - Sorbitol.
  - Magnesium citrate.
  - Magnesium sulfate.
  - *Effects are the result of osmotic action.*
- No evidence-based indication for routine use in poisoned patients.
- May be used in conjunction with another therapy, most commonly AC.
- Side effects.
  - Abdominal cramping.
  - Nausea.
  - Vomiting.
  - Hypotension, transient.
  - Electrolyte disturbances.
    - Especially with administration of multiple doses.
- Contraindications.
  - Absence of bowel sounds, recent bowel or abdominal surgery.
  - Intestinal perforation or obstruction.
  - Hypotension.
  - Renal failure.
  - Heart block.

Whole-Bowel Irrigation

- Uses osmotically balanced polyethylene glycol electrolyte solution to rapidly empty the contents of the GI tract.
  - Typically within 2 to 6 hours.
- Isotonic, nonabsorbable solution.
  - Does *not* result in electrolyte disturbances that can be associated with cathartic agents.
- Indications.
  - Iron tablets.
  - Heavy metals.
    - Lead paint chips or pellets.
  - Lithium.
  - Sustained-release tablets.
  - May also be used in body packers.
    - Individuals who swallow packets of illegal/illicit drugs.
- Monitoring.
  - Abdominal radiographs, serial.
    - Since most of these substances are radiopaque, radiographs can track the progress of the substance.
- Contraindicated.
  - Unprotected airway.
  - Hemodynamic instability.
  - Bowel obstruction.
  - Ileus.
  - Bowel perforation.

- Intractable vomiting.
- Do not administer if the substance is adsorbed by AC.
  - May interfere with the adsorptive properties of AC.

Common Diagnostic Testing

Lara G. Smith

Screening

- Frequently confirms what was determined by a detailed history and physical examination.
- A negative screening does not mean that there has not been an ingestion.
- Testing for specific agents allows:
  - Determination of anecdote (if available).
  - Determination of expected symptoms.

Urine Testing

- Many drugs/toxins and their metabolites accumulate in the urine.
  - Increases the sensitivity of detection.
- May remain positive after the symptoms of the substance have waned.
  - A positive screening does not always correlate with the degree of symptoms.
- Variable detection due to timing of collection related to ingestion and specific gravity of specimen.

Serum Testing

- Detection and quantification (when available) provides a better correlation with the current clinical state of the patient.
- Less sensitive for exposure history.
  - May no longer be detected in the serum.
- More invasive than urine testing.

Serum and Urine Panel Testing

- Available in most institutions.
  - May vary in testing composition.
  - Familiarity with the toxins included on institution-specific panels is essential.
- Beneficial due to high frequency of multidrug ingestions.
- Specific testing on drug panels is often selected using:
  - Common locally ingested agents.
  - Agents with available antidotes.
  - Availability of STAT (special tertiary admissions testing).
- Examples of panels:
  - Serum overdose panel.
    - Acetaminophen.
    - Salicylate.
    - TCAs.
    - Barbiturate level.
    - Phenobarbital level.

- Alcohol panel.
  - Ethanol.
  - Methanol.
  - Isopropanol.
  - Acetone.
    - *Does not include ethylene glycol and propylene glycol.*
- Urine drugs of abuse panel.
  - Qualitative (rather than quantitative) urine detection.
  - Benzoylecgonine (metabolite of cocaine).
  - Opiates.
  - Benzodiazepines.
  - Amphetamines.
  - Methadone.
  - Barbiturates.
  - Phencyclidine.

- Other studies that may be of benefit in cases of toxic ingestion include:
  - Blood gas analysis.
  - Electrolytes with blood glucose.
  - Liver function testing.
  - Renal function panel.
  - Complete blood counts.
  - EKG.
  - Urinalysis with pH.

Herbal Supplementation Toxicity

- See Table 13.3.

TABLE 13.3   Common Herbal Supplements: Toxicity

Supplement	Indication	Interactions/Toxicity
Ginkgo biloba	Memory difficulty. Intermittent claudication. Tinnitus. Sexual dysfunction. Asthma.	Increased bleeding risk. Intensified bleeding risk if taken with an anticoagulant or antiplatelet medication. May result in slowed metabolism of medications metabolized through cytochrome P450 pathway.
Ginseng	Improving overall health. Increasing sense of well-being. Blood glucose regulation. Improving stamina. Improving mental and physical performance. Treating erectile dysfunction. Controlling blood pressure.	Rarely associated with adverse events or drug interactions in short term. May be associated with headaches, insomnia, and diarrhea. May lower blood glucose levels. *Use with caution in patients with diabetes.* Long-term use associated with mastalgia. Not recommended for use with caffeine due to stimulant effects.
St. John's wort	Depression. Anxiety. Sleep disturbances.	Interacts with many medications, especially antidepressants (e.g., serotonin syndrome), oral contraceptives, cyclosporine, digoxin, warfarin, phenytoin, phenobarbital.
Kava-kava	Sleeping aid. Stress reliever. Muscle relaxant.	May potentiate sedation when taken in conjunction with sedative-hypnotic agents. Hepatotoxicity; sales restricted in some countries after case reports of hepatotoxicity.
Garlic	Infections. Hypertension. Colic. Cancer.	Contact dermatitis. Gastroenteritis. Nausea/vomiting. Possesses antiplatelet effects; may interfere with antiplatelet or anticoagulation medications by increasing risk of bleeding.

1. A child presents to the ED lethargic and hypotensive and is suspected to have consumed antifreeze. What treatment would likely be indicated?
   a. Gastric decontamination.
   b. Fomepizole.
   c. Hemodialysis.
   d. Sodium bicarbonate.

Answer: **B**

Fomepizole is indicated for known or suspected ethylene glycol or methyl alcohol intoxication to inhibit alcohol dehydrogenase production, a source of significant toxicity. Antifreeze is most likely an ethylene glycol exposure and is often ingested by toddlers because of its attractive color and sweet taste. Gastric decontamination is not indicated. Hemodialysis can be considered if prolonged fomepizole treatment is needed and persistent acidosis develops. Sodium bicarbonate administration is increasingly debated.

2. A teenager is found unconscious after attending a party and is suspected to have been intoxicated. Which one of the following laboratory tests requires frequent monitoring?
   a. Glucose.
   b. Liver function.
   c. Methanol levels.
   d. Electrolytes.

Answer: **A**

Ethanol intoxication can cause profound hypoglycemia, and is often delayed in presentation. Liver function tests also require intermittent monitoring, but not with the same frequency as glucose. Methanol is a different type of alcohol than ethanol. Electrolytes need frequent monitoring only in the presence of persistent vomiting and diarrhea.

3. Which of the following is the most effective treatment of acetaminophen overdose?
   a. Whole-bowel irrigation.
   b. NAC.
   c. Hemodialysis.
   d. Syrup of ipecac.

Answer: **B**

NAC is the antidote for an acetaminophen overdose, and other therapies are usually not warranted. There is an algorithm that assists in determining if treatment with NAC is indicated. AC can also be used if administered soon after the ingestion (ideally <1 hour after the ingestion).

4. A child ingested a toxic amount of acetaminophen. What is the peak time for the effects of this toxicity to develop?
   a. Immediately.
   b. Within 24 hours.
   c. 24 to 48 hours.
   d. >72 hours.

Answer: **D**

The peak toxicity for an acetaminophen overdose occurs at 72 hours postingestion. In severe cases, encephalopathy, liver failure, coagulopathy, and even death may occur.

5. Which of the following best describes the course of acetaminophen toxicity?
   a. Delayed onset, slow progression.
   b. Rapid onset, rapid progression.
   c. Variable progression.
   d. Slow onset, rapid progression.

Answer: **A**

The clinical course of acetaminophen overdose is a delayed onset with a slow progression. Initial symptoms of acetaminophen toxicity are nonspecific, including malaise and nausea. Peak hepatotoxicity, leading to hepatocellular necrosis and liver failure in some patients, occurs between 72 and 96 hours after the ingestion.

6. At a preoperative evaluation visit, a teenager discloses his use of ginkgo biloba to improve his mental acuity. Discontinuing the gingko biloba prior to surgery is recommended due to which of the following risks associated with its use?
   a. Interactions with inhaled anesthetics.
   b. Anemia.
   c. Increased bleeding risks.
   d. Hyperkalemia.

Answer: **C**

Discontinuation of gingko biloba prior to surgery is recommended due to the potential for increasing bleeding risks. Interactions with inhaled anesthetics, anemia, and hyperkalemia have not been associated with gingko biloba use.

7. Which of the following is a limitation to the use of herbal supplements in the pediatric population?
   a. Lack of government regulation.
   b. Poor availability to the public.
   c. Increased bleeding risks.
   d. Useful only in juvenile idiopathic arthritis.

Answer: **A**

(continues on page 382)

Use of herbal supplementation is not uncommon in pediatrics. Use of these agents is influenced by word of mouth, chronic medical problems, skepticism or lack of results from traditional medications, and dissatisfaction with current regimen. It has been estimated that as many as 20% to 40% of children and adolescents take dietary or herbal supplements.

8. Which of the following factors can increase the incidence of lactic acidosis with metformin overdose?
    a. Prior ingestion of metformin.
    b. Preexisting renal insufficiency.
    c. Isolated cardiac pathology.
    d. Preexisting hypoglycemic state.

Answer: **B**

Preexisting renal insufficiency can increase incidence of lactic acidosis with metformin overdose because of its primary renal excretion (90% eliminated unchanged in the urine). Metformin should not be administered to a child with renal function under the normal limit for age. Measure baseline renal function annually when treating patients with this medication.

9. Which of the following laboratory studies is needed to evaluate a patient with a metformin overdose?
    a. CBC with differential and C-reactive protein.
    b. Hepatic function panel and pyruvate level.
    c. Lactic acid level and pH level.
    d. Insulin level and serum sodium level.

Answer: **C**

Metformin reduces blood glucose by reducing the absorption of glucose from the GI tract, decreasing hepatic gluconeogenesis, and increasing peripheral glucose utilization. Lactic acidosis is a well-described occurrence in metformin overdose, though the mechanism of hyperlactemia in toxicity is not well understood.

10. What are the most common symptoms associated with a calcium channel blocker ingestion?
    a. Hypertension, tachycardia, agitation.
    b. Tachypnea, fever, excessive salivation.
    c. Hypotension, bradycardia, altered mental status.
    d. Laryngospasm, constipation, coma.

Answer: **C**

Calcium channel blocking agents (e.g., amlodipine, verapamil, diltiazem) bind to the L-type, slow channels in cell membranes. This results in reduced inflow of calcium into the cell and inhibition of depolarization of pacemaker cells and produces relaxation of coronary smooth muscle vasculature. Side effects of calcium channel blocking agent toxicity include hypotension, bradycardia, bradydysrhythmias, ileus, seizure, coma, and noncardiogenic pulmonary edema.

11. A 2-year-old boy arrives at the ED after being found with an open bottle of his caregiver's prescription metoprolol. The caregiver did not see anything in his mouth, but he was "chewing something" when she walked into the room. She called his parents, who told her to take him to the ED. Upon further questioning, she reveals she refilled her metoprolol prescription "a few weeks ago" but did not remember how many pills were left before the child opened the bottle. She hands you the bottle with nine pills left. Which of the following is your first step?
    a. Administer AC (1 g/kg) via nasogastric tube.
    b. Call the pharmacy where the prescription was refilled and find out the exact date it was last refilled.
    c. Assess the child's airway, breathing, and circulation.
    d. Administer 20 cc/kg normal saline bolus.

Answer: **C**

After a known or suspected ingestion, the first step is to assess the patient's airway, breathing, and circulation to ensure emergency interventions are not indicated. Ingestion of metoprolol, a β-blocker antihypertensive agent, is commonly associated with hypotension, bradycardia, bronchospasm, and death.

12. A 4-year-old presents to the ED with her mother, who states, "I think she took some of my propranolol." The child told her mother that she "didn't like the candy" in her mother's purse approximately 30 minutes prior to presentation. The mother then discovered that 3 to 4 of her 60-mg extended-release tablets were missing from her prescription bottle. Your first assessment of the child reveals an awake, alert girl in no apparent distress, with a heart rate of 103 beats per minute and a blood pressure of 95/48 mmHg. Knowing that this child most likely ingested some propranolol tablets, which of the following is the next step in your management plan?
    a. Obtain an EKG.
    b. Administer AC (1 g/kg) either by mouth or via nasogastric tube.
    c. Obtain serum electrolytes.
    d. Administer 20 cc/kg normal saline bolus.

Answer: **B**

Rationale: After assuring that the patient's airway, breathing, and circulation are stable, the next step is to administer AC based on the time frame provided by the child's mother. AC is most effective when administered soon after the ingestion, ideally <1 hour after the ingestion.

13. When evaluating a child with altered mental status, a pungent garlic odor is noted on his breath. This child has most likely ingested which of the following agents?
    a. β-Blocker.
    b. Opioid.
    c. Ginseng.
    d. Organophosphate.

Answer: **D**

Organophosphate ingestions often result in a pungent garlic body odor after ingestion.

14. A 13-year-old boy presents to the ED with confusion, drowsiness, slurred speech, and nausea. His vital signs are normal for his age, he has no signs of respiratory depression, and he has the ability to protect his airway. He states that he found a handful of pills that belonged to a friend and took them. What is the most likely class of medication ingested?
    a. Opioid.
    b. Benzodiazepine.
    c. β-Blocker.
    d. Neuraminidase inhibitor.

Answer: **B**

Benzodiazepine ingestion causes CNS depression, including confusion, drowsiness, and slurred speech. Respiratory depression is uncommon, especially in mild to moderate toxicity. It is not uncommon for vital signs to be within normal parameters. Narcotic ingestions have a higher likelihood of causing respiratory depression. β-Blockers cause bradycardia, hypotension, arrhythmias, hypoglycemia, and hypothermia. Neuraminidase inhibitors are associated with nausea and vomiting.

15. A 6-year-old girl is brought to the ED by her mother, who states that she swallowed an unknown amount of a family member's lorazepam. The patient is drowsy, but able to answer questions appropriately. She has a cough and a gag. Vital signs include a heart rate of 90 beats per minute, respiratory rate of 18 breaths per minute, blood pressure of 65/40 mmHg. Which of the following interventions is indicated first in the management of this patient?
    a. Administer flumazenil.
    b. Administer 20 mL/kg normal saline bolus.
    c. Administer AC.
    d. Intubate for respiratory depression.

Answer: **B**

Administer a bolus for hypotension. Flumazenil is only indicated in iatrogenic oversedation or respiratory depression. AC is generally indicated with co-ingestions and more severe symptoms. This patient is not exhibiting signs of respiratory depression or inability to protect her airway, so she should not be intubated at this time.

16. When admitting a 10-year-old patient with mild benzodiazepine toxicity, which of the following clinical presentations would you anticipate?
    a. Bradycardia, hypotension, tachypnea, irritability, liver failure.
    b. Respiratory depression, inability to protect airway, comatose, bradycardia, hypotension.
    c. Confusion, fatigue, ataxia, nausea, normal vital signs.
    d. Tachycardia, tachypnea, hypertension, diaphoresis.

Answer: **C**

CNS depression, including drowsiness, fatigue, memory loss, ataxia, and slurred speech, is the hallmark symptom of benzodiazepine toxicity. Vital signs are generally normal for age with mild benzodiazepine toxicity. Respiratory depression rarely occurs and only in severe toxicity.

17. A 15-year-old boy is brought to the ED by family members with complaints of headache, nausea, and dizziness. He reports that after school he was working in the garage with a kerosene heater to keep warm. Which of the following is the most appropriate diagnostic test for this adolescent?
    a. Chest radiography.
    b. Arterial blood gas analysis.
    c. A 12-lead EKG.
    d. CT of head.

Answer: **B**

The arterial blood gas analysis will provide the CO level to confirm presence of toxic levels of COHb in this adolescent with exposure to kerosene gas in a closed space. A normal COHb level is <2% in an otherwise healthy nonsmoker. Chest radiography is generally not required unless there is respiratory deterioration or requirement for intubation. A 12-lead EKG and CT of the head are generally not needed in the initial evaluation of CO poisoning.

18. A 17-year-old girl is brought to the ED with confirmed CO poisoning. Her presenting arterial blood gas measurements are pH 7.15, $Paco_2$ 80, Pao_2 85, bicarbonate 18 mEq/L, and COHb of 35%. She is somnolent, with a respiratory rate of 10 breaths per minute on a nasal cannula at 2 L per minute. What is the most appropriate intervention?
    a. Place her on a non-rebreather face mask.
    b. Transport her on nasal cannula $oxygen_2$ to hyperbaric O_2 treatment tank.
    c. Immediate endotracheal intubation.
    d. Administer sodium bicarbonate 50 mEq IV.

Answer: **C**

CO causes severe lethargy. A low respiratory rate and blood gas that indicates acidosis and hypercarbia are evidence that the adolescent is in respiratory failure and requires intubation prior to hyperbaric oxygen therapy.

19. A 3-year-old arrives to the ED with multiple episodes of emesis after drinking lamp oil he found in the garage. Which of the following is this child most at risk for developing?
    a. Gastritis.
    b. Aspiration pneumonitis.
    c. Dehydration.
    d. Renal insufficiency.

Answer: **B**

Vomiting, in conjunction with a hydrocarbon ingestion, places this patient at a high risk of developing aspiration pneumonitis. The thinner viscosity of the lamp oil can make it easier for it to be distributed into smaller airways, increasing the risk of more diffuse disease.

20. Which of the following is a muscarinic symptom of cholinergic excess?
    a. Weakness.
    b. Constipation.

(continues on page 384)

c. Lacrimation.
d. Mydriasis.

Answer: **C**

Muscarinic symptoms of cholinergic excess include salivation, lacrimation, urination, defecation, GI cramps, and emesis (mnemonic = SLUDGE).

CASE STUDY

A 3-year-old boy is brought to the ED by his grandmother after she had difficulty awakening him from his afternoon nap. He was acting normally that day, with no illness symptoms or sick contacts. When asked about the events of the day, the grandmother noted that the child had been playing with her purse, which contained her medications, including clonidine for hypertension.

The boy's vital signs on presentation included a heart rate of 100 beats per minute, respiratory rate of 19 breaths per minute, blood pressure of 75/40 mmHg, oxygen saturation of 96% on room air. He is sleeping, but easily arousable on examination.

---

21. What would be the first step in managing this child after ensuring that his respiratory status is stable?
    a. A 12-lead EKG.
    b. Chest radiography.
    c. Normal saline bolus 20 mL/kg.
    d. Head CT.

Answer: **C**

The patient's blood pressure is below the 5th percentile for age. With the possibility of a clonidine ingestion, the blood pressure should be treated aggressively because of the risk of deterioration if not addressed promptly.

22. What symptoms can be anticipated when a child experiences an accidental clonidine ingestion?
    a. Bradycardia, CNS depression.
    b. Bradycardia, hyperactivity.
    c. Tachycardia, CNS depression.
    d. Tachycardia, hyperactivity.

Answer: **A**

The most commonly noted symptoms of clonidine overdose include bradycardia, hypotension, CNS depression, and respiratory depression.

23. The majority of pediatric poisonings occur in which location?
    a. School.
    b. Friend's house.
    c. Home/residence.
    d. Grandparent's home/extended family residence.

Answer: **C**

The overwhelming majority of pediatric poisonings occur in the child's home/residence.

24. When managing an adolescent after an acetaminophen ingestion, which of the following serial laboratory studies will be obtained?
    a. Liver function test.
    b. Renal function panel.
    c. Arterial blood gas analysis.
    d. Cardiac troponin test.

Answer: **A**

Many laboratory tests will be needed when evaluating a child after a significant acetaminophen ingestion; however, acetaminophen is metabolized in the liver and toxic ingestions lead to hepatocellular injury and liver failure. Serial liver function tests are needed to monitor trends to determine the course of therapy and overall patient plan.

25. When discussing complementary medicine strategies with an adolescent who consumes three to four cola beverages per day, you recommend avoiding which of the following complementary therapies?
    a. Gingko biloba.
    b. Ginseng.
    c. St. John's wort.
    d. Peppermint oil.

Answer: **B**

Due to its stimulant effects, it is recommended that ginseng not be combined with caffeine.

26. An adolescent presents to the ED with an intentional acetaminophen overdose. He ingested acetaminophen off and on from 2 p.m. to 3:30 p.m. and presented to the hospital at 4 p.m. What time should the first acetaminophen level be obtained?
    a. 4 p.m.
    b. 5 p.m.
    c. 6 p.m.
    d. 7 p.m.

Answer: **C**

An acetaminophen level should be drawn 4 hours from the initial ingestion of the medication. In this case, the ingestion began at 2 p.m., so 4 hours later is 6 p.m. If the history is unreliable, an acetaminophen level may be warranted immediately upon presentation.

27. A child presents to the ED several hours after ingesting a significant amount of cold and flu medication in a suicide attempt. You anticipate administering which of the following therapies?
    a. NAC.
    b. Flumazenil.
    c. AC.
    d. Calcium gluconate.

Answer: **A**

Many over-the-counter cough, cold, and pain reliever medications contain acetaminophen. An ingestion of a toxic amount of acetaminophen results in a depletion of bodily stores of glutathione and resultant excess metabolism into toxic substances, resulting in hepatocellular necrosis and liver failure. Acetaminophen toxicity is treated with NAC.

CASE STUDY

A 3-year-old girl is brought to the ED with seizure-like activity. She was found playing with an insecticide container earlier in the day on the family farm, but was not suspected of drinking the solution. On examination, her heart rate is 140 beats per minute, blood pressure 125/85 mmHg, temperature 37°C, respiratory rate 36 breaths per minute, and oxygen saturation 90% on room air. Her pupils are pinpoint and bilaterally equal in size. She is unresponsive to painful stimuli, has copious oral secretions, and has diffuse wheezing bilaterally. She was also incontinent of urine. During the evaluation, the child experiences a generalized tonic–clonic seizure. You suspect organophosphate poisoning and administer one dose of lorazepam (Ativan) to stop the seizure activity.

28. In addition to giving lorazepam, which of the following is the next best step in evaluation and treatment of this child?
a. Obtain an emergent head CT and EEG.
b. Give a single dose of pralidoxime, but atropine is contraindicated in presence of tachycardia.
c. Administer atropine in repeated doses until there is improvement in bronchial secretions.
d. Consult a toxicologist and wait for his or her recommendations.

Answer: **C**

Administer atropine in repeated doses until there is improvement in bronchial secretions. Bradycardia commonly occurs with organophosphate poisoning secondary to cholinergic excess at muscarinic receptors. However, because of nicotinic effects, there can be either tachycardia or bradycardia. Atropine is required to reverse the muscarinic effects. Often, large doses of atropine are required and are tailored to drying of secretions. Head CT and EEG can be considered to evaluate for head trauma and other causes of seizures. However, with the high suspicion of organophosphate toxicity, treatment with atropine to manage secretions takes precedence.

29. Which of the following antidotes used for organophosphate poisoning will prevent aging of cholinesterase?
a. Atropine.
b. Ativan.
c. Pralidoxime.
d. Succinylcholine.

Answer: **C**

Organophosphates bind to and inactivate acetylcholinesterase. Over time, the enzyme becomes phosphorylated, a process referred to as aging. Pralidoxime works by preventing aging and reactivating the enzyme. Atropine is indicated in organophosphate poisonings; however, it does not impact cholinesterase aging.

30. A 16-year-old girl presents to the ED after taking an undisclosed amount of unidentified tablets in the home. Her symptoms of gastric upset, hematemesis, and tinnitus support an ingestion of which of the following agents?
a. Acetaminophen.
b. Camphor.
c. Dextromethorphan.
d. Salicylate.

Answer: **D**

Salicylate ingestions commonly present with findings of nausea, vomiting, hematemesis, gastric pain, tinnitus or changes in hearing, tachypnea, tachycardia, dehydration, and fever. Severe salicylate ingestions are also associated with metabolic acidosis, seizures, delirium, coma, and death.

CASE STUDY

A 15-year-old girl lives with her mother and is normally a "straight A student." Her mother notices that she has not been acting like herself since she woke up this morning, dressing inappropriately after a shower. She complains that her mother took her cell phone, even though it is on her dresser. When her mother tries to talk to her, she has a generalized tonic–clonic seizure lasting approximately 5 minutes. The mother calls the emergency medical service and the girl is taken to the hospital. In ED, she is noted to have a temperature of 37°C, heart rate of 140 beats per minute, blood pressure of 130/90 mmHg, respiratory rate of 18 breaths per minute, and an oxygen saturation of 100% on room air. She is agitated and speaking incoherently. Her pupils are 7 mm bilaterally equal and not reactive to light. Her mucous membranes are dry. No focal neurologic deficits are noted. Her mother reports that she gives herbal products like yerba mate and Echinacea to keep the patient healthy. Urine and serum drug screens, including a TCA screen, are negative. The EKG demonstrates a prolonged QTc interval, but is otherwise normal.

31. The clinical presentation is consistent with which of the following?
a. Viral encephalitis.
b. TCA overdose.
c. Echinacea toxicity.
d. Diphenhydramine toxicity.

Answer: **D**

This patient has symptoms consistent with anticholinergic syndrome. TCA overdose is a possibility, but in the absence of hypotension, metabolic acidosis, normal QRS duration, and negative TCA screen, it is less likely than a diphenhydramine overdose.

32. Which study will confirm this diagnosis in this patient?
a. Lumbar puncture.
b. Co-oximetry of an arterial blood sample.

(continues on page 386)

c. No confirmatory diagnostic test is necessary.

d. Lactic acid level.

Answer: **C**

No confirmatory diagnostic test is necessary for this patient's management. Diphenhydramine levels cannot be measured and the diagnosis is based on history and clinical presentation. A lumbar puncture would be indicated if there was history consistent with acute infectious process. Co-oximetry would be indicated if there was history concerning for CO poisoning (e.g., smoke inhalation).

CASE STUDY

A 15-year-old boy presents to the ED following a witnessed ingestion of bath salts. On physical examination, he is diaphoretic and cool peripherally, with a blood pressure of 150/95 mmHg and a heart rate of 125 beats per minute.

33. Which organ system are you most concerned about after a bath salt ingestion?

a. Neurologic.

b. Cardiac.

c. Pulmonary.

d. Endocrine.

Answer: **B**

His symptoms point to a cardiac etiology that could originate from coronary vasospasm associated with bath salts ingestion.

34. To evaluate for cardiac damage following ingestion of bath salts, the initial evaluation should include which of the following?

a. Cardiac MRI.

b. A 12-lead EKG.

c. Echocardiography.

d. Cardiac CT.

Answer: **B**

The initial evaluation of coronary involvement includes a 12-lead EKG to evaluate for ST segment changes. This rapid and noninvasive test provides excellent information about cardiac stain and ischemia.

Recommended Reading

Bronstein, A. C., Spyker, D. A., Cantilena, L. R., Rumack, B. H., & Dart, R. C. (2012). 2011 Annual report of the American Association of Poison Control Centers' National Poison Data Systems: 29th annual report. *Clinical Toxicology, 50,* 911–1164.

Buckley, N. A., Juurlink, D. N., Isbister, G., Bennett, M. H., & Lavonas, E. J. (2011, April 13). Hyperbaric oxygen for carbon monoxide poisoning. *Cochrane Database Systematic Review,* (4), CD002041. doi:10.1002/14651858.CD002041.pub3.

Burda, A. M., Kubic, A., & Wahl, M. (2012). Toxicologic emergencies. In K. Reuter Rice & B. Bolick (Eds.), *Pediatric acute care: A guide for interprofessional practice* (pp. 1111–1134). Burlington, MA: Jones & Bartlett Learning.

Joshi, P. (2006). Toxidromes and their treatment. In B. P. Fuhrman & J. Zimmerman (Eds.), *Pediatric critical care* (3rd ed., pp. 1521–1531). Philadelphia, PA: Mosby Elsevier.

Kruse, J. A. (2012). Methanol and ethylene glycol intoxication. *Critical Care Clinics, 28,* 661–711.

Morey-Mas, P., Visser, M. H. M., Winkelmolen, L., & Touw, D. J. (2013). Clinical toxicology and management of intoxications with synthetic cathinones ("bath salts"). *Journal of Pharmacy Practice, 26*(4), 353–357.

National Institute of Health. National Center for Complementary and Alternative Medicine (NCCAM). (2013). *Echinacea.* Retrieved from http://nccam.nih.gov/health/echinacea/ataglance.htm?nav=gsa

National Institute of Health. National Center for Complementary and Alternative Medicine (NCCAM). (2013). *Gingko.* Retrieved from http://nccam.nih.gov/health/ginkgo

Sedation and Analgesia

Sedation and Analgesia

Shari Simone & Lauren Sorce

Introduction

- Managing pain and anxiety in children undergoing diagnostic or therapeutic procedures or to maintain comfort and safety while mechanically ventilated can be challenging.
- Decisions regarding pain and sedation management must include a comprehensive evaluation of the child's acute and chronic medical conditions, emotional and cognitive capabilities, and age, as well as inclusion of appropriate assessment data and comprehensive knowledge of agents and their potential risk factors.

Pain

- Defined as an unpleasant, subjective, sensory, and emotional experience associated with actual or potential tissue damage.
- Classification.
  - *Nociceptive*: acute pain defined as either somatic (e.g., skin, bone, or connective tissue) or visceral (e.g., internal organs).
  - *Neuropathic*: pain due to nerve damage.
  - *Functional*: pain due to the abnormal presence of, or inappropriate activation of, abnormal pain pathways within the nervous system.
  - *Acute*: short lived and occurs with an injury or near the injured tissue due to an adverse chemical, thermal, or mechanical stimulus.
  - *Chronic*: any pain (e.g., nociceptive, neuropathic, or functional) that lasts longer than 1 month.
- Evaluation.
  - Critical to the management of pain in acutely and critically ill children.
  - Tools include self-report, observation, and physiologic-based instruments.
  - Examples include *FACES* and numeric rating scale self-report tools and the *face, legs, activity, cry, and consolability (FLACC)* behavioral scale.
- Agents and reversal (Table 14.1).

- Local anesthetics.
  - Topical.
    - Can be used for minor painful procedures or as adjunct medication for invasive procedures.
    - Allow 30 to 60 minutes for skin penetration with a duration of effect <4 hours.
    - Systemic absorption may occur; monitor for lidocaine toxicity if used over significant body surface area.
    - Examples include lidocaine/prilocaine (EMLA™) and lidocaine (LMX™) creams.
  - Intradermal.
    - Can be used for minor painful procedures or adjunct medication for invasive procedure.
    - Action is within 1 to 2 minutes with duration <1 hour.
    - Examples include intradermal lidocaine and buffered lidocaine 1% in jet injector.
- Procedural pain management considerations.
  - Purpose: use of sedative, analgesic, and dissociative medications to provide anxiolysis, amnesia, analgesia, sedation, and motor control during painful or unpleasant diagnostic or therapeutic procedures.
  - Definitions.
    - *Minimal sedation*: state of sedation that provides anxiolysis.
    - *Moderate sedation*: drug-induced depressed consciousness, but patient is able to respond purposefully to verbal commands or light physical stimulation.
    - *Deep sedation*: drug-induced depressed consciousness from which patient is not easily aroused, and has partial or complete loss of protective reflexes.
    - *General anesthesia*: drug-induced loss of consciousness; patient is not arousable even to painful stimuli.
  - Presedation evaluation includes the following:
    - *Length of procedure*: influences choice of short-acting versus long-acting medications.
    - *Painful versus nonpainful procedure*: influences selection of agents (e.g., choosing a sedative for diagnostic study versus analgesic and sedative for painful procedure).
    - *Location of procedure*: Availability of resources influences choice of agents and number of doses administered.

TABLE 14.1 Sedatives, Analgesics, and Neuromuscular Blocking Agents and Available Reversal Agents

Medication	Dosing	Significant Side Effects
Sedatives		
Midazolam	***Anxiolysis or amnesia:*** *Neonatal:* IV/IM: 0.05–0.1 mg/kg/dose over 5 min. *Child:* IV: 0.025–0.15 mg/kg/dose. IM: 0.1–0.15 mg/kg/dose, maximum dose 10 mg. Intranasal: 0.2–0.3 mg/kg/dose. *Adult:* IM: 0.07–0.0.8 mg/kg/dose. IV: 0.02–0.04 mg/kg/dose. ***Procedural Sedation:*** *Neonatal:* IV/IM: 0.05–0.1 mg/kg/dose over 5 min. *Child:* IV: 0.025–0.15 mg/kg/dose. IM: 0.1–0.15 mg/kg, maximum dose 10 mg. Intranasal: 0.2–0.3 mg/kg/dose. *Adult:* 0.5–2 mg IV. ***Mechanical Ventilation:*** *Neonatal gestational age 32 wk:* IV continuous infusion: 0.03 mg/kg/hr *Neonatal gestational age >32 wk:* IV continuous infusion: 0.06 mg/kg/hr. *Child:* IV continuous infusion: Load with 0.05–0.2 mg/kg/dose. Infusion: 0.06–0.12 mg/kg/hr. *Adult:* IV continuous infusion: Load with 0.01–0.05 mg/kg/dose. Infusion: 0.02–0.1 mg/kg/hr. *Titrate medications to achieve goal sedation.*	Hypotension, bradycardia, cardiac arrest, respiratory depression or arrest.
Lorazepam	***Sedation:*** *Child:* IV/PO: 0.02–0.1 mg/kg/dose every 4–8 hr. *Adult:* PO: 1–10 mg/day divided in 2–3 doses. Preoperative: IV: 0.04 mg/kg/dose, maximum dose 4 mg. IM: 0.05 mg/kg/dose, maximum dose 4 mg. ***Procedural sedation:*** *Child:* PO/IV/IM: 0.02–0.09 mg/kg/dose. *Adult:* PO: 1–10 mg/day divided in 2–3 doses. Preoperative: IV: 0.04 mg/kg/dose, maximum dose 4 mg. IM: 0.05 mg/kg/dose, maximum dose 4 mg. ***Mechanical Ventilation:*** *Child:* IV/PO: 0.02–0.1 mg/kg every 4–8 hr. Infusion: 0.025–0.2 mg/kg/hr (Tobias, 1995). *Titrate medications to achieve goal sedation.*	Respiratory depression, apnea, bradycardia, and circulatory collapse. High dose or long-term use of parenteral formulation may result in toxicity (lactic acidosis, osmotic gap, and renal failure) as related to formulation with polyethylene glycol.

TABLE 14.1	Sedatives, Analgesics, and Neuromuscular Blocking Agents and Available Reversal Agents (*Continued*)	
Medication	**Dosing**	**Significant Side Effects**
Diazepam	***Procedural Sedation:*** *Child:* PO: 0.2–0.3 mg/kg/dose. IV: 0.05–0.1 mg/kg/dose. ***Sedation/anxiolysis:*** PO: 0.12–0.8 mg/kg/day divided every 6–8 hr. IV/IM: 0.04–0.3 mg/kg/dose to maximum 0.6 mg/kg within 8 hr. ***Adolescent Sedation:*** PO: 10 mg. IV: 5 mg, may repeat 2.5 mg. ***Adult Sedation:*** PO/IV/IM: 2–10 mg/day 3–4 times per day. *Intubated patient:* IV: 0.03–0.1 mg/kg every 30 min to 6 hr.	Sudden hypotension, cardiac arrest, laryngospasm, and apnea or respiratory depression may result from rapid IV push. Use with caution in neonates: parenteral and rectal gel formulations contain benzoic acid, benzyl alcohol, and sodium benzoate.
Etomidate	***Procedural sedation:*** *Child:* IV: 0.1–0.3 mg/kg/dose. *Adult:* IV: 0.2–0.6 mg/kg/dose for *anesthesia* induction.	Apnea, laryngospasm, bradycardia, tachycardia, hypertension, hypotension, and myoclonus. Adrenal suppression may result after a single dose.
Pentobarbital	***Procedural sedation:*** *Child:* IM: 2–6 mg/kg/dose, maximum dose 100 mg/dose. IV: 1–2 mg/kg/dose, repeat 1–2 mg/kg every 3–5 min until desired state to maximum 6 mg/kg. *Infant:* IV 1–3 mg/kg/dose to maximum of 100 mg until asleep. PO: <4 y/o: 3–6 mg/kg/dose, maximum dose 100 mg. 4 y/o: 1.5–3 mg/kg/dose, maximum dose 100 mg. *Adolescent:* IV: 100 mg prior to procedure. ***Hypnotic:*** *Child:* IM: 2–6 mg/kg/dose. *Adult:* IV: 100 mg every 1–3 min, total dose 500 mg. IM: 150–200 mg. ***Failed sedation in intubated infants, children, and adolescents:*** 1 mg/kg/hr IV continuous infusion.	Respiratory depression, apnea, laryngospasm, arrhythmias, bradycardia, hypotension, syncope, and angioedema.
Analgesics		
Morphine	***Pain management:*** *Neonatal:* PO: 0.08 mg/kg/dose. IV/IM: 0.05–0.1 mg/kg/dose. *Infants ≤6 mo:* PO: 0.08–0.1 mg/kg/dose. IV: 0.025–0.03 mg/kg/dose. *Infants >6 mo, Child, and Adolescent:* PO: 0.2–0.5 mg/kg/dose every 4–6 hr PRN.	Respiratory depression, severe hypotension, syncope, peripheral vasodilation, orthostatic hypotension, noncardiogenic pulmonary edema, CNS depression, increased intracranial pressure, and histamine release.

(Continued)

TABLE 14.1   Sedatives, Analgesics, and Neuromuscular Blocking Agents and Available Reversal Agents (*Continued*)

Medication	Dosing	Significant Side Effects
	If patient weight >50 kg, dose 15–20 mg every 3–4 hr. IV/IM/SQ: 0.05 mg/kg/dose: range, 0.1–0.2 mg/kg/dose. If patient weight >50 kg, dose 5–8 mg every 3–4 hr. *Adults:* 10–30 mg every 4 hr PRN (variable according to formulation). IV continuous infusion: *Neonatal:* 0.01mg/kg/hr. *Child <50 kg:* 0.01–0.04 mg/kg/hr, titrate as needed. *Child 50 kg:* 1.5 mg/hr. *Adult:* 0.8–10 mg/hr. Epidural continuous infusion: *Child:* 0.001–0.005 mg/kg/hr. *Adult:* Dose varies based on specific medication. *May titrate to effect.*	
Hydromorphone	*Infants >6 mo and >10 kg:* PO: 0.03 mg/kg/dose every 4 hr PRN. IV: 0.01 mg/kg/dose every 3–6 hr PRN. IV continuous infusion: 0.003–0.005 mg/kg/hr. *Children and Adolescents <50 kg:* PO: 0.03–0.08 mg/kg/dose every 3–4 hr PRN. IV: 0.015 mg/kg/dose every 3–6 hr PRN. *Children and Adolescents >50 kg:* PO: 1–2 mg/dose every 3–4 hr PRN. IV: 0.2–0.6 mg/dose every 2–4 hr PRN. IM/SQ: 0.8–1 mg every 4–6 hr PRN. Rectal: 3 mg every 4–8 hr PRN. *Adults:* PO: 2–4 mg/dose every 4–6 hr PRN; may titrate dose to effect. IV: 0.2–1 mg/dose every 2–3 hr PRN. IM/SQ: 0.8–1 mg every 3–4 hr PRN. Rectal: 3 mg every 6–8 hr PRN. *May titrate to effect.*	Respiratory depression, especially in patients with preexisting respiratory conditions. Hypotension (may be exaggerated in patients with hypovolemia), orthostatic hypotension, peripheral vasodilation, CNS depression, increased intracranial pressure, and histamine release.
Fentanyl	***Sedation/analgesia:*** *Neonates and young infants:* IV: 1–4 µg/kg/dose, may repeat every 2–4 hr. IV continuous infusion: 0.5–1 µg/kg/hr; titrate to effect. *Children:* IV: 1–2 µg/kg/dose. IV continuous infusion: 1–3 µg/kg/hr; titrate to effect. *Adolescent:* IV: 0.5–1 µg/kg/dose, may repeat at 30–60 min; or 25–50 µg, may repeat 4–5 times with 25 µg. IV continuous infusion: 1–2 µg/kg/hr; titrate to effect. ***Pain Management (unlabeled use):*** *Adult:* IV: 50–100 µg/dose every 1–2 hr PRN. *Intubated Adult:* IV continuous infusion: 50–700 µg/hr. *May titrate to effect.*	May cause life-threatening respiratory depression and/or hypotension. Chest wall rigidity, orthostatic hypotension, arrhythmia, syncope, bradycardia, and CNS depression.

TABLE 14.1	Sedatives, Analgesics, and Neuromuscular Blocking Agents and Available Reversal Agents (*Continued*)	
Medication	**Dosing**	**Significant Side Effects**
Methadone	***Pain management:*** *Children:* IV: 0.1 mg/kg/dose every 4 hr for 2–3 doses, titrate to every 6–12 hr as needed (weaning may be required with long-term therapy due to tissue accumulation). PO/IM/SQ: 0.1 mg/kg/dose every 4 hr for 2–3 doses, titrate to every 6–12 hr as needed. Maximum dose: 10 mg/dose. *Adult:* PO: 2.5–10 mg interval range every 8–12 hr. IV/IM/SQ: 2.5 mg every 8–12 hr. Iatrogenic narcotic dependency: individualize dosing for patient.	Life-threatening respiratory depression, prolonged QT interval or torsade de pointes, death, cardiac arrhythmias, increased intracranial pressure, and histamine release.
Dexmedetomidine	***Sedation (ICU/Procedural):*** *Child:* IV load: 0.5–1 µg/kg/dose. IV continuous infusion: 0.2–0.7 µg/kg/hr. Use caution with continuous infusions >24 hr as no randomized controlled trial has been done evaluating this application in children. ***ICU sedation:*** *Adult:* 1 µg/kg IV load over 10 min with infusion 0.2–0.7 µg/kg/hr. ***Procedural sedation:*** *Adult:* 0.5–1 µg/kg IV load with 0.2–1 µg/kg/hr during procedure.	Respiratory acidosis, pulmonary edema, bradycardia, sinus arrest, hypotension, and hypertension.
Clonidine	*Child* PO: 2 µg/kg/dose every 4–6 hr; increase over days as needed to range 2–4 µg/kg/dose. Epidural: 0.5 µg/kg/hr; titrate to effect. Transdermal: Convert oral dosing to patch.	When combined with stimulants, patients may suffer serious cardiovascular events or sudden death Hypotension, CHF, and sedation.
Ketamine	***Sedation:*** *Child:* PO: 6–10 mg/kg/dose 30 min preprocedure. IM: 3–7 mg/kg/dose. IV: 0.5–2 mg/kg/dose. IV continuous infusion: 5–20 µg/kg/min; titrate to effect. *Adult:* IM: 2–4 mg/kg/dose. IV: 0.2–0.75 mg/kg/dose. IV continuous infusion: 2–7 µg/kg/min.	Respiratory depression, laryngospasm, hypersalivation, tachycardia, hypertension, hypotension, increased cerebral blood flow, and postanesthetic delirium.
Propofol	***Anesthesia:*** *Child:* IV: 2.5–5 mg/kg/dose over 20–30 s, then 125–150 µg/kg/min for 10–15 min, decrease to goal level of sedation (usual dose is 125–150 µg/kg/min). ***Adult ICU sedation:*** IV: 100–150 µg/kg/min or 0.5 mg/kg/dose, then continuous infusion 0.3–3 mg/kg/hr.	Continuous infusion of propofol in children has led to propofol infusion syndrome (severe metabolic acidosis, hyperkalemia, lipemia, rhabdomyolysis, hepatomegaly, cardiac failure, and kidney failure); not recommended to use this way. Significant hypotension, bradycardia, hypothermia, and respiratory depression in the patient without an artificial airway.

(Continued)

TABLE 14.1   Sedatives, Analgesics, and Neuromuscular Blocking Agents and Available Reversal Agents (*Continued*)

Medication	Dosing	Significant Side Effects
Neuromuscular Blocking Agents *must be prepared for airway management when dosing*		
Succinylcholine	*All age groups:* IM: 3–4 mg/kg/dose (not to exceed 150 mg) *Infants:* IV: 2 mg/kg/dose *Child:* IV: 1 mg/kg/dose *Adult:* IV: 0.6 mg/kg/dose ***RSI:*** *Adult:* IV: 1–1.5 mg/kg/dose	Apnea, asystole, hypotension, arrhythmias, and myoglobinuria. Rhabdomyolysis when used in patients with undiagnosed myopathy. May trigger malignant hyperthermia.
Cisatracurium	*Children 1–23 mo:* IV: 0.15 mg/kg/dose over 5–10 s *Children 2–12 y/o:* IV: 0.1–0.15 mg/kg/dose over 5–10 s IV continuous infusion: 1–4 µg/kg/min *Children >12 y/o:* IV: 0.15–0.2 mg/kg/dose IV continuous infusion: 1–4 µg/kg/min ***RSI:*** *Adults:* IV: 0.15–0.2 µg/kg/min IV continuous infusion: 1–3 µg/kg/min	Bronchospasm, hypotension, and flushing. May get acute quadriplegic myopathy syndrome or myositis ossificans with prolonged use.
Pancuronium	*Neonates and infants:* IV: 0.1 mg/kg/dose IV continuous infusion: 0.4–0.6 µg/kg/min *Children:* IV: 0.15 mg/kg/kg Continuous infusion: 0.5–1.7 µg/kg/min *Adolescents and Adults:* IV: 0.15 mg/kg/dose every 30–60 min PRN IV continuous infusion: 0.4–0.6 µg/kg/min	Bronchospasm, wheezing, increased blood pressure and cardiac output, tachycardia (use with caution in patients with baseline tachycardia or risk for tachyarrhythmias). Excessive salivation and profound muscle weakness. May get acute quadriplegic myopathy syndrome or myositis ossificans with prolonged use.
Rocuronium	***RSI:*** *Children:* IV: 0.6–1.2 mg/kg/dose IV continuous infusion: 7–12 µg/kg/min *Adult:* IV: 0.6–1.2 mg/kg/dose IV continuous infusion: 4–16 µg/kg/min	Bronchospasm, increased pulmonary vascular resistance, hypertension, hypotension, tachycardia, and shock.
Vecuronium	*Neonate:* IV: 0.1 mg/kg/dose *Infant (7 wk–1 y):* IV: 0.1 mg/kg/dose IV continuous infusion: 1–1.5 µg/kg/min *Child:* IV: 0.1 mg/kg/dose IV continuous infusion: 1.5–2.5 µg/kg/min *Adult:* IV: 0.1 mg/kg/dose IV continuous infusion: 0.8–1.7 µg/kg/min	Bradycardia, circulatory collapse, and edema. May get acute quadriplegic myopathy syndrome or myositis ossificans with prolonged use.

TABLE 14.1 Sedatives, Analgesics, and Neuromuscular Blocking Agents and Available Reversal Agents (Continued)

Medication	Dosing	Significant Side Effects
Reversal Agents		
Flumazenil (benzodiazepine reversal agent)	*Child:* Initial dose: 0.01 mg/kg over 15 s, may repeat 0.01 mg/kg after 45 s, then every minute for maximum cumulative dose 0.05 mg/kg for maximum dose 1 mg *Adult:* 0.2 mg over 15 s, repeat 0.2 mg after 45 s, then every 60 s up to total 1 mg. Maximum dose 3 mg in 1 hr	Black Box Warning: High-risk patients (physically dependent on benzodiazepines, repeated doses of parenteral benzodiazepines, overdose, mixed-drug overdose, severe hepatic impairment) may have seizures when flumazenil is used. May result in seizures in patients dependent on medication Patients may experience resumption of sedation after flumazenil has worn off.
Naloxone (Narcotic reversal agent)	***Total reversal of narcotic effect:*** *Infant, child 5 y/o:* IV: 0.1 mg/kg/dose *Child >5 y/o:* 2 mg/dose PALS guidelines recommend 2–3 times the IV dose via IM, SQ, or ET route *Adult:* 0.4–2 mg/dose every 2–3 min ***Post anesthetic narcotic reversal:*** *Infant, child, adolescent:* IV: 0.001–0.005 mg/kg/dose and titrate to effect *Adult:* IV 0.1–0.2 mg every 2–3 min	May precipitate withdrawal. Hypertension, hypotension, ventricular arrhythmias, cardiac arrest.
Neostigmine (nondepolarizing neuromuscular blocking reversal agent)	*Infant:* IV: 0.025–0.1 mg/kg/dose *Child:* IV: 0.025–0.8 mg/kg/dose *Adult:* 0.5–2.5 mg (do not exceed total dose 5 mg)	Administer with atropine or glycopyrrolate to limit salivation Bronchoconstriction, laryngospasm, dyspnea, respiratory arrest, bradycardia, asystole, AV block, agitation, seizures, and salivation.

PO, per os (oral); IV, intravenous; IM, intramuscular; SQ, subcutaneous; PR, per rectum; CHF, congestive heart failure; CNS, central nervous system; NMBA, neuromuscular blocking agent; RSI, rapid-sequence intubation; PALS, pediatric advanced life support
Data obtained from http://online.lexi.com except where cited.

- *Obtaining patient "AMPLE" history.*
  - Allergies.
  - Medications: current medications, previous sedation/anesthetic history.
  - Past medical history: general health, risk factors for sedation, airway problems, hepatic or renal dysfunction.
  - Last meal: NPO status, volume status.
  - Events leading up to scenario: reason for sedation.
- *Preprocedure NPO status:* Table 14.2 presents the generally accepted fasting guidelines endorsed by the American Academy of Pediatrics (AAP) and American Association of Anesthesiologists (ASA).
- *Preprocedure physical examination:* should include airway, lung sounds, heart sounds, and neurologic examination.

TABLE 14.2 Preprocedure Fasting Guidelines

Pre-procedure Fasting Guidelines	
Diet	Minimal Fasting Time Period (hr)
Clear liquids	2
Human breast milk	4
Infant formula or milk	6
Solid food	8

From American Society of Anesthesiologists.

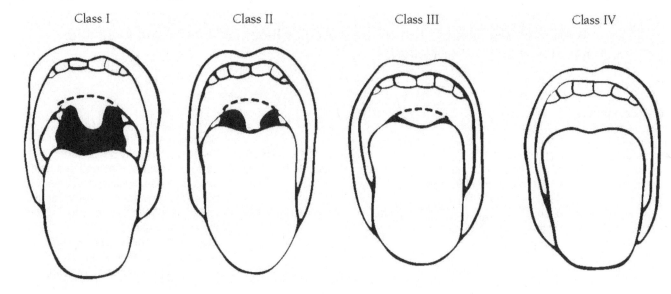

Class I   Class II   Class III   Class IV

FIGURE 14.1 • **The Mallampati Classification.**

- Mallampati classification (Figure 14.1): used in combination with other screening tools to evaluate airway for degree of intubation difficulty.
  - Classifies the size of the tongue by opening the mouth as wide as possible and examining the oropharynx to determine the degree of visualization of uvula and tonsillar pillars.
- ASA Physical Status classification (Table 14.3): categorizes patients based on general health status to determine suitability for sedation.
  - Anesthesiologist consult recommended if the patient has an ASA classification of 3 or has significant risk factors that may result in airway or hemodynamic compromise with the administration of moderate sedation.
- For more information on difficult airway, see Section 4.
- Agent selection considerations in addition to the preprocedure assessment factors.
  - *Mechanism of action of the drug*: primarily sedative or analgesic properties.
  - *Pharmacokinetics of the drugs*: including duration and route of administration. Intravenous (IV) route is usually the preferred route and provides the ability to more easily titrate the medication to the desired effect.
  - *Dose response*: Important to avoid repeated administration of medications before the peak effect of a previous dose has been reached, as can result in an excessive total drug effect over time.
  - Recognize the risks associated with the use of combinations of medications (e.g., the use of an opioid and a benzodiazepine increases the risk of respiratory depression above that seen when either is used as single agent).
- Moderate sedation agents.
  - Local (lidocaine) and topical (EMLA™, LMX™ cream) anesthetics aid in decreasing pain perception and are used as adjunct measures for invasive procedures.

TABLE 14.3   ASA Physical Status Classification System

ASA Class	Description	Suitability for Sedation
P1	Normal healthy patient.	Excellent.
P2	Patient with mild systemic disease.	Generally good.
P3	Patient with severe systemic disease.	Intermediate to poor; consider benefits to relative risks.
P4	Patient with severe systemic disease that is a constant threat to life.	Poor; benefits rarely outweigh risks.
P5	Moribund patient who is not expected to survive without the operation.	Extremely poor.

ASA, American Association of Anesthesiologists

- Oral sucrose demonstrated to be safe and effective in reducing signs of distress associated with minor, painful procedures in neonates and moderately effective in infants up to 6 months of age.
- Single agents are often used for diagnostic procedures; however, moderate sedation for therapeutic procedures is often best achieved with a combination of a benzodiazepine and an opioid.
- Procedure.
  - Completion of presedation institutional documentation.
  - Application of cardiorespiratory monitors.

- Equipment includes oxygen, bag-mask ventilation, suction, airway adjuncts, advanced airway equipment, and resuscitation equipment.
- "Time out" procedure performed by sedation nurse and nurse practitioner/health care provider.
- Monitoring includes vital signs, oxygen saturation, level of consciousness, and pain and sedation scores before and at regular intervals during procedure, including before and after all sedation administered.
- Capnography should be considered for long procedures or when access to the patient is limited (e.g., MRI).
- Documentation includes vital signs, medications with doses and times, supportive measures, and any significant events.
- Discharge criteria.
  - Monitor until patient fully recovered and sedation risks no longer exist.
  - No evidence-based set of clinical indicators exist for safe discharge following procedural sedation, but general criteria includes stable vital signs, pain well controlled, return to baseline level of consciousness, nausea and/or vomiting controlled, and patient adequately tolerating oral intake to maintain hydration.
- Postoperative pain management.
  - A variety of analgesic medications can be used for postoperative pain management and may include nonopioids, nonsteroidal anti-inflammatory drugs (NSAIDs), opioids, and regional analgesia.
  - The approach to management is based on severity of pain experienced.
    - Mild pain: nonopioid analgesics (e.g., acetaminophen and NSAIDs).
    - Moderate pain: lower-potency opioid (e.g., oxycodone), with or without nonopioids.
    - Severe pain: higher-potency opioid (e.g., morphine, fentanyl, or hydromorphone), with or without nonopioids.
  - Patient-controlled analgesia (PCA) commonly used to control moderate-to-severe postoperative pain by administering small preset doses of an IV analgesic medication via a programmed delivery system.
    - Pump activation: primarily by the patient; however, caregiver- or nurse-controlled analgesia may be used in patients who are cognitively or physically unable to activate pump.
  - Commonly prescribed opioids include morphine, hydromorphone, and fentanyl.
  - Epidural analgesia is also frequently used to control surgical pain.
    - Infusions commonly have a combination of an anesthetic and opioid (e.g., bupivacaine with fentanyl).
    - Most common complication is respiratory depression because the level of anesthesia is too high or used in combination with IV analgesia.
  - Adverse effects of PCA and epidural infusions are presented in Table 14.4.
  - Caudal block is a regional anesthetic technique to provide analgesia below the umbilicus when severe pain is expected only for 24 hours postoperatively.
  - Important to incorporate age-appropriate nonpharmacologic pain strategies.

TABLE 14.4	Patient-Controlled Analgesia and Epidural Infusion Adverse Effects and Treatment
Adverse Effect	**Treatment**
Respiratory depression	• Decrease PCA dosing. • Increase the lockout interval. • Decrease/discontinue the basal rate if present. • Low-dose naloxone 2–10 µg/kg/dose IV.
Apnea	• Assist ventilation as needed. • Stop infusion. • Reverse the opioid with naloxone 0.1 mg/kg/dose IV (maximum dose: 2 mg).
Pruritus	• Administer antihistamine (i.e., diphenhydramine). • Consider low-dose naloxone 2–10 µg/kg/dose IV. • Consider changing the opioid (e.g., hydromorphone causes a lesser degree of pruritus than morphine). • Consider adding an NSAID.
Nausea and vomiting	• Administer antiemetic (e.g., ondansetron). • Consider changing the opioid or decreasing the dose and adding an NSAID.
Constipation	• Stool softener and stimulant daily and adjusted as needed (e.g., docusate plus senna or polyethylene glycol).
Urinary retention	• Common side effect with epidural opioid infusion. • Consider decreasing opioid dosage. • Bladder catheterization.

PCA, patient-controlled analgesia; IV, intravenous; NSAID, nonsteroidal anti-inflammatory drug

- Chronic pain management.
  - Patients with a history of chronic pain who present with an acute process require an interdisciplinary approach for optimal pain management.
  - Consider consulting pain (pain team or anesthesiologist), pharmacy, neurology, and psychiatry for optimal pharmacologic management.
  - Consider PCA infusion for acute on chronic pain control and around-the-clock (ATC) NSAID (e.g., sickle cell crisis).
  - Consider ATC opioid combination analgesic (e.g., oxycodone and acetaminophen) or opioid ATC for moderate pain management.
  - If on chronic opioids, patient will require increased doses to adequately control acute pain.
  - Continue adjunctive home medications if possible (e.g., tricyclic antidepressant or anticonvulsant).

- Consider consulting child life, complementary, and alternative medical therapists and psychiatry for optimal nonpharmacologic management.
- Pain management in critical illness.
  - Patients with critical illness are subject to a variety of painful experiences, including invasive therapies.
  - Identification of a desired pain score can facilitate pharmacological therapy.
  - Frequent assessment of pain is required to ensure if pain is present and how the child is responding to the interventions provided. Utilizing appropriate developmental pain scales is critical.
  - Critically ill and hemodynamically unstable children need careful medication selection to reduce the risk of further decompensation.
  - Narcotics are a mainstay of pain management in critically ill children.
  - Integrating parent/caregiver participation in nonpharmacologic approaches to pain is important.
  - Management strategies.
    - Continuous infusions.
      - Continuous infusions maintain steady-state therapy, but must be titrated based on individual patient and degree of illness.
      - May be used in combination with PCA, but assessment of sedation level is critical.
    - ATC schedule.
      - Consider ATC scheduling for critically ill children who have limited vascular access, always assuring pain goal is met.
      - If using more than one type of pain relief medication within the same class (e.g., hydrocodone and morphine), alternate times to reduce risk of oversedation and/or periods of break-through pain.
      - Consider transition to as-needed medications as pain subsides.

Sedation

- Definitions.
  - *Anxiety*: state of apprehension that develops in response to stress and includes physiologic, behavioral, emotional responses.
  - *Agitation*: an exaggerated physical, physiologic, behavioral, and emotional state involving excessive, often nonpurposeful motor activity.
  - *Delirium*: state of acute brain dysfunction characterized by four features: 1) inattention and disturbance in consciousness, 2) change in cognition (e.g., memory deficits, disorientation, language disturbances), 3) acute onset, and 4) fluctuating course. Symptoms may include agitation, lethargy, or confusion.
  - *Risk factors*: 1) *predisposing factors*: psychiatric disease, genetic disposition, chronic neurologic disorders; 2) *precipitating factors*: sleep deprivation, oversedation, poorly controlled pain, immobilization, electrolyte imbalances, and infection.

- Assessment.
  - Assessment is critical for optimal sedation in acute and critically ill children.
  - Sedation tools include *Ramsey Sedations Scale*, *Comfort scale*, and *State Behavioral Scale*.
  - Delirium is not easily recognized in children and can be mistaken for behavioral issues or oversedation.
  - Delirium tools are still in development. Pediatric Confusion Assessment Method is currently the most commonly used tool (see Section 6).
- Agents and reversal (see Table 14.1).
- Procedural or diagnostic sedation is the delivery of sedating or dissociative medications to produce a state of depressed consciousness, with or without opioid analgesics.
- Sedation selection considerations to facilitate nonpainful procedure or diagnostic imaging.
  - Benzodiazepine (midazolam is commonly used): short-acting, anxiolytic, amnestic, hypnotic, skeletal muscle relaxant, with no analgesic activity, useful to decrease anxiety associated with procedure.
  - Barbiturate (pentobarbital is commonly used): long-acting sedative than benzodiazepine, useful for sedation prior to diagnostic imaging.
  - Dexmedetomidine is a selective α2 agonist with potent sedative and analgesic properties; use is increasing but must be administered as a continuous infusion.
- Sedation selection considerations to facilitate painful procedure.
  - Benzodiazepine: For antegrade amnesia and sedation in combination with an opioid.
  - Ketamine: Dissociative anesthetic that has analgesic, amnesic, and sedative properties, useful for sedation for painful procedure.
  - Etomidate: Rapidly acting sedative with no analgesic activity, useful for urgent procedures (e.g., intubation).
  - Propofol is a general anesthetic agent that may be used for painful procedural sedation in the intensive care setting or under the guidance of an anesthesiologist/anesthesia provider.
- Sedation for mechanically ventilated children.
  - Critically ill and intubated children are likely to require sedation during their illness in order to facilitate ventilator synchrony, tolerance of immobility, and reduction of metabolic demands during critical illness.
  - Special attention to kidney and hepatic insufficiencies in relation to the medication pharmacokinetics is important to avoid oversedation.
- Management strategies.
  - Continuous infusions.
    - Continuous infusions maintain steady-state therapy and are titrated based on desired sedation; however, monitoring is needed to avoid oversedation.
  - ATC schedule.
    - Consider ATC scheduling for critically ill children who have limited vascular access.
    - Ensure that the patient achieves the desired sedation score to reduce the risk of agitation or undersedation.

TABLE 14.5 **Pharmacologic Treatment for Delirium**

Agent	Route and Dosing	Side Effects	Comments
Antipsychotics			
Haldol (Haloperidol)	IV, IM, or PO. IV loading dose: 0.15–0.25 mg/kg IV. Maintenance: 0.05–0.5 mg/kg/d.	Prolonged QTc interval and risk of torsades de pointes, extrapyramidal symptoms, hypotension, sedation, dystonia, neuroleptic malignant syndrome.	Haldol is less sedating and has fewer anticholinergic effects than other antipsychotics. IV form has less QT effects. Obtain baseline EKG and monitor at intervals. Obtain baseline electrolytes and monitor at intervals. Must be cognizant of multiple drug interactions and potential for increased side effects.
Geodon (Ziprasidone)	PO: start at 20 mg twice a day; IM can be administered for acute delirium (10 mg).		
Zyprexa (Olanzapine)	PO: 2.5–5-mg starting dose. Maximum dose = 20 mg.		
Risperidal (Risperidone)	PO: <50 kg: 0.25 mg increase by 0.25 mg/wk. >50 kg: 0.5 mg increase by 0.5 mg/wk. Maximum = 3 mg/d.		
Associated Agitation			
Lorazepam (Ativan)	IV: 0.05–0.1 mg. Maximum starting dose = 2 mg.	Respiratory depression, sedating.	May provoke delirium symptoms.
Dexmedetomidine (Precedex)	IV: 1 µg/kg 10–15 min, continuous infusion 0.2–0.7 µg/kg/hr.	Bradycardia, hypotension.	Risk of tolerance after 5 d, must be weaned off.

PO, per os (oral); IV, intravenous; IM, intramuscular; QTc, corrected QT interval

- Consider transition to as-needed medications as illness improves and need for sedation is reduced.
- Treatment for Delirium.
  - Nonpharmacologic and pharmacologic management.
    - Promote normal circadian rhythm—normal sleep, consistent orientation, family involvement, adherence to patient routines, minimal restraints when possible and early rehabilitation.
    - Psychiatry consult guides pharmacologic strategies (Table 14.5).

Weaning Narcotics and Sedatives

- Introduction.
  - Continuous use of sedative and analgesic agents for several days increases the risk of tolerance, dependence, and withdrawal, which vary among patients and can be affected by agent, age of patient, cognitive state, and medical conditions.

- Predominant manifestations include central nervous system effects, sympathetic hyperactivity, and gastrointestinal disturbances.
- Definitions.
  - *Tolerance* is a decrease in a drug's effect over time or the need to increase the dose to achieve the same effect.
  - Dependence is the continued need for the drug's administration to prevent withdrawal.
  - *Withdrawal* is a constellation of physical symptoms that occurs when an opioid or benzodiazepine is abruptly discontinued in a patient who has developed tolerance.
- Strategies to prevention withdrawal syndrome.
  - Sedation and analgesic agents should be weaned as soon as deemed possible based on the patient's improving status.
  - Patients receiving <5 days of sedation agents can be weaned from these agents fairly rapidly.
  - Pediatric patients receiving sedation and/or analgesic agents 5 days are at risk for withdrawal.

- Withdrawal is seen in 100% of pediatric patients receiving opioids or benzodiazepines for > 9 days and will require a slow sedation taper.
  - Sedation-weaning strategies should consider factors such as single versus multiple drug tolerance and total infusion days.
  - Equipotent conversion of IV to oral medications.
- Treatment of breakthrough withdrawal.
  - Tapering adjustments for repeated withdrawal symptoms or if symptoms consistent with oversedation.
- Assessment of withdrawal syndrome.
  - Frequent assessment and aggressive treatment of withdrawal symptoms using pharmacologic, environmental, and nursing care approaches are critical for optimal outcomes.
  - Assessment tools include neonatal assessment scale for infants <1 month and the Withdrawal Assessment Tool (WAT) for infants and children.
- Treatment of withdrawal syndrome.
  - Patients who have received opioids or other sedative agents for 5 days, benefit from switching from IV agents to ATC long-acting oral agents.
  - The most common conversions of IV to oral agents are fentanyl to methadone and midazolam to diazepam.
    - The conversion between these medications must take into account differences in drug potency, half-life, and bioavailability. For example, fentanyl is 100 times more potent than methadone but the half-life of methadone is 75 to 100 times as long as fentanyl and oral methadone bioavailability is approximately 75% of IV fentanyl.
    - Appropriate conversion may be guided by a pharmacist or anesthesiologist.
  - If symptoms of withdrawal are observed during the weaning process, an IV dose of "rescue" morphine (0.05–0.1 mg/kg) or lorazepam (0.05–0.1 mg/kg) should be administered for opioid or benzodiazepine withdrawal.
  - The most common adjunctive therapy to smooth sedation titration and minimize withdrawal is the use of clonidine.
    - Clonidine is an $\alpha2$-adrenergic medication that is available orally or as a transdermal patch.
    - PO starting dose ranges from 3 to 5 $\mu g/kg/day$.
    - Transdermal patch is available in 100 μg and 200 μg concentrations, with peak effect reached in 72 hours and remains potent for a total of 7 days.
    - Adverse effects include sedation, bradycardia, and hypotension.

Neuromuscular Blocking Agents

- Classification.
  - Depolarizing or agonist neuromuscular blocking agent (NMBA) produces muscle paralysis through binding with acetylcholine receptor, allowing for muscle contraction and then paralysis.
  - Nondepolarizing or antagonist NMBA produces muscle paralysis through competitive binding at the acetylcholine receptor site and does not allow for depolarization.
- Agents and reversal (see Table 14.1).
- Indications.
  - Primarily used to reduce metabolic demand, facilitate therapeutic and diagnostic procedures, facilitate muscle control, and promote ventilator synchrony.
- Monitoring.
  - Utilize minimum effective dose to reduce the risk of inadvertent prolongation of NMBA.
  - Identify changes in kidney and liver functions and reduce NMBA doses or change medication to one whose pharmacokinetics are independent of kidney and liver functions (e.g., cisatracurium) to reduce inadvertent prolongation of NMBA.
  - Ensure daily monitoring of depth of muscle blockade to reduce the risk of excessive blockade.
  - Use train of four (TOF) or medication holiday for NMBA monitoring when using a continuous infusion.
    - TOF use of a nerve stimulator delivering four rapid-sequence electrical stimuli to a nerve.
      - Most common nerves used are the facial and ulnar nerves.
      - Desired number of elicited twitches is at least 1/4.
      - Patients who have 0/4 twitches are maximally muscle blocked and may be at risk for prolonged neuromuscular blockade beyond the desired goal.
    - Medication holiday—stopping the NMBA infusion and awaiting for first muscle movement.
      - Depending on the pharmacokinetics of the medication, the time to muscle twitch will vary.
      - Patients whose time to first twitch is outside of known pharmacokinetics of the medication should have the dose of the NMBA decreased when it is restarted.
      - Patients whose time to first twitch is sooner than the known pharmacokinetics may resume the medication at the original dose, provided the goal of neuromuscular blockade is being achieved.

CASE STUDY

JB, a previously healthy 3-year-old with respiratory failure secondary to respiratory syncytial virus (RSV) bronchiolitis and pneumonia, is intubated and mechanically ventilated. He requires central line access to support hemodynamics and administer fluid resuscitation. He has required sedation and NMBAs to facilitate ventilation secondary to bronchospasm for the first 2 days. As his disease plateaus, he is treated with continuous infusions of pain and sedation medications. A transpyloric tube is placed for nutritional support, and he intermittently cries with stimuli and hands-on care. He is extubated on hospital day 8. His sedation and pain medications are stopped on hospital day 9, and he transfers out of the intensive care unit on hospital day 10.

The first four questions refer to this scenario.

1. JB requires pain management related to airway pain from the endotracheal tube. Which of the following agents would best meet his needs?
   a. Morphine.
   b. Tylenol.
   c. Methadone.
   d. Fentanyl.

Answer: **D**

Fentanyl is a synthetic narcotic that works by binding to the mu receptors. Unlike morphine, it is not associated with histamine release, making it useful in children with bronchospasm and those with hemodynamic instability. Careful dosing is required as it is 50 to 100 times more potent than morphine. Methadone is not a good option because repeat dosing is required to reach the full pharmacodynamics effect.

2. JB is requiring a NMBA to facilitate ventilator synchrony. His recent laboratory values indicate an elevated BUN (blood urea nitrogen) and creatinine. Which of the following NMBAs is the best choice for him?
   a. Pancuronium.
   b. Cisatracurium.
   c. Vecuronium.
   d. Succinylcholine.

Answer: **B**

Cisatracurium is a nondepolarizing NMBA. It is metabolized by Hoffman degradation. Therefore, evolving acute kidney injury will not impact the pharmacokinetics of this medication.

3. On hospital day 10, the bedside nurse calls to inform the provider that JB is sneezing, irritable, diaphoretic, febrile, vomiting and has loose stools. Based on this information, the likely cause is

   a. Hospital-acquired infection.
   b. Respiratory distress.
   c. Withdrawal syndrome.
   d. Feeding intolerance.

Answer: **C**

Sneezing, irritability, diaphoresis, fever, vomiting, and loose stools are symptoms of withdrawal. Children exposed to opioids and/or benzodiazepines for 5 days are at risk for withdrawal syndrome, which becomes evident between 8 and 48 hours after the medications are discontinued. Monitoring children for withdrawal symptoms using an assessment tool (e.g., Withdrawal Assessment Tool 1) is critical to identifying and subsequently treating withdrawal symptoms.

4. In addition to methadone, the best choice of medications to use for this child to treat withdrawal symptoms includes:
   a. Clonidine 2 µg/kg/dose every 4 to 6 hours.
   b. Valium 5 mg/kg/day divided every 12 hours.
   c. Clonidine patch 1 mg/kg.
   d. Ativan 0.5 mg/kg/dose every 4 hours.

Answer: **A**

Clonidine is an antihypertensive that has a sedative effect in children and can be administered in either an oral or a patch format. Clonidine provides a nice adjunct to the use of methadone or a benzodiazepine for withdrawal symptoms. It is important to monitor blood pressure with the use of clonidine.

5. The most common nerves used for TOF stimulation are:
   a. Facial and ulnar nerves.
   b. Facial and trigeminal nerves.
   c. Ulnar and vagus nerves.
   d. Vagus and trigeminal nerves.

Answer: **A**

TOF testing is used to measure the degree of neuromuscular blockade with a nerve stimulator. This type of assessment assists in preventing complications of prolonged neuromuscular blockade and allows for minimal medication administration. The facial and ulnar nerves are most commonly used for TOF evaluation.

6. When converting IV fentanyl to oral methadone, the most important information to remember is:
   a. Methadone has a much shorter half-life than fentanyl.
   b. Methadone dose is equivalent to fentanyl.
   c. Fentanyl is 100 times more potent than methadone.
   d. Fentanyl has a much longer half-life than methadone.

Answer: **C**

(continues on page 400)

When planning the conversion of IV morphine or fentanyl to oral methadone, it is most important to remember that fentanyl is 100 times more potent than methadone, but methadone has a much longer half-life than fentanyl.

7. A 3-year-old with respiratory failure has required sedation with fentanyl and midazolam continuous infusions for the past 3 days and has been comfortable with stable ventilator settings. Today he is irritable, moving about, opening his eyes, and breathing against the ventilator, with a drop in his oxygen saturations. The most likely explanation for this activity is that the child is:
   a. experiencing dependence to the IV fentanyl.
   b. experiencing tolerance to the current dosing of medications and needs increased dosing.
   c. showing signs of ventilator-associated pneumonia.
   d. showing signs of improvement in status, indicating he is ready for weaning.

Answer: **B**

Tolerance is a decrease in effects of sedation and/or analgesics and is an indication that the medication needs to be increased. *Dependence* is the term used to describe a continuing need for the drug's administration to prevent withdrawal symptoms.

8. Chest wall rigidity is a side effect associated with which of the following circumstances?
   a. Administering morphine intravenously too quickly.
   b. Administering fentanyl too quickly.
   c. Weaning a fentanyl drip by more than 20%.
   d. Weaning midazolam drip by more than 10%.

Answer: **B**

When administering fentanyl by IV push, it is important to infuse it according to the manufacturers' instructions, because if given too quickly, chest wall rigidity can occur, which will prohibit effective ventilation. If chest wall rigidity occurs, it is treated with narcotic antagonists or NMBAs.

9. Which of the following are the most likely symptoms of delirium in a 13-year-old who has been in the intensive care unit for 3 weeks following significant trauma?
   a. Increased need for narcotics for pain, excessive sleep, and inability to speak in clear sentences.
   b. Increased need for narcotics for pain, increased oxygen requirement, and inability to recognize his mother.
   c. Agitation, inability to recognize his mother, and inability to speak in clear sentences.
   d. Excessive sleep, agitation, and increased oxygen requirement.

Answer: **C**

Delirium is a state of acute brain dysfunction characterized by four features: 1) inattention and disturbance in consciousness; 2) change in cognition (i.e., memory deficits, disorientation, language disturbances); 3) acute onset; and 4) fluctuating course.

Symptoms may include agitation, lethargy, or confusion, and in this case, include agitation, memory loss, and inability to speak in clear sentences.

10. Which of the following is a most important process for evaluating and managing pain in acutely ill children?
    a. Administering a developmentally appropriate pain scale.
    b. Using a PCA to administer postoperative pain medication.
    c. Maintaining a cardiac and respiratory monitor to determine fluctuations in vital signs.
    d. Administering pain medication within an hour of a request.

Answer: **A**

When managing pain in an acutely ill child, it is most important to continually evaluate their pain level with the use of a developmentally appropriate pain scale tool. There are many of these tools available and they can be used even in premature infants. It is important to understand the reliability and validity of the tool being used and to use the tool repeatedly through the child's pain experience.

11. Which of the following agents is a general anesthetic that may be used for painful procedural sedation in the intensive care setting and in many states must be used under the guidance of an anesthesiologist?
    a. Etomidate.
    b. Succinylcholine.
    c. Propofol.
    d. Ketamine.

Answer: **C**

Propofol is a general anesthetic that is administered intravenously and can be used for procedural sedation or for short-term support of an intubated, ventilated patient. Rules governing the use of propofol are typically state determined. Propofol is usually considered a drug that must be given or administered under the supervision of an anesthesiologist.

12. Which of the following medications is a sedative with amnesic properties?
    a. Fentanyl.
    b. Pentobarbital.
    c. Ketamine.
    d. Midazolam.

Answer: **D**

Midazolam is a benzodiazepine that is used for sedation and has significant amnesic effects.

13. Which of the following medications is both a sedative and an analgesic and must be administered in a continuous infusion?
    a. Midazolam.
    b. Pentobarbital.
    c. Dexmedetomidine.
    d. Succinylcholine.

Answer: **C**

Dexmedetomidine can be administered alone or in combination with other analgesics and sedatives to assist in achieving sedative effects. It is considered an α2 agonist with both analgesic and sedative properties. Unfortunately, there have been no randomized control trials with this medication in children; so caution must be used as to the length of therapy.

14. A child with an ASA physical status classification of P1:
    a. Is an excellent candidate for sedation.
    b. Is a poor candidate for sedation and must be monitoring very closely.
    c. Is only being sedated because the child will not survive without the surgical intervention.
    d. Has a chronic medical condition that will likely cause complications with sedation.

Answer: **A**

The ASA (American Association of Anesthesiologist) physical status classification scale was developed to assist in determining the status of patients prior to surgery, thus offering information on anesthesia risk. The scale is self-explanatory and the classes are from P1–P5, with a patient that is deemed P1 the most fit candidate for sedation.

15. A 6-year-old has had an extensive orthopedic surgery and is being managed with a morphine PCA pump for pain control. He is stable and comfortable, but experiencing itching constantly. What would be the best option for managing this side effect?
    a. Decreasing the dose of morphine until the itching subsides.
    b. Adding a continuous infusion of naloxone.
    c. Adding a clonidine patch.
    d. Changing the PCA medication to fentanyl.

Answer: **B**

Narcotics such as morphine, especially delivered in a continuous or short-interval schedule can cause significant itching as a side effect. A child whose pain is well controlled should not have the medication changed, but have the itching addressed. Adding a naloxone infusion or administering Benadryl would be two options for managing the side effect.

16. A 2-year-old is being managed on BiPAP (bilevel positive airway pressure) for status asthmaticus with severe hypoxia. He was being given small doses of midazolam to assist with initiating the therapy and keeping the mask on his face. Despite a backup rate on the BiPAP machine, he suddenly has no respiratory effort. In addition to supporting him with bag-mask ventilation, what other therapy is warranted?
    a. Narcan.
    b. Flumazenil.
    c. Rocuronium in preparation for intubation.
    d. Pancuronium in preparation for intubation.

Answer: **B**

The use of sedation agents can result in respiratory depression and arrest. In addition to supporting ventilation, flumazenil is the benzodiazepine reversal agent that should be administered for this child prior to attempting intubation and ventilation.

Recommended Readings

American Society of Anesthesiologists Task Force on Sedation and Analgesia by Non-Anesthesiologists. (2002). Practice guidelines for sedation and analgesia by non-anesthesiologists. *Anesthesiology, 96*(2), 1004–1017.

Anand, K. J. S., Wilson, D. F., Berger, J., Harrison, R., Meert, K. L., Zimmerman, J., . . . Nicholson, C. (2010). Tolerance and withdrawal from prolonged opioid use in critically ill children. *Pediatrics, 125*, e1208–e1225.

Anghelescu, D., Ross, C., Oakes, L., & Burgoyne, L. (2008). The safety of concurrent administration of opioids via epidural and intravenous routes for postoperative pain in pediatric oncology patients. *Journal of Pain and Symptom Management, 35*(4), 412–419.

Arenas-Lopez, S., Riphagen, S., Tibby, S., Durward, A., Tomlin, S., Davies, G., & Murdoch, I. (2004). Use of oral clonidine for sedation in ventilated pediatric intensive care patients. *Intensive Care Medicine, 30*(10), 1625–1629.

Cunliffe, M., McArthur, L., & Dooley, F. (2004). Managing sedation withdrawal in children who undergo prolonged PICU admission after discharge to the ward. *Pediatric Anesthesia, 14*(1), 293–298.

Franck, L., Harris, S., Soentenga, D., Amling, J., & Curley, M. (2008). The Withdrawal Assessment Tool-1 (WAT-1): An assessment instrument for monitoring opioid and benzodiazepine withdrawal symptoms in pediatric patients. *Pediatric Critical Care Medicine, 9*(6), 573–580.

Greco, C., & Berde, C. (2005). Pain management for the hospitalized pediatric patient. *Pediatric Clinics of North America, 52*, 995–1027.

International Association of the Study of Pain. (2007). *Pain terminology.* Retrieved from http://www.iasp-pain.org

Ista, E., van Dijk, M., Gamel, C., Tibboel, D., & de Hoog, M. (2008). Withdrawal symptoms in critically ill children after long-term administration of sedatives and/or analgesics: A first evaluation. *Critical Care Medicine, 36*(8), 2427–2432.

Krauss, B., & Green, S. (2006). Procedural sedation and analgesia in children. *Lancet, 367*(4), 766–780.

Lexicomp Online. (2013). *Lexi-drug book.* Retrieved from http://online.lexi.com

Mace, S., Brown, L., Francis, L., Godwin, S., Han, S., & Howard, P., . . . Clark, R. M. (2008). Clinical policy: Critical issues in the sedation of pediatric patients in the emergency department. *Journal of Emergency Nursing, 34*(3), e33–e107.

Playfor, S., Jenkins, I., Boyles, C., Choonara, I., Davies, G., Haywood, T., . . . Wolf, A. (2006). Consensus guidelines on sedation and analgesia in critically ill children. *Intensive Care Medicine, 32*(8), 1125–1136.

Robertson, R., Darsey, E., Fortenberry, J., Pettignano, R., & Hartley, G. (2000). Evaluation of an opiate-weaning protocol using methadone in pediatric intensive care unit patients. *Pediatric Critical Care Medicine, 1*(2), 119–123.

Siddappa, R., Fletcher, J., Heard, A., Kielma, D., Cimino, M., & Heard, C. (2003). Methadone dosage for prevention of opioid withdrawal in children. *Pediatric Anesthesia, 13*(1), 805–810.

Simone, S., & Sorce, L. (2012). Analgesia, paralytics, sedation, and withdrawal. In K. Reuter-Rice & B. Bolick (Eds.), *Pediatric acute care: A guide for interprofessional practice* (pp. 151–187). Burlington, MA: Jones & Bartlett Learning.

Smith, H. A. B., Fuchs, D. C., Pandharipande, P. P., Barr, F. E., & Ely, E. W. (2009). Delirium: An emerging frontier in the management of critically ill children. *Critical Care Clinics, 25*, 593–614.

Tobias, J.D. (1995). Lorazepam versus midazolam for sedation. *Critical Care Medicine, 23*(6), 1151–1152.

Gastrointestinal Disorders

Appendicitis

Sarah A. Martin

Background

- Appendicitis is the most common reason for abdominal surgery in children in the United States.
- Although it can occur at any age, it is most commonly diagnosed between 10 and 12 years of age and occurs more often in males than females.
- Perforation rates may be as high as 60% in children <5 years of age and 100% in infants.

Definition

- A progressive inflammatory process of the appendix, which is a finger-like structure projecting from the cecum, which is usually located in the right lower quadrant. The function of the appendix is not known.

Etiology/Types

- Appendicitis is thought to occur from the occlusion of the appendiceal lumen with an appendicolith or fecalith (feces which has formed a stone), lymph node proliferation, ingested foreign body, tumor, or parasitic infection.
- The trajectory of appendicitis has been described as acute progressing to suppurative with further progression to gangrenous, and eventual perforation, and finally abscess formation.
- Two major types: nonperforated or acute, and perforated.
- Perforated appendix results in increased morbidity, with the diagnosis often made upon presence of an intra-abdominal abscess on diagnostic imaging.

Pathophysiology

- Initially, there is occlusion of the appendiceal lumen, which blocks mucus and bacterial drainage, causing distension, and raising the appendiceal intraluminal pressure.
- Appendiceal distension causes stimulation of the 8th to 10th visceral afferent thoracic nerve, leading to periumbilical pain.
- Increased intraluminal pressure impairs appendiceal perfusion with eventual gangrene, leading to perforation.

Clinical Presentation

- The classic clinical presentation consists of the report of periumbilical pain with progression to right lower quadrant pain (McBurney point) accompanied by anorexia and eventually vomiting and diarrhea.
- Nearly 50% of children will have atypical presentations.
- A recent systematic review of clinical prediction rules for children with acute abdominal pain concluded that the Pediatric Appendix Score and the Modified Alvarado score were the most validated (Kulik, Uleryk, & Maguire, 2013).
- Common signs and symptoms include: fever (more common with perforation), decreased activity level, point tenderness at McBurney point (anatomic marker for the usual location of the appendix, which is one third the distance along a line from the umbilicus to the right anterior iliac spine), and rebound tenderness related to peritonitis associated with perforation.
  - Rebound tenderness: an increase in pain with the release of pressure rather than the application of pressure.
- Specific signs of appendicitis.
  - Psoas sign—Concomitant irritation of the psoas muscle and associated pain will be present with passive extension or flexion of the right lower extremity.
  - Obturator sign—If appendix lies on the obturator internus muscle, pain may be present with internal rotation of the right thigh.
  - Rovsing sign—Pain reported in the right lower quadrant with palpation of the left lower quadrant.

Diagnostic Evaluation

- Laboratory.
  - Complete blood count (CBC).
    - Leukocytosis with a white blood cell (WBC) count >10,000 to 15,000 cells/mm^3, and bandemia.
  - Complete metabolic panel may be done to evaluate for other abnormalities (e.g., dehydration, liver abnormalities).

- Urinalysis for presence of a urinary tract infection.
- Pregnancy test in appropriate-age female adolescents.
- Radiologic evaluation.
  - Ultrasound.
    - Pros: no radiation exposure, portable, fast, diagnostic for gynecologic disease.
    - Cons: study limited by appendix position, bowel gas pattern, obesity (not recommended if BMI > 25 in adults), operator experience.
    - Diagnostic indicators: noncompressible, fluid filled, >6 mm in diameter, and wall that is irregular or >2 mm thick; following perforation, appendix may not be visible or may see focal periappendiceal or pelvic fluid collections.
  - Computed tomography (CT).
    - Pros: most sensitive test.
    - Cons: exposure to ionizing radiation with potential for radiation-induced malignancies, use of contrast, possible sedation.
    - Diagnostic indicators: Distended appendiceal diameter >7 mm in maximal diameter, appendiceal wall thickening, surrounding fat stranding and a calcified appendicolith (target sign) or regional lymph node enlargement may be appreciated (Figure 15.1).

Management

- Equivocal examination findings.
  - Serial abdominal examination.
  - NPO, intravenous (IV) fluid administration, antipyretics, and analgesia as indicated.
  - Diet challenge as supported by response to hydration.
  - Children with viral illness usually improve with IV hydration; however, children with appendicitis do not.
- Acute nonperforated.
  - Administer antibiotics.

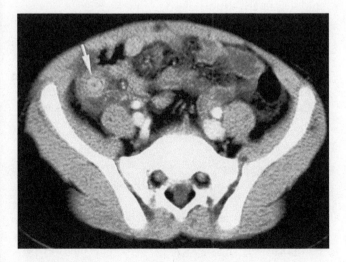

FIGURE 15.1 • **CT Acute Appendicitis.** CT of a 12-year-old boy with right lower quadrant pain shows a thick, dilated appendix (*arrow*) with enhancing walls. There is surrounding inflammation.

- Antibiotic coverage targeted toward bacterial flora in the appendix (*Escherichia coli*, Streptococcus group *milleri*, anaerobes, and *Pseudomonas aeruginosa*).
- Appendectomy.
  - Laparoscopic or open appendectomy.
  - Generally performed within 6 to 24 hours while patients receiving IV antibiotics and fluids.
- Postoperative care.
  - Acute: appendicitis; no postoperative antibiotics.
  - Gangrenous: IV antibiotics.
  - Diet advancement as tolerated.
  - IV analgesia transitioned to oral as tolerated.
- Perforated.
  - Nonoperative management.
    - Antibiotic therapy is generally prescribed for 5 to 7 days depending on patient response. Ceftriaxone and Flagyl for perforated appendix have proven to be adequate.
    - Interventional radiology abscess drainage, if feasible.
    - Consider placement of a percutaneously inserted central venous catheter at the time of abscess drainage.
    - Prolonged ileus may require parenteral nutrition (PN).
    - Interval appendectomy approximately 6 to 8 weeks later.
  - Operative management.
    - If child does not improve with nonoperative management (remains febrile, persistent pain), operative management indicated.

Abdominal Mass

Sarah A. Martin

Background

- Although the majority of abdominal masses in children are benign conditions (e.g., organomegaly, constipation, umbilical hernia), approximately one third of the cancers in children <16 years of age are intra-abdominal in origin.
- Benign cystic masses and the most common malignant abdominal masses including neuroblastoma, Wilms tumor, and hepatoblastoma will be described.
  - Additional information on common malignant tumors can be accessed after registering at the St. Jude Children's Research Hospital "Cure4Kids" site at https://www.cure4kids.org/ums/home/ and in Section 10 (Hematology and Oncology).

Types of Masses

- Benign cystic lesion.
  - Uncommon in children.
  - Types of cystic abdominal masses; choledochal cyst, polycystic kidney disease, duplication cyst, cystic teratoma.

- Neuroblastoma is the most common extracranial tumor in children, age at presentation is 18 months, with the prevalence greatest in children <4 years (85%).
- Wilms tumor is the most common renal tumor and the fifth most common pediatric malignancy, with a common presentation age of 1 to 5 years.
- Hepatoblastoma is the most common malignant liver tumor with a mean age at diagnosis 1 year, occurring in the right lobe of the liver and associated with extreme prematurity, very low birth weight, Beckwith–Wiedemann syndrome, Gardner syndrome, and familial adenomatous polyposis disease.

Clinical Presentation

- Presentations are variable, and commonly, a mass is noted incidentally by a parent, caregiver, or health professional with an asymptomatic child.
- General symptoms include: abdominal pain, abdominal distension, constipation, and anorexia.
- Tumor-specific symptoms: Refer to Chapter 10 for details of malignant abdominal masses.

Diagnostic Evaluation

- Radiologic—After the diagnosis of a mass is made (clinical examination, abdominal flat plate, ultrasound, CT), consider obtaining any additional imaging at a referral center with pediatric oncology, surgery, and radiology to minimize radiation exposure and optimize the required evaluation for the suspected lesion.
- Tumor-specific imaging.
  - Neuroblastoma—CT preferred diagnostic test, coarse calcifications present in 90% of the cases; may detect liver metastases.
  - Wilms tumor—Ultrasound may confirm the site of origin, and a CT is used to better characterize the mass, evaluate the other kidney, and detect vascular invasion.
  - Hepatoblastoma—CT is done to evaluate for tumor extent and vascular involvement. An ultrasound, if done, will evaluate for the inferior vena cava and hepatic veins.

Laboratory

- CBC, comprehensive metabolic panel, α-fetoprotein, serum ferritin, and tumor markers as indicated by suspected lesion. See tumor-specific oncological studies in section 10.
- Pathology.
  - A tissue sample of lesion is needed for diagnosis and confirmation by pathology.

Management

- Benign cystic lesions.
  - Surgical excision as appropriate.
- Malignant masses.
  - Based on staging/grading, tumor size, and vessel involvement.
  - Will include biopsy, tumor resection, chemotherapy.

Biliary Atresia

Sarah A. Martin

Background

- The incidence of biliary atresia (BA) is 1:10,000 live births with approximately 300 new cases diagnosed each year in the United States.

Definition

- BA is absence or obstruction (due to fibrosis) of the biliary tree, (extrahepatic) leading to intrahepatic bile duct obstruction and proliferation.

Etiology/Types

- Specific etiology remains unknown and thought to be more than one type of this diagnosis.
- Davenport (2012) contends there are four types: (1) syndromic BA and associated malformations (i.e., BA splenic malformation syndrome, cat-eye) and random malformations (e.g., esophageal atresia (EA), jejunal atresia, malrotation), (2) cystic BA—cystic change in an obliterated biliary tract, (3) cytomegalovirus-associated BA, in which the infants have positive serology, (4) isolated BA (largest group of infants).
- Proposed nongenetic etiologies: infection, intrauterine infection, toxin exposure.

Pathophysiology

- There is obstruction of bile flow from the liver due to an inflammatory process.
- Fibrosis or scarring obliterates the ducts and prevents bile from being transported from the liver to the gastrointestinal (GI) tract.
- Resultant cirrhosis and the eventual development of liver failure.

Clinical Presentation

- Physical examination findings: jaundice, acholic stool, and dark urine.
- Laboratory findings: Fractionated bilirubin will reveal a conjugated hyperbilirubinemia, elevated liver transaminases from hepatocellular injury, and additional studies may be done to evaluate for other infectious causes (e.g., TORCH infections, viral hepatitis) and metabolic causes of cholestatic jaundice.

Diagnostic Evaluation

- Radiologic evaluation.
  - Abdominal ultrasound: gallbladder noted to be absent or small.
  - Hepatobiliary scintigraphy, in which there is no excretion of the isotope detected in the intestine.
  - Confirmatory cholangiogram is done at the time of laparotomy/laparoscopy for surgical intervention.

Management

- Kasai procedure or portoenterostomy.
  - Best results in children <2 months of age in experienced hands.

- Excision of the extrahepatic biliary tract and anastomosis of a Roux-en-Y limb to the jejunal limb at the porta hepatis.
- The goal of the procedure is to reestablish bile flow as evident by pigmented stool in the immediate postoperative period.
- Deemed a successful operation if conjugated bilirubin level is <2 mg/dL at 3 months postop; long-term outcome is variable with a small percentage of children achieving lasting drainage that is effective.
- Complications: bacterial cholangitis.
- Medical therapy for children with chronic disease.
  - Nutrition.
    - Require 130% to 150% of the recommended daily allowance, and many require 150 kcal/kg/day to achieve appropriate growth.
    - May require formulas with increased medium chain triglycerides as they do not require bile acids for digestion (e.g., breastmilk, Pregestimil, or Portagen).
    - Supplement with fat-soluble vitamins (A, D, E, and K).
    - Supplemental nocturnal feeds with a nasogastric (NG) tube may be necessary for growth failure.
- Treatment of cholestasis.
  - Clinical symptoms include worsening jaundice and pruritis.
  - Pharmacologic therapy: actigal (decreases bile viscosity), questran (removes bile salts), phenobarbital (stimulates bile flow).
  - Bathing and skin comfort measures.
- Treatment of portal hypertension.
  - Hepatosplenomegaly—Patients may sequester platelets with resultant thrombocytopenia.
  - Varices—Collateral vessels from the increased portal venous pressure in the esophagus and rectum. Treatment is controversial and requires treatment of hypovolemia with an acute bleed, administration of H2 blocker or proton pump inhibitor, and endoscopy for variceal banding or ligation.
  - Ascites—accumulation of fluid in the abdomen from increased capillary pressures and low oncotic pressure from decreased serum protein levels (low albumin and total protein). Possible fluid restriction, albumin infusion, use of diuretics (aldosterone antagonist).
- Liver transplantation.

PEARL
- *BA is the most common indication for liver transplantation.*

Cholecystitis/Cholelithiasis

Sarah A. Martin

Background

- There is an increase in gallbladder disease in children mainly attributed to improved diagnostic modalities (ultrasound) and the obesity epidemic.

- Known spectrum of gallbladder disease ranging from biliary colic/dyskinesia, cholelithiasis, acute acalculous cholecystitis, choledocholithiasis, and cholangitis.
- Acute cholecystitis is often attributed to the presence of gallstones; however, there are a myriad of etiologies that contribute to gallstone disease for which the patient may or may not develop cholecystitis or experience an acute illness but undergo cholecystectomy as an elective procedure.

Definition

- Cholecystitis is inflammation of the gallbladder, which is most commonly caused by gallstones. However, there are two types of disease: acalculous or calculous, depending on the presence of cholelithiasis.
- Cholelithiasis (presence of gallstone[s]).
  - Four types of gallstones.
  - Cholesterol—70% to 100% cholesterol; associated with obesity and insulin resistance; most commonly seen in adolescents and adults.
  - Black pigment—calcium bilirubinate (calcium salts of unconjugated bilirubin); associated with hemolytic disease and PN administration.
  - Brown pigment—calcium bilirubinate and fatty acids and are associated with biliary tract infections.
  - Calcium carbonate—related to transient cystic duct obstruction.

Etiology/Types

- Acalculous is most commonly caused by sepsis or a severe infection.
- Calculous from nonhemolytic cholelithiasis; formation of gallstones in the absence of a hemolytic disease.
  - Obesity.
  - PN.
  - History of an ileal resection (e.g., in infants with necrotizing enterocolitis, atresia, volvulus).
  - Cystic fibrosis.
  - Medications (e.g., ceftriaxone and furosemide).
  - Oral contraceptives.
  - Pregnancy.
- Calculous, from hemolytic cholelithiasis; bile in these patients has an increased amount of unconjugated bilirubin, leading to the formation of gallbladder sludge, resulting in an increased risk of cholelithiasis.
  - Sickle cell disease, thalassemia, spherocytosis, Gilbert syndrome.

Pathophysiology

- Stasis within the gallbladder.
- Sludge formation and inflammation that may lead to obstruction and further inflammation in the presence of gallstones.
- Bile stasis and bacterial overgrowth lead to the release of lysolecithin (phospholipid) and other proinflammatory agents, exacerbating the inflammatory response.
- Pain is attributed to the increased pressure within the gallbladder.

Clinical Presentation

- Acalculous—fever, vomiting, right upper quadrant pain, and positive Murphy sign (pain on deep inspiration when the inflamed gallbladder is palpated).
- Calculous—with cholelithiasis—"silent stones" that are recognized incidentally on imaging but without symptoms.
- Range of presentation with fever, right upper quadrant/abdominal pain, positive Murphy sign, vomiting.

Diagnostic Evaluation

- Laboratory.
  - Liver transaminases, bilirubin, and WBC count may be elevated; obtain amylase and lipase.
- Radiologic evaluation.
  - Ultrasound; thickened gallbladder that contains debris; gallstones may or may not be present (Figure 15.2).
  - Endoscopic retrograde cholangiopancreatography (ERCP) can be done to evaluate the pancreas and common bile duct with possible stone removal, if present.
  - Magnetic resonance cholangiopancreatography can be done with no radiation exposure to define and evaluate the biliary structures; however, this is strictly diagnostic, and there can be no intervention.

Management

- Acalculous.
  - Supportive care and antimicrobials for self-limiting cases.
  - Cholecystectomy for progressive gallbladder distension or clinical deterioration.
- Calculous.
  - ERCP may be indicated if a stone is present with common bile duct dilation prior to a cholecystectomy.
  - Surgery may be delayed to allow for resolution of the inflammation.
  - Cholecystectomy; either by an open or laparoscopic technique.
  - Hospital stay of 1 to 2 days following a laparoscopic procedure, and 2 to 4 days if an open procedure is performed.

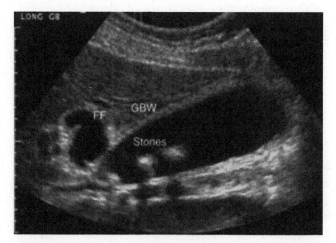

FIGURE 15.2 • **Ultrasound Cholelithiasis.** Right upper quadrant abdominal ultrasound revealing cholelithiasis.

- Discharge criteria include tolerating diet, pain well controlled with oral analgesia, without fever.

Esophageal Atresia

Deiadra J. Garrett

Background/Definition

- Esophageal atresia (EA) is a congenital defect in which there is interruption of the continuity of the esophagus; the esophagus ends in a blind pouch; usually associated with tracheoesophageal fistula.
- EA occurs in about 1 in 3,000 to 4,500 live births; duodenal atresia occurs in 1 in 5,000 to 10,000 live births.
- In 50% to 75% of children with EA, at least one other anomaly is present.

Etiology/Types: Five Types of EA

- Type A—EA without fistula.
- Type B—EA with proximal fistula.
- Type C—EA with distal fistula; most common type.
- Type D—EA with proximal and distal fistulas.
- Type E—Tracheoesophageal fistula without atresia.

Clinical Presentation

- Newborn with excessive oral secretions, drooling, accompanied by coughing, choking, or sneezing.
- Feeding can cause cyanosis, choking, and emesis.

Diagnostic Evaluation

- Failure to pass NG or orogastric tube into the stomach.
- Chest radiograph—anteroposterior and lateral, which demonstrates NG tube coiled in upper esophagus.
- Assess for VACTERAL (Vertebral, Anorectal, Cardiac, Tracheoesophageal, Renal, and Limb anomalies) association.

Management

- Surgery.
  - Separate tracheoesophageal fistula, if present.
  - Establish esophageal continuity.

Duodenal Atresia

Deiadra J. Garrett

Definition/Background

- Obstruction of proximal duodenum secondary to failure of recanalization.
- Associated with Trisomy 21; approximately 30% of patients with duodenal atresia will have Trisomy 21.

Clinical Presentation

- Bilious emesis in the first hours of life.

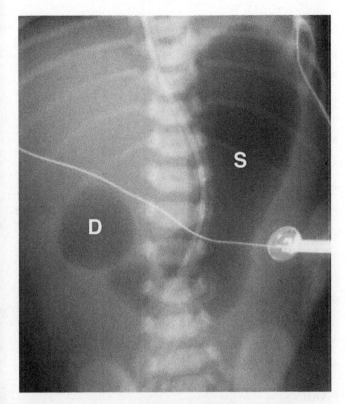

FIGURE 15.3 • **Radiograph Duodenal Atresia.**
Supine radiograph demonstrates gas in the stomach (S) and markedly dilated duodenal bulb (D), producing the double bubble sign. The remainder of the abdomen is gasless.

Diagnostic Evaluation

- Abdominal radiograph—double bubble sign representing the stomach and proximal duodenum (Figure 15.3).

Management

- Surgery.
  - Duodenoduodenostomy (bypass obstruction).
  - Malrotation is treated with a Ladd procedure.

Gastrointestinal Foreign Body Ingestion

Erin M. Garth

Background/Definition

- Entrance of a foreign body into the GI tract via the mouth.

Etiology/Types

- Esophageal.
- Gastric/Intestinal.

Clinical Presentation

- Esophageal: dysphagia, emesis, food refusal, salivation, coughing, choking, gagging, or asymptomatic.

- Gastric/intestinal: typically present after a witnessed or reported event.
  - May present with peritoneal signs if ingestion has led to intestinal perforation.

Diagnostic Evaluation

- Anteroposterior radiograph of chest and/or abdomen.

Management

- Esophageal: endoscopy for removal of foreign body.

Special Considerations

- Batteries/sharp objects—Prompt endoscopy for removal with special consideration to button batteries; can cause mucosal injury within 1 hour. Observe for esophageal perforation.
- Gastric/intestinal: conservative management. Majority of foreign bodies that have entered into the stomach will pass through the intestine.
- Magnets—Ingestion of ≥2 magnets increases the risk of perforation and obstruction. Prompt surgical intervention warranted.
- Sharp objects—Open safety pins warrant removal. All other sharp objects (e.g., glass, straight pins) can be managed conservatively with weekly assessments.

Gastroesophageal Reflux

Lori Stern

Background

- Occurs when reflux is associated with symptoms or complications.
- Risk factors: neurologic impairment, obesity, repaired EA or other congenital esophageal disease, cystic fibrosis, hiatal hernia, repaired achalasia, family history of gastroesophageal reflux disease (GERD).

Definition

- Gastroesophageal reflux: the movement of gastric contents into the esophagus.
- GERD: the symptoms or complications of gastroesophageal reflux.

Etiology

- Primary cause is transient relaxation of the lower esophageal sphincter, which allows gastric contents to move into the esophagus.

Clinical Presentation

- Poor weight gain, feeding aversion.
- Unexplained crying, choking, or coughing.
- Sleep disturbances.
- Gagging.
- Regurgitating.
- Dental erosion (older child).

- Dystonic head positioning (Sandifer syndrome).
- Abdominal or chest pain (older child).

Diagnostic Evaluation

- Upper GI: evaluates for anatomical malformations; not sensitive or specific for GERD.
- pH probe: measures lower esophageal acidity over 24 hours; helpful in measuring esophageal acidity exposure, but does not establish relationship with symptoms or disease in most cases; does not measure nonacid reflux.
- Combined multiple intraluminal impedance study and pH monitoring: measures both acid and nonacid exposure and is superior to pH monitoring alone in establishing a temporal relationship with symptoms and disease.
- Endoscopy and biopsy: not sensitive for diagnosis of GERD, but can exclude other esophageal complications or disorders such as eosinophilic esophagitis.
- Radionuclide scintigraphy (milk scan): not specific for diagnosis of GERD; useful in measuring gastric emptying.
- Empiric trial of acid suppression: Expert opinion suggests an empiric trial of a proton pump inhibitor in the older child or adolescent with typical symptoms for up to 4 weeks is justified, though not specific for diagnosis of GERD.

Management

- Nonpharmacologic.
  - Infants.
    - Elevate head of crib 30°; can use reflux wedge, avoidance of overfeeding, upright position for 30 minutes after feeding.
    - Consider a 1-to-2 week trial of hypoallergenic formula.
    - Increase caloric density of formula, or consider tube feeding if poor weight gain.
  - Child or adolescent.
    - Elevated head of bed, left-sided positioning, avoidance of caffeine, chocolate, fatty or spicy foods, carbonated beverages.
    - Small frequent meals, avoid eating 2 to 3 hours before bedtime.
    - Lose weight if overweight.
- Medical management.
  - H2 blockers are generally first-line choice, especially for infants.
  - Proton pump inhibitors; not indicated for infants <1 year of age.
  - Prokinetic agents can be used to promote stomach emptying.
- Surgical management.
  - Nissen fundoplication—the fundus of the stomach is wrapped around the lower esophagus to improve function of the lower esophageal sphincter.
  - Complication rates are higher in neurologically impaired children.
  - Due to the risk of complications, usually reserved for those children with multiple pneumonia episodes felt to be related to aspiration and those with intractable reflux unresponsive to medical therapy.

Gastroenteritis

Background/Definition

- Acute gastroenteritis is defined as "nonspecific inflammation of the gut".
- Most commonly describes a transient viral infection of the GI tract.
- Can also be bacterial or parasitic.

Etiology

- Viral.
  - Rotavirus, adenovirus, astrovirus, calcivirus, coronavirus, sapovirus, parvovirus.
- Bacterial.
  - *Salmonella, Shigella, Yersinia, Campylobacter, E. coli O157:H7, Yersinia, Aeromonas, Bacillus cereus, Clostridium difficile.*
- Parasitic.
  - Cryptosporidium, Giardia, Enteromonas hominis.

Pathophysiology

- Transmitted via fecal–oral route. Person to person, contaminated food/water, and/or fomites.
- Viral.
  - Lysis of mucosal enterocytes leads to a dysfunctional brush border and causes malabsorption.
  - Some viral infections (e.g., rotavirus) interfere with calcium channels and lead to loss of sodium and water.
  - Stimulation of the enteric nervous system leads to increased electrolyte secretion and intestinal water loss.
- Bacterial.
  - Toxin production by organism. Toxins bind to enterocyte receptors, which leads to increased fluid secretion, loss of water, stool, and electrolytes.
- Parasitic.
  - Organisms invade GI mucosal epithelial cells → villous atrophy → malabsorption.

Clinical Presentation

- History often includes travel, sick contacts, recent antibiotic use.
- Vomiting, diarrhea, and fever are the hallmark symptoms, but all three may not be present.
- Normal bowel movement but with increased frequency and larger water content.
- Stool output of >3 bowel movements/day.
  - Acute diarrhea ≤14 days.
  - Persistent diarrhea >14 days.
  - Chronic diarrhea >30 days.
- Symptoms may also include myalgias, headaches, and/or fatigue.
- Refer to Section 8 (Fluid and Electrolytes) for classification, evaluation and assessment of dehydration.

Diagnostic Evaluation

- Diagnosis can be made from the history and physical examination.

- For diarrhea that is bloody and/or persistent, obtain:
  - Stool cultures, including *E. coli* O157:H7 (shiga-toxin producing strain), consider rapid rotavirus testing.
  - Basic metabolic panel for electrolyte disturbances, CBC.

Management

- Minimal to no clinical dehydration.
  - Manage at home with supportive care.
  - Oral rehydration solution (ORS) for maintenance hydration.
  - Continue age-appropriate diet.
- Mild to moderate dehydration in acute care setting.
  - Oral rehydration therapy.
    - Rehydration (ORS) over 3 to 4 hours + replacement fluids for ongoing losses.
    - Maintenance (ORS).
    - Resume age-appropriate diet as soon as losses have been replaced and vomiting subsides.
    - Observation until signs of dehydration are resolved and caregivers demonstrate efficient delivery of oral rehydration therapy for home management.
- Severe dehydration in acute or intensive-care setting.
  - IV fluid replacement.
  - Stool replacement in addition to maintenance IV fluids.
  - Replacement of electrolytes and buffer if acidotic.
  - ORS via mouth or NG tube once patient is stable.
- Antibiotics may be indicated in certain bacterial infections; *contraindicated* in *E. coli* O157:H7.
- Antipyretics and antiemetics can be useful as supportive care.
  - Do not recommend home use of antiemetics as persistent vomiting would require further investigation.
- Hand hygiene is of paramount importance in preventing spread of disease.

PEARLS

- *Antidiarrheal medications often contain aspirin, which contributes to Reye syndrome and should be avoided.*

Gastrointestinal Bleeding

Background/Definition

- Can be divided into upper GI tract and lower GI tract bleeding.
- Division is anatomically made by the ligament of Treitz (division between the duodenum and the jejunum).
- Always abnormal.

Etiology

- Upper GI tract.
  - Lesions of the GI mucosa.
    - Ulcers (gastric or duodenal); Helicobacter pylori is one possible cause.
  - Esophageal varices.
    - Liver disease.

- Lower GI tract.
  - Infectious colitis: the most common cause of lower GI bleeding is infection.
  - Colonic polyps.
  - Allergic colitis/milk-protein enteropathy.
  - Anal fissure.
  - Inflammatory bowel disease (IBD).
    - Crohn disease, ulcerative colitis.
  - Ischemia.
    - Intussusception.
    - Any lesion that obstructs intestinal blood flow (e.g., tumor).
  - Meckel diverticulum.

Pathophysiology

- Upper GI tract.
  - Gastritis, duodenitis.
    - Nonsteroidal anti-inflammatory drugs use, Helicobacter pylori infection, prolonged NPO status.
  - Esophageal varices.
    - Liver disease with portal hypertension.
- Lower GI tract.
  - Colitis: infectious, inflammatory, ischemic, allergic.
  - Polyps: rarely cancerous in children; most common are juvenile polyps and familial polyposis syndromes.
  - Meckel diverticulum (ectopic gastric mucosa): most common in school-aged child.
  - Anal fissure: associated with constipation.

Clinical Presentation

- Upper GI tract.
  - Hematemesis/bright red blood from gastric tube.
  - Coffee-ground emesis/output from gastric tube.
- Lower GI tract.
  - Melena: hemoccult positive stool with black, tarry appearance.
  - Hematochezia—important to differentiate painful versus painless.
    - Painful: streaks of blood on top of stool or bright red blood mixed into stool.
    - Painless: bright red blood per rectum.

Diagnostic Evaluation

- Upper GI bleed.
  - Hemodynamically unstable.
    - Labwork: CBC, PT/PTT, blood type and cross-match, basic metabolic panel, panel for disseminated intravascular coagulation.
    - Consider urgent upper endoscopy with biopsies to locate source of bleed.
    - Consider gastric lavage.
  - Hemodynamically stable.
    - Labwork: CBC, basic metabolic panel.
    - Upper endoscopy with biopsies.
- Lower GI bleed.
  - Hemodynamically unstable.

- Lab work: CBC, PT/PTT, blood type and cross-match, basic metabolic panel, panel for disseminated intravascular coagulation.
- Upper endoscopy and colonoscopy with biopsies.
- Consider tagged red blood cell (RBC) scan.
  - Must be bleeding briskly for scan to detect source of bleed.
- Infectious stool studies.
- Hemodynamically stable.
  - Laboratory evaluation: CBC, basic metabolic panel.
  - Infectious stool studies.
  - Upper endoscopy and colonoscopy with biopsies.

Management

- Hemodynamically unstable (*upper & lower GI bleeds*).
  - Obtain IV access and administer fluid volume.
  - Initial fluids: normal saline, lactated Ringer solution, and/or packed RBCs (PRBCs).
  - NPO.
  - Proton pump inhibitor; intravenously.
  - Consider octreotide for bleeding esophageal varices; may also require banding via upper endoscopy.
  - Consider vitamin K administration if coagulopathy noted.
- Hemodynamically stable upper GI bleed.
  - Proton pump inhibitor.
  - Treat infectious etiology if identified (i.e., *Helicobacter pylori*).
- Hemodynamically stable lower GI bleed: management is dependent on etiology.
  - Meckel diverticulum: surgical consult/evaluation.
  - Colonic polyps: colonoscopic removal with snare.
  - IBD: gastroenterology consult.
  - Treat infectious etiology if identified.

Hepatitis

Erin M. Garth

Background

- Liver provides many functions in the body, including (1) metabolism of glucose, lipid, nitrogen, drugs, and toxins; (2) Synthesis of albumin and coagulation factors; (3) formation of bile and bile acids.

Definition

- Inflammation or death of hepatocytes. Process can be self-limiting or can cause fibrosis and cirrhosis, leading to chronic liver disease or hepatic failure.

Etiology/Types

- Idiopathic.
- Viral.
  - A—fecal–oral; common in child care centers; contaminated food/water.
  - B—blood, saliva, semen, transplacental; infants especially susceptible.
  - C—mother to infant, blood, saliva, semen (0.1%–2% of children in the United States).
  - Cytomegalovirus (CMV), HIV, Epstein–Barr virus (EBV).
- Bacterial.
  - Sepsis, urinary tract infection.
- Toxins—alcohol, drugs: acetaminophen, nonsteroidal anti-inflammatory drugs, ACE inhibitors, nicotinic acid, isoniazid, sulfonamides, erythromycin; griseofulvin and fluconazole.
- Autoimmune.
- Metabolic/Genetic—α1-antitrypsin deficiency, Tyrosinemia, Galactosemia, Hypothyroidism, Progressive familial intrahepatic cholestasis.
- Steatohepatitis and Nonalcoholic steatohepatitis.
- Secondary to comorbidity—(e.g., cardiac, thyroid).
- PN–associated cholestasis.

Pathophysiology

- Hepatocellular injury can be due to functional or obstructive pathways.
- Viral—Errors in RNA transcription lead to different genotypes.
- Congenital disorders lead to abnormal development or malfunctioning of hepatocytes, biliary tree.

Clinical Presentation

- Asymptomatic with abnormalities in laboratory values.
- Acute or chronic symptoms: chronic condition can present with acute changes.
- General symptoms: fever, malaise, anorexia, nausea, vomiting, abdominal pain, diarrhea. jaundice, joint pains, low-grade fever.
- Physical examination findings: jaundice, hepatomegaly, abdominal tenderness.

Diagnostic Evaluation

- Liver function tests are not true tests of liver function. These tests are indirect markers of hepatobiliary disease.
- Laboratory evaluation.
  - AST, ALT, total/conjugated bilirubin, fractionated alkaline phosphatase, GGT, PT/PTT, INR, complete metabolic profile, ammonia, α1-antitrypsin.
  - Fractionated alkaline phosphatase and GGT can help distinguish if source is liver or other muscle/tissue etiology.
  - Rapid decrease in AST/ALT with increased coagulation and bilirubin suggests worsening hepatic failure.
  - Clotting factors, especially factor V, can help distinguish between liver disease and malnutrition (e.g., vitamin K deficiency).
  - Disease types based on lab values.
- Viral—ALT > AST; peak 7 to 14 days; resolve 6 weeks.
  - A—Hep A IgM.
  - B—Hep B IgM core antibody.
  - C—Hep C antibody or RNA.
- Autoimmune—immunoglobulin >3 g/dL; high protein-to-albumin ratio.
- Alcoholic—AST 2X>ALT.
- Drug—ALT and AST >10, 1000 IU/L.

- Steatohepatitis—ALT/AST less than 4 × upper limit of normal; need to evaluate for other conditions (e.g., infection, coagulopathies).
- Imaging.
  - Abdominal ultrasound with Doppler.
- Liver biopsy.

Management

- Asymptomatic.
  - Serial laboratory evaluation, monitor for symptoms.
- Symptomatic.
  - Supportive care—hydration, bowel rest, trend laboratory values.
  - Severe symptoms of nausea, vomiting, and persistent abnormal values may require hospitalization.
  - Antivirals—if chronic and symptomatic; treatment efficacy depends on genotype.
  - Autoimmune—steroids.
  - Education—avoid sharing toothbrush, razor, personal items with blood.
  - Prevention via washing fruits and vegetables, good hand hygiene.

PEARLS

- *Vaccination is available and part of the recommended immunization schedules for Hepatitis A and B.*
- *A diagnosis of Hepatitis A does not lead to chronic infection.*

Hepatic Failure

Tonya A. Schneidereith

Background/Definition

- Clinical manifestation of acute and severe hepatic injury with many causes.
- Acute hepatic failure occurs rapidly; children lose hepatic function and become critically ill within days.
- Viewed as multisystemic disorder.
- Accounts for 10% to 15% of pediatric liver transplants.

Etiology

- Metabolic—Wilson disease, inborn errors of metabolism, mitochondrial chain disorders.
- Infectious—Hepatitis A, B, and C, human herpes virus-6, EBV, adenovirus.
- Toxic/Drug-induced—acetaminophen, sodium valproate.
  - Drug-induced liver failure is most common cause in the United States.
  - Acetaminophen is responsible for most cases of drug-induced liver failure.
- Autoimmune—giant cell hepatitis.
- Vascular—venoocclusive disease, Budd–Chiari syndrome.
- Undetermined.

Pathophysiology

- Hepatocytes die in large numbers, leading to multisystem organ failure, hepatic encephalopathy, and cerebral edema.

Clinical Presentation

- Varies according to etiology.
- Can include lethargy, failure to thrive, jaundice, hepatomegaly.
- Encephalopathy can be late sign.

Diagnostic

- Liver-specific blood tests.
- In neonates, includes tests for inborn errors of metabolism and viral infections.
- Key is to establish etiology of liver failure to direct therapy.

Management

- Intensive-care management until liver function is restored or transplant performed.
- Care is supportive to minimize effects of metabolic disorders, hemorrhage and digestive tract bleeding, cardiopulmonary failure, renal failure, and cerebral edema.
- Liver transplant if indicated (See Liver Transplantation in this section).

Hyperbilirubinemia

Erin M. Garth

Background

- Bilirubin results from catabolism of RBCs or other heme-containing molecules and from erythropoiesis.

Definition

- Elevated blood bilirubin levels.
- Unconjugated/indirect levels suggest hemolytic cause.
- Conjugated/direct is more indicative of hepatobiliary disease.

Etiology/Types: Indirect or Direct Hyperbilirubinemia

Indirect Hyperbilirubinemia

- Pathophysiology.
  - Physiologic (newborns): increased erythrocyte breakdown, enzyme deficiency, increased extrahepatic circulation.
  - Pathologic: hemolytic anemia from infection, G6PD deficiency, ABO incompatibility, Gilbert syndrome, Crigler–Najjar syndrome, hyperthyroidism; drugs: amitriptyline, ketonazole.
- Clinical presentation.
  - Encephalopathy and seizures (in more severe cases).
  - Jaundice of skin, sclera.
  - Mild lethargy, poor feeding.
- Diagnostic evaluation.
  - Total and direct bilirubin, blood type and Rh of infant and mother, CBC, reticulocyte count, Direct Coombs' Test, G6PD, urinalysis, urine culture.

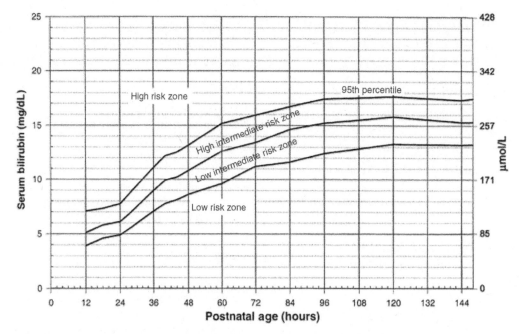

FIGURE 15.4 • **Nomogram for Designation of Risk of Developing Hyperbilirubinemia.** (From Bhutani, V. K., Johnson, L. H., & Sivievri, E. M. (1999). Predictive ability of a predischarge hour-specific serum bilirubin for subsequent significant hyperbilirubinemia in healthy term and near-term newborns. *Pediatrics*, *103*(1), 6–14 , with permission.)

- Neonates: Refer to Bhutani nomogram (Figure 15.4), which estimates risk based on hour of life total bilirubin.
- Gilbert syndrome <5 mg/dL; Crigler–Najjar syndrome >5 mg/dL.
- Management.
  - Phototherapy.
  - Maintain sufficient PO intake (especially in breastfed babies).
- Long-term complication of untreated neonatal hyperbilirubinemia.
  - Kernicterus—Bilirubin-induced brain dysfunction as a result of bilirubin deposition into gray matter of brain.
  - Irreversible.

Direct Hyperbilirubinemia

- Pathophysiology.
  - Anatomic/obstruction—BA, choledochal cyst, gallstones/sludge, Cystic Fibrosis.
  - Infectious (inflammation)—sepsis, urinary tract infection, viral.
  - Metabolic/Genetic (bile duct paucity)—Alagille syndrome, Down syndrome, α1-antitrypsin.
- Clinical presentation.
  - Jaundice, hepatomegaly, acholic stools, fatigue, fever, lethargy, neurological changes.
- Diagnostic evaluation.
  - Total/conjugated bilirubin.
    - Total bilirubin less than 5 mg/dL + direct bilirubin greater than 1.0 mg/dL is considered abnormal.

- Total bilirubin greater than 5 mg/dL + direct bilirubin more than 20% of the total is considered abnormal.
- ALT, AST, GGT, urinalysis, urine culture, blood culture, viral studies—CMV, EBV, hepatitis A/B/C.
- Management.
  - Fat malabsorption—medium chain triglyceride (MCT) supplement (Pregestimil/Alimentum, MCT oil).
  - Improve bile flow—Ursodiol.
  - Manage pruritis—topical emollients and diphenhydramine or hydroxyzine.

PEARLS

- *Physiologic: total bilirubin ≥14 mg/dL; resolves in 2 weeks.*
- *Hyperbilirubinemia in children >2 weeks of age requires further investigation.*
- *Direct bilirubin level ≥1.5 mg/dL → requires further evaluation.*

Ileus

Kelly Finkbeiner

Background/Definition

- An ileus is a nonmechanical obstruction of the intestines.
- It is a disruption of peristalsis that can be partial or complete, results in dilation of proximal intestines.

Etiology

- Postoperative ileus is a functional obstruction seen after most intestinal surgeries.
- Most common cause of an ileus is from manipulation of the intestines during surgery.
- Peritonitis or abdominal trauma can lead to prolonged ileus.
- Opioid use causes a decrease in GI activity resulting in decreased peristalsis.

Clinical Presentation

- Abdominal distension, absent or hypoactive bowel sounds, increased pain and vomiting.

Diagnostic Evaluation

- Abdominal radiograph.

Management

- Bowel rest and decompression with a nasal gastric tube.
- Adequate postoperative pain management with nonnarcotic medications.
- Routine postoperative care to include ambulation and time.

Inflammatory Bowel Disease (Crohn Disease and Ulcerative Colitis)

Kelly Finkbeiner

Background

- IBD is an umbrella term for Crohn disease and ulcerative colitis, which are inflammatory processes of the GI tract with very similar presentations.
- IBD fluctuates between periods of remission and exacerbation.
- The difference between Crohn disease and Ulcerative Colitis is based on the location and characteristics of the inflammation.

Definition

- Crohn Disease: inflammatory process that can affect any portion of the GI tract. Most commonly affects the terminal ileum. The inflammation is in the *entire* lumen of the intestines.
- Ulcerative colitis: inflammatory process that affects the *colon and rectum*. The inflammation is in the mucosal layer of the intestinal wall.

Etiology

- The exact etiology is not fully understood, but both genetic and environmental factors may be involved.
- First-degree relatives of patients with IBD are 3 to 20 times more likely to develop inflammatory bowel; affects males and females equally.
- Most commonly diagnosed between 15 and 30 years of age with a second peak between 50 to 80 years of age.

Pathophysiology

- Genetic predisposition is "turned on" by the environmental factor and causes an excessive immune response resulting in chronic intestinal inflammation. Some environmental influences that may increase risk of IBD are smoking, oral contraception, infectious colitis, or infectious agents.
- The normal GI tract is stimulated, causing physiologic inflammation of the intestinal tract; however, some environmental or genetic factors then cause this inflammation to become pathologic in IBD.

Clinical Presentation

- The clinical presentation for IBD can differ, depending on the intestinal location affected and severity of inflammation.
  - Crohn disease: pain, diarrhea, weight loss, perirectal inflammation with fistula.
  - Ulcerative colitis: bloody, watery diarrhea, weight loss, tenesmus, and urgency.

Diagnostic Evaluation

- Labs: CBC, erythrocyte sedimentation rate, C-reactive protein (CRP), albumin, liver function test, and GGT.
- IBD serology: identifies markers specific to IBD.
- Stool studies for infectious etiology of diarrhea.
- Endoscopy of the intestinal tract with biopsy and histology; gold standard diagnosis of IBD.

Management

- The goal of all treatment is to maintain remission.
- Remission is the clinical relief of symptoms, normalization of inflammatory markers, and normalization of histologic changes and mucosal healing.
- IBD requires a holistic approach to care with all aspects of the patient being considered.
- Mental health must be addressed in relation to dealing with a chronic condition.
- Induction of remission.
  - Corticosteroids are used as first-line therapy for induction and remission after an IBD flare-up. During induction of remission, all maintenance medications are continued because they have the ability to induce remission or help the action of the corticosteroids.
  - Exclusive PN for 8 weeks with bowel rest. This therapy has a similar remission rate as corticosteroids with less side effects.
  - Biologic agents (e.g., Infliximab) are used for severe inflammation or refractory to other treatments to help induce remission.
- Maintenance of remission.
  - Immunosuppressive medications are used to maintain remission because of slow onset of action.
  - Aminosalicylates reduce inflammation to maintain remission in mild UC and Crohn disease.
  - Immunosuppressive therapy should be started while still on steroid treatments; steroids are then tapered.
  - Supplementary nutrition with any treatment. Probiotics are useful as adjunct therapy.
  - Antibiotics have a role in treating perirectal fistula or abscess in Crohn disease.

- Surgical intervention is appropriate for patients with refractory disease, uncontrolled GI bleeding, bowel perforation, or stricture causing an obstruction, with bowel resection being the last option.
- Total colectomy in UC with J-pouch is the surgical treatment of refractory disease, toxic megacolon, perforation, or severe colitis. In UC, a total colectomy can be curative.
- Resection of a stricture or area of colitis in Crohn disease is the surgical treatment. In severe cases when the intestines become perforated, an ostomy is required.

Intussusception
Kelly Finkbeiner

Background

- Intussusception is the most common cause of intestinal obstruction in infants and children. It can lead to intestinal death and high morbidity if untreated.

Definition

- Intussusception is the telescoping of one intestinal segment into the adjacent bowel, which causes an obstructive process.
- The ileocecal region of the bowel is most commonly affected. It most commonly starts in the distal ileum and passes through the ileocecal valve into the colon.
- The telescoping of the intestines can cause the mesentery to be twisted, decreasing blood supply, and causing tissue death.
- Decreased perfusion to the intestines causes sloughing of the tissue, which presents with "currant jelly" stool (late sign).

Etiology

- Incidence is 1 per 2,000 infants/children, with 65% of cases occurring in children <1 year of age.
- Slight increase among white males.
- Lead point intussusception occurs most commonly in children 5 to 14 years of age.

Types

- Idiopathic—most common type of intussusception; most common in infants and young children. Exact etiology is unknown. Association with a recent upper respiratory tract infection or gastroenteritis can occur; etiology is hypertrophy of lymphoid tissue in the intestinal wall.
- Lead point—has an identifiable cause or abnormality in the intestinal mucosa. Most common lead points are Meckel diverticulum. Other lead points include polyps, the appendix, cyst, carcinoid tumors, foreign bodies, hemangioma, non-Hodgkin's lymphoma, intestinal hematomas, and Henoch–Schonlein purpura.
- Postsurgical intussusception—Typically seen after abdominal or chest surgery. The etiology is decreased motility after anesthesia. Postsurgical intussusception should be considered in a surgical patient who is not progressing as expected and continues to have significant nasal gastric tube output, or unexplained pain.
- Recurrent intussusception is possible.

Clinical Presentation

- Healthy, well-nourished infant or child with abdominal pain that can be crampy or brief, and severe colicky pain that causes the infant or child to retract the legs up to the abdomen.
- Emesis and bloody stools, described as "currant jelly" stool, are a late sign.
- Lethargy is a late sign and may indicate that bowel is compromised.

Diagnostic Evaluation

- Abdominal radiograph or ultrasound.
- Air or Barium enema—both diagnostic and therapeutic.

Management

- Air enema or barium enema.
- Surgical reduction—laparoscopic or open reduction.
- Antibiotic administration prior to reducing intussusception using an enema is standard practice of some surgeons.
- Postreduction care for nonsurgical patients.
  - Clear liquids after a short period of intestinal rest and advanced to an age-appropriate diet quickly. Monitor for perforation or recurrence. Observe for a period of time from 4 to 24 hours to ensure no perforation or recurrence. Risk of recurrence is higher after a nonsurgical reduction.
- Postreduction care for surgical patient—Standard surgical care including close monitoring for perforation and recurrence.
  - Surgical patients have a longer recovery period and will require analgesia and postoperative follow-up.
  - Recurrence may happen 24 hours to years after reduction.
  - Average occurrence rate is 10% with approximately 1/3 occurring in the first 24 hours after reduction. Recurrence is not as common with surgical reduction.

Liver Transplantation
Louise M. Flynn

Background

- End stage liver disease requires liver transplantation for patient survival.
- The first liver transplant with extended survival was done in 1967.
- With the development of immunosuppressive medications, long-term graft and recipient survival has been achieved.

Definition

- Liver transplantation—replacement of native liver with healthy liver from donor for treatment of end stage liver disease.
- Donated livers may be whole or segment; donors may be deceased or living (left lateral segment or right lobe).

Etiology

- End stage liver disease has multiple causes.
- In children, the most common disease leading to liver transplantation is BA.
- Other causes include inborn metabolic disorders of the liver, autoimmune hepatitis, hepatic tumors (e.g., hepatoblastoma, hepatocellular carcinoma), Wilson disease, toxin/drug-induced, viral hepatitis, fulminant liver failure.

Immediate Postoperative Concerns

- Rejection.
- Infection; CMV, EBV, fungal infection. Also at increased risk for other bacterial and viral infections.
- Bile leaks: occurs early. Fever, abdominal pain, peritoneal irritation, may note bile in closed suction drain (e.g., Jackson-Pratt). May self-seal, or reoperation may be required.
- Hepatic artery thrombosis: noted by rise in liver functions, diagnosed by vascular ultrasound. Requires emergent reoperation and/or retransplant.
- Portal vein thrombosis: rare, abnormal liver noted, diagnosed by vascular ultrasound, may result in ascites.
- Fluid balance.

Intermediate/Long-Term Concerns

- Infection.
- Lymphoproliferative disease (associated with EBV; reduce immunosuppressive therapy).

Diagnostic Evaluation

- Frequent lab monitoring (with focus on synthetic function and liver enzymes).
- Ultrasound with vascular Doppler.

Management

- Initiate immunosupression therapy (e.g., tacrolimus, cyclosporine, steroids, basiliximab, antithymocyte).
- Prophylactic antibiotic/antiviral medications (Cytogam, ganciclovir, or valganciclovir for CMV; trimethoprim-sulfamethoxazole for Pneumocystis jiroveci prophylaxis; nystatin, clotrimazole troches, or fluconazole for candida/fungal infection prophylaxis).
- Close monitoring for infection (include monitoring of CMV and EBV polymerase chain reaction).
- Fluid management to ensure adequate graft perfusion.
- Anticoagulants (aspirin) to prevent vascular thrombosis.
- Close assessment/monitoring for postoperative complications including bile leaks, bleeding, and infections.

Malrotation/Volvulus

Rita Tracewell

Background

- Intestinal malrotation occurs in approximately one in 500 live births; equally in males and females.

- Approximately 60% of children with malrotation present in the first month of life, 20% present between 1 month and 1 year of age, and the remainder present after the first year of age.
- Malrotation may occur as an isolated condition, but is usually found in combination with other congenital anomalies.
- As many as 70% of children with intestinal malrotation will also have congenital malformations; however, when the intestinal malrotation is associated with volvulus, the anomaly is usually the patient's only disorder.

Definition

- Asymptomatic anatomical variant that occurs as a result of incomplete rotation of the intestine during fetal development.
- Volvulus occurs when small bowel twists around the superior mesenteric artery, resulting in vascular compromise to large portions of the midgut.
- Midgut volvulus may lead to widespread intestinal ischemia and progress rapidly to necrosis of the bowel, perforation, shock respiratory failure, and death.

Pathophysiology

- At approximately the fourth week of embryonic life, the gut begins to change from a straight-line structure to an elongated tube herniating into the umbilical cord.
- The upper portion of this structure, the duodenojejunal loop, develops into duodenum and jejunum. The lower portion, the cecocolic loop, later becomes the terminal ileum, cecum, and colon.
- As the developing bowel rotates in and out of the abdominal cavity, the superior mesenteric artery, which supplies blood to this section of the gut, acts as an axis.
- Upon reentering the abdominal cavity, the duodenum moves to the region of the ligament of Trietz, and the colon that follows is directed to the left upper quadrant. The cecum subsequently rotates counterclockwise within the abdominal cavity and comes to lie in the right lower quadrant. The duodenum becomes fixed to the posterior abdominal wall before the colon is completely rotated. After rotation, the right and left colon and the mesenteric root become fixed to the posterior abdomen. These attachments provide a broad base of support to the mesentery and the superior mesenteric artery, preventing twisting of the mesenteric root and kinking of the vascular supply.
- Abdominal rotation and attachments are complete by 3 months' gestation.

Etiology

- Malrotation occurs when the bowel fails to rotate after it returns to the abdominal cavity.
- The most common type occurs with incomplete rotation of 180° instead of the normal 270° rotation, and involves failure of the cecum to move into the right lower quadrant.

Clinical Presentation

- Presentation is usually in the first year of life with symptoms of acute or chronic bowel obstruction. Infants present within the first week of life with bilious emesis and acute bowel obstruction. Older infants present with episodes of recurrent colicky abdominal pain. Children may present with recurrent episodes of vomiting, abdominal pain, or both.

- Occasionally, patients may present with malabsorption or protein-losing enteropathy associated with bacterial overgrowth. Symptoms are caused by intermittent volvulus or duodenal compression by Ladd bands or other adhesive bands affecting the small and large bowel.
- 25% to 50% of adolescents with malrotation are asymptomatic.
- Symptomatic adolescents present with acute intestinal obstruction of history of recurrent episodes of abdominal pain with less frequent vomiting and diarrhea.
- Patients of all ages, with a rotational anomaly, can develop volvulus without preexisting symptoms.

Diagnostic Evaluation

- CBC, type and screen, and electrolytes should be obtained.
  - Electrolyte imbalances are expected secondary to vomiting and third spacing of fluid into the bowel and abdominal cavity.
  - Pooling of blood into the for intestine causes anemia.
- Flat and upright or lateral decubitus view abdominal radiographs are adequate to evaluate intestinal obstruction. The diagnosis of malrotation cannot be made on plain films alone.
- An upper GI (UGI) series is the preferred study to evaluate the position of the ligament of Trietz.
  - If malrotation exists, UGI will show abnormal position of the ligament of Trietz, partial obstruction of the duodenum, with a spiral or corkscrew appearance, and proximal jejunum in the right abdomen.
  - When volvulus is present, the barium column is noted to end in a peculiar beaking effect and pathognomonic for a volvulus. (Figure 15.5).

Management

- Malrotation is treated surgically with the Ladd procedure, which involves a midline laparotomy incision for adequate visualization of the intestines and related structures. The intestines are taken out of the abdominal cavity and untwisted, if a twist is present. Any Ladd bands overlying the cecum or duodenum are removed. The purpose of the Ladd procedure is not to return the bowel to a normal configuration, which is anatomically impossible, but to minimize future risk of volvulus by widening the mesentery, and placing the bowel in a nonrotation position.
- All patients with volvulus or suspected volvulus and systemic decompensation should proceed to the operating room for an emergent laparotomy.
- Preoperative management includes cardiopulmonary and circulatory resuscitation. A gastric decompression tube should be placed, along with the administration of broad-spectrum antibiotics, to cover gut flora.

PEARL

- *Bilious vomiting in a neonate is highly suspicious for malrotation with volvulus until proven otherwise.*

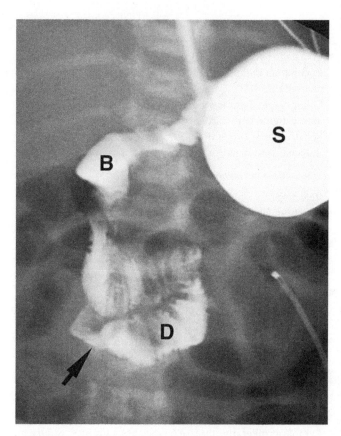

FIGURE 15.5 • **Upper GI Midgut Volvulus.** Malrotation with intermittent midgut volvulus. UGI image from an infant with intermittent abdominal pain and bilious vomiting shows malrotation. The duodenojejunal junction is inferior to the duodenal bulb *(B)*. There is abrupt termination *(arrow)* of the duodenum *(D)* secondary to volvulus stomach *(S)*.

Meckel Diverticulum

Rita Tracewell

Background/Definition

- The most common congenital abnormality of the small intestine, caused by an incomplete obliteration of the omphalomesenteric duct (also called the vitelline duct or yolk stalk).
- Occurs in 2% of the population, located within 2 feet of the ileocecal junction, measures 2 inches in length and about 2 cm in diameter, has two types of ectopic mucosa (gastric and pancreatic).
- Incidence is 2:1 male-to-female ratio.

Pathophysiology

- The yolk sac develops on approximately day 10 in the inner mass of the embryo and expands to become both the primitive gut and the cavity of the chorion (which gives rise to the placenta). A passage, known as the omphalomesenteric duct, is created. After supplying nourishment to the embryo, the yolk sac usually disappears between the fifth and ninth weeks of pregnancy. If the omphalomesenteric duct persists, it becomes a protuberant sac known as Meckel diverticulum.

Clinical Presentation

- The three most common presentations of a symptomatic Meckel diverticulum are lower GI bleeding, intestinal obstruction, and abdominal pain.
- The most common symptom manifested in children is painless GI bleeding.
- Bleeding results from ulceration of the adjacent ileal mucosa by the acid secretions of the gastric or pancreatic tissue found in the diverticulum, and is present in 25% to 56% of children with symptomatic lesions.
- Bleeding can be minimal, with dark, tarry stools, or it may be significant, with a more reddish stool. There may also be copious bright red blood from the rectum and no stool.

Diagnostic Evaluation

- The "gold standard" for diagnosing Meckel diverticulum is the Meckel scan or scintigraphy. The injected isotope, technetium pertechnetate, is readily absorbed by gastric mucosa and appears anywhere gastric mucosa exists in the body.
- Fifty percent of symptomatic Meckel diverticula have ectopic gastric or pancreatic cells within them.
- The scan should be repeated if results are negative but suspicion remains high.
- The scan is highly accurate, with 95% specificity and 85% sensitivity.

Management

- Preoperatively.
  - Children who have painless bleeding usually stop bleeding spontaneously, allowing for the Meckel scan and surgery to be performed electively.
  - Children with active bleeding require fluid resuscitation provided as PRBCs, and stabilization before going to the operating room.
  - Patients with obstructive symptoms require rapid resuscitation to expedite operative intervention and to avoid ischemic bowel resection.
- Operative procedure.
  - The open diverticulectomy operative procedure remains the traditional approach through a transverse right lower quadrant incision, or at the location seen on the Meckel scan. Once resected, the diverticulum can be opened and evaluated for ulcers.
  - An appendectomy is performed to avoid future diagnostic dilemmas.

PEARL

- *Although the hallmark of Meckel diverticulum is painless rectal bleeding, other symptoms may predominate. Bowel obstruction, appendicitis-like symptoms, or an acute abdomen with bleeding may represent a symptomatic Meckel diverticulum.*

Necrotizing Enterocolitis

Tonya A. Schneidereith

Background/Definition

- Necrotizing Enterocolitis (NEC) is a disease confined mostly to premature infants.
- Incidence has increased with improved NICU technology.
- Premature infants are more likely to be colonized by pathogenic bacteria, potentially leading to compromised intestinal barrier and NEC.

Etiology

- Most common GI emergency of premature infants.
- Approximately 1:1,000 live births.
- Black males account for highest incidence.

Pathophysiology

- Severe inflammatory disorder that can involve any portion of GI tract, which typically involves the ileum and proximal colon and believed to be an inflammatory response to injury.
- Initial issues arise from injury to immature intestinal epithelium, bacterial translocation, and immune response.
- Can result in bacterial overgrowth and progression through full-thickness intestinal wall and subsequent perforations.

Clinical Presentation

- Nonspecific, but can include apnea, bradycardia, temperature instability, lethargy, mottling, and increased ventilatory support requirements.
- May have difficulties with feeding, increased abdominal girth, bloody stools, palpable mass, or color change on the abdominal wall.

Diagnostic

- Laboratory data are nonspecific; may have thrombocytopenia, increased CRP, and metabolic acidosis.
- Hallmark sign is pneumotosis intestinalis on abdominal radiograph. May also show dilated loops of bowel that do not change on repeated abdominal radiographs (fixed loops), intrahepatic portal venous air, and ascites (Figure 15.6).
- Obtain supine and left lateral decubitus films for possible pneumoperitoneum.

Management

- Bowel rest: gastric decompression with NG tube.
- Blood, urine, and sputum cultures prior to the initiation of antibiotics.
- Broad-spectrum antibiotics targeting intestinal organisms for approximately 7 to 14 days (e.g., ampicillin and cefotaxime; plus anaerobic coverage for infants more than several weeks of age [e.g., flagyl] or other regimen based on institution and provider preference).
- Surgery for bowel perforation.
- Most common complication is short bowel syndrome, when not enough bowel is present to absorb necessary nutrients.

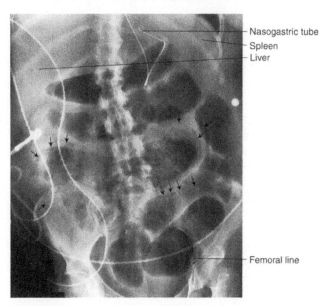

Nasogastric tube
Spleen
Liver

Femoral line

FIGURE 15.6 • **Radiograph Pneumatosis Intestinalis.** Abdomen anteroposterior supine radiograph. Pneumatosis intestinalis (air in the bowel wall). There is widespread bubbly air within the small intestine walls (*arrows*).

Prevention

● Feeding infants with breast milk, and standardized feeding protocols may decrease likelihood of developing NEC.
● Preliminary evidence shows reduced incidence of NEC in infants treated with probiotics.

PEARLS
● *5% of NEC cases can recur.*
● *Mortality of NEC has been estimated to be between 10% and 50%.*

Pyloric Stenosis
Tonya A. Schneidereith

Background/Definition

● One of the most common causes of vomiting in infants.
● Vomiting secondary to gastric outlet obstruction from hypertrophied pyloric muscle and subsequent gastric outlet obstruction.

Etiology

● Onset of symptoms generally between 2 and 8 weeks of age.
● Peak occurrence 3 to 5 weeks of age.
● Increased incidence in families.

Pathophysiology

● Not clearly understood.
● Related to a multitude of factors, including genetic, environmental, and mechanical.

● Hypertrophy of pylorus muscle leads to narrowing between the stomach and duodenum; resultant irritation and swelling lead to a complete obstruction.

Clinical Presentation

● Initially, the infant appears well with feedings; may vomit occasionally.
● As obstruction worsens, emesis becomes forceful, projecting up to 3 feet from the infant.
● Emesis is nonbilious.
● Infant appears fretful, hungry, and fails to gain weight as the obstruction worsens.

Diagnostic

● Dehydration may lead to metabolic acidosis.
● Vomiting may lead to metabolic alkalosis.
● Common findings with chemistries are hypochloremia, hypokalemia, and hyperbilirubinemia.
● Peristaltic waves may be visualized across the abdomen.
● Olive-sized mass may be palpated in right upper quadrant.
● Diagnosis confirmed with abdominal ultrasound.

Management

● Restore fluid and electrolyte balance.
● Once stable, pyloromyotomy performed, either open or laparoscopically.
  ● Pyloromyotomy splits the pyloric muscle to increase diameter and gastric emptying.
● Feedings can begin once gastric contents are able to empty into the duodenum, usually 6 hours postop.

Short Bowel Syndrome
Tonya A. Schneidereith

Background/Definition

● Decreased ability to digest and absorb nutrients necessary to maintain growth, hydration, and electrolyte homeostasis.
● Also known as short gut syndrome or intestinal failure.

Etiology

● Typically results from a bowel resection due to necrotizing enterocolitis, intestinal atresia, gastroschisis, and malrotation with volvulus.
● Leads to need for prolonged PN, usually more than 3 months.

Pathophysiology

● The pathophysiology is related to the location of bowel removed. The inability to absorb certain nutrients is secondary to the types of bowel lost in the resection.
● Jejunal resections can lead to decreased cholecystokinin and gastric hypersecretion.
● Ileocecal valve resection can lead to overgrowth of bacteria in the small intestine.

- Ileal resection can lead to malabsorption, steatorrhea, secretory diarrhea, and decreased transit time.
- Colonic resection can lead to increased gastric emptying.
- The child with 35 cm or more of residual bowel will have greater success weaning from TPN.

Clinical Presentation

- Can be divided into three phases.
- Acute phase: lasts approximately one month after resection. Characterized by watery ostomy output. Requires IVF and TPN to maintain hydration and electrolyte balance. May benefit from H2 blockers or proton pump inhibitors.
- Recovery phase: begins after a few weeks and can last for a few months. Diarrhea and ostomy output decrease. Enteral nutrition slowly advanced, while TPN gradually decreased.
- Maintenance phase: Enteral feeds are tolerated, and TPN is discontinued. Oral feedings are often started in this stage.

Management

- Goals are to optimize nutrition, facilitate growth, minimize fluid and electrolyte losses, and maximize enteral absorption.
- TPN to provide calories and nutrients.
- Special considerations include careful monitoring of serum bicarbonate (lost in stool or stoma output) and sodium (lost or poor absorption). May need to increase acetate in TPN to balance bicarbonate losses.
- May require proton pump inhibitors postoperatively due to hypergastrin state.
- Consider medications to promote motility. These may include erythromycin or azithromycin.
- Requires vigilance to prevent catheter-associated central line infections.

Diagnostic Testing
Air and Barium Enema
Dieadra J. Garrett

Definition

- Injection of air or barium in rectum to assess colon.

Indications

- Used to assess colon for etiology of obstruction, some problems include intestinal atresia and Hirschsprung disease.
- Diagnostic and therapeutic in children with intussusception; air or barium enema.

Limitations

- Should not be performed in patients who have signs of peritonitis.

Postprocedural Considerations

- Perforation, bleeding.

Endoscopy
Dieadra J. Garrett

Definition

- Use of an endoscope to assess upper or lower intestine.

Indications

- Esophagogastroduodenoscopy (EGD).
  - Assesses esophagus, stomach, and first portion of duodenum for pathology.
  - Aids in treating patients with abdominal pain, vomiting, failure to thrive, gastroesophageal reflux disease (GERD), and removal of foreign bodies.
- Colonoscopy.
  - Assesses colon for pathology and biopsy and can be used to remove polyps.

Limitations

- Often requires general anesthesia in pediatric patients.
- Not able to visualize entire small bowel; proximal duodenum can be visualized on EGD and terminal ileum during colonoscopy.

Diagnostic Information

- Can directly visualize the tissue and offer medical or surgical treatment.

Post- and Intraprocedural Complications

- Hemorrhage, perforation.

Endoscopic Retrograde Cholangiopancreatography
Dieadra J. Garrett

Definition

- Using an endoscope with fluoroscopy to visualize the biliary and pancreatic ducts.

Indications

- Assess for cause of biliary or pancreatic duct obstruction.
- Remove gallstones from common bile duct and perform a sphincterotomy.
- Biopsy tissue for further testing.

Limitation

- Often requires general anesthesia, and technically challenging in small children.

Diagnostic Information

- Identifies source of biliary or pancreatic pathology.
- Useful in patients with biliary obstruction where stones can be extracted, stents can be placed, and a sphincterotomy can be performed.

Postprocedural Complications

● Perforation, pancreatitis, hemorrhage.

Kidneys, Ureter, Bladder Radiograph

Dieadra J. Garrett

Background

● The kidneys, ureter, bladder (KUB) is a useful radiograph in the setting of GI disease. The ability to differentiate between bone, organ, and air is important when evaluating for constipation, gas, obstruction, and perforation.

Definition

● KUB is a plain frontal supine radiograph of the abdomen that visualizes from the diaphragm to the bladder. A KUB will aid in observation of calcifications, gas patterns, feces, or free peritoneal air.

Etiology/Types

● Useful study in detecting GI conditions as well as assessment of indwelling devices (e.g., NG tubes, jejunal tubes).

Clinical Indications

● Abdominal pain with suspected constipation to perforation, nausea, vomiting, ileus.

Abdominal Ultrasound

Dieadra J. Garrett

Background

● A reliable method of imaging that does not require radiation, which can be used to evaluate the liver to the spleen and from the kidneys to the pelvis.

Definition

● Abdominal ultrasound uses high-frequency sound waves via a probe that travels through tissue. The sound waves are reflected, scattered, and then modified and processed into an image. By use of mathematical algorithms, images, or cine movies, a "real-time" image is produced.
● The "B-mode" or "brightness-modulated" mode is used to image the abdomen by producing a two-dimensional gray-scale image of tissue.
● Abdominal ultrasound can produce images of the bowel that are specific and diagnostic.

Clinical Indications

● Useful in the evaluation of clinical presentations of.
  ● Abdominal pain, suspected appendicitis, pyloric stenosis, intussusception.

1. A 14-year-old female with a history of Crohn's disease is complaining of abdominal pain on presentation to the emergency department (ED). An order for a KUB will be most helpful in determining the presence of which of the following?
   a. Ascites.
   b. Colonic thrombosis.
   c. Free air.
   d. Small bowel mass.

Answer: **C**

Crohn disease results in ulcerations of the large and small intestines. Inflammation of the intestinal tract can cause fissures to the lymphoid tissue that may lead to perforation and free air. The KUB can diagnose free air as well as feces that may be the cause of abdominal pain in a patient with this diagnosis

2. A 14-year-old patient has a diagnosis of choledocholithiasis and increased liver and pancreatic enzymes. The next step in management is to obtain:
   a. ERCP.
   b. Meckel scan.
   c. EGD.
   d. Liver biopsy.

Answer: **A**

An ERCP, otherwise known as endoscopic retrograde cholangio-pancreatography, can be done to evaluate the pancreas and common bile duct with possible stone removal, if present.

3. A 13-year-old patient underwent an ERCP and sphincterotomy for a common bile duct stone and now has pancreatitis. This can be explained by:
   a. Nature of disease.
   b. Known complication of ERCP.
   c. Obstruction during the procedure.
   d. Stone still blocking the common bile duct.

Answer: **B**

Pancreatitis, perforation of the gall bladder or bowel, and hemorrhage are potential complications of an ERCP

4. A 6-year-old child is complaining of acute abdominal pain that radiates to the right lower quadrant. An abdominal ultrasound is ordered. Requirements for the ultrasound are:
   a. IV access with a fluid bolus prior to the ultrasound.
   b. IV access with no fluid bolus.
   c. No prior preparation is necessary.
   d. Oral contrast of 15 mL/kg, to be ingested 1 hour prior to ultrasound.

Answer: **C**

Ultrasound is safe, inexpensive, and typically available in most institutions. The advantage of ultrasound over CT is absence of radiation and no need for oral contrast prior to study. Ultrasound of the abdomen can evaluate organs of the abdominal quadrants (biliary tree, liver, pancreas), spleen, and kidneys as well as bladder and bowel. There is strong support for the use of ultrasound as the initial radiologic measurement to evaluate the abdomen.

A previously healthy, afebrile 6-year-old boy presented to the ED with a 2-day history of abdominal pain and bloody stools. Pain is described as crampy and isolated to the left side of his abdomen. Parents describe bright red blood and passing of clots per rectum, as well as episodes of melena. History indicated no sick contacts, no recent travel, and no previous history of GI bleeding. The child is well-hydrated, pale, but nontoxic. Heart rate was 120 to 140 beats per minute, with a resting blood pressure of 104/45 mmHg. He had a soft, nondistended abdomen with pain on palpation of the left lower quadrant. No peritoneal signs were noted. A recent hemoglobin was 10 g/dL, and is now 7 g/dL. Electrolytes, kidney and liver function tests, WBC count, and coagulation studies are all normal. In the ED, the patient received a fluid bolus and a PRBC transfusion. Stools were sent for culture, electron microscopy, and ova and parasites. The patient was admitted to the general pediatric ward, on the pediatric surgery service, for further evaluation and treatment.

5. Based on the presentation, what is the most likely diagnosis?
   a. Appendicitis.
   b. Meckel Diverticulum.
   c. Ileus.
   d. Intussusception.

Answer: **B**

Meckel diverticulum presents typically with painless rectal bleeding and no other symptoms. Crampy pain and a decreased hemoglobin are other signs of Meckel.

Intussusception is typically seen in in infants and children <3 years of age. The absence of peritoneal signs, normal appetite, and absence of fever make a diagnosis of appendicitis less likely. A child with a midgut volvulus presents with vomiting, absence of rectal bleeding, and is typically more ill-appearing. Bloody stools, drop in hemoglobin, an acute onset of abdominal pain, and absence of peritoneal signs make a Meckel diverticulum the most likely diagnosis for this child.

(continues on page 422)

6. The most important diagnostic test for a child with painless or acute rectal bleeding will include:
   a. Liver function tests, amylase, lipase.
   b. Upper GI series.
   c. Endoscopy and biopsy.
   d. Meckel nuclear medicine scan.

Answer: **D**

A Meckel scan is the gold standard diagnostic study to determine the presence of Meckel diverticulum. The isotope administered for a Meckel scan is readily absorbed by gastric and pancreatic mucosa, which is contained in 50% of patients with symptomatic Meckel diverticulum. The test is highly accurate and noninvasive. Typically, if the scan is positive, surgery is planned. If the scan is negative, it warrants repeating, especially with classic symptoms.

7. Which is the appropriate procedure to treat a child with a positive Meckel scan?
   a. Appendectomy.
   b. Air contrast enema reduction in fluoroscopy.
   c. Open diverticulectomy.
   d. Colectomy.

Answer: **C**

The operative procedure to correct Meckel diverticulum is a diverticulectomy. A bowel resection may be necessary if the child's bowel experienced ischemic compromise.

8. Acute cholecystitis is best characterized by which of the following clinical findings?
   a. Fever, right upper abdominal pain, elevated WBC count, and bilirubin level.
   b. Fever, abdominal pain, and a palpable gallstone.
   c. Diffuse abdominal pain, elevated WBC count, and elevated cholesterol level.
   d. Epigastric pain, vomiting, and elevated amylase and lipase level.

Answer: **A**

Fever, right upper abdominal pain, elevated WBC count and bilirubin level are the most common signs and symptoms for the patient with acute cholecystitis. Gallstones are not palpable and are almost always diagnosed following radiologic imaging. Diffuse abdominal pain would more likely be present with peritonitis that is associated with a bowel perforation or appendicitis. Epigastric pain, vomiting, and elevated amylase and lipase level are more commonly appreciated in patients with pancreatitis.

The next three questions are from the following case:
A 6 year-old-female is brought to the ED with a chief complaint of abdominal pain and vomiting. She has vomited 12 times (nonbloody, nonbilious) since the onset of illness 24 hours ago and continues to complain of diffuse abdominal pain and is unable to keep any liquids down. Her urine output is significantly decreased. She has not had fever, diarrhea, dysuria, coughing, or other upper respiratory tract infection symptoms. There have been no sick contacts or recent travel.

Past medical history is significant for two previous episodes of severe abdominal pain associated with two to three episodes of vomiting that spontaneously resolved. The first episode occurred at 3 years of age, and the second at 5 years of age.
Examination
Vital Signs: temperature 37.2°C, heart rate 105 beats per minute, respiratory rate 30 breaths per minute, blood pressure 108/68 mmHg. She is moderately ill-appearing; pale with sunken eyes, and moist oral mucus membranes. Abdomen is soft with diffuse mild tenderness. Bowel sounds are decreased. No costovertebral angle tenderness and no rashes or lesions. During the examination, the child has an episode of bilious emesis with increasing complaints of abdominal pain and abdominal distension. On reevaluation, her heart rate is 140 to 155 beats per minute, and blood pressure 85/50 mmHg.

9. This child's symptoms most likely are caused from which of the following conditions?
   a. Intussusception.
   b. Viral Gastroenteritis.
   c. Malrotation/Volvulus.
   d. Appendicitis.

Answer: **C**

A diagnosis of gastroenteritis is not high on the differential, given the symptoms are not typical of a viral illness. Appendicitis cannot be excluded; however, there is no history of fever or diarrhea, both common symptoms seen in both viral gastroenteritis and appendicitis. The patient's past medical history of abdominal pain and vomiting with spontaneous resolution best fits a diagnosis of malrotation with intermittent volvulus.

10. What diagnostic test(s) should be ordered to support the suspected diagnosis?
    a. Barium enema.
    b. UGI series.
    c. CT of abdomen and pelvis.
    d. Flat and upright plain abdominal radiographs.

Answer: **B**

An UGI series is the gold standard for diagnosing malrotation and will demonstrate abnormal position of the ligament of Treitz, partial obstruction of the duodenum, with a spiral or corkscrew appearance, and proximal jejunum in the right abdomen. A barium enema will not indicate an abnormal location of the ligament of Trietz. A CT and plain abdominal films may show an obstruction, but not malrotation.

11. What interventions should be instituted based on the patient's change in examination?
    a. IV fluids at maintenance rate, morphine IV for analgesia, repeat vital signs in 1 hour.
    b. Increase IV fluid rate to 1.5 times maintenance, order stat abdominal radiograph, broad-spectrum antibiotics.

c. NG tube for gastric decompression, placement of urinary catheter, 20 mL/kg normal saline fluid boluses, broad-spectrum antibiotics, type and screen, chemistries.

d. Normal saline fluid bolus, morphine IV for analgesia, stat abdominal CT.

Answer: C

A child with acute presentation of midgut volvulus requires immediate and aggressive fluid resuscitation to correct hypovolemia and metabolic imbalance. A NG tube for gastric decompression should be placed, along with a foley catheter, to measure accurate urine output. Broad-spectrum antibiotics should be ordered to avoid bacterial translocation through the necrotic bowel wall. Type and screen for PRBC transfusion and chemistries to monitor hypovolemia and metabolic imbalances. Prepare patient for emergent laparotomy; Ladd procedure and possible bowel resection.

12. A previously healthy toddler presents with 2-day history of watery stools, occurring 6 times per day, fever to 38.5°C, and nonbloody/nonbilious vomiting with foods/liquids. On examination, he is irritable, appears thirsty, and his heart rate is 160 beats per minute. Which of the following should be done FIRST?

a. Admit to hospital for IV fluids.

b. Obtain stool studies.

c. Administer 50 to 100 mL/kg ORS over 2 to 4 hours.

d. Order a one-time dose of loperamide.

Answer: C

History and examination findings for this child indicate mild to moderate dehydration. ORS is the appropriate first step for rehydration.

13. A school-aged child is admitted for a 4-day history of diarrhea, which became bloody in the last 24 hours. Which of the following diagnostic studies should be recommended as follow-up once the child is discharged home?

a. Basic metabolic panel and sedimentation rate.

b. Basic metabolic panel and CBC.

c. Sedimentation rate and CBC.

d. Liver function tests and sedimentation rate.

Answer: B

A rare, but serious, late sequelae of *E. coli* gastroenteritis is hemolytic uremic syndrome (HUS), and *E. coli* gastroenteritis must be considered with any episode of acute onset of bloody stools. HUS is characterized by a triad of hemolytic anemia, thrombocytopenia, and acute renal dysfunction. Appropriate monitoring for HUS includes renal function tests and a CBC.

14. An adolescent presents with a 2-day history of fever, vomiting, and nonbloody diarrhea. The patient's younger siblings are at home with similar symptoms. Physical examination reveals right lower quadrant discomfort with rebound tenderness. The first diagnostic study should include:

a. Abdominal CT.

b. Infectious stool studies.

c. Basic metabolic panel.

d. Urinalysis.

Answer: A

Despite presenting symptoms and sick contacts in the home, acute gastroenteritis rarely presents with focal tenderness on examination. Examination findings provide red flags for acute appendicitis, so an abdominal CT is the most important diagnostic study for this child.

15. What would be the first diagnostic test for a 12-month-old child who presents with colicky abdominal pain that started 4 hours ago?

a. Barium enema.

b. Air enema.

c. Abdominal ultrasound.

d. Abdominal radiograph.

Answer: C

A barium or air enema would be both diagnostic and therapeutic if the symptoms were certain to be intussusception, but an abdominal ultrasound is the gold standard diagnostic test for intussusception and should be completed prior to going to radiology for a barium or air enema. It is more appropriate to do an ultrasound, which is much less invasive than a barium or air enema as an initial diagnostic study.

16. An 8-month-old infant is 5 days postop from a liver transplant for BA. She received a whole organ from a deceased donor. After an episode of hypotension, she was noted to have an elevation in her liver enzymes. What imaging study should be ordered?

a. Abdominal CT.

b. Abdominal ultrasound with vascular Doppler.

c. Abdominal radiograph.

d. MR cholangiogram.

Answer: B

The clinical findings indicate the possibility of a hepatic artery thrombosis, which will be visible on ultrasound with vascular Doppler study. Once diagnosed, the child should be taken to the operating room emergently for thrombectomy.

17. At what point is surgical reduction indicated for an intussusception?

a. After two recurrent intussusception events.

b. Inability to reduce the intussusception after three attempts.

c. When the patient is diagnosed with an intussusception.

d. After five recurrent intussusception events.

Answer: B

The only indication for surgical reduction of an intussusception in an infant is the inability to reduce the intussusception nonsurgically. Surgical backup should be in place prior to the radiology procedure, but is done only if the barium or air enema is unsuccessful after three attempts or if there are any concerns for perforation.

(continues on page 424)

18. Discharge teaching for a family of a 9-month-old who had an intussusception reduced by barium enema should include what important information about recurrence?
    a. Once the intussusception is reduced, it will not recur.
    b. The largest risk of recurrence is in the first 24 hours.
    c. Recurrence is less likely if the intussusception was reduced by barium enema.
    d. If a recurrence occurs, it must be surgically reduced.

Answer: **B**

It is very important to educate families about what the signs of intussusception are so that they will quickly return with any concerns. The greatest chance of recurrence is in the first 24 hours. Recurrence is less likely if the intussusception is reduced surgically, not by barium enema. As long as the intussusception is easily reduced by barium enema, a barium enema will be attempted no matter the number of recurrences of intussusception.

19. A 15-year-old girl has had unintentional weight loss over the past 3 months, diarrhea that has become bloody, and urgency to have bowel movements. Based on just these symptoms, what is the most probable diagnosis?
    a. Ulcerative colitis.
    b. Crohn's disease.
    c. Gastroenteritis.
    d. Diverticulitis.

Answer: **A**

These symptoms would be associated with a diagnosis of ulcerative colitis because of the long-term weight loss, bloody stool, and the urgency seen with this disease. Gastroenteritis is not associated with weight loss or urgency. In Crohn disease, the diarrhea is not typically bloody.

20. In addition to careful history taking, what would be the next step in making this diagnosis of ulcerative colitis?
    a. Abdominal CT.
    b. Endoscopy with biopsy.
    c. CBC, basic metabolic profile (BMP), CRP, erythrocyte sedimentation rate, and stool studies.
    d. IBD serology markers.

Answer: **C**

An abdominal CT may identify some abdominal complaints, but would not be helpful in diagnosing ulcerative colitis. Endoscopy with biopsy would make the diagnosis, but is very invasive and requires a bowel prep and anesthesia, so it would not be the first choice. A CBC, BMP, CRP, ESR, and stool studies would be easy and provide information quickly so that you could proceed in the appropriate direction.

21. Which treatment for ulcerative colitis allows for the greatest chance of remission in patients with refractory UC?
    a. Total colectomy with J-pouch.
    b. Enteral nutrition for 8 weeks.
    c. Corticosteroids.
    d. Aminosalicylates.

Answer: **A**

A total colectomy with J-pouch created surgically is the only therapy that allows complete remission or cure of UC because the diseased colon is being removed. The other therapies are appropriate to induce or maintain remission; however, in refractory disease, a colectomy would be an appropriate treatment.

22. A 17-year-old female with a history of Crohn's disease presents with abdominal pain, weight loss, and frequent stool. She is currently only on an aminosalicylate. She was weaned off the corticosteroids 4 months ago. Which of the following would be the best treatment for her?
    a. Total colectomy with J-pouch.
    b. Enteral nutrition for 8 weeks.
    c. Corticosteroids.
    d. Increasing dose of Aminosalicylate.

Answer: **C**

A total colectomy with J-pouch is never indicated in a patient with Crohn's disease. The use of enteral nutrition would be appropriate in this patient; however, it can be difficult for patients at this age and with minor symptoms. Corticosteroids may be a better treatment for her lifestyle. Adjusting the dose of aminosalicylates will not induce remission, but may help to maintain remission longer once she is stable and weaning off corticosteroids

The next three questions pertain to this scenario:
A 10-year-old male underwent a laparoscopic appendectomy for perforated appendicitis with extensive peritonitis. He is currently postoperative day #2, drinking clear liquids, and taking hydrocodone and acetaminophen for pain control. On morning rounds, it is noted that his abdomen is distended and he is having more pain then on previous examinations. He has one episode of vomiting as the team finishes rounds.

23. What is the most likely finding based on history and physical examination?
    a. Mechanical small bowel obstruction.
    b. Postoperative ileus.
    c. Normal postoperative course.
    d. Intra-abdominal abscess.

Answer: **B**

The most common early symptoms of a postoperative ileus are abdominal distension and worsening pain. Vomiting is a late sign of an ileus.

24. What is the most appropriate management to relieve the patient's symptoms?
    a. Nothing; symptoms will resolve on their own.
    b. NPO, place a NG tube.
    c. NPO, IV fluids, and increase narcotic dose.
    d. Continue IV antibiotics and increase narcotic dose.

Answer: **B**

An ileus will resolve over time, but if the patient is allowed to drink or eat, he would become more distended and would eventually start vomiting, which could prolong the ileus. If vomiting develops, it is appropriate to place an NG tube. Pain management with narcotics will slow down the intestines, causing the ileus to potentially persist longer.

25. What is the best description of the expected findings of an ileus on an abdominal radiograph?
    a. Dilated bowel with air fluid levels.
    b. Gasless bowel.
    c. Dilated bowel with decompressed proximal bowel.
    d. Extremely dilated bowel throughout the abdomen.

Answer: A

The radiograph of a child with an ileus usually demonstrates mildly dilated bowel with air fluid levels since air and fluid are not moving through the intestines. On the abdominal radiograph, the air rises, and the fluid stays at the bottom, resulting in the appearance of a straight line between the gas and the fluid. If extreme dilation or proximal bowel decompression were present, mechanical obstruction would be of more concern.

26. A 5-week-old infant with jaundice since birth is exclusively breastfed and growing well. Parents report 1 week of clay-colored stools and dark urine. TORCH screen was obtained and is normal. Laboratory studies reveal ALT 300 IU/L, AST 250 IU/L, total bilirubin 6 mg/dL, and a conjugated bilirubin 2.5 mg/dL. What is the next step in management?
    a. Arrange hospital admission for urgent liver biopsy.
    b. Repeat liver function tests in 2 weeks.
    c. Obtain abdominal ultrasound.
    d. Initiate phototherapy.

Answer: C

Physiologic jaundice is most often resolved at 2 weeks of age, so high bilirubin levels at this time are abnormal. Phototherapy is the treatment for unconjugated hyperbilirubinemia. Ultrasound is the first step in further evaluation for hyperbilirubinemia in this infant. The patient will likely need liver biopsy and may require hospitalization, depending on imaging results.

27. A one-and-a-half-year-old status post Kasai procedure for BA presents at 8 weeks of age with congestion, malaise, and frequent stools. On physical examination, the child is afebrile, weight is down 2 kg (3 percentile for age), no jaundice, +hepatomegaly, ALT 120 IU/L, AST 134 IU/L, total bilirubin 1 mg/dL, and CBC within normal limits. What additional evaluation is indicated?
    a. Reweigh in one week after resolution of acute illness.
    b. Urinalysis and culture.
    c. Complete metabolic profile, 25-DOH, fecal fat studies.
    d. Repeat CBC and liver function tests.

Answer: C

The child's surgical history puts him at risk for malabsorption and poor weight gain, so ordering a metabolic panel, vitamin D level, and fecal fat study is most reasonable.

28. An obese adolescent with type 2 diabetes mellitus presents to the ED with a 3-day history of abdominal pain and bilious emesis. Laboratory studies reveal ALT 420 IU/L and AST 399 IU/L. This patient is at risk for which hepatic condition?
    a. Hepatitis C.
    b. Nonalcoholic steatohepatitis.
    c. Wilson Disease.
    d. Gilbert Syndrome.

Answer: B

These laboratory values, patient history, and physical findings are most consistent with nonalcoholic steatohepatitis.

29. The parent of a 3-month-old with trisomy 21 reports the infant has had 2 weeks of fussiness and poor PO intake. Current weight is 4.5 kg. Initial bloodwork reveals total bilirubin 4.2 mg/dL and direct bilirubin 0.8 mg/dL. What is the next step in evaluation?
    a. Metabolic screen for G6PD.
    b. Reassure caregivers that labs are within normal limits.
    c. Referral to subspecialty gastroenterology.
    d. Abdominal ultrasound.

Answer: B

Minimally elevated total bilirubin level can be indicative of mild dehydration, and at this point, no further evaluation needs to take place. The infant should be followed for weight checks and feeding assessment.

30. A 17-year-old previously healthy female presents with several weeks of fatigue and low-grade fever. On examination, she has lymphadenopathy, jaundice, and hepatomegaly, and is found to have multiple tattoos. Laboratory results include ALT 1, 393 IU/L, AST 1142 IU/L, Total bilirubin 5 mg/dL, amylase 100, lipase 79. What is the most likely diagnosis?
    a. Autoimmune hepatitis.
    b. Choledocholithiasis.
    c. Viral hepatitis.
    d. IBD.

Answer: C

Lymphadenopathy suggests an infectious origin. Tattoos are a risk factor for hepatitis A, B, C, so further studies should be obtained to include antigens for hepatitis.

31. A 6-week-old who was born at 31 weeks' gestation and spent a long time in the NICU for feeding difficulties presents with lethargy and fever. Parents report three wet diapers in the past 24 hours. Jaundice and hepatomegaly are noted on physical examination. What is the first step in management?
    a. Referral to Gastroenterology specialist.
    b. Urinalysis, urine culture, CBC.
    c. Initiate IV fluids.
    d. Obtain transaminase and bilirubin levels.

Answer: C

(continues on page 426)

In the initial evaluation of an ill infant, it is important to address hydration status. Despite the need to obtain laboratory sampling and perhaps a gastroenterology consult, it is important to reestablish hydration as the most immediate concern.

32. A previously healthy school-aged child presents to the ED with hematemesis. Vital signs are as follows (Table 15.1): What is the *first* intervention in managing this child?

TABLE 15.1 Vital Signs

Heart Rate	145 beats/minute
Respiratory Rate	28 breaths/minute
Blood Pressure	80/40 mmHg
Temperature	37.2°C
Hemoglobin	7.2 mg/dL

   a. Administer PRBCs.
   b. Administer 20 mL/kg isotonic crystalloid fluids IV.
   c. Consult Gastroenterology.
   d. Order tagged RBC scan.

Answer: **B**

The patient is hemodynamically unstable, so you must start with ABCs. Airway is open, patient is breathing, but circulation is inadequate, as evidenced by hypotension and tachycardia. The history makes hypovolemia secondary to acute blood loss the most likely etiology, so PRBCs will be needed, but for immediate volume repletion, the first step is always isotonic crystalloid IV fluids.

33. A previously healthy and hemodynamically stable adolescent presents with a 2-day history of hematochezia and diarrhea. The patient's mother has Crohn's disease. What diagnostic test will help determine the *most* likely etiology of the symptoms?
   a. Colonoscopy.
   b. Basic metabolic panel.
   c. Stool culture.
   d. Abdominal CT.

Answer: **C**

Infection is the most common cause of colitis worldwide. Despite the family history of IBD, the acute onset of symptoms makes an infectious etiology much more likely. If symptoms persist, colonoscopy may be indicated, but it should not be done first. Basic metabolic panel would help evaluate for HUS, which is a sequela, but not an etiology of bloody diarrhea. An abdominal CT may be indicated if symptoms persist or if there is severe abdominal pain, but would not be the first-line diagnostic study for this patient.

34. An exclusively breastfed 2-month-old presents with blood streaks in the stool for 2 to 3 weeks. Stools are otherwise yellow and seedy, and are easily passed 2 to 3 times per day. Physical examination reveals a hemodynamically stable infant who is gaining 30 g/day. What is the best *initial* recommendation?
   a. Switch to an amino acid–based/elemental formula.
   b. Order a glycerin suppository.
   c. Order an H-2 blocker.
   d. Eliminate milk and soy from mother's diet.

Answer: **D**

The most likely diagnosis for this infant is allergic colitis or milk-protein enteropathy. As the child is well-appearing and growing at a normal rate, it is best to promote ongoing breastfeeding with a trial of an elimination diet instead of switching immediately to an elemental formula. There is no evidence to support that an H-2 blocker improves allergic colitis. The stooling history reveals no signs of constipation, so a glycerin suppository would not be helpful.

35. A 3-month-old infant with no significant medical history presents with small volume feeding, arching, and pulling away from the bottle during feeds. He is not vomiting, but has increased crying throughout the day. The infant is continuing to demonstrate appropriate weight gain. The best initial management for this infant would be:
   a. Order a 24-hour pH probe study.
   b. Order a combined multiple intraluminal impedance study and pH probe.
   c. Start overnight NG feeds at a very slow rate.
   d. Start a trial of an H-2 blocker.

Answer: **D**

Since the child is demonstrating appropriate growth and is otherwise healthy, the least invasive step would be to start a trial of an H-2 blocker such as ranitidine for 2 to 3 weeks to see if symptoms improve. A pH probe does not measure nonacid reflux, and although a pH probe and manometry study will provide the best information, it is expensive and invasive. Overnight feedings are not indicated in this case since the child is growing well and because an NG tube can stimulate reflux in some cases.

Recommended Readings

Abraham, C., & Cho, J. H. (2009). Inflammatory bowel disease. *The New England Journal of Medicine, 361*(21), 2066–2078.

Al-Tokhais, T., Hsieh, H., Pemberton, J., Elnahas, A., Puligandla, P., & Flageole, H. (2012). Antibiotics administration before enema reduction of intussusception: Is it necessary? *Journal of Pediatric Surgery, 47,* 928–930.

American Academy of Pediatrics. Subcommittee on Hyperbilirubinemia. (2004). Management of hyperbilirubinemia in the newborn infant 35 or more weeks of gestation. *Pediatrics, 114*(1), 297–316.

Amin, S. C., Pappas, C., Iyengar, H., & Maheshwari, A. (2013). Short bowel syndrome in the NICU. *Clinics in Perinatology, 40*(1), 53–68.

Askew, N. (2010). An overview of infantile hypertrophic pyloric stenosis. *Paediatric Nursing, 22*(8), 27–30.

Bansal, S., Banever, G. T., Karrer, F. M., & Partrick, D. A. (2012). Appendicitis in children less than 5 years old: Influence of age and presentation of outcome. *The American Journal of Surgery, 204,* 1031–1035.

Bishop, C. A., & Carter, M. E. (2013). Appendicitis. In N. T. Browne, L. M. Flanigan, C. A. McComisky, & P. Pieper (Eds.), *Nursing care of the pediatric surgical patient* (pp. 407–416). Burlington, MA: Jones & Bartlett Learning.

Chiang, M. (2013). Solid tumors. In N. T. Browne, L. M. Flanigan, C. A. McComisky, & P. Pieper (Eds.), *Nursing care of the pediatric surgical patient* (pp. 447–469). Burlington, MA: Jones & Bartlett Learning.

Committee on Infectious Diseases, American Academy of Pediatrics. (2011). *Redbook.* Elk Grove, IL: Author.

Critch, J., Day, A. S., Otley, A., King-Moore, C., Teitelbaum, J. E., & Shashidhar, H. (2012). Use of enteral nutrition for the control of intestinal inflammation in pediatric Crohn's disease. *Journal of Pediatric Gastroenterology and Nutrition, 54,* 298–305.

Day, A. S., Ledder, O., Leach, S. T., & Lemberg, D. A. (2012). Crohn's and colitis in children and adolescents. *World Journal of Gastroenterology, 18*(41), 5862–5869.

Devictor, D., Tissieres, P., Durand, P., Chevret, L., & Debray, D. (2011). Acute liver failure in neonates, infants, and children. *Expert Reviews in Gastroenterolgty & Hepatology, 5*(6), 717–729.

Dominguez, K. M., & Moss, L. (2012). Necrotizing enterocolitis. *Clinics in Perinatology, 39,* 387–401.

Davenport, K. P., Blanco, F. C., & Sandler, A. D. (2012). Pediatric malignancies: Neuroblastoma, Wilm's tumor, hepatoblastoma, rhabdomyosarcoma, and sacroccygeal teratoma. *Surgical Clinics of North America, 92,* 745–767.

Davenport, M. (2012). Biliary atresia: Clinical aspects. *Seminars in Pediatric Surgery, 21,* 175–184.

Flanigan, L. M. (2013). Biliary atresia and choledochal cyst. In N. T. Browne, L. M. Flanigan, C. A. McComiskey, & P. Pieper (Eds.), *Nursing care of the pediatric surgical patient* (3rd ed., pp. 435–446), Sudbury, MA: Jones & Bartlett Learning.

Herwig, K., Brenkert, T., & Losek, J. D. (2009). Enema-reduced intussusception management. Is hospitalization necessary? *Pediatric Emergency Care, 25*(2), 74–77.

Hricik, D. (Ed.). (2011). *Primer on transplantation.* Singapore: Wiley-Blackwell.

Ingoe, R., & Lange, P. (2007). The Ladd's procedure for correction of intestinal malrotation with volvulus in children. *Association of Perioperative Registered Nurses Journal, 85,* 300–308.

Jung, S. A. (2012). Differential diagnosis of inflammatory bowel disease: What is the role of colonoscopy? *Clinical Endoscopy, 45*(3), 254–262.

Kerr, C. L. (2012). Appendicitis. In K. Reuter-Rice & B. N. Bolick (Eds.), *Pediatric acute care: A guide for interprofessional practice* (pp. 478–481). Burlington, MA: Jones & Bartlett Learning.

Kulik, D. M., Uleryk, E. M., & Maguire, J. L. (2013). Does this child have appendicitis? A systematic review of clinical prediction rules for children with acute abdominal pain. *Journal of Clinical Epidemiology, 66,* 95–104.

Leyva-Vega, M., & Haber, B. (2010). Biliary atresia. In W. P. Bishop (Ed.), *Pediatric practice gastroenterology* (pp. 330–340). New York, NY: McGraw-Hill.

Mack, C. L., Gonzalez-Peralta, R. P., Gupta, N., Leung, D., Narkewicz, M. R., Roberts, E. A., . . . Schwarz, K. B. (2012). NASPGHAN practice guidelines: Diagnosis and management of Hepatitis C infection in infants, children, and adolescents. *Journal of Pediatric Gastroenterology and Nutrition, 54,* 838–855.

McConnie, R. M. (2011). Hepatitis. In K. Reuter-Rice & B. N. Bolick (Eds.), *Pediatric acute care: A guide for interprofessional practice* (pp. 503–507). Burlington, MA: Jones & Barlett Learning.

Modi, B. P., & Jaksic, T. (2012). Pediatric intestinal failure and vascular access. *The Surgical Clinics of North America, 92*(3), 729–743.

Mouat, L. (2012). Cholecystitis. In K. Reuter-Rice & B. N. Bolick (Eds.), *Pediatric acute care: A guide for interprofessional practice* (pp. 489–491). Burlington, MA: Jones & Bartlett Learning.

Pepper, V. K., Stanfill, A. B., & Pearl, R. H. (2012). Diagnosis and management of pediatric appendicitis, intussusception, and meckel diverticulum. *Surgical Clinics of North America, 92,* 505–526.

Piercce, J., & Rodriguez, K. (2012). Abdominal mass. In K. Reuter-Rice & B. N. Bolick (Eds.), *Pediatric acute care: A guide for interprofessional practice* (pp. 481–484). Burlington, MA: Jones & Bartlett Learning.

Romero, J. R., & O'Connor, J. A. (2010).Viral hepatitis. In W. P. Bishop (Ed.), *Pediatric practice gastroenterology* (pp. 341–355). New York, NY: McGraw-Hill.

Russell, T. L. (2011). Indirect hyperbillirubinemia in the neonate. In K. Reuter-Rice & B. N. Bolick (Eds.), *Pediatric acute care: A guide for interprofessional practice* (pp. 528–535). Burlington, MA: Jones & Bartlett Learning.

Schupp, C. J., Klingmuller, V., Strauch, K., Bahr, M., Zovko, D., Hannmann, T., & Loff, S. (2010). Typical signs of appendicitis in ultrasonography mimicked by other diseases? *Pediatric Surgery International, 26,* 697–702.

Stoops, M. M., & Slusher, J. A. (2013). Splenectomy and cholecystectomy. In N. T. Browne, L. M. Flanigan, C. A. McComiskey, & P. Pieper (Eds.), *Nursing care of the pediatric surgical patient* (3rd ed., pp. 417–431). Sudbury, MA: Jones & Bartlett Learning.

Svensson, J., & Makin, E. (2012). Gallstone disease in children. *Seminars in Pediatric Surgery, 21,* 255–265.

Veereman-Wauters, G., & Wenzl, T. G. (2009). Pediatric gastroesophageal reflux clinical practice guidelines: Joint recommendations of NASPGHAN* and ESPGHANY. *Journal of Pediatric Gastroenterology and Nutrition, 49,* 498–547.

Wise, B. V. (2012). Liver failure. In K. Reuter-Rice & B. N. Bolick (Eds.), *Pediatric acute care: A guide for interprofessional practice* (pp. 557–560). Burlington, MA: Jones & Bartlett Learning.

Yu, E. L. (2012). Inflammatory bowel disease. In K. Reuter-Rice & B. Bolick (Eds.), *Pediatric acute care: A guide for interprofessional practice* (pp. 549–555). Burlington, MA: Jones & Bartlett Learning.

Kidney and Genitourinary Disorders

General Renal Principles

- Kidney function is indicated by the glomerular filtration rate (GFR).
- The kidneys of children reach adult GFR at approximately 1 year of age, but measured GFR vary by age.
- GFR can be estimated (eGFR) with the patient height, serum creatinine, and a constant (Schwartz equation).
  eGFR mL/minute/1.73 m^2 = (k)(height)/serum creatinine
  - k = constant of 0.413 for all ages/genders.
  - Height is measured in centimeters.
  - Serum creatinine is measured in mg/dL.
  - Renal blood flow is dependent on intravascular volume and adequate cardiac output with oxygenated blood.
- Fractional excretion of sodium.
  - Equation used to determine whether kidney dysfunction is only a result of hypoperfusion to kidney.
  - Results.
    - <1% prerenal (e.g., hypovolemia, sepsis, congestive heart failure).
    - >1% intrinsic (e.g., acute tubular necrosis, glomerulonephritis [GN]).
    - >4% postrenal (e.g., obstruction, urolithiasis).
- BUN-to-creatinine ratio.
  - Normal ratio is 10:1 to 20:1.
  - Elevated ratios are often associated with shock or dehydration with acute kidney failure. Also may result from nephrolithiasis or gastrointestinal or pulmonary hemorrhage.
  - Low ratios are often associated with rhabdomyolysis, syndrome of inappropriate antidiuretic hormone secretion, lung disease, malignancy, low dietary protein intake, or certain medications.

Acute Renal Failure

Andrea M. Kline-Tilford

Background/Definition

- Also known as acute kidney failure.
- Multifactorial process.

Definition

- An abrupt cessation or significant decline in the kidney's ability to eliminate waste products, regulate acid–base balance, and regulate electrolyte balance.

Pathophysiology

- Damage to renal epithelium results in secretion of vasoactive compounds (e.g., angiotensin, prostaglandins, nitric oxide, and endothelin).
- Released vasoactive compounds result in increased vascular resistance and decreased blood flow, ultimately tubular damage. GFR is reduced and urine output decreases.

Etiology

- Many etiologies, including hemolytic uremic syndrome (HUS), shock, and GN.
- Classified as prerenal, intrinsic renal, and postrenal.
- Prerenal is the most common.
- Highest mortality rates are associated with multiorgan system failure; however, complete recovery of kidney function occurs in some patients.

Evaluation

- Medication history (e.g., nephrotoxic agents).
- Vital signs (e.g., blood pressure, heart rate, temperature).
- Fluid balance: urine output.
- Serum electrolytes and complete blood count (CBC).
- Consider hepatic panel if concern for hepatorenal syndrome.
- Chest radiography if accompanied by respiratory symptoms.

Management

- Fluid management: judicious (e.g., restore intravascular volume or diuresis depending on clinical status). Aggressive hydration may result in fluid overload, pulmonary edema, and respiratory compromise.
- Calculation of fractional excretion of sodium may help guide fluid management.
- Fluid management with urine output replacement and calculated insensible losses may be warranted.

Box 16.1 Common Etiologies of Acute Renal Failure in Children

Prerenal Kidney Disease

- Dehydration/depleted intravascular volume.
- Distributive volume issues/decreased effective intravascular volume.

Intrinsic Kidney Disease

- Acute tubular necrosis.
- Ischemia/hypoxia in kidneys.
- Medication-/drug-induced.
- Infection (e.g., HUS, poststreptococcal GN).
- Interstitial nephritis.
- GN.
- Renal artery or vein thrombosis.
- Vascular lesions.
- Endogenous toxins (e.g., myoglobin).
- Exogenous toxins (e.g., methanol, ethylene glycol).
- Idiopathic.

Obstructive Uropathy

- Bilateral ureteral obstruction.
- Kidney obstruction.

Specific Genetic Conditions Associated with Acute Renal Failure

- Polycystic kidney disease.
- Alport syndrome.
- Nephrotic syndrome (focal segmental glomerulosclerosis, membranoproliferative GN).
- Systemic lupus erythematosus (SLE).
- Diabetes.

Box 16.2 Presenting Signs and Symptoms of Acute Renal Failure

- Oliguria/Anuria.
- Edema.
- Electrolyte abnormalities.
- Decreased appetite.
- Nausea.
- Fatigue.
- Shortness of breath.
- Hypertension.
- Confusion.

- Hyponatremia is common. Risk for seizure activity if serum sodium <125 mEq/L. Treat with hypertonic saline solution (e.g., 3% saline administration).
- Hyperkalemia may be life-threatening (e.g., ventricular tachycardia, ventricular fibrillation).
  - EKG findings in hyperkalemia may include peaked T waves, prolongation of PR interval, widening of QRS complex, flattening of P waves.
  - Imperative to reduce extracellular potassium level and stabilize the cardiac cell membrane to avoid ventricular tachycardia/fibrillation. Glucose, sodium bicarbonate, insulin, and albuterol shift potassium into the cells.
  - Calcium chloride can stabilize the cardiac cell membrane.
  - Sodium polystyrene can exchange potassium and sodium in the colon.
  - Emergent dialysis is often indicated for serum potassium levels >7 mEq/L.
- Hypertension therapy: avoid angiotensin-converting enzyme (ACE) inhibitors. Goal is normal blood pressure for gender and height.
- Adjust medications that are renally excreted; consult a pharmacist.
- Renal supportive therapies may be indicated. See more information on renal supportive therapies later in this section.

Urinary Tract Infection

Andrea M. Kline-Tilford

Definition

- Bacterial or fungal infection in any part of the urinary tract (e.g., urethra, ureters, bladder, kidney).
- Migration to the kidney results in pyelonephritis (e.g., upper urinary tract infection [UTI]).

Background

- Accounts for as many as 5% to 14% of all pediatric emergency department (ED) visits.
- Common cause of hospitalization for infants and young children.
- Uncircumcised males have the highest incidence in the first 3 months of life.
- Genetic predisposition and history of dysfunctional voiding or elimination (e.g., encopresis) are associated with higher rates of UTI.
- In otherwise healthy children, UTI may indicate an underlying abnormality in the urinary tract (e.g., vesicoureteral reflux (VUR) disease; varying degrees of severity).

Etiology

- Most common etiology is colonic organisms.
- Commonly associated with gram-negative bacteria (e.g., *Escherichia coli*, *Klebsiella* species, and *Pseudomonas aeruginosa*), gram-positive bacteria (e.g., *Enterococcus*, *Staphylococcus aureus*, group B streptococcus).
- Has also been associated with *Candida*, adenovirus, and herpes simplex virus.

Pathophysiology

- Invasion of microorganisms (bacteria or fungi most commonly) into urethra, ascending the urinary tract to the bladder.
- Pathogen infiltrates the mucosa of the bladder, resulting in an inflammatory response.

Clinical Presentation

- Infants/Young children: fever, irritability/fussiness, decreased appetite, lethargy or changes in activity level, jaundice, and/or weight loss.
- Preschool/Young school age: abdominal pain, nausea/vomiting, and urinary frequency.
- Older children: urinary frequency, dysuria, urgency, suprapubic pain, and/or nausea/vomiting.

Evaluation

- Evaluate history for UTIs, structural abnormalities of the urinary tract, bubble baths, voiding/elimination dysfunction, sexual activity, maltreatment risk.
- Physical examination: evaluate for sacral dimple, costovertebral angle, or suprapubic tenderness.
- Urinalysis: presence of leukocyte esterase, nitrites, >5 white blood cells (WBCs), or bacteria/hpf.
- Urine culture: identifies pathogen and evaluates antibiotic sensitivity/resistance.
  - More than 50,000 colony-forming units/mL of a single organism and pyuria represent UTI in appropriately obtained specimens.
  - Must consider collection method/route and clinical presentation.
  - Urinalysis *and* urine culture are recommended to determine the presence of a UTI.
- Imaging.
  - Ultrasound: evaluates anatomy, kidney size/shape, and for evidence of hydronephrosis. Can also be used to evaluate for areas of inflammation and signs of pyelonephritis. Indications: UTI in children 2 months to 2 years of age.
  - Voiding cystourethrography: If renal and bladder ultrasound show hydronephrosis, scarring, or other evidence of high-grade VUR or obstructive uropathy, as well as in other atypical or complex clinical circumstances. Also indicated in all infants 2 months of age to 2 years with recurrence of febrile UTI.
  - Dimercaptosuccinic acid (DMSA) scintigraphy: Nuclear medicine scan used to evaluate for renal scarring.

Management

- Antibiotic therapy, tailored to specific organism when culture and sensitivities are available.
  - Duration of therapy determined by patient age, severity of illness, local resistance patterns, associated underlying disorders.
  - Uncomplicated UTI duration of therapy is 7 to 10 days; some studies support shorter duration of 2 to 4 days of therapy.
  - Complicated UTI therapy is generally 14 days.
  - Trimethoprim–sulfamethoxazole, amoxicillin–clavulanate, cefixime are acceptable selections for initial oral therapy.
  - Ceftriaxone, cefotaxime, gentamicin are acceptable selections for initial parenteral therapy.
  - In general, oral antibiotics are equally effective as parenteral therapy.
- Discomfort/fever: acetaminophen.
- Hospitalization is recommended when children are unable to tolerate oral medications or maintain adequate hydration, failure to improve on outpatient therapy, evidence of sepsis/septic shock, or underlying medical conditions that may complicate the management of UTI.
- Patient family education: signs of UTI, hygiene, limiting bubble baths, constipation prevention, urination after intercourse if sexually active.
- Close clinical follow-up after 7 to 10 days of antimicrobial therapy to evaluate for recurrent UTI.

PEARLS

- *Underlying urinary tract abnormalities are important to recognize early so that they do not lead to renal scarring.*
- *Prophylactic antibiotics do not reduce the risk of recurrent UTI, even in cases of mild-to-moderate VUR.*

Pyelonephritis

Samantha Lee

Definition

- Bacterial infection of the upper urinary tract caused by an ascending infection originated in the lower urinary tract.

Most Common Etiologies

- Gram-positive bacteria: *Enterococcus* spp. and *Staph. aureus*.
- Gram-negative bacteria: *E. coli*, *Klebsiella* spp., *Proteus* spp., *P. aeruginosa*, *Serratia* spp., and *Enterobacter aerogenes*.

Background

- 60% to 65% of children with febrile UTI also have acute pyelonephritis.
- Most cases of acute pyelonephritis respond readily to antibiotics.

Pathophysiology

- Bacterial invasion into the upper urinary tract with patchy interstitial inflammation and collections of neutrophils, leading to tubular necrosis.

Clinical Presentation

- Fever, lethargy.
- Tachycardia, tachypnea, dehydration.
- Pain (abdominal, suprapubic, flank, and/or costovertebral).
- Odorous urine.

Diagnostic Evaluation

- Urinalysis: rapid detection of leukocyte esterase and nitrites.
- Urine culture with sensitivities: critical for determining organism and appropriate antibiotic therapy.
- Basic metabolic panel: evaluation of kidney function.
- CBC with differential: evaluation of WBC count and differential.

- Blood culture: Positive culture indicates bacteremia.
- C-reactive protein: elevated, indicating an inflammatory process.
- Erythrocyte sedimentation rate: elevated, indicating an inflammatory process.
- Renal ultrasound for children 2 to 24 months of age.

Management

- Intravenous (IV) antimicrobial therapy.
- Hydration.
- Renal ultrasound.
- Voiding cystourethrography (VCUG): in some cases.
  - VCUG is typically reserved for children with recurrent febrile UTI who have evidence of abnormalities on ultrasound.

Nephritis
Samantha Lee

Definition

- Inflammation within the kidney.

Etiology/Types

- Primary (acute poststreptococcal GN, most common form) (see next section).
- Secondary.
- Hereditary.

Pathophysiology

- Deposits of immunoglobulins, complement, and cell-mediated immune reactions lead to inflammation and injury.

Clinical Presentation

- History of recent throat infection, decreased urine output, dark urine, fatigue, headache.
- Rash on buttocks and posterior legs, arthralgia, and weight loss (symptoms of secondary GN).
- Elevated blood pressure.
- Edema.
- Other signs of fluid overload/congestive heart failure.

Diagnostic Evaluation

- Electrolyte panel, creatinine, BUN, CBC with differential, urinalysis with urine culture and sensitivities, and throat culture.
- If acute poststreptococcal GN is suspected, a serum antistreptolysin-O (ASO) titer should be checked.
- To assess for systemic disease, autoimmune panels such as serum complement levels (C3, C4), lupus serologies, anti-DNase B, perinuclear antineutrophil antibody (P-ANCA), cellular antineutrophil cytoplasmic antibody (C-ANCA), and IgA are useful.
- Low serum C3 levels are indicative of secondary GN.

Management

- Antibiotic: penicillin, first line.

- Treatment of hypertension or acute renal insufficiency.
  - Judicious fluid management.
  - Sodium-restricted diet.
  - Diuretics.
  - Calcium channel antagonists, vasodilators, or ACE inhibitors.
- For secondary forms of GN.
  - Corticosteroids and cyclophosphamide to counteract the inflammatory process.

Acute Poststreptococcal Glomerulonephritis
Tamara L. Hill

Background/Definition

- Caused by a prior infection with specific nephritogenic strains of a beta-hemolytic streptococcus of the throat or skin.
- Most common glomerular cause of hematuria.

Etiology/Types

- Commonly follows group A streptococcal pharyngitis during the cold weather months and streptococcal skin infections or pyoderma during warm weather months.

Clinical Presentation

- Sudden onset of gross hematuria, edema, hypertension, and renal insufficiency.

Diagnostic Evaluation

- Urinalysis: red blood cells—often associated with red blood cell casts, proteinuria, and polymorphonuclear leukocytes.
- Elevated ASO titer.
- Complement level: C3 level initially decreased; returns to normal 6 to 8 weeks after presentation (sometimes sooner).
- Throat culture positive for group A streptococcus can confirm diagnosis.

Management

- Penicillin: a 10-day course.
- Cephalosporins or macrolide antibiotics can be used in patients with penicillin allergy.
- Acute renal insufficiency: furosemide.
- Hypertension: antihypertensive agents and sodium restriction.

Renal Artery/Vein Thrombosis
Samantha Lee & Andrea M. Kline-Tilford

Definition

- Formation of a thrombus in the renal artery or vein.

Background

- Relatively rare.

- Most commonly associated with asphyxia, sepsis, shock, dehydration, hypercoagulable state, indwelling umbilical catheter, or maternal diabetes in newborns/infants.
- Also associated with nephrotic syndrome, congenital heart disease, inherited hypercoagulable state (e.g., Factor V Leiden deficiency), sepsis, exposure to contrast agents, or after kidney transplantation in children.

Pathophysiology

- Clot formation as a result of endothelial cell injury or hypercoagulable/sludging state. Thrombus forms in the intrarenal circulation; may extend to inferior vena cava or main renal vein.
- Renal artery thrombus: acute occlusion of the renal artery due to thrombus formation, leading to renal infarction and irreversible loss of renal function.

Clinical Presentation

- Abrupt onset of hematuria.
- Flank mass, unilateral or bilateral.
- Flank pain.
- Oliguria.
- Hypertension.

Diagnostic Evaluation

- Doppler ultrasound of kidneys is diagnostic.
- Ultrasound: enlarged kidney(s) (early stages), atrophic kidney(s) (late stages).
- Radionuclide study: minimal or no function in the affected kidney(s).
- Abdominal CT: filling defect during venous phase after contrast administration.
- Magnetic resonance venography may also be used; avoid administration of contrast.
- Microangiopathic hemolytic anemia; thrombocytopenia in some cases.

Management

- Monitor and maintain fluid and electrolyte balance.
- Blood pressure monitoring; antihypertensive agents.
  - If refractory to pharmacologic therapy, may require nephrectomy.
- Treatment with anticoagulants (e.g., heparin) or thrombolytics (e.g., streptokinase, recombinant tissue plasminogen activator) is common, but controversial.
- Inferior vena cava thrombus may require thrombectomy.
- Treat underlying disease (e.g., nephrotic syndrome), if indicated.

Complications

- Pulmonary embolism, renal atrophy (affected side).

Renal Tubular Acidosis

Samantha Lee

Background

- Result of an inherited or acquired defect that affects the kidneys' ability to filter bicarbonate or excrete ammonia.

- Sickle cell anemia can be a genetic cause of renal tubular acidosis (RTA).
- Acquired causes: certain medications, obstructive uropathy, and autoimmune diseases.
- Often associated with presence of a UTI.

Definition

- A relatively uncommon clinical syndrome characterized by defects in the renal tubules as a result of failure to maintain a normal serum bicarbonate level despite the consumption of a regular diet and normal metabolism and acid production.

Pathophysiology

- Defects in renal tubules lead to a hyperchloremic metabolic acidosis, with a normal to moderately decreased GFR and normal anion gap.

Etiology/Types

- Type I RTA (distal): decrease in acid excretion.
- Type II RTA (proximal): failure of bicarbonate reabsorption with decreased ammonium absorption.
- Type IV RTA: aldosterone deficiency or impairment of its effects, resulting in reduced potassium excretion, hyperkalemia, and acidosis.
- Types I and II are most common in children.

Clinical Presentation

- Polyuria.
- Polydipsia.
- Preference of savory foods.
- Hypokalemia.
- Refractory rickets.
- Metabolic acidosis.

Presentation of Specific Types

- Type I RTA: linked to multiple genetic disorders (sensorineural hearing loss and nephrocalcinosis); failure to thrive or short stature, anorexia, vomiting, and dehydration.
- Type II RTA: failure to thrive, hyperchloremic acidosis with hypokalemia, and rarely nephrocalcinosis; rickets or osteomalacia may indicate Fanconi syndrome.
- Type III RTA: no longer used as a classification; now thought to be a combination of types I and II.
- Type IV RTA: Hypertension common if child has underlying Gordon syndrome, renal parenchymal disease, or mineralocorticoid dysfunction.

Diagnostic Evaluation

- Serum and urine electrolytes.
- Fractional excretion of bicarbonate and urine pH.
- Urine glucose and protein, calcium-to-creatinine ratio.
- 24-hour urine sample (i.e., citrate, calcium, potassium, and oxalate).
- Radiographies of long bone or wrists for evaluation of rickets.
- Abdominal ultrasound (kidneys).
- Genetic or chromosomal evaluation.

Management

- Emergency or impatient management for children with hyperchloremic, non–anion gap acidosis requiring bicarbonate replacement intravenously.
- Slow rehydration and electrolyte replacement, sodium bicarbonate or citrate, diuretic, phosphate replacements in children with rickets.

PEARL

- *Without proper therapy, chronic acidity in the blood results in growth retardation, nephrolithiasis, bone disease, and chronic renal failure.*

Hemolytic Uremic Syndrome

Tamara L. Hill

Background/Definition

- HUS is the most common cause of acute renal failure (ARF) in children <4 years of age.
- Characterized by the simultaneous occurrence of microangiopathic hemolytic anemia, thrombocytopenia, and uremia.

Etiology

- Divided into Shiga-toxin-associated HUS and non–Shiga-toxin-associated HUS based on clinical presentation.
- Shiga-toxin-associated HUS occurs after a prodromal episode of bloody diarrhea caused by *E. coli* infection.
- Non–Shiga-toxin-associated HUS is distinguished by absence of diarrhea or Shiga-toxin-producing *E. coli* infection, but with microangiopathic hemolytic anemia, thrombocytopenia, and uremia.

Clinical Presentation

- Gastroenteritis with fever, vomiting, diarrhea, abdominal pain, and diarrhea that begins as watery but then becomes bloody.
- Physical examination: dehydration, edema, petechiae, hepatosplenomegaly, and marked irritability.

Diagnostic Evaluation

- Hemoglobin level is commonly 5 to 9 g/dL.
- Peripheral blood smear reveals helmet cells, burr cells, and fragmented red blood cells.
- Reticulocyte count is moderately elevated.
- Coombs test result is negative.
- Significant leukocytosis with the leukocyte count greater than 300,000/mm³.

Management

- Supportive care.
- Aggressive management of fluids, electrolytes, and nutrition.
- Control of hypertension and early initiation of dialysis have been associated with a decrease in mortality.

Nephrotic Syndrome

Tamara L. Hill & Samantha Lee

Background/Definition

- Kidney filtration disorder in which too much protein is filtered out of the blood, leaking into the urine.
- Results in proteinuria, edema, and hyperlipidemia.

Etiology

- Idiopathic (90%).
- Believed to have immunopathogenesis.
- Genetic disorders.
- Secondary causes include infection, drugs, immunologic/allergic disorders, association with malignant disease, glomerular filtration.

Box 16.3 Causes of Childhood Nephrotic Syndrome

Idiopathic
- Minimal change disease.
- Focal segmental glomerulosclerosis.
- Membranoproliferative GN.
- IgA nephropathy.

Secondary
- Diabetes.
- Henoch–Schönlein purpura.
- Hepatitis B or C.
- SLE.
- Malignancy.
- Vasculitis.
- Streptococcal infection.
- Human immunodeficiency syndrome.
- Congenital syphilis, toxoplasmosis, cytomegalovirus, rubella.
- Malaria.
- Certain medications: penicillamine, gold, nonsteroidal anti-inflammatory medications, interferon, mercury, pamidronate, lithium.

Genetic
- Nail–patella syndrome, Pierson syndrome, and others.

Pathophysiology

- Injury to the basement membrane epithelial cells (podocytes) which causes collapse of the podocyte structure, spacing, and fracture of the protein barrier, allowing negatively charged proteins to move free across this disrupted filtration membrane.
- Results in proteinuria, edema, and decreased circulating albumin causing increased interstitial edema.
- Increased synthesis of lipoproteins and decreased lipid catabolism.
  - Hyperlipidemia.

Clinical Presentation

- Edema: most notably, periorbital edema.
- Frothy or foamy urine.
- Sudden increase in weight with edema.
- Hypertension.
- Hypoalbuminemia.
- Hyperlipidemia.

Diagnostic Evaluation

- Urine dipstick to determine proteinuria (rapid).
- 24-hour urine collection (ideal).
- CBC with differential.
- Complete metabolic panel with serum albumin.
- Serum C3/C4 complement.
- Antinuclear antibody.
- Hepatitis B and C.
- HIV testing.
- Immunologic studies (IgG, IgM, IgE).
- Kidney biopsy.

Management

- High-dose steroids (prednisone 2 mg/kg/day for 6 weeks divided into three doses).
- Treatment continues until patient is in remission (3 days with zero-trace protein via urine dipstick).
- Once proteinuria is resolved, maintenance dose of steroids—2 mg/kg every other morning, then tapered off over 6 weeks.
- If no remission after initial treatment, patient is considered steroid-resistant. Begin cytotoxic medications such as cyclosporine A, cyclophosphamide, or chlorambucil.
- Supportive therapy includes ACE inhibitors, statins, and diuretics, and restricting dietary sodium to 1,500 to 2,000 mg/day.

PEARL

- *Hallmark of nephrotic syndrome is massive proteinuria and decreased circulating albumin levels.*

Henoch-Schönlein Purpura Nephritis

Tamara L. Hill

Background/Definition

- Systemic vasculitis of the small vessels.
- Henoch–Schönlein purpura nephritis and IgA nephropathy are similar in renal pathologic findings, but systemic findings are noted only in the former.
- Occurs at any age from infancy to adulthood, but is overwhelmingly a childhood disease.
- Approximately 14 to 15 cases per 100,000 population.

Etiology/Pathophysiology

- Unknown.
- Appears to be mediated by the formation of immune complexes containing IgA within the skin, intestines, and glomeruli.

Clinical Presentation

- Symptoms usually present 1 to 3 weeks after an upper respiratory tract infection or gastrointestinal infection (e.g., Epstein–Barr virus, parvovirus B19, *Helicobacter pylori* infection, *Yersinia* infection, *Shigella* infection, *Salmonella* infection), or environmental allergen exposure (e.g., medications, foods, insect bites).
- Raised, nonblanching, purpuric rash, most prominent on the buttocks and lower legs.
- Abdominal pain.
- Arthralgias.
- GN.
- Presentation may be acute or insidious.

Diagnostic Evaluation

- Clinical presentation.
- Gross hematuria.
- Urinalysis: microscopic or gross hematuria and proteinuria.
- CBC: leukocytosis with eosinophilia, thrombocytosis.
- D-dimer: increased.
- Prothrombin time and activate partial thromboplastin time: decreased.
- IgA levels: may be increased.
- Stool guaiac test: occult blood.
- Kidney biopsy findings are indistinguishable from those of IgA nephropathy.

Management

- Resolves spontaneously in >90% of patients.
- Symptomatic management of systemic complications is the treatment of choice.
- Prednisone 1 to 2 mg/kg/day for 14 days in some cases (more severe).
- Plasmapheresis, high-dose IV immunoglobulin (IVIG), and immunosuppressant therapy may be needed for refractory cases.

PEARL

- *As many as one third of patients may have recurrence of symptoms.*

IgA Nephropathy

Tamara L. Hill

Background/Definition

- IgA nephropathy, also known as Berger disease or Berger nephropathy, is a renal disorder characterized by IgA antibodies affecting the kidneys, resulting in hematuria and proteinuria.
- The most common form of chronic glomerular disease.

Etiology

- Unknown.

Clinical Presentation

- Gross hematuria following a respiratory infection.
- May be associated with edema of hands and feet.

Diagnostic Evaluation

- Urinalysis: gross hematuria and proteinuria.
- Serum BUN and creatinine levels are elevated.

Management

- Primary goal is prevention or delay of chronic renal failure.
- Primary treatment is blood pressure control; antihypertensives.
- Immunosuppressive therapy with alternate-day corticosteroids or more intensive multidrug regimens may be beneficial.
- ACE inhibitors are effective in reducing proteinuria.

Polycystic Kidney Disease

Tamara L. Hill

Background/Definition

- Markedly enlarged kidneys with numerous cysts throughout the cortex and medulla.
- Fourth leading cause of kidney failure.

Etiology/Types

- There are two types:
  - Autosomal recessive polycystic kidney disease (ARPKD).
  - Autosomal dominant polycystic kidney disease (ADPKD).
    - ADPKD is the most common type of hereditary kidney disease.
- Both types are caused by gene defects of PKD1 or PKD2.

Clinical Presentation

- ARPKD: presents in the neonate as bilateral flank masses during the neonatal or early infancy period.
- ADPKD: presents in the fourth or fifth decade of life with bilateral flank masses, hypertension, abdominal masses, abdominal pain/discomfort, and UTIs. ADPKD affects many organs, and cysts may be found in the liver, pancreas, spleen, and ovaries.

Diagnostic Evaluation

- Confirmed by the presence of enlarged kidneys (ultrasound; CT or MRI may be used if ultrasound results are equivocal) with bilateral macrocysts.

Management

- Treatment for both types is primarily supportive.
- Control of hypertension; fluids and electrolytes are essential.
  - ACE inhibitors and angiotensin II receptor antagonists are agents of choice.
- Prompt treatment of UTIs and avoidance of dehydration.
- Avoidance of contact sports.
- Routine ultrasound and serum chemistry monitoring (e.g., annually, more frequently depending on clinical status).

PEARL

- *It is not uncommon for an otherwise healthy individual, especially older adult to have one, two, or three cysts in a kidney, without associated clinical problems or underlying polycystic kidney disease (PKD).*

Membranoproliferative Glomerular Nephritis

Tamara L. Hill

Background/Definition

- Membranoproliferative glomerular nephritis (MPGN) is the most common cause of GN in older children and adults.
- This form of nephritis results in ongoing glomerular injury that leads to glomerular destruction and end-stage renal disease.

Etiology/Types

- Autoimmune disease (e.g., SLE, scleroderma, Sjögren syndrome, sarcoidosis).
- Malignancy (e.g., leukemia, lymphoma).
- Infectious (e.g., hepatitis B, hepatitis C, endocarditis, malaria).

Clinical Presentation

- Nephrotic syndrome.
- Gross hematuria or asymptomatic microscopic hematuria.
- Proteinuria.
- Renal function may be normal or decreased.
- Hypertension is common.
- Serum complement 3 (C3) may be low.

Diagnostic Evaluation

- Kidney biopsy is the gold standard for diagnosis.

Management

- Systemic steroids for children and antiplatelets for adults.
- Additional therapies include plasmapheresis and plasma infusion.

Testicular Torsion

Deiadra J. Garrett

Definition/Background

- Twisting of the spermatic cord causing compromised blood flow to testicle.
- Occurs in 1:4,000 males <25 years of age.

Types

- Two types:
  - Intravaginal: spermatic cord twists around the tunica vaginalis.

- May occur at any age.
- Accounts for 90% of testicular torsion cases.
- Typically, it is a congenital malformation resulting in abnormal fixation allowing the epididymis, spermatic cord, and testicle to hang freely in the scrotal sac.
  - This allows the structures to twist within the tunica vaginalis.
  - Usually a bilateral deformity ("bell clapper" deformity).
- Extravaginal: spermatic cord twists proximal to the tunica vaginalis (entire scrotal contents).
  - Occurs perinatally during the descent of the testes; may present at birth.

Predisposing Factors

- Trauma.
- Testicular tumor.
- Testicles lying in horizontal plane.
- History of cryptorchidism and increasing testicular volume.

Clinical Presentation

- Occurs in children <3 years of age and after puberty most commonly.
- Sudden onset of pain involving the testis; usually unrelenting.
- Testis is enlarged and tender.
- Absence of cremasteric reflex.
- Affected testicle higher in the scrotum.

Diagnosis

- Ultrasound.
  - Absence of blood flow to the involved testis; twisting of spermatic cord.

Treatment

- Emergent surgical exploration.
  - Manual detorsion of testis.
  - Affix testis to scrotal wall to prevent recurrence (orchiopexy).
  - In most cases, contralateral testis will also be explored and fixed with nonabsorbable suture to prevent future torsion.
  - In general, 4- to 8-hour window before irreversible testicular injury.
  - If testicle cannot be salvaged, it is removed (orchiectomy).
- IV fluids, NPO, analgesia when preparing for operating room.
- If loss of testis, support from child life, social/spiritual support may be beneficial.

Ovarian (Adnexal) Torsion
Deiadra J. Garrett

Definition

- Twisting of adnexal structures compromising blood flow to the ovary.
- Usually associated with a cyst or mass.

Clinical Presentation

- Peaks in adolescence.
- Acute onset of abdominal pain caused by ischemia.
  - More common on right side.
- Nausea and vomiting.

Diagnosis

- Can be challenging.
- Doppler ultrasound is definitive study.
  - Assess for absence of blood flow in the involved ovary or associated ovarian cyst or mass.
  - False-negative results are possible depending on the severity of torsion.
- Abdominal CT or MRI is reserved for patients with nondefinitive findings on ultrasound and intermittent symptoms.
- CBC to evaluate for anemia.
- Urinalysis to evaluate for UTI.
- β-hCG to evaluate for pregnancy.

Treatment

- Medical emergency.
- Emergent surgical exploration.
  - Detorsion of involved ovary.
  - Cystectomy, if indicated.
  - Rarely is oophorectomy indicated; ovary can often be salvaged for up to 24 hours after the onset of abdominal pain.

Priapism
Andrea M. Kline-Tilford

Definition/Background

- Painful, sustained erection not associated with sexual arousal, lasting ≥30 minutes.
- Occurs in as many as 27% of males with sickle cell disease.

Etiology

- Stasis in erectile tissue (e.g., erythrocyte sickling and vascular sludging) of corporeal bodies.
- Most commonly associated with sickle cell disease.
- Spinal cord injury, trauma, and leukemic infiltration are less common associations.
- Medication exposure (e.g., erectile dysfunction medications, cocaine, marijuana, and ecstasy) has also been described.

Clinical Presentation

- History: sickle cell disease, trauma, medication exposure.
- Onset often during sleep.
- Frequency increases with age.

Diagnostic Evaluation

- Painful erection.
- Inspect level of rigidity and tenderness.

Management

- Warm sitz baths.
- Analgesics.
- Aggressive hydration.
- Urology consultation of erection lasting 4 hours.
  - Aspiration of blood from corpora and irrigation with saline or dilute adrenergic solution.
  - Surgical management with a shunt may be considered in refractory cases.
- Simple or exchange transfusion may be considered in children with sickle cell disease.
- Hematology consult if associated with sickle cell disease.

PEARL

- *Embarrassment may delay seeking medical attention.*

Renal Supportive Therapies

Continuous Renal Replacement Therapy

Mary C. Caverly

Background

- Slow continuous hemodialysis and hemofiltration for critically ill patients used to treat fluid overload, ARF, chronic renal failure, life-threatening electrolyte imbalances, intoxications (molecule size dependent), and concomitant sepsis and/or multiorgan failure.
- Only used in the critical care setting.

Definition

- An extracorporeal blood purification therapy intended to substitute for impaired renal function over an extended period of time.
- Therapy is administered continuously, for 24 hours per day.
- May be administered for days or weeks, but is not a long-term therapy.

Clinical Presentations Commonly Necessitating the Use of Continuous Renal Replacement Therapy

- Sepsis with hemodynamic instability; may be used for cytokine removal.
  - Reduces hemodynamic instability.
  - Allows precise volume control.
  - Toxin removal.
  - Effective control of uremia, hypophosphatemia, hyperkalemia.
- Acute kidney injury: estimated creatinine clearance decreased by 50%, urine output <0.5 mL/kg/hour × 16 hours (RIFLE criteria).
- Fluid overload: hypervolemia with pulmonary edema or respiratory failure refractory to diuretic therapy.
- Uremia with encephalopathy: removal of urea and toxins.
- ARF: estimated creatinine clearance decreased by 75% or urine output <0.3 mL/kg/hour for 24 hours or anuric for 12 hours (RIFLE criteria).

- Intoxication: Molecular size must be able to be cleared by filter for effective treatment.

Benefits

- Fluid removal; urea, creatinine, and potassium clearance; toxin clearance.

Complications

- Hypotension, hypothermia, bleeding, electrolyte imbalance, central line infection (hemodialysis catheter), and vessel thrombus.
  - Consider packed red blood cells transfusion prior to start of continuous renal replacement therapy (CRRT) (especially if ≤10 kg).
  - Hyperthermia unit may be added to CRRT machine to warm the blood being returned to the patient.

Preparation for CRRT

- Placement of hemodialysis catheter (e.g., temporary or permanent).
  - Internal jugular or subclavian vein: temporary or permanent catheter.
  - Femoral vein: temporary access only, difficult to maintain due to hip flexion; accessible vessel to cannulate, but limited by patient movement once in place (Table 16.1).

During CRRT

- Maintenance of anticoagulation.
  - Sodium citrate.
    - Combines with calcium ion to render clotting factors inactive within the filter.
    - Citrate processed through the liver.
    - Must have continuous infusion of calcium outside of the circuit to maintain normal calcium levels.
    - Prior to initiating sodium citrate in the CRRT circuit, the patient's ionized calcium should be ≥1.1 mmol/L.
    - Benefits: minimal bleeding risks and extended filter life.
    - Risks.
      - Metabolic alkalosis.
        - Citrate is buffered into bicarbonate.
        - Treatment: eliminate acetate and bicarbonate sources.
      - Citrate lock.
        - Rising total calcium with dropping ionized calcium.
        - Delivery of citrate exceeds hepatic metabolism and CRRT clearance.
        - Increase dialysis by 20% to 30%.
        - Decrease or stop citrate for 3 to 4 hours and restart at 70% of prior rate.
      - Hypocalcemia, hypernatremia, hyperglycemia.
        - Must monitor CRRT ionized calcium levels, and serum ionized and total calcium, sodium, and glucose levels.
  - Heparin.
    - Acts indirectly at multiple sites in both intrinsic and extrinsic coagulation pathways to prolong coagulation.

TABLE 16.1 Selection of Renal Replacement Therapy Method*

Slow Continuous Ultrafiltration	Continuous Venovenous Hemofiltration	Continuous Venovenous Dialysis	Continuous Venovenous Hemodiafiltration
• Removal of free water from blood.	• Plasma and metabolites are removed from blood via ultrafiltration. • Employs convection method: Solutes pass across the semipermeable membrane along with the solvent in response to a positive membrane pressure.	• Plasma and metabolites are removed from blood via dialysis. • Employs diffusion method: Solutes are transported across a semipermeable membrane, moving from areas of higher concentration to lower concentration. • Effective small molecule clearance (e.g., urea, creatinine, phosphorus, and uric acid).	• Plasma and metabolites are removed from blood via filtration and dialysis. • Uses replacement fluid to limit the increased blood viscosity within the hemodialysis filter. • Blood volume reconstituted by IV fluid as replacement fluid with desirable electrolytes. • Replacement fluid is not returned to the patient. • Most efficient solute clearance.

*Each method requires a hemodialysis catheter

- Goal is to achieve activated clotting time (ACT) 180 to 220 milliseconds, commonly used to maintain the circuit.
- Benefits: may be used in liver failure.
- Risks: bleeding.
- Monitoring: anticoagulation (ACT, protime, and pro-thrombin time).

Hemodialysis

Mary C. Caverly

Background

- Dialysis is prescribed when medical interventions fail to manage disease resulting from kidney injury.
- Kidney dysfunction results in electrolyte imbalance, anasarca, and accumulation of uremic toxins.

Definition

- Hemodialysis is a substitute for native kidney function.
- Blood and dialysis fluid enter hemodialysis filter in a counter-current approach.
- This maximizes the concentration gradient between the blood and dialysis fluid.
- Typically, hemodialysis will run for 3 to 4 hours each session.

Indications for Hemodialysis

- Hypervolemia: respiratory compromise, heart failure, hypertension, hyponatremia, and/or anasarca.
- Electrolyte abnormalities: hyperkalemia, hyperphosphatemia, hypocalcemia, and/or acidosis.
- Symptomatic azotemia or uremia: confusion, bradycardia, platelet dysfunction, pericardial effusion.
- Asymptomatic azotemia or uremia (i.e., acute or chronic renal failure).
- Toxicity of non–protein-bound medications, poisons, or ammonia.

- Malnutrition: decreased intake due to volume restriction, increased metabolic demands, catabolic metabolism, or malabsorption.

Treatment and Requirements

- Placement of hemodialysis catheter: short-term hemodialysis catheter, tunneled hemodialysis catheter (internal jugular or superior vena cava), or arteriovenous fistula or graft—internal vascular access surgical connection joining an artery and vein for hemodialysis use.
- Hemodialysis treatment.
  - Blood flow rate typically 150 to 350 mL/minute with dialysis at 500 mL/hour.
  - Requires at least 7 Fr catheter to allow appropriate blood flow rate.
  - Ideally, patient weight is >10 kg.
  - Requires anticoagulation during therapy (typically with sodium citrate).
  - Hemodynamic stability required prior to initiation.
- Hemodialysis treatment requirements.
  - Inpatient (acute and critical care) or outpatient facility.
  - Hemodialysis technician.

Benefits and Complications

- Benefits: fluid removal, urea, creatinine, potassium, and toxin clearance (most effective dialysis).
- Complications.
  - Disequilibrium syndrome.
    - Dialysis-induced cerebral edema.
    - Symptoms: nausea, headache, confusion, and seizures.
    - Treatment: mannitol infusion (poorly cleared by dialysis) and short session with low blood flow rate without ultrafiltration.
  - Hypotension.
    - Caused by rapid removal of fluid from intravascular space.
    - Symptoms: prior to hypotension, tachycardia, nausea, "crampy" abdominal pain, and emesis.

- Treatment: small fluid boluses, decrease in ultrafiltration.
- If shock occurs, treat with fluid and discontinue dialysis.
- Bleeding.
- Electrolyte imbalance.
  - Pre- and postdialysis weights.
  - Fluid, electrolyte, and hemodynamic monitoring.
- Catheter infection.
- Vessel thrombosis.
  - Heparinize catheter after use.
- Baroreceptor dysfunction (may happen with chronic renal failure).
  - Symptoms: bradycardia.
  - Treatment: atropine or epinephrine to restore perfusion.

Peritoneal Dialysis

Mary C. Caverly

Background

- Dialysis using the peritoneal cavity to substitute for native kidney function.
- May be used in the acute care or home setting.

Definition

- Hyperosmolar dialysate solution is infused into the peritoneal cavity to facilitate the removal of electrolytes, toxins, and free water.
- Uses the peritoneal space as the semipermeable membrane filter.
- Solutes move from the intravascular space into the peritoneal space over a prescribed period of time (dwell time) and then are passively drained into an external drainage collection system.

Equipment and Treatment

- Tenckhoff catheter.
  - Percutaneous or surgically inserted flexible single-lumen catheter allows for peritoneal dialysis fluid to flow into the peritoneal space, dwells for a prescribed period of time, and then drains into an external collection bag.
  - Healing takes approximately 2 weeks.
  - Typical volumes of 10 mL/kg/cycle may be used immediately after insertion; after peritoneal lining is healed, 20 to 40 mL/kg/cycle may be used.
- Cycler machines.
  - May be used in the acute care and home setting.
  - CCPD—continuous cycling peritoneal dialysis via machine.
    - Nighttime-only therapy or nighttime and periodic day treatment.
    - 8 to 10 cycles with dwell times of 30 to 45 minutes.
  - CAPD—continuous ambulatory peritoneal dialysis.
    - Maximize fluid and toxin removal.
- Peritoneal dialysis fluid (1.5%, 2.5%, 4.25% glucose solution).
  - Dialysis fluid is hyperosmolar (to serum) and contains a high concentration of carbohydrates.

- Promotes ultrafiltration.
- Higher the percentage of carbohydrate solution, greater the volume of fluid removed.

Peritoneal Dialysis Benefits, Complications, and Contraindications

Benefits

- Fluid removal; urea, creatinine, and potassium clearance.
- Clearance of toxins.
- Treatment may be provided at home, outpatient, or inpatient.
- May be used in neonates and infants.

Complications

- Abdominal discomfort.
- Peritonitis.
- Electrolyte imbalance, hyperglycemia, protein loss.
- Inguinal/abdominal hernia.
- Respiratory compromise.
- Long-term peritoneal fibrotic tissue may limit functional dialysis.
- Peritoneum may lose its selectivity over time (decreased clearance, increased proteinemia).
- Contraindicated in patients with significant abdominal pathology.

Management

- Patient weight prior to and immediately after therapy.
- Must end therapy with drain cycle.
- Monitor fluid, electrolytes, and hemodynamic status.
- Access peritoneal catheter using aseptic or sterile technique.
- Monitor for sepsis; may treat peritonitis by adding antibiotics to dialysis fluid.

Kidney Biopsy

Definition

- Microscopic evaluation of kidney tissue.

Indications

- Diagnostic evaluation of kidney disease.
- Evaluation of rejection after kidney transplant; guides immunosuppression therapy.
- Detection of primary or metastatic kidney malignancy.

Method

- Most commonly performed percutaneously; needle inserted through skin, through tissue, and into kidney.
  - May be performed blindly (landmarks) or with the assistance of imaging guidance using ultrasound, CT, or fluoroscopy.
- Occasionally, may be performed through an open procedure.

Contraindications/Relative Contraindications

- Coagulation disorders: increased risk of procedural bleeding.
- Operative kidney tumors (may result in dissemination of malignant cells to surrounding tissue).

- Hydronephrosis: risk of perforating large renal pelvis, resulting in urine leak requiring surgical repair.
- UTI: risk of disseminating infection.

Potential Complications

- Hemorrhage: kidney is highly vascular.
- Unintended puncture of surrounding organ (e.g., liver, lung, bowel, inferior vena cava).

Preprocedure Evaluation/Plan

- NPO per institutional policy.
- Coagulation studies, CBC, type and cross/type, and screen.
- Sedation may not be required in older cooperative children; however, often indicated in young children.

Postprocedure

- Pressure over puncture site for approximately 20 minutes, followed by pressure dressing.
- Limited movement/activity for 24 hours after procedure.
- Monitor for signs/symptoms of hemorrhage.
- Evaluate abdomen for signs of hemorrhage or bowel perforation.

Kidney Transplant

Tresa E. Zielinski

Indications

- Irreversible kidney failure.
- Most common etiologies are congenital, urologic, and inherited disorders.
- Evaluation may begin when the estimated creatinine clearance is <60 mL/minute/1.73 m^2.
- If circumstances allow, transplantation prior to dialysis requirement is ideal to avoid associated morbidities.

Contraindications

- Malignancy, chronic illness with shortened life expectancy, severe brain damage, inability to improve quality of life.

Evaluation

- Diagnosis of kidney failure/end-stage disease and evaluation for multisystem involvement.
  - Laboratory sampling.
  - Anti-human leukocyte antigen antibodies and panel-reactive antibodies: evaluated for sensitization to determine which donor antigens should be avoided to prevent rejection.
  - Radiologic evaluation.
    - Ultrasound: evaluate for urinary tract abnormalities.
    - Echocardiogram.
    - Electrocardiogram.
  - Invasive studies.
    - Cardiac catheterization, in select patients.
    - Angiogram, in select patients.
- Discussion of prognosis and appropriateness of transplantation.

- Psychosocial evaluation (e.g., family's ability to adhere to posttransplant therapies and follow-up appointments, readiness for transplant, religious or cultural beliefs that may impact transplantation, evaluation of resources, and barriers to transplantation).

Donor Selection

- Deceased or living donors may be used.
- Live donors are preferred, with improved graft survival unless high suspicion of recurrent disease.
- Live donors: focus on overall donor health. Must be ≥18 years of age unless an identical twin. May be exceptions with the evaluation by an ethics team.

Preparing for Transplantation

- Goal to achieve optimal physical and mental health state prior to transplant, with financial planning.

Donor Evaluation (Living Donors)

- Preliminary laboratory sampling: blood type, human leukocyte antigen typing, crossmatch.
  - Referral to unbiased physician.

Posttransplant

- Maintenance immunosuppression.
  - Calcineurin inhibitor, usually in conjunction with a second agent such as an antiproliferative agent (e.g., mycophenolate mofetil) or mTOR inhibitor (e.g., rapamune).
  - Calcineurin inhibitors are nephrotoxic; levels require monitoring.

Cadaveric Kidney Differences

- Graft function: Poor initial graft function is more common. Can indicate acute tubular necrosis. Dialysis may be required in the first few weeks after transplant; typically only temporary.
- Starting of immunosuppression often differs between living and cadaveric donors.

Rejection

- Must always be considered on the differential diagnosis of transplant patients.
- Presentation varies.
- Common signs/symptoms include hypertension, fever, proteinuria, oliguria, or graft nonfunction.
- Definitive diagnosis is through biopsy.

Signs and Symptoms of Rejection

- Hyperacute: minutes to hours after transplant.
- Acute: 3 to 90 days after transplant.
- Chronic: >60 days after transplant.

Posttransplant Infection

- Signs and symptoms.
  - Fever.
    - Days: atelectasis.
    - Weeks: foreign objects.

- 2 to 6 weeks: fungal.
- 6 to 8 weeks: viral.
- Elevated WBC count.
- Primary versus reactivation versus reinfection.
  - Epstein–Barr virus (DNA virus of the herpes virus family).
    - Signs and symptoms: mononucleosis-like syndrome, hepatitis syndrome.
      - Epstein–Barr virus posttransplant lymphoproliferative disease occurs in 23% to 50% seronegative recipients and in 1% to 2% seropositive recipients.
    - Primary infection typically worse than reactivation.
  - Cytomegalovirus (DNA virus of the herpes virus family).
    - Signs and symptoms.
      - Fever, leukopenia/thrombocytopenia, mononucleosis-like syndrome, hepatitis, enteric ulceration, pneumonia.
  - *Pneumocystis carinii pneumonia.*
  - Varicella zoster.
    - Mortality 5% to 15%, related to visceral dissemination, primarily pneumonitis.
    - Symptoms.
      - Fever, abdominal pain, rash; new lesions may occur for 5 to 7 days up to 2 weeks, degree of WBC count suppression correlates with visceral dissemination and mortality.
    - If exposure is known within 96 hours, varicella zoster immune globulin (VZIG) will reduce severity of clinical disease, pneumonitis, and death.
  - Hepatitis.
    - 50% mortality rate.
    - 100% transmission rate between seronegative recipients and seropositive donors.
- Respiratory syncytial virus.
- Fungal infections.
- Posttransplant lymphoproliferative disease.
  - Mortality 33% to 58%; 85% of cases are caused by Epstein–Barr virus.
  - Allograft loss approximately 60%.
  - Treatment: cessation of immunosuppression.

Patient and Family Education

- Avoid aminoglycosides/nephrotoxic drugs.
- No live immunizations.

Renal Ultrasound

Mary C. Caverly

Background

- Used to create images of soft tissue structures.
- Cannot be used to image bone or gas-filled organs.
- When used in conjunction with Doppler, it can evaluate venous and arterial flow.

Definition

- Use of high-frequency sound waves transformed into pictures.
- Renal ultrasound specifically can determine kidney size, shape, and location.
- Indicated for the evaluation of:
  - Gross structural abnormalities, fluid collections (e.g., abscess, cysts, infection), solid mass (e.g., tumors), calculi, duplication anomalies, inflammation (e.g., hydronephrosis, hydroureters).
  - Kidney size, location, shape.
  - Venous and arterial blood flow to kidney.
  - Bladder (e.g., thickening or abnormality).
  - Fluid collection (e.g., guide needle during aspiration/sampling).

Procedure

- Noninvasive, no radiation.
- Best results when patient is quiet, not moving.
- In some cases, NPO 4 to 8 hours prior to examination.

Voiding Cystourethrogram

Mary C. Caverly

Background

- Diagnostic study to identify VUR.

Definition

- Invasive radiologic procedure using fluoroscopy and radionuclide to evaluate flow of urine.
- Identifies abnormalities of bladder and urethra, and grades level of VUR, if present.

Indications for VCUG

- Should not be performed routinely after the first febrile UTI.
- If renal and bladder ultrasound show hydronephrosis, scarring, or other evidence of high-grade VUR or obstructive uropathy, as well as in other atypical or complex clinical circumstances.
- Infants 2 months of age to 2 years with recurrence of febrile UTI.
- Females >2 years of age with their first UTI.
- Females <5 years of age with febrile UTI.
- Recurrent pyelonephritis.
- Suspected urinary obstruction or stricture—bilateral hydronephrosis.
- Suspected bladder trauma or rupture.

Procedure

- Insertion of urinary catheter; radionuclide instilled into bladder and catheter removed.
- Fluoroscopy used to evaluate the flow of urine.
- Retrograde flow represents presence of VUR.
- Extravasation of urine outside of bladder represents bladder rupture.

- Obstructed flow represents urethral strictures or posterior urethral valves.

Preparation

- Child life therapy to help prepare the child for the examination.
- Distraction techniques; sedation may be required.

Dimercaptosuccinic Acid Scan

Mary C. Caverly

Background

- DMSA scan evaluates the size, shape, and position of the kidneys.
- It also detects scarring in the kidneys caused by infection.
- A static examination.

Definition

- Nuclear medicine scan of the kidneys using a radioactive tracer that localizes in the kidney; used to identify parenchymal damage and renal scarring.

Indications for Dimercaptosuccinic Acid

- Identification of renal scarring after pyelonephritis or UTI.
- Evaluation of acute pyelonephritis.
- May also be used to evaluate for certain masses or vasculitis.

Study Method

- Tracer attaches to functioning renal cortex.
- Identifies renal scarring.
- Identifies extent of parenchymal damage.
- Timing after infection controversial.

Procedure

- IV catheter is inserted and radioactive tracer injected—technetium-99m (DMSA).
  - Short-acting, eliminated in urine.
- Scan occurs 2 to 4 hours after injection of radioactive tracer.

Preparation

- Child life—to help prepare the child for the examination.
- Distraction techniques; sedation may be required.

1. A preschooler attended an outdoor camp, where the child sustained several insect bites and a bee sting. The next morning, the child was irritable with abdominal pain and periorbital edema. A urinalysis revealed 3+ protein and serum albumin <2.5 g/dL. What is the *most* likely initial treatment?
   a. STAT epinephrine.
   b. STAT furosemide (Lasix).
   c. Steroid therapy.
   d. Immunosuppressive therapy.

Answer: **C**

While rare, insect bites have been associated with nephrotic syndrome. Patients with nephrotic syndrome exhibit proteinuria, periorbital edema, and low serum albumin from third-spacing. First-line therapy is corticosteroid administration.

2. Which one of the following is the best indication of kidney function following transplant?
   a. Urine output.
   b. Urine specific gravity of 1.010.
   c. Central venous pressure of 6 mmHg.
   d. Hypertension.

Answer: **A**

The best indication of a successful kidney transplant is the formation of adequate urine output. Other chemical studies (BUN, creatinine, others) can be used to suggest a successful kidney transplant.

3. Fever that develops in a child 7 weeks after kidney transplantation is most likely indicative of which of the following?
   a. Bacterial infection.
   b. Medication reaction.
   c. Viral infection.
   d. Likely incidental.

Answer: **C**

Timing of fever following kidney transplant is important in determining the source. Fever 6 to 8 weeks after kidney transplant is most commonly associated with a viral process. Fever days after transplant is more commonly associated with atelectasis, 1 to 2 weeks after transplant is associated with a foreign object (e.g., central venous catheter), and 2 to 6 weeks after transplant is often associated with a fungal infection.

4. A 5-year-old boy presents to the ED with complaints of sharp flank pain, decreased urine output, and "dark-colored urine." History includes wrestling with an older brother 2 days earlier. On examination, a firm flank mass is noted. Which of the following diagnostic tests would be most predictive of the cause of these symptoms?
   a. Urinalysis.
   b. CBC.
   c. Abdominal radiography.
   d. Angiography.

Answer: **D**

In this case, renal artery thrombosis should be on the list of differentials. An angiography is positive in nearly every case. Renal artery thrombosis can lead to renal infarct and subsequent loss of renal function. It is imperative to evaluate for this pathology.

5. A 3-week-old female infant presents with decreased urine output. She normally has six to eight wet diapers per day; however, in the past 2 days she has only had two wet diapers. Parents report finding a "lump" in the infant's lower right back. Newborn history reveals hospitalization in the neonatal intensive care unit for the first week of life with discharge home on day of life 14. What is the most important first step in management?
   a. Administer a 0.9% normal saline bolus.
   b. Initiate a heparin infusion.
   c. Call a nephrologist.
   d. Initiate broad-spectrum antibiotics.

Answer: **A**

This infant's history is concerning for a renal artery occlusion, leading to hypoperfusion of the kidney and decreased urine output. It is important to determine whether this infant had an umbilical arterial catheter placed in the neonatal intensive care unit. History of an umbilical arterial catheter is associated with high risk of a renal artery occlusion. Administering a fluid bolus will help to evaluate and treat for dehydration while other imaging tests are in process.

6. A 2-month-old infant is born to a diabetic mother. His initial glucose was 25 mg/dL, and the level stabilized over the next 24 hours, allowing him to be discharged home on day of life 5. At the 2-month visit, the primary care provider notes a new abdominal mass on palpation with a history which suggests decreased urine output. The infant is diagnosed with hydronephrosis on abdominal ultrasound. What should the family be told about the prognosis?
   a. This is a normal variant.
   b. Infant should be evaluated for a renal vascular thrombosis.
   c. Infant should be evaluated for a UTI.
   d. Infant will need further cardiac evaluation.

Answer: **B**

(continues on page 444)

Hydronephrosis can occur as the result of several underlying pathophysiologic occurrences that impair flow of urine out of the kidney(s). Some etiologies include urinary tract structural abnormalities, nephrolithiasis, and renal artery thrombosis. A new abdominal mass along with decreased urine output is concerning for a renal vascular thrombosis.

7. Which of the following antibiotics is the standard therapy for treatment of acute poststreptococcal GN?
   a. Amoxicillin.
   b. Penicillin V.
   c. Cephalexin.
   d. Bactrim.

Answer: **B**

Penicillin V is the drug of choice for treatment of poststreptococcal GN, except for patients allergic to penicillin. Ampicillin or amoxicillin is often used, but these drugs have no microbiologic advantage over penicillin V.

8. An otherwise healthy 2-year-old presents with a 4-day history of diarrhea and pallor. Diarrhea began as yellow mucus, but then became bloody during the last 2 days. Laboratory studies reveal a BUN of 49 mg/dL, creatinine of 3.88 mg/dL, and hemoglobin of 7.2 g/dL. The caregiver mentions they attended a family cookout 2 days before the diarrhea began. Which of the following is the *most* likely cause?
   a. Gastroenteritis.
   b. Irritable bowel disease.
   c. HUS.
   d. Abdominal lymphoma.

Answer: **C**

Yellow mucous diarrhea that becomes bloody, associated with elevated BUN/creatinine, anemia, and thrombocytopenia after ingesting raw meat, is a classic presentation of HUS.

9. Which of the following organisms is *most* commonly associated with HUS?
   a. *Giardia lamblia.*
   b. *E. coli* OH157:H7.
   c. *Clostridium difficile.*
   d. *Helicobacter pylori.*

Answer: **B**

The precise etiology of HUS is unknown; however, it has most commonly been associated with *E. coli, Salmonella, Shigella,* and *Streptococcus* pneumonia infections.

10. What is the primary treatment for IgA nephropathy?
    a. Antihypertensive agents.
    b. Anticoagulation therapy.
    c. Nonsteroidal anti-inflammatory agents.
    d. Diuretic agents.

Answer: **A**

The ultimate goal in the treatment of IgA nephropathy is to prevent or delay chronic renal failure, and the primary treatment is blood pressure control.

11. Which of the following is the preferred treatment for PKD in order to preserve kidney function?
    a. Removal of renal cysts.
    b. Management of blood pressure.
    c. Immunosuppressive therapy.
    d. Dialysis.

Answer: **B**

Management of blood pressure is critical in PKD because the rate of disease progression in PKD correlates with the presence of hypertension. Renal function will be seriously affected over time if blood pressure is not managed.

12. A 15-year-old girl is currently receiving hemodialysis 3 times per week for the last 6 months. She arrives in the ED with complaints of fever, nausea, and vomiting. Laboratory studies have been obtained and electrolytes are unremarkable, BUN is 150 mg/dL, and creatinine is 3.5 mg/dL. Current vital signs are a temperature of 39.4°C, heart rate of 134 beats per minute, blood pressure of 94/43 mmHg, and oxygen saturation of 98% on room air. A fluid bolus is in progress. What is the most important next step in managing this adolescent?
    a. Start second normal saline fluid bolus of 20 mL/kg.
    b. Administer ceftriaxone and vancomycin.
    c. Start a dopamine drip.
    d. Call for hemodialysis.

Answer: **B**

Symptoms suggestive of an infectious process need to be addressed with broad-spectrum antibiotics initiated within the first 30 minutes of suspected sepsis.

13. A 4-year-old girl is in ARF and her most recent laboratory results include a serum creatinine level of 3.1 mg/dL. Which medication does not require a dose adjustment based on renal function?
    a. Ranitidine.
    b. Fluconazole.
    c. Acetaminophen.
    d. Vancomycin.

Answer: **C**

Acetaminophen is primarily metabolized through the liver and does not require dose adjustments in cases of ARF (except in cases of hepatorenal syndrome). Dosing adjustment is not necessary in acute or chronic renal dysfunction or impairment. Ranitidine, fluconazole, and vancomycin require dosage adjustment in ARF.

14. Diagnosis of MPGN is made by which of the following methods?
    a. Renal ultrasound.
    b. Renal biopsy.

c. Renal CT.

d. Renal MRI.

Answer: B

The diagnosis of MPGN is made by renal biopsy. Indications for biopsy include nephritic syndrome in children >10 years of age with significant proteinuria, microscopic hematuria, and hypo-complementation, lasting longer than 8 weeks.

15. A 2-month-old female infant presents to the ED with diffuse anasarca, most notably periorbital edema. Laboratory values were as follows: hemoglobin 10 g/dL, total serum protein 4.4 g/dL, albumin 1.5 g/dL, and 3+ urine albumin. Renal biopsy showed mesangial proliferation with sclerosis in glomeruli. What is the most likely diagnosis?

a. Acute kidney failure.

b. Congestive heart failure.

c. Nephrotic syndrome.

d. Pyelonephritis.

Answer: C

This infant is displaying classic signs of nephrotic syndrome. These patients typically present with edema—most notably, periorbital edema. Laboratory values will reveal hypoalbuminemia with high urine protein. The sclerosis in the glomeruli is the result of accumulation of proteins and compensatory hypertrophy.

16. First-line therapy for a patient who presents with dependent edema, hypoalbuminemia, and 3+ proteinuria is:

a. High-dose steroids (2 mg/kg/day) for 1 week.

b. IV albumin for 3 days.

c. IV albumin for 6 weeks.

d. High-dose steroids (2 mg/kg/day) for 6 weeks.

Answer: D

First-line therapy for nephrotic syndrome is high-dose steroids (2 mg/kg/day or 60 mg/m^2/day) for 6 weeks. Treatment continues until patient is in remission, which typically takes 4 to 6 weeks. Remission is defined as 3 consecutive days with no trace protein via urine dipstick or a urine protein/creatinine ratio less than 0.2.

17. In nephrotic syndrome, the amount of protein in the urine is often directly correlated with which of the following?

a. Severity of podocyte injury or malfunction.

b. Amount of protein ingested by the patient.

c. Patient's diuretic regimen.

d. Age of the patient.

Answer: A

In patients with nephrotic syndrome, the podocytes, or basement membrane epithelial cells, are damaged, missing, or fused together. Injury to these epithelial cells causes disruption of the protein barrier, thus allowing proteins to freely move across the filtration membrane into the urine.

18. A 12-year-old Caucasian boy presents with a 4-day history of "dark urine" and "puffy eyes." Two weeks earlier, he had a sore throat and fever. He improved with no treatment. On examination, he is hypertensive, has periorbital edema, and is nontoxic appearing. Urinalysis reveals moderate blood and protein. What is the most reliable laboratory test to confirm the diagnosis?

a. CBC.

b. Serum ASO titer.

c. C-reactive protein.

d. Blood culture.

Answer: B

This child has signs and symptoms most consistent with acute post-streptococcal GN. The most important laboratory test is measurement of an ASO titer. It is positive in approximately 60% of patients with acute poststreptococcal GN. Confirming the diagnosis also requires confirmatory evidence of invasive streptococcal infection (e.g., group A beta-hemolytic streptococci) on throat culture.

19. An 11-year-old presents with a 3-week history of flu-like symptoms, chest pain, hemoptysis, blood-tinged diarrhea, and decreased urine output. There is a strong family history of SLE. Serum laboratory values are as follows: sodium 140 mEq/L, potassium 5 mEq/L, chloride 105 mEq/L, HCO 16 mEq/L, BUN 22 mg/dL, creatinine 1.62 mg/dL, uric acid 8 mg/dL, creatine kinase 700 g/L, random urine creatinine 300 mg/dL, urine protein 66 mg/dL, urinalysis significant for large amounts of blood, and 100 mg/dL protein. Which of the following confirmatory tests would be most helpful in the diagnosis?

a. Erythrocyte sedimentation rate, C3, and C4.

b. Coagulation panel, C3, and C4.

c. ANA, anti-double-stranded DNA, and anti-Smith antibodies.

d. ANA, C3, and C4.

Answer: C

Symptoms including chest pain, hemoptysis, blood-tinged diarrhea, flu-like symptoms, and decreased urine output could be consistent with a diagnosis of lupus nephritis. A strong family history of SLE would also indicate the need to consider testing, and this diagnosis should be high on the differential. ANA, anti-double-stranded DNA, and anti-Smith antibodies are the most sensitive tests for SLE. It is one of many secondary causes of GN.

20. A 6-year-old boy presents to the ED with a 12-hour history of vomiting, right upper quadrant pain, chills, increasing lethargy, and fever. He appears lethargic and has diffuse abdominal pain and right costovertebral angle pain and tenderness. A urinalysis reveals pyuria. Which antimicrobial regimen would be most beneficial?

a. Ceftriaxone.

b. Gentamicin and metronidazole.

c. Cefazolin.

d. Tobramycin.

Answer: A

Pyuria along with symptoms of vomiting, right upper quadrant pain, chills, increasing lethargy, and fever are consistent with pyelonephritis. Until culture and sensitivities are definitive, it is beneficial

(continues on page 446)

to start with a broad-spectrum antimicrobial. Gram-negative bacteria are the most common pathogens in pyelonephritis.

21. A 5-month-old child has poor weight gain, currently at less than 5th percentile on the growth chart, height at 10th percentile, and head circumference at 50th percentile. He feeds via bottle, and seems to take a sufficient volume. Screening laboratory results are as follows: sodium 140 mEq/L, potassium 4 mEq/L, chloride 110 mEq/L, bicarbonate 15 mEq/L, BUN 16 mg/dL, creatinine 0.3 mg/dL, and urine pH 9.0 from a urinalysis. Which of the following is the most appropriate therapy for this child?
    a. IV steroids.
    b. Oral supplementation of potassium chloride.
    c. Dialysis.
    d. Oral supplementation with sodium bicarbonate (Bicitra).

Answer: **D**

Indications of RTA include poor growth, high chloride and low bicarbonate on electrolyte panel with high urine bicarbonate. The child's small size is significant for failure to thrive, which is associated with RTA. Oral bicarbonate supplementation would be necessary to correct his electrolyte derangements.

22. Which of the following describes the classic signs and symptoms of type II RTA?
    a. Periorbital edema, proteinuria, and metabolic acidosis.
    b. Decreased urine output, rash on face and neck, and failure to thrive.
    c. Failure to thrive, metabolic acidosis, and hypokalemia.
    d. Elevated blood pressure, tachypnea, and gallop rhythm.

Answer: **C**

The typical clinical presentation of type II RTA includes infants with failure to thrive, hyperchloremic acidosis, and hypokalemia. This type of RTA is associated with more generalized proximal tubular dysfunction and Fanconi syndrome.

23. Which of the following values are needed to calculate a patient's estimated GFR?
    a. Weight and height.
    b. Weight and serum creatinine.
    c. Serum potassium and serum creatinine.
    d. Height and serum creatinine.

Answer: **D**

GFR can be estimated (eGFR) with the patient height, serum creatinine, and a constant (Schwartz equation).
eGFR mL/minute/1.73 m2 = (k)(height)/serum creatinine
- k = constant of 0.413 for all ages/genders.
- Height is measured in centimeters.
- Serum creatinine measured in mg/dL.

24. A 1-year-old female infant presents with her second febrile UTI. Which of the following studies is recommended?
    a. Renal ultrasound.
    b. Abdominal CT.
    c. VCUG.
    d. Bladder volume measurement scan.

Answer: **C**

VCUG is indicated for any child aged 2 to 24 months with recurrence of a febrile UTI. A renal ultrasound is recommended with the first documented UTI in this age group and VCUG is recommended if there are significant abnormalities as described in the American Academy of Pediatrics clinical practice guideline. An abdominal CT and bladder volume measurement scan are not indicated at this time.

25. Which of the following presentations would warrant immediate renal replacement therapy?
    a. Ingestion of acetaminophen.
    b. Severe dehydration with no urine output and a potassium level of 7.0 mEq/L.
    c. Significant overhydration with 3 mL/kg/hour of urine output and potassium level of 5.5 mEq/L.
    d. Ingestion of calcium channel blocker.

Answer: **B**

CRRT is used to manage overhydration in situations where kidney function is questioned, and also to filter electrolytes such as potassium. Acetaminophen is metabolized in the liver, so dialysis would not be effective, and calcium channel blocker ingestion can be managed by administering calcium. High potassium is life-threatening, and without urine output, the child should receive CRRT emergently.

Recommended Readings

Egging, D. (2012). Pelvic pain. In K. Reuter-Rice & B. Bolick (Eds.), *Pediatric acute care: A guide to interprofessional practice* (pp. 852–856). Burlington, MA: Jones & Bartlett Learning.

Jandeska, S. (2012). Dialysis and renal replacement therapy. In K. Reuter-Rice & B. Bolick (Eds.), *Pediatric acute care: A guide to interprofessional practice* (pp. 826–830). Burlington, MA: Jones & Bartlett Learning.

Jandeska, S. (2012). Physiology and diagnostics. In K. Reuter-Rice & B. Bolick (Eds.), *Pediatric acute care: A guide to interprofessional practice* (pp. 816–820). Burlington, MA: Jones & Bartlett Learning.

Jordan, S. C., Vo, A. A., Peng, A., Toyoda, M., & Tyan, D. (2006). Intravenous gammaglobulin (IVIG): A noval approach to improve transplant rates and outcomes in highly HLA-sensitized patients. *American Journal of Transplantation, 6*, 459–466.

Haut, C. (2012). Urinary tract infection. In K. Reuter-Rice & B. Bolick (Eds.), *Pediatric acute care: A guide to interprofessional practice* (pp. 864–867). Burlington, MA: Jones & Bartlett Learning.

Haut, C., Kitchen, B., & Jandeska, S. (2012). Renal tubular acidosis. In K. Reuter-Rice & B. Bolick (Eds.), *Pediatric acute care: A guide for interprofessional practice* (pp. 861–864). Burlington, MA: Jones & Bartlett Learning.

Kewalramani, A. L. (2012). Testicular torsion. In K. Reuter-Rice & B. Bolick (Eds.), *Pediatric acute care: A guide to interprofessional practice* (pp. 824–826). Burlington, MA: Jones & Bartlett Learning.

Kidney Disease Improving Global Outcomes. (2009). KDIGO clinical guideline for the care of kidney transplant recipients. *American Journal of Transplantation, 9*(Suppl. 3), 1–65.

Kitchen, B. (2012). Kidney insufficiency. In K. Reuter-Rice & B. Bolick (Eds.), *Pediatric acute care: A guide to interprofessional practice* (pp. 836–841). Burlington, MA: Jones & Bartlett Learning.

Kitchen, B. (2012). Nephrolithiasis. In K. Reuter-Rice & B. Bolick (Eds.), *Pediatric acute care: A guide to interprofessional practice* (pp. 845–849). Burlington, MA: Jones & Bartlett Learning.

Kramer, J. E. (2012). Priapism. In K. Reuter-Rice & B. Bolick (Eds.), *Pediatric acute care: A guide to interprofessional practice* (pp. 823–824). Burlington, MA: Jones & Bartlett Learning.

LaPoint-Rudow, D., Ohler, L., & Shafer, T. (Eds.). (2006). *A clinician's guide to donation and transplantation.* Lenexa, KS: Applied Measurement Professionals.

Montgomery, R. A. (2010). Renal transplantation across HLA and ABO antibody barriers: Integrating paired donation into desensitization protocols. *American Journal of Transplantation, 10,* 49–57.

Parker, A. L. (2012). Nephrotic syndrome. In K. Reuter-Rice & B. Bolick (Eds.), *Pediatric acute care: A guide to interprofessional practice* (pp. 849–852). Burlington, MA: Jones & Bartlett Learning.

Parker, A. L. (2012). Pyelonephritis and nephritis. In K. Reuter-Rice & B. Bolick (Eds.), *Pediatric acute care: A guide to interprofessional practice* (pp. 856–861). Burlington, MA: Jones & Bartlett Learning.

Pickering, L. K., Baker, C. J., Kimberlin, D. W., & Long, S. S. (2012). *American Academy of Pediatrics: 2012 Report of the committee on infectious diseases* (29th ed.). Elk Grove Village, IL. American Academy of Pediatrics.

Porter, C. C., & Avner, E. D. (2011). Renal vein thrombosis. In R. M. Kliegman, R. E. Behrman, H. B. Jenson, & B. F. Stanton (Eds.), *Nelson textbook of pediatrics* (17th ed.). Philadelphia, PA: W. B. Saunders.

Schrier, R. W. (2007). *Diseases of the kidney & urinary tract.* Philadelphia, PA: Wolters Kluwer Health/Lippincott Williams & Wilkins.

Subcommittee on Urinary Tract Infection and Steering Committee on Quality Improvement and Management. (2011). Urinary tract infection: Clinical practice guideline for the diagnosis and management of the initial UTI in febrile infants and children 2 to 24 months. *Pediatrics, 128*(3), 595–610.

Tredger, J. M., Brown, N. W., & Dhawan, A. (2006). Immunosupppression in pediatric solid organ transplantation: Opportunities, risks, and management. *Pediatric Transplantation, 10,* 879–892.

U.S. Department of Health and Human Services: Organ procurement and transplantation. Retrieved from: http://optn.transplant.hrsa.gov/

Vogt, B., & Avner, E. (2011). Renal failure. In R. M. Kliegman, R. E. Behrman, H. B. Jenson, & B. F. Stanton (Eds.), *Nelson textbook of pediatrics* (17th ed., pp. 2206–2210). Philadelphia, PA: W. B. Saunders.

Zielinski, T. E. (2012). Kidney transplantation. In K. Reuter-Rice & B. Bolick (Eds.), *Pediatric acute care: A guide to interprofessional practice* (pp. 841–845). Burlington, MA: Jones & Bartlett Learning.

Immunologic and Rheumatologic Disorders

Anaphylaxis

Kimberly L. DiMaria & Cheryl N. Bartke

Background

- Anaphylaxis occurs most commonly among children and adolescents.
- Although the incidence of allergies and severe allergic reactions is on the rise, the estimated lifetime prevalence of anaphylaxis rate remains low at 0.05% to 2%.
- Fatal cases of anaphylaxis are rare.

Definition

- A potentially life-threatening systemic reaction to an allergen or trigger that primarily affects the mucocutaneous, hemodynamic, and respiratory systems.

Etiology

- Most common triggers are food (e.g., eggs, shellfish, nuts), medications (e.g., antibiotics, nonsteroidal anti-inflammatories), and stinging.
- Can occur through a variety of mechanisms, which are classified into the following categories:
  - Immunologic IgE-mediated/IgE-dependent/type I hypersensitivity reaction.
  - Immunologic non-IgE-mediated/IgE-independent.
  - Nonimmunologic/direct mast cell activation.
  - Idiopathic.
- An allergen, such as radiocontrast, can precipitate an anaphylactic response through more than one mechanism, either an IgE-mediated response or a direct mast cell activation (i.e., causing histamine release).
- Regardless of the mechanism, the clinical manifestations and initial management are identical.

Pathophysiology

- Antigen-specific IgE is formed when an individual who is genetically susceptible is exposed to an allergen or trigger.
- When that person is subsequently exposed to the same allergen, mast cell activation occurs rapidly because the antigen-specific IgE has already bound to the mast cells via IgE receptors, making the cascade of inflammatory reactions rapid.
- Activation of mast cells and basophils triggers a rapid release of various inflammatory and newly formed mediators, including histamine, tryptase, leukotrienes, prostaglandins, platelet-activating factor, and various cytokines.
- Mediators affect various target organs, including the heart, lungs, vasculature, gastrointestinal tract, and skin.
- Heart rate, myocardial contractility, coronary blood flow, and electrical conduction through the sinoatrial and atrioventricular nodes are affected by the release of histamine and platelet-activating factor, causing decreased cardiac output and possible myocardial ischemia.
- Bronchospasm and increased mucus production in the lungs can occur as a result of mediator release.
- Vasodilation and increased vascular permeability lead to hypotension, distributive shock, and eventually impaired oxygen delivery.
- Increased vascular permeability of the airways and intestinal tract causes laryngeal edema and gastrointestinal upset.
- Mucocutaneous symptoms of flushing, angioedema, urticaria, and pruritus occur as a result of histamine release.

Clinical Presentation

- Rapid onset: minutes to hours.
- Hives, itching, abdominal pain, emesis, stridor, wheezing, shortness of breath, laryngeal edema, hypotension, and shock.
- If not treated promptly, can lead to cardiorespiratory collapse and death.

Diagnostic Evaluation

- Clinical diagnosis based on pathopneumonic symptomology.
- No specific laboratory test can confirm the diagnosis of anaphylaxis.
- However, plasma histamine levels, serum total tryptase levels, and serum IgE levels, if measured during or following an anaphylactic episode, are all elevated.

- Skin testing is indicated to confirm allergens or triggers.
  - Care should be taken to ensure that testing is carried out in a health care facility that can manage anaphylaxis, should the patient develop a reaction to a trigger.

Management

- ABC assessment.
- Additional key examination components include pulmonary, neurologic, and skin examinations, and frequent vital signs.
- Discontinue exposure to trigger/allergen if possible (e.g., a patient receiving intravenous [IV] chemotherapy).
- Epinephrine administration, intramuscular/subcutaneous; should not be delayed if anaphylaxis is suspected.
  - Delays in administration are associated with worse outcomes.
  - Administration should occur promptly on recognition of mild anaphylaxis symptoms; it is not necessary to wait until potentially life-threatening symptoms develop.
  - 0.01 mg/kg of 1:1,000 (1 mg/mL) into vastus lateralis muscle.
    - Maximum dose: 0.3 mg for children; 0.5 mg for adults.
    - If possible, inject with an autoinjector.
  - *Epinephrine is the only effective treatment for anaphylaxis.* It will decrease laryngeal edema, treat hypotension and shock, cause bronchodilation, and increase cardiac output by increasing heart rate and myocardial contraction.
  - There is no absolute contraindication of epinephrine administration for treatment of anaphylaxis.
  - Repeat the dose every 5 to 15 minutes as needed.
  - An estimated 20% of patients will require multiple doses of epinephrine.
  - May consider initiating IV epinephrine infusion.
- Place patient in a recumbent or supine position with lower extremities elevated above the heart.
- Administer oxygen; secure airway if necessary.
- Obtain IV access and administer 0.9% normal saline.
  - 30 to 40 mL/kg often required to treat hypotension.
- Consider administration of adjunctive medications after epinephrine administration.
  - H_1-antihistamine: diphenhydramine.
  - Nebulized β-agonist: albuterol.
  - Glucocorticoids: methylprednisolone IV or prednisone PO.
  - H_2-antihistamine: ranitidine.

PEARLS

- *The key to successful management of anaphylaxis is the prompt recognition of the signs and symptoms and the administration of epinephrine.*
- *If in doubt about whether or not a patient is experiencing an allergic/anaphylactic reaction, administer epinephrine.*
- *Symptoms of anaphylaxis are variable, depending on the individual. Additionally, the same person may have different manifestations of anaphylaxis from one episode to another.*
- *Providers should consider mastocytosis or clonal mast cell disorder as an underlying diagnosis for idiopathic anaphylaxis.*

Immunodeficiencies
Megan Trahan

Definition

- A group of genetic disorders that affect components of innate and adaptive immune systems and ultimately lead to susceptibility to infection.

Etiology/Types

- Humoral.
  - Isolated immunoglobulin deficiency (IgM, IgA, or IgG subclass).
  - X-linked agammaglobulinemia.
  - Common variable immunodeficiency.
  - Transient hypogammaglobulinemia of infancy.
  - Hyper-IgM syndrome.
- Cellular.
  - 22q11.2 Deletion syndrome.
- Combined antibody and cellular defects.
  - Severe combined immunodeficiency (SCID).
  - Wiskott–Aldrich syndrome.
  - Ataxia telangiectasia syndrome.
- Phagocytic.
  - Chronic granulomatous disease (CGD).
  - Hyper-IgE syndrome.
  - Leukocyte adhesion deficits.
- Complement.
  - Early complement defect (C2, C3, or C5).
  - Late complement defect.

Pathophysiology

- Humoral: antibody production or function.
  - X-linked, autosomal recessive, or autosomal dominant inheritance, if known.
- Cellular.
  - 22q11.2 Deletion: t-cell deficiency secondary to thymic aplasia or hypoplasia.
- Combined antibody and cellular.
  - SCID: multiple subtypes, some deficiency of T cells, B cells, and/or natural killer cells.
  - Autosomal recessive inheritance.
- Phagocytic.
  - Oxidative dysfunction of polymorphonuclear leukocytes and monocytes, leading to inability to kill phagocytosed bacteria and fungi.
- Complement.
  - Complement proteins may be absent or reduced in number.

Clinical Presentation

- Common warning signs of primary immunodeficiency (Table 17.1).
- In addition to infection, it may present with autoimmune diseases or lymphoid malignancy.
- Evaluate for syndromes associated with primary immunodeficiency (e.g., 22q11 deletion [DiGeorge syndrome] or ataxia telangiectasia).

TABLE 17.1 Warning Signs of Primary Immunodeficiency

10 Warning Signs of Primary Immunodeficiency

≥4 new ear infections within 1 y	Recurrent, deep skin or organ abscesses.
≥2 sinus infections within 1 y	Persistent thrush in mouth or fungal infection on skin.
≥2 mo on antibiotics with little effect	Need for IV antibiotics to clear infections.
≥2 pneumonias within 1 y	≥2 deep-seated infections including septicemia.
Failure of an infant to gain weight or grow normally	A family history of primary immunodeficiency.

Adapted from Jeffery Modell Foundation. (2013). *10 warning signs of primary immunodeficiency*. Retrieved from http://www.info4pi.org/aboutPI/index.cfm?section=aboutPI&content=warningsigns

- Evaluate immune organs: tonsils, spleen, and lymph nodes.
- Specific disease types and common presentations.
  - Humoral: sinopulmonary infections with encapsulated organisms.
  - Combined (SCIDs): failure to thrive, respiratory tract or gastrointestinal infections, candidal skin infections, *Pneumocystis jiroveci* pneumonia.
  - Phagocytic (CGD): infection with catalase-positive organisms (*Escherichia coli, Pseudomonas, Klebsiella, Serratia, Salmonella, Candida,* and *Aspergillus*).
  - Complement.
    - Early complement defects: sepsis.
    - Late complement defects: Neisseria infections.

Diagnostic Evaluation

- Complete blood count (CBC): evaluate for anemia, thrombocytopenia, lymphopenia, or neutropenia.
- Quantitative immunoglobulins (IgG, IgA, IgM, IgE).
- Total protein and albumin.
  - Low total protein with normal albumin suggests immunoglobulin deficiency.
- Antibody titers to vaccinations.
- Complement activity (CH50, C3, and C4).
- Nitroblue tetrazolium dye test: evaluate for CGD.

Management

- Depends on specific immunodeficiency.
- Treat infection with appropriate antimicrobial based on suspected or confirmed organism.
- Administer leukocyte-poor *Cytomegalovirus* (CMV)-negative blood when blood product administration is necessary.
- Consider postexposure prophylaxis for varicella zoster.
- Avoid live virus vaccines.

General Treatment

- Humoral.
  - IV immunoglobulins (IVIG) or subcutaneous immunoglobulin.
  - Antibiotic prophylaxis.
  - Do not require vaccines as they cannot make antibodies.
- Cellular: bone marrow transplant depending on severity.
- Combined antibody and cellular.
  - Strict isolation.
  - Bone marrow transplant.
  - IV immunoglobulin (IVIG).
  - Pneumocystis prophylaxis (e.g., trimethoprim–sulfamethoxazole).
- Phagocytic.
  - Treat infection.
  - Trimethoprim–sulfamethoxazole prophylaxis.
  - Recombinant gamma interferon.
- Complement.
  - Prevention of infection with vaccines.
  - Prompt treatment of infection.

Juvenile Idiopathic Arthritis

Jan A. Odiaga

Background

- Juvenile idiopathic arthritis (JIA) encompasses a complex group of disorders comprising several clinical entities with the common feature of arthritis.
- Each subtype of JIA is characterized by a different mode of presentation, disease course, and outcome.

Definition

- The diagnosis of JIA requires the persistence of arthritis for >6 weeks in a child <16 years of age in whom there is no other identified cause for arthritis.
- Currently, seven subtypes have been identified by stratification criteria.

Etiology/Types

- See Table 17.2.

Pathophysiology

- Underlying cause and pathogenesis of JIA remain unclear.
- JIA is a heterogeneous disorder, and the subtypes have varying clinical and laboratory features that may reflect distinct immunopathogenic processes.
- The pathogenesis for each subtype is undoubtedly multifactorial and likely triggered by environmental stimuli in genetically susceptible individuals.

Clinical Presentation

- Clinically characterized by joint effusion, joint line tenderness and warmth, restricted range of movement, and limitation of movement secondary to pain.

TABLE 17.2 Types and Features of Juvenile Idiopathic Arthritis

JIA Subtype	Age & Gender	Typical Joint Involvement	Occurrence of Uveitis	Other Features
Oligoarticular • Persistent • Extended	Early childhood. F > M.	≤4 joints. Large joints: knees, ankles, wrist. Persistent disease: never >4 joints affected. Extended disease: involves >4 joints after first 6 mo of disease.	Common (30%), especially if ANA-positive. Usually asymptomatic.	ANA 60%–80% positive.
Polyarticular (RF-negative)	2 peaks: 2–4 y of age and 6–12 y of age. F > M.	≥5 joints. Symmetric.	Common (15%).	ANA 25% positive. Cervical spine abnormalities and TMJ.
Polyarticular (RF-positive)	F > M Late childhood/ early adolescence.	Symmetric small and large joints. Erosive joint disease.	Rare (<1%).	ANA 75% positive. Rheumatoid nodules.
Systemic	M = F Throughout childhood.	Poly or oligoarticular.	Rare (<1%).	Daily (quotidian) fever for 2 weeks. Evanescent rash. Lymphadenopathy. Hepatosplenomegaly. Serositis.
Enthesitis-related arthritis	M > F Late childhood/ adolescence.	Weight-bearing joint, especially hip and intertarsal joints. History of inflammatory back pain or sacroiliac joint tenderness.	Symptomatic acute uveitis (~7%).	Enthesitis. HLA-B27-positive. Axial involvement (including sacroiliitis). Family history of HLA-B27-associated disease.
Psoriatic arthritis	F > M 2 peaks: 2–4 y of age and 9–11 y of age.	Asymmetric or symmetric small or large joints.	Common (10%).	Nail pits, onycholysis. Dactylitis. Psoriasis. Family history psoriasis.
Undifferentiated				Does not fulfill criteria for any above category or fulfills criteria for >1 category.

F, Female; M, Male; ANA, Antinuclear antibodies; RF, Rheumatoid actor; TMJ, Temporomandibular joint disorder

- The common feature of all the subtypes of JIA is arthritis.
- Joint inflammation results in pain, loss of function, and morning stiffness.
- The distribution of joint involvement varies between subtypes of JIA.
- Systemic symptoms typically occur in systemic and polyarticular subtypes and can include fatigue, weight loss, anemia, anorexia, or fever. Growth abnormalities can complicate JIA and result in short stature or localized growth disturbance such as bony overgrowth, prematurely fused epiphyses, and limb length discrepancies (refer to Table 17.2).

Diagnostic Evaluation

- No single laboratory test can diagnose JIA.
- Diagnosis is based on history and physical examination.
- Physical examination focuses on the presence of any joint swelling, pain, and range of motion, flexibility, abnormal gait pattern, and activity limitations.
- Laboratory analysis should include antinuclear antibody (ANA), rheumatoid factor, and anti–cyclic citrullinated peptide; a positive ANA test does not confirm a diagnosis of JIA but may be prognostic for uveitis.

Management

- Pain management and maintenance of functional mobility.
- Dietary/herbal supplements.
  - Calcium and vitamin D supplementation.
- Pharmacologic therapy.
  - Anti-inflammatory drugs: corticosteroids—oral and intra-articular injections.
  - Immunomodulatory therapy with disease-modifying anti-rheumatic drugs.
  - Tumor necrosis factor α inhibitors.
  - Interleukin (IL) inhibitors.
  - T-cell- and B-cell-targeted therapy.
- The goal of treatment in JIA is disease remission provided by a family-centered interdisciplinary team approach.
- The minimum standards of care for children with arthritis are (1) early recognition of JIA and access to specialist and multidisciplinary care; (2) access to information, treatment options, and support; (3) empowering patients and caregivers; and (4) a planned, coordinated transition to adult care.

Kawasaki Disease

Kelly A. Swain

Background

- A small- to medium-vessel vasculitis.
- Affects 9.1 to 32.5 per 100,000 children annually, with a small male predominance.
- Most commonly affects patients under the age of 4 years, with a peak incidence between 18 months and 2 years of age.

Definition

- An inflammation of the blood vessels that can lead to necrosis and arterial aneurysms, more specifically coronary artery aneurysms.

Diagnostic Criteria

- Specific criteria, in addition to fever for 5 days, must be met for the diagnosis of classic (4–5 criteria) or atypical or incomplete Kawasaki (2 criteria).
  - Bilateral painless bulbar conjunctival injection: without exudate.
  - Changes in lips and oral cavity: injected oral mucosa, dry/cracked lips, strawberry tongue.
  - Polymorphous exanthema.
  - Cervical lymphadenopathy (≥1.5 cm): typically unilateral.
  - Changes in extremities (e.g., palms of hands and/or soles of feet). Acute: erythema and edema; convalescent: peeling/desquamation.
- Other findings.
  - Cardiovascular: heart murmur, congestive heart failure, pericardial effusion, ECG changes (e.g., arrhythmias, abnormal Q waves, prolonged PR or QT intervals, ST segment changes), and enlarged cardiac silhouette on chest radiograph, myocardial infarction, and arterial aneurysms throughout the body, including the coronaries.

- Gastrointestinal: abdominal pain, diarrhea, nausea and/or vomiting, hepatitis.
- Musculoskeletal: arthritis.
- Pulmonary: upper respiratory tract symptoms, pulmonary infiltrate.
- Genitourinary: sterile pyuria.
- Joint: arthralgias, arthritis.
- Skin: perineal rash; transverse furrows of fingernails (Beau lines).
- Laboratory abnormalities.
  - Leukocytosis; increased neutrophils, erythrocyte sedimentation rate (ESR), C-reactive protein (CRP), platelets, serum transaminases, and γ-glutamyl transferase; hypoalbuminemia, anemia.
- Sudden-onset high fever: typically the first presenting sign.

Etiology

- Unknown.
- Hypothesized infectious and genetic components may play a role.

Clinical Presentation

- Presence of fever for at least 5 days and 2 (incomplete/atypical) to 5 classic clinical criteria.
- There are three phases:
  - Acute phase: weeks 1 to 2.
  - Subacute phase: weeks 2 to 4.
  - Convalescent phase: weeks 3 to 8.

Diagnostic Evaluation

- There are no specific tools or diagnostic tests that confirm Kawasaki disease; however, some are used to help determine/support the diagnosis.
  - Laboratory.
    - Inflammatory markers: elevated CRP and ESR.
    - CBC: leukocytosis, neutrophilia, eosinophilia, anemia, and thrombocytosis.
    - Metabolic panel: hypoalbuminemia, hypokalemia, elevated transaminases and GGT, elevated pancreatic enzymes.
    - Coagulation factors: elevated fibrinogen.
  - Radiographic.
    - Chest radiography: Cardiomegaly may be present.
  - Echocardiography.
    - Coronary abnormalities, including dilation, stenosis, aneurysms, and/or decreased ventricular function or infarction.

Management

- Prompt diagnosis is key.
- IV immunoglobulin (IVIG) 2 g/kg.
- Aspirin (ASA) 80 to 100 mg/kg/day divided every 6 hours and weaned with defervescence.
- Long-term therapy: Treatment is tailored to the risk level identified and includes:
  - Risk level I: no coronary involvement. ASA for 6 to 8 weeks with counseling follow-up every 5 years.
  - Risk level II: coronary artery dilation with resolution by 8 weeks. ASA for 6 to 8 weeks with counseling follow-up every 3 years.

- Risk level III: coronary aneurysm measuring 3 to 6 mm. ASA until resolution of aneurysm and limited activity for 8 weeks if <10 years of age. Stress test every 2 years and prior to admission into sports for those >10 years of age. Annual echocardiography and angiography if abnormal stress test is observed.
- Risk level IV: nonobstructive coronary aneurysm measuring >6 mm and/or multiple complex aneurysms. Long-term ASA in addition to anticoagulation therapy. Annual stress test, biannual echocardiography and ECG in addition to a cardiac catheterization on a biannual or annual basis. No high-impact sports. Counseling.
- Risk level V: obstructed coronary aneurysms. All recommendations included in risk level IV in addition to β-adrenergic blocking agents.

Systemic Lupus Erythematosus

Kelly A. Swain

Background

- An autoimmune connective tissue and small vessel vasculitis affecting multiorgan systems.
- Affects 0.5 to 0.6 per 100,000 children per year with a higher incidence in females that increases with age.
- Non-whites are affected more frequently and with increased severity.

Definition/Pathophysiology

- An autoimmune chronic inflammation of the blood vessels and connective tissue affecting multiorgan systems.
- HLA class II alleles DR2 and DR3 as well as complement deficiencies of C2 or C4 contribute to the development of systemic lupus erythematosus (SLE).

Diagnostic Criteria

- American College of Rheumatology Criteria modified from Chang and Hsu, 2012, for classification of systemic lupus erythematosus: 4 criteria from the list that follows indicate 96% sensitivity and between 96% and 100% specificity in pediatric lupus.
  - Malar or discoid rash.
  - Photosensitivity.
  - Oral and/or nasal mucocutaneous ulcerations.
  - Arthritis.
  - Nephritis with proteinuria >0.5 g/day; cellular casts.
  - Encephalopathy—seizures.
  - Psychosis.
  - Pleuritis or pericarditis.
  - Cytopenia.
  - Positive immunoserology: double-stranded DNA antibodies and anti-Smith antibodies.
  - Anti-nuclear antibodies (ANA).

Etiology

- Hypothesized hormonal, environmental, and genetic components may play a role.

Clinical Presentation

- Acute or subtle presentation within the following systems:
  - Pulmonary: pneumonitis, pleural effusion, atelectasis, infection causing respiratory distress, hemorrhage, and decreased pulmonary function tests.
  - Cardiovascular: pericarditis, myocarditis, endocarditis, and Libman–Sacks endocarditis manifested by cardiomegaly, murmur, friction rub, dysrhythmias, and heart failure.
  - Renal (75% of children have renal disease): hematuria, proteinuria, and nephrotic syndrome.
  - Gastrointestinal: autoimmune hepatitis, protein-losing enteropathy, pancreatitis, steroid-induced fatty liver, and Budd–Chiari syndrome manifested by abdominal pain, nausea and vomiting, ascites, and hepatomegaly.
  - Hematology: (>60% have cytopenia) anemia, lymphopenia, leukopenia, thrombocytopenia, thrombosis, and stroke.
  - Musculoskeletal: arthritis and arthralgias.
  - Endocrine: hypothyroidism, delayed puberty, and irregular menses.
  - Neurology: headaches (most common), seizures, psychosis, transverse myelitis, and CNS vasculitis.

Diagnostic Evaluation

- Diagnosis of SLE requires 4 of the 11 diagnostic criteria over time.
- Considered a periodic disease, and therefore, not all criteria may be met at one single time.
- Laboratory evaluation for cytopenias, hemolytic anemia, inflammatory markers, serologies for SLE, autoimmune hepatitis, as well as thyroiditis aid in the diagnosis in addition to presenting signs.
- Presentation often includes fatigue, rash, fever, and arthritis.

Management

- Based on symptoms and organs affected.
- Therapies include induction and maintenance therapy.
- Sunscreen >30 SPF to help control and prevent rash, corticosteroids, immunomodulators (tacrolimus), steroid-sparing agents (e.g., methotrexate, azathioprine, and mycophenolate), nonsteroidal anti-inflammatories, and hydroxychloroquine.
- Remission therapy can include cyclophosphamide or mycophenolate mofetil, and rituximab.
- Immunizations must be kept current, including pneumococcus, meningococcus, and *Haemophilus influenzae* type B.
- Hypertension must be treated aggressively.

PEARLS

- *Some medications can cause symptoms that resemble SLE (e.g., anticonvulsants, isoniazid, minocycline, and hydralazine). Symptoms resolve when the medication is discontinued.*
- *Neonatal lupus is a transient syndrome that is passed to neonates by mothers (who most often are undiagnosed) via the placenta and is often associated with heart block (unresolving), rash, thrombocytopenia, abnormal liver function, and Coombs positive hemolytic anemia.*

1. A 10-year-old girl presents with a daily fever for approximately 10 days which occurs late in the afternoon and is accompanied by a rash. The rash is a discrete, salmon-pink macule of different sizes. It migrates to different locations on skin, including her trunk and proximal extremities, but rarely persists in one location more than 1 hour. She has been complaining of knee and hip pain for 6 weeks that seems to resolve and spontaneously reappear, limiting her ability to play soccer. She has no history of travel and her immunizations are up-to-date. What is the most likely differential diagnosis?
   a. Acute lymphocytic leukemia.
   b. Lyme disease.
   c. Kawasaki disease.
   d. Systemic JIA.

Answer: **D**

Acute lymphocytic leukemia is the most common cancer in children, peaking between 2 and 5 years of age. Pain is acute and often wakes a child from sleep. Lyme disease is associated with an initial rash described as a migratory "bull's-eye rash" with flu-like symptoms. Systemic JIA is typically associated with fever accompanied by an erythematous evanescent rash that appears during fever, lymphadenopathy, hepatomegaly or splenomegaly, and serositis. Kawasaki disease is characterized by fever, rash, conjunctival injection, cervical lymphadenitis, inflammation of the lips and oral cavity, and erythema and edema of the hands and feet.

2. Which one of the following is the most important step in the management of a child with suspected anaphylactic shock?
   a. Monitor the patient closely.
   b. Administer a histamine (H_2) blocker.
   c. Place the patient in a recumbent position.
   d. Administer epinephrine.

Answer: **D**

Although all the choices may be included in the treatment plan, the best answer is to administer epinephrine. If anaphylaxis is suspected and the patient is in shock, rapid administration of epinephrine is imperative to intervene with the cascade. Patients will require monitoring, positioning, and may require adjunctive administration of an H_2 blocker. However, administration of epinephrine is life in the management of anaphylactic shock.

3. Which of the following two mechanisms can precipitate an anaphylactic response?
   a. IgE-mediated, mast cell activation.
   b. IgE-mediated, mast cell downregulation.
   c. IgG-mediated, mast cell activation.
   d. IgG-mediated, mast cell downregulation.

Answer: **A**

Antigen-specific IgE is formed when an individual who is *genetically prone/predisposed/susceptible* is exposed to an allergen or trigger. When the individual is subsequently exposed to the same allergen, mast cell activation occurs rapidly because the antigen-specific IgE has already bound to the mast cells via IgE receptors, making the cascade of inflammatory reactions rapid. The activation of mast cells and basophils triggers a rapid release of various inflammatory and newly formed mediators including histamine, tryptase, leukotrienes, prostaglandins, platelet-activating factor, and cytokines. Anaphylaxis is IgE-mediated and mast cell activated.

4. An 8-year-old African American girl is evaluated for complaints of fatigue, shortness of breath, rash, and cough for 3 weeks. A chest radiograph reveals small bilateral pleural effusions, pneumonitis, and cardiomegaly. Which of the following diagnosis should be considered in this child?
   a. Mycoplasma (e.g., walking) pneumonia.
   b. SLE.
   c. Cardiomyopathy.
   d. Localized scleroderma.

Answer: **B**

A diagnosis of SLE is made by meeting at least 4 out of 11 criteria that are set forth by the American College of Rheumatology. SLE must be considered in early stages of presentation to prevent risk for increased organ damage when diagnosed late.

5. A 17-year-old with the diagnosis of SLE is admitted with chest pain, fatigue, dyspnea, and tachycardia. A murmur is noted on auscultation. Which of the following should be considered?
   a. "Shrinking lung" syndrome.
   b. Libman–Sacks endocarditis.
   c. Sepsis.
   d. Pericarditis.

Answer: **B**

Libman–Sacks endocarditis is a form of nonbacterial endocarditis that should be considered in patients with SLE when a murmur is noted on examination. In conjunction with cardiac symptoms, the murmur may indicate progression of mitral valve disease.

6. A child with a recently diagnosed seizure disorder, on anticonvulsant therapy, presents with malar rash, thrombocytopenia, fatigue, and complaints of joint pain. Which of the following is the most likely explanation?
   a. Kawasaki disease.
   b. Drug-induced lupus erythematosus.

c. JIA.

d. Allergic reaction.

Answer: **B**

Anticonvulsant therapy and other medications such as isoniazid, procainamide, and infliximab can produce SLE symptoms as an autoimmune response to therapy. The symptoms resolve once the medication is discontinued. This presentation is not consistent with Kawasaki disease, JIA, or an allergic reaction.

7. A 12-year-old girl with a known complement deficiency presents to the emergency department with an isolated fever of 100.4°F. She appears clinically well. Which of the following management strategies is best for this patient?

a. Order acetaminophen and discharge the patient.

b. Initiate a septic workup and initiate antibiotics.

c. Prepare for bone marrow transplantation.

d. Prepare for administration of IL inhibitors.

Answer: **B**

Patients with known complement disorders require a thorough infectious evaluation and antibiotic administration, ideally after cultures obtained, when presenting with a fever. Delay in antibiotic administration can increase the risk for morbidity and mortality in these patients with compromised immune systems. Bone marrow transplantation and IL inhibitors are not indicated in this child.

8. Which of the following management strategies is indicated in patients with complement deficiencies?

a. Avoid annual influenza vaccine.

b. Bone marrow transplant.

c. Administration of all vaccines per CDC guidelines.

d. Monthly gamma globulin infusions.

Answer: **C**

Patient with complement deficiencies must receive all vaccines per CDC guidelines. These patients also require prompt evaluation and antibiotic evaluation when experiencing signs/symptoms of infection. Bone marrow transplant and monthly gamma globulin infusions are not indicated in these patients.

9. A 15-month-old female toddler is seen in clinic with fever of 104°F for 2 days, generalized morbilliform rash, and an otherwise normal examination. Which of the following is the most appropriate course of action?

a. Prescribe antipyretics and request follow-up in 3 days if no resolution of fever and/or rash.

b. Prescribe antipyretics and reassure parents the most likely cause is viral, with fever and rash resolving spontaneously.

c. Obtain a urinalysis, urine culture, and CBC.

d. Obtain cerebrospinal fluid (CSF) and blood cultures.

Answer: **A**

Prompt recognition is key to the diagnosis and treatment of Kawasaki disease. Typical and atypical classifications require 2 to 6 criteria be met, which include fever for at least 4 days in addition to the other manifestations. Antipyretics should be prescribed for comfort as well as for control of high fever, and reevaluation should be completed after 4 days of persistent fever to evaluate for other potential causes of fever and rash. Laboratory studies can assist in the evaluation of Kawasaki disease when the fever persists for 4 or more days.

10. A 4-year-old is seen in the emergency department with a history of fever for 1 week up to 106°F, conjunctivitis, complaints of generalized pain, nausea, and vomiting. The clinician suspects Kawasaki disease. Which of the following tests should be ordered first to assist in determining the diagnosis?

a. Chest radiography, pancreatic function tests, and CSF cultures.

b. CBC; blood, urine, and CSF cultures.

c. Echocardiography, urine and blood cultures.

d. CBC; liver and pancreatic function tests and inflammatory markers.

Answer: **D**

Laboratory findings consistent for Kawasaki disease include elevated CRP and ESR, thrombocytosis, anemia, elevated transaminases, as well as pancreatitis. Aseptic meningitis is also seen, although less frequently. Echocardiography should be completed to evaluate for coronary aneurysms and to rule out pericardial effusion, although the absence of coronary abnormalities does not rule out Kawasaki disease. Echocardiography will be needed if the laboratory evaluation and clinical signs suggest Kawasaki disease; however, it is not needed in this stage of the evaluation.

Recommended Readings

Anas, N., Newton, D., Perkin, R., & Swift, J. (2008). *Pediatric hospital medicine: Textbook of inpatient management* (2nd ed.). Philadelphia, PA: Lippincott Williams & Wilkins.

Chang, J. (2012). Juvenile idiopathic arthritis. In K. Reuter-Rice & B. Bolick (Eds.), *Pediatric acute care: A guide to interprofessional practice* (pp. 691–699). Burlington, MA: Jones & Bartlett Learning.

Chang, J., & Hsu, J. (2012). Systemic lupus erythematosus. In K. Reuter-Rice & B. Bolick (Eds.), *Pediatric acute care: A guide to interprofessional practice* (pp. 700–704). Burlington, MA: Jones & Bartlett Learning.

Ferdman, R. M. (2012). Anaphylaxis. In K. Reuter-Rice & B. Bolick (Eds.), *Pediatric acute care: A guide to interprofessional practice* (pp. 667–678). Burlington, MA: Jones & Bartlett Learning.

Gowdie, P. J., & Tse, S. M. (2012). Juvenile idiopathic arthritis. *Pediatric Clinics of North America, 59*(2), 301–327. doi:10.1016/j.pcl.2012.03.014.Pediatr

Jeffery Modell Foundation. (2013). *10 Warning signs of primary immunodeficiency.* Retrieved from http://www.info4pi.org/aboutPI/index.cfm?section=aboutPI&content=warningsins

Jordan, M. B., Allen, C. E., Weitzman, S., Filipovich, A. H., & McClain, K. L. (2011). How I treat hemophagocytic lymphohistiocytosis. *Blood, 118*(15), 4041–4052.

Lieberman, P., Camargo, C. A., Bohlke, K., Jick, H., Miller, R. L., Sheikh, A., & Simons, F. E. R. (2006). Epidemiology of anaphylaxis: Findings of the American College of Allergy, Asthma and Immunology Epidemiology of Anaphylaxis Working Group. *Annals of Allergy, Asthma, & Immunology, 97,* 596–602.

Lieberman, P., Nicklas, R. A., Oppenheimer, J., Kemp, S. F., Lang, D. M., Bernstein, D. I., . . . Wallace, D. (2010). The diagnosis and management of anaphylaxis practice parameter: 2010 Update. *Journal of Allergy & Clinical Immunology, 126,* 477–480.e1–e42.

McIntire, S., & Rosen, P. (2007). Rheumatology. In H. Davis & B. Zitelli (Eds.), *Atlas of pediatric physical diagnosis* (5th ed., pp. 266–270). Philadelphia, PA: Mosby.

Mosier, R. (2012). Vasculitis. In K. Reuter-Rice & B. Bolick (Eds.), *Pediatric acute care: A guide to interprofessional practice* (pp. 705–709). Burlington, MA: Jones & Bartlett Learning.

Newburger, J. W., Takahashi, M., Gerber, M. A., Gewitz, M. H., Tani, L. Y., Burns, J. C., . . . Taubert, K. A. (2004). Diagnosis, treatment, and long-term management of Kawasaki disease: A statement for health professionals from the committee on rheumatic fever, endocarditis, and Kawasaki disease, council on cardiovascular disease in the young, American Heart Association. *Pediatrics, 114,* 1708–1733.

Reid, B. (2012). Immunodeficiencies. In K. Reuter-Rice & B. Bolick (Eds.), *Pediatric acute care: A guide to interprofessional practice* (pp. 705–709). Burlington, MA: Jones & Bartlett Learning.

Simons, F. E. R. (2010). Anaphylaxis. *Journal of Allergy & Clinical Immunology, 125,* S161–S181.

Simons, F. E. R., Ardusso, L. R. F., Bilo, M. B., Dimov, V., Ebisawa, M., El-Gamal, Y. M., . . . Worm, M. (2012). 2012 Update: World Allergy Organization guidelines for the assessment and management of anaphylaxis. *Current Opinion in Allergy Clinical Immunology, 12,* 389–399.

Simons, F. E. R., Ardusso, L. R. F., Bilo, M. B., El-Gamal, Y. M., Ledford, D. K., Ring, J., . . . Thong, B. Y. (2011). World Allergy Organization anaphylaxis guidelines: Summary. *Journal of Allergy & Clinical Immunology, 127,* 587–593.e1–e22.

Weiss, J. (2012). Pediatric systemic lupus erythematosus: More than a positive antinuclear antibody. *Pediatrics in Review, 33,* 61–73.

Heent

Airway Malacia

Marisa Mize & Cathy Haut

Choanal Atresia

Background

- Choanal atresia is a congenital abnormality which is either unilateral (most common) or bilateral resulting in one or both nares being partially or completely occluded.
- Occurs in 1 per 5,000 to 8,000 live births; twice as common in females.
- Often seen in association with other developmental anomalies such as CHARGE syndrome and Treacher Collins syndrome.

Pathophysiology

- Nasal airway obstruction or occlusion.

Etiology/Types

- Unilateral: more common type, occurs in 60% to 75% of cases.
- Bilateral: life-threatening due to the obligatory nasal breathing of infants.

Clinical Presentation

- Respiratory distress shortly after birth as neonate has obligatory nasal breathing pattern.
- Noisy breathing, poor feeding, nasal drainage or discharge, and cyclic breathing when crying.

Diagnostic Evaluation

- Close mouth and auscultate at nares to determine if neonate is able to breathe through the nose.
- Passage of thin, flexible catheter into nares.
- Flexible nasal endoscopy or computed tomography (CT) can be used.

Management

- Initial observation.
- Surgical repair accomplished with transnasal puncture, transnasal endoscopic approach, or transpalatal approach.

- Both types of surgery include stenting or opening the narrowed passage.

Laryngomalacia

Marisa Mize & Cathy Haut

Background

- Most common congenital laryngeal anomaly; 70% of children with stridor; most common form of noninfectious stridor.
- Can present as mild intermittent or life-threatening.
- Can be associated with sleep-disordered breathing and obstructive sleep apnea.

Definition

- Inward collapse of the arytenoid cartilages and subglottic tissue due to excess mucosa and abnormal or reduced laryngeal tone causing stridor in young infants.
- Symptoms become apparent after the first 2 weeks of life, or delayed at 1 to 2 months of life and usually disappear by 12 to 18 months of age.

Etiology/Types

- Congenital (may outgrow within the first year of life).
- Gastroesophageal reflux and neurologic abnormalities may combine to cause airway compromise.

Pathophysiology

- Inspiratory stridor in the crying infant is often caused by laryngeal cartilages, which collapse due to lack of rigidity.
- Laryngomalacia affects the supraglottic structures, which include portions of the larynx above the level of the vocal cords.
- The infantile epiglottis is also longer than that of older children, which may predispose to posterior placement,

and the cartilage is more pliable, also impacting the collapsibility of the airway the collapsibility of the airway.

Clinical Presentation

- Inspiratory stridor.
- Symptoms worsen when infant is crying, agitated, feeding, has an intercurrent respiratory illness, or positioned prone.
- Coughing, choking and emesis with feedings, and slow or difficult oral intake may be noted.
- May result in hypoxia and hypercapnia.

Diagnostic Evaluation

- History and physical examination.
  - High-pitched, low-pitched, or vibratory stridor.
  - Suprasternal retractions.
  - Position changes impact examination; worse when neck is flexed or in prone position.
- Flexible fiber-optic laryngoscopy indicating:
  - A tightly curled, omega-shaped epiglottis.
  - Retroflexion (posterior displacement) of epiglottis.
  - Short aryepiglottic folds.
  - Redundant, prolapsing arytenoid mucosa and cartilage.
- Airway fluoroscopy.
  - Laryngeal collapse on inspiration.

Management

- Observation.
- Surgical intervention is indicated for failure to gain weight; procedure involves laser excision of tissue collapsing into glottis during expiration.

Tracheomalacia
Marisa Mize & Cathy Haut

Background

- Tracheomalacia (TM) is the most common congenital anomaly of the trachea; more common in premature infants.
- Some cases are associated with tracheobronchial fistula.
- Incidence of congenital form is approximately 1 in 1,500 children.
- More common in children requiring prolonged mechanical ventilation, bronchopulmonary dysplasia, or chronic pulmonary disease.
- Approximately half of patients have gastroesophageal reflux.
- Occurs in 20% to 60% of children with cardiovascular abnormalities.
- Often associated with feeding problems.

Definition

- Upper airway lacking cartilaginous rigidity, resulting in impedance on exhalation.

Etiology/Types

- TM: floppy cartilaginous involvement limited to the trachea.
  - Primary: congenital.
  - Secondary: acquired (e.g., prolonged intubation).
- Tracheobronchomalacia: floppy cartilaginous involvement of the trachea and mainstem bronchi; more severe form of malacia.

Pathophysiology

- TM: weakness of the cartilaginous structure of the trachea.
  - Frequently a result of a reduction and/or atrophy of the longitudinal elastic fibers of the pars membranacea, or impaired cartilage integrity.
  - Results in an airway that is softer and more susceptible to collapse. Various degrees of collapse occur, contributing to airway obstruction.

Clinical Presentation

- Symptoms may appear in the first weeks of life, though commonly delayed 2 to 3 months.
- Expiratory stridor and cough are the most frequently occurring symptoms.
- Symptoms worsen with agitation, crying, feeding, or upper airway infections.
- May be asymptomatic with sleep or when quietly awake.
- Harsh, barky cough.
- Respiratory distress with visible collapse of upper airway during exhalation.
- Noisy medium- to high-pitched breathing.

Diagnostic Evaluation

- History is an important part of determining diagnosis.
  - Physical examination: homophonous expiratory wheeze (intrathoracic forms), intercostal retractions, worse during intercurrent respiratory illnesses.
- Flexible bronchoscopy (tracheal collapse >50% on exhalation is diagnostic): may also be used to determine the level of positive end-expiratory pressure required to overcome airway collapse (e.g., positive end-expiratory pressure titration). Performed during spontaneous respiration.
- CT (with inspiratory and expiratory phases): provides evaluation of aortic arch anatomy/airway compression, presence of vascular ring.
- Fluoroscopy: evaluates underlying anatomy.
- Laryngoscopy: laryngomalacia.
- Barium testing: identifies external compression from esophagus due to vascular malformation.

Management

- Observation (most cases); symptom resolution at or before 18 months of age.
- Tracheostomy and continuous positive pressure or mechanical ventilation for children with severe disease.
- Aortopexy may be required in severe cases; suspends the anterior trachea, reducing airway compression.

- *As the child grows, trachea becomes larger and cartilage becomes more rigid, resulting in improvement or resolution of symptoms.*
- *Avoid β_2 agonists; smooth muscle relaxation effects may worsen tracheal airway collapse.*

Epiglottitis

Lisa Genualdi

Background/Definition

- Epiglottitis is an acute severe inflammation of the epiglottis; results in repositioning of the epiglottis posteriorly, which can result in airway obstruction.
- Potential for complete airway obstruction.
- An airway emergency.
- Access to an experienced anesthesiologist is important.

Epidemiology/Etiology

- Most often occurs in children aged 1 to 5 years, with a slight male predominance.
- Incidence of epiglottitis has decreased dramatically since the *Haemophilus influenzae* (Hib) vaccine.
- Other causative agents include *Staphylococcus aureus*, group A streptococcus, and *Streptococcus pneumoniae*.

Clinical Presentation

- Sudden onset of symptoms.
- Rapid progression to total airway obstruction.
- Toxic appearance, agitation, with fever and severe sore throat and dysphagia.
- Clinical signs of airway obstruction include muffled voice, drooling, and tripod sitting position.

Diagnostic Evaluation

- Lateral neck radiography will reveal enlarged epiglottis and distention of the hypopharynx ("thumb sign") or postlingual triangle and loss of the vallecular air space (Figure 18.1).
- Direct laryngoscopy will reveal a beefy red, swollen epiglottis, and aryepiglottic folds.

Management

- Noxious stimuli must be avoided to maintain airway patency.
- Endotracheal intubation may be required by a pediatric anesthesia or otolaryngology specialist.
- Obtain blood culture when airway is secure or the airway is no longer critical.
- Initiate empiric antimicrobial therapy: third-generation cephalosporin or vancomycin plus a third-generation cephalosporin if penicillin-resistant pneumococci or methicillin-resistant *Staph. aureus* is suspected. Antimicrobial therapy for 7 to 10 days.

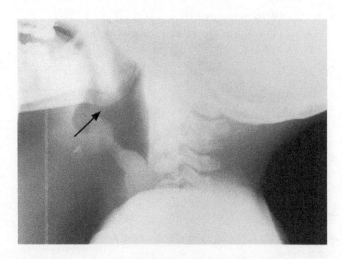

FIGURE 18.1 • **Epiglottitis Thumb Print Sign.** Epiglottitis thumb sign on inspiratory soft tissue lateral neck radiograph, suggesting epiglottitis.

Mastoiditis

Lisa Genualdi

Definition

- An inflammation of the mastoid process of the temporal bone.
- Can be a complication of acute otitis media (AOM).

Epidemiology/Etiology

- Most common causative organisms are *Strep. pneumoniae* and group A streptococcus.
- *Staph. aureus*, *H. influenzae*, and *Pseudomonas aeruginosa* are also reported.
- First stage: acute mastoiditis with periostitis—spread of infectious process through the mastoid emissary veins and into the periosteum.
- Second stage: acute coalescent mastoiditis—infiltration and demineralization of bone and breakdown of proteinaceous organic components.
- Can spread into the cerebral vasculature, cranium, regional soft tissue, or other intratemporal spaces.

Clinical Presentation

- Acute mastoiditis presents with findings of AOM, including erythema, dullness, and bulging of the tympanic membrane along with tenderness and swelling of the mastoid process.
- Findings include postauricular changes, erythema, tenderness, edema, and fluctuance.
- External auditory canal may be edematous and sagging.
- Systemic signs and symptoms include lethargy, irritability, fever, poor feeding, facial weakness and neurologic signs, lymphadenopathy, and rhinorrhea.
- In children >18 months of age, postauricular swelling pushes the pinna up and out.
- Infants have the appearance of the ear being pushed down by postauricular swelling.

- Acute coalescent mastoiditis.
  - Triad of otalgia, auricular proptosis, and a bulging, erythematous, tympanic membrane.

Diagnostic Evaluation

- Clinical evaluation.
- CT: imaging study of choice; confirms mastoid filling, presence of periosteal abscess, or destruction of bony separations of the mastoid.
- Magnetic resonance imaging (MRI): for patients with signs of increased intracranial pressure or intracranial complications such as dural venous sinus thrombosis or epidural abscess.
- Blood culture.
- Lumbar puncture if suspicion for central nervous system infection.

Management

- Antibiotic therapy.
  - Outpatient: acute mastoiditis without periosteitis.
    - Oral antibiotics (high-dose amoxicillin).
  - Inpatient: no resolution of illness with oral antibiotics, or concern for complications associated with mastoiditis.
    - Broad-spectrum intravenous antibiotics (may require meningitic dosing if suspicion for central nervous system involvement).
  - Duration of therapy is based on clinical signs of recovery.
- Acute mastoiditis with periostitis.
  - If abscess, may require surgical drainage, or tympanostomy tube for continued middle ear drainage.
- Coalescent mastoiditis.
  - May require mastoidectomy.
- Consulting services to consider if extension of infection to central nervous system.
  - Neurosurgery.
    - Critical care, infectious disease, hematology.

PEARLS

- *Complications include:*
  - *Thrombosis of the lateral or sigmoid venous sinus, labyrinthitis, osteomyelitis.*
- *Central nervous system conditions can also be associated, including epidural or subdural empyema, abscess, or meningitis.*

Orbital Cellulitis

Dana L. Lerma

Definition

- Acute infectious process with an inflammatory component involving the posterior tissues of the orbital septum.
- The globe is not involved.

Etiology/Types

- Orbital cellulitis is less common than periorbital cellulitis.
- The median age of hospitalized children is 7.5 years, though more prevalent in younger children.
- Most commonly caused by bacterial sinusitis, although other causes include ophthalmic or paranasal sinus surgery, orbital trauma (particularly involving foreign bodies), dental or middle ear infection, or dacryocystitis. Less commonly, caused by vascular seeding of an endogenous infection.
- *Staph. aureus* and *Streptococcus* are the two most common causative organisms.
- Increased incidence in winter season.

Pathophysiology

- Results from direct extension of paranasal sinus infection that readily spreads through the lamina papyracea, the thin medial wall of the orbit, causing erythema and edema of the eyelid and surrounding tissue.

Clinical Presentation

- Marked erythema and edema of the eyelid and surrounding skin, tenderness to palpation, and pain without palpation are common.
- Systemic symptoms include fever, fatigue, and headache.
- Edema and inflammation of the extraocular muscles, proptosis, painful or limited eye movements, and diplopia may also be present.
- More advanced infections include optic nerve edema, along with an abnormal pupillary response, and in severe cases, leads to visual impairment and blindness.

Diagnostic Evaluation

- CT of the orbits and paranasal sinuses, with and without contrast.
- Blood cultures and complete blood count (CBC) with differential.
- Lumbar puncture should be considered in the presence of meningeal signs or if central nervous system dysfunction is suspected.

Management

- Hospital admission.
- High-dose intravenous antibiotics (typically vancomycin and a second- or third-generation cephalosporin) until the patient is afebrile and orbital and dermatologic changes improve (generally 3–5 days), after which a 2- to 3-week course of oral antibiotics (generally cephalosporin) is continued. Adjust antibiotics based on culture results.
- Daily ophthalmologic examination; more frequent examinations may be required with severe cases.
- Repeat CT with acute changes in vision, extraocular motility, or pupillary reaction.
- Surgical drainage indicated in abscess not responding to initial antibiotic therapy.
- Ophthalmology consultation for examination and management.
- Otolaryngology consult; most common source of infection is sinusitis.

- *Early and adequate treatment greatly improves outcome of patients with orbital cellulitis.*
- *Parents should be instructed to notify provider immediately with signs of recurrence of disease to prevent further complications.*

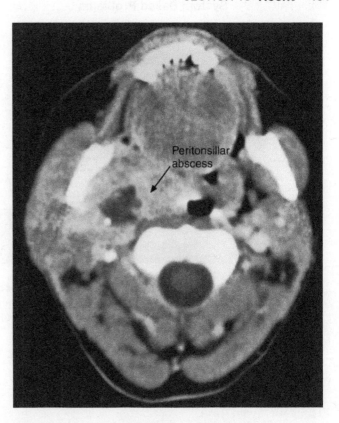

FIGURE 18.2 • **Peritonsillar Abscess Neck CT.** CT of a patient with a peritonsillar abscess (*arrow*).

Peritonsillar Abscess

Lisa Genualdi

Pathophysiology

- A local cellulitis that progresses first to phlegmon, then abscess, although suppurative adenitis is the most common presentation.
- Location includes the superior, middle, or inferior tonsillar poles. Superior tonsillar pole is most prevalent.
- May extend to upper airway obstruction.

Epidemiology/Etiology

- Most common deep neck infection in children; occurs more frequently in adolescents.
- Infections are typically polymicrobial. Common pathogens include *Strep. pyogenes*, *Staph. aureus*, and *Haemophilus* species.

Presentation

- Recent history of pharyngitis or snoring, fever, severe sore throat, dysphagia, unilateral pain, trismus, neck swelling, drooling, muffled voice, ear pain on affected side, tripod positioning and anterior cervical lymphadenopathy, swollen tonsils with uvula deviation.
- Concerning findings include drooling, tripod positioning, and swollen tonsils.

Diagnostic Evaluation

- CBC with leukocytosis.
- Blood culture, but rarely positive.
- Throat culture: evaluate for group A streptococcus.
- Neck abscess incision and drainage with culture.
- CT with IV contrast: determines extent of infection and differentiates abscess from cellulitis (Figure 18.2).

Management

- Avoid noxious stimuli.
- Surgical drainage: consider if abscess is larger than 2 cm or if failure to respond to IV antibiotics.
- IV empiric antimicrobial therapy with ampicillin–sulbactam or clindamycin.
- Consider providing coverage for resistant organisms (e.g., vancomycin); follow culture.
- Once afebrile with clinical improvement, antibiotics can be changed to oral agents.

Retropharyngeal Abscess

Lisa Genualdi

Pathophysiology

- Abscess formation occurs following trauma to the pharynx or by primary infection.
- Infection can be isolated to a single lymph node, extend to the abscess wall, or rupture and spread purulent material throughout the retropharyngeal space.

Epidemiology/Etiology

- Most often occurs in children 1 to 5 years of age.
- Infections are usually polymicrobial.
- Common pathogens include *Strep. pyogenes*, *Staphy. aureus*, and *Haemophilus* species.

Presentation

- History associated with retropharyngeal abscess (RPA) may include endotracheal intubation, oral foreign object, dental procedures, recent infection of any structures that drain into the retropharyngeal space.
- Fever, sore throat, dysphagia, unilateral pain, trismus, neck swelling, and drooling are symptoms of an RFA.
- Other findings include muffled voice, chest pain with mediastinal extension of infection, tripod positioning, anterior

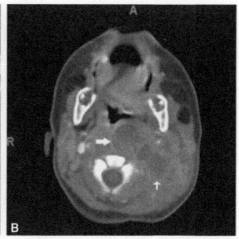

FIGURE 18.3 • **Retropharyngeal Abscess Lateral Neck Radiograph and CT.**
A: A lateral neck radiograph demonstrating retropharyngeal abscess *(arrow)*. **B:** A CT of neck with contrast demonstrating a retropharyngeal abscess *(large arrow)* and smaller, contiguous parapharyngeal abscess *(small arrow).*

cervical lymphadenopathy, lateral compression of the posterior pharynx, and a fluctuant mass.

Diagnostic Evaluation

- CBC with differential; leukocytosis.
- Blood culture is rarely positive.
- Lateral neck X-ray.
- CT with IV contrast to identify extent of infection and differentiate abscess from cellulitis (Figure 18.3).

Management

- Noxious stimuli should be avoided.
- Chest radiograph to evaluate for mediastinal expansion.
- Lateral neck radiograph may help differentiate RPA from epiglottitis.
- Endotracheal intubation by a pediatric anesthesia or otolaryngology specialist is required in cases of complete airway obstruction.
- Surgical drainage is required for airway compromise:
  - Abscess >2 cm, or failed response to IV antibiotics within 24 hours.
- IV empiric antimicrobial therapy for coverage of aerobic and anaerobic organisms.
- Once patient is afebrile with clinical improvement antimicrobial therapy can be changed to oral agent.

Tracheitis

Lisa Genualdi

Background/Definition

- Bacterial infection of the larynx, trachea, or bronchi which causes an inflammatory process resulting in formation of adherent mucopurulent pseudomembranes inside the airways.

- Secretions result in subglottic regional narrowing and airway compromise.
- Subglottic, hypopharyngeal, and esophageal stenosis, acute respiratory distress syndrome, and multiple organ dysfunction syndrome are complications.

Pathophysiology

- A diffuse inflammatory process of the larynx, trachea, and bronchi with adherent or semi-adherent mucopurulent membranes within the trachea at the cricoid cartilage level which can cause acute airway obstruction secondary to subglottic edema.

Epidemiology/Etiology

- Occurs in children 3 weeks to 16 years of age, with mean age of 4; male predominance 2:1.
- Typically occurs in fall and winter seasons, with history of preceding viral infection or trauma.
- Most common pathogens include *Staph. aureus* and community-acquired MRSA.
- *Moraxella catarrhalis, H. influenzae* type b, *Klebsiella,* and *Pseudomonas aeruginosa* have also been implicated as pathogens.
- Causative anaerobes include *Peptostreptococcus, Bacteroides,* and *Prevotella.*

Presentation

- Upper and lower respiratory tract infection, fever, cough, stridor, respiratory distress, and copious, tenacious secretions.
- Presents acutely with high fever, toxic appearance, leukocytosis, stridor, and bark-like cough.
- Subacute presentation.
  - Several-day history of croup-like symptoms.
  - Tracheitis can be initially diagnosed as croup.
  - Lower respiratory tract disease presents with concurrent viral pathology.

Diagnostic Evaluation

- Lateral neck radiography.
  - Differentiates tracheitis from epiglottitis, croup, and RPA.
- Blood culture is rarely positive.
- White blood cell count may not be elevated.
- Aerobic and anaerobic tracheal aspirates.
- Laryngotracheobronchoscopy may be considered for definitive diagnosis if endotracheal intubation is not required.
- Purulent secretions (culture).
- Erythematous trachea.
- Air leak syndrome occurs in some patients.

Management

- Maintain airway patency and avoid noxious stimuli which can lead to obstruction.
- Endotracheal tube intubation for imminent airway obstruction.
- Positive pressure ventilation can be complicated by thick secretions.
- Empiric IV antimicrobial therapy.
- Once afebrile, antimicrobial therapy is transitioned to oral agents.

Vocal Cord Dysfunction/Paralysis

Marisa Mize & Cathy Haut

Background

- Vocal cord dysfunction (VCD).
  - Characterized as abnormal adduction of the vocal cords during the respiratory cycle (especially during the inspiratory phase) that produces airflow obstruction at the level of the larynx.
  - Symptoms often mimic asthma.
  - Causes include exercise, psychological conditions, airborne irritants, rhinosinusitis, gastroesophageal reflux disease, or use of certain medications (e.g., antihistamines).
- Vocal cord paralysis (VCP).
  - May be caused by a variety of mediastinal disease entities, including neoplastic, inflammatory, and vascular conditions,

complication of thoracic surgery, or can be the presenting symptom of another disease process.
  - Can be either congenital or acquired and presents with inspiratory stridor.
  - Children can phonate with the thyroid muscle serving as the tensor of the vocal cords.
  - Children with brain stem compression, such as Arnold–Chiari malformation, may present with signs and symptoms of VCP.

Definition

- The recurrent branch of the superior laryngeal nerve, originating from the 10th cranial nerve, is positioned such that the vocal cords are in paramedian or median position.

Etiology/Types

- Congenital, unilateral or bilateral, left- or right-sided.
- Associated with brain stem compression (Arnold–Chiari malformation), or can be a complication from thoracic surgery.

Clinical Presentation

- Inspiratory stridor, or expiratory wheezing.
- Symptoms may mimic asthma; may be diagnosed with asthma and be unresponsive to therapy.

Diagnostic Evaluation

- Observation.
- Flexible laryngoscopy is considered the gold standard for the diagnosis of VCD.
- Chest radiography.
- Fluoroscopy.
- Axial CT of the neck can identify ipsilateral pyriform sinus dilation, medial rotation, thickening of the aryepiglottic fold, and ipsilateral laryngeal ventricle dilatation.

Management

- Removal of precipitating factors, speech therapy, and anticholinergic medications.
- Supportive care, decompression if presence of Arnold–Chiari malformation, arytenoidopexy, tracheostomy.

1. A 2-day-old neonate has been noted to have difficulty feeding with coughing and increased work of breathing. Based on this information, which of the following should be considered high on the differential list?
   a. Congenital heart disease.
   b. Choanal atresia.
   c. Pleural effusion.
   d. Respiratory distress syndrome.

Answer: **B**

Choanal atresia is a congenital malformation that can be indicated by increased work of breathing. Newborns are obligate nose breathers at birth and will struggle to eat with obstruction of one or both nares. The difficulty in breathing is most noticeable when the infant is eating.

2. A 15-year-old has a 3-day history of sore throat, fever, trismus, and dysphagia. She presents to the emergency room today with unilateral neck swelling. A CBC reveals a white blood cell count of 24,000/mm³. Which of the following is the most likely diagnosis?
   a. Epiglottitis.
   b. Bacterial tracheitis.
   c. Peritonsillar abscess.
   d. Croup.

Answer: **C**

Differentiating between bacterial tracheitis, peritonsillar abscess, and croup includes careful history taking and assessment of current symptoms. Epiglottitis is a medical emergency. It is uncommon since the development of the *H. influenzae* vaccine and includes rapid onset of high fever, dysphagia, severe sore throat, and rapidly progressing upper airway obstruction (drooling, tripod sitting position). Croup usually presents with stridor, mild cough, and low-grade fever and is typically limited to young children. Bacterial tracheitis is a diffuse inflammatory process of the larynx, trachea, and bronchi that causes difficulty breathing and usually high fever. Peritonsillar abscess is bacterial in origin and more common in adolescents with symptoms including severe sore throat, trismus, and dysphagia, with a recent history of pharyngitis.

3. An 18-month-old has just completed a course of amoxicillin for AOM and returns with high fever and irritability. She has unilateral postauricular edema, erythema, and tenderness. Which of the following is the most likely diagnosis?
   a. Ear trauma.
   b. AOM.
   c. Mastoiditis.
   d. RPA.

Answer: **C**

Mastoiditis is an inflammation of the mastoid process of the temporal bone which can be a complication of AOM. Common presenting symptoms include fever, postauricular edema, erythema, and tenderness, and a sagging external auditory canal.

4. Treatment of choice for acute mastoiditis without periosteitis includes:
   a. Standard antibiotic therapy administered for AOM.
   b. Broad-spectrum IV antibiotic therapy.
   c. Broad-spectrum IV antibiotic therapy at meningitic dosing.
   d. Antibiotic therapy is not necessary.

Answer: **A**

IV antibiotic therapy is necessary for children who are ill-appearing, have a periosteal abscess, or have been refractory to oral antibiotic therapy. The majority of patients diagnosed with mastoiditis will have recently taken oral antibiotics for AOM without resolution of illness. If there is concern of central nervous system involvement, meningitic dosing of broad-spectrum IV antibiotics is required. Delayed treatment of mastoiditis can lead to complications such as labyrinthitis, osteomyelitis, and central nervous system involvement.

5. A 4-year-old who has up-to-date immunizations is admitted with orbital cellulitis. Pending final culture results, what organisms should be suspected, and what antibiotics would be appropriate to prescribe?
   a. *Staph. aureus* and *Streptococcus;* IV Flagyl and IV vancomycin.
   b. *Staph. aureus* and *Streptococcus;* IV ceftriaxone and IV vancomycin.
   c. *Staph. aureus* and *H. influenzae;* oral amoxicillin and clindamycin.
   d. *Staph. aureus* and *H. influenzae;* IV ceftazidime and oral clindamycin.

Answer: **B**

Staph. aureus and *Streptococcus* are the two most common causative organisms of orbital cellulitis. *H. influenzae* should primarily be suspected in patients who are not immunized. The appropriate initial antibiotic therapy is IV vancomycin and a second- or third-generation cephalosporin, such as ceftriaxone.

6. A 6-month-old infant with laryngomalacia continues to gain weight, but has significant stridor when crying. The appropriate intervention is:
   a. Surgical excision by laser.
   b. Observation and reevaluation in 1 month.
   c. Racemic nebulization twice a day.
   d. Treatment for GERD.

Answer: **B**

Infants with laryngomalacia often have prolapse of the arytenoid tissues, which can partially cover the glottis and impede airflow, thus, create stridor. As the infant grows, these cartilages become stronger and the stridor disappears.

7. The *most* common organisms isolated when children are diagnosed with epiglottitis include:
   a. *H. influenzae* type b, *Staph. aureus*, group A streptococcus, and *Strep. pneumoniae*.
   b. Parainfluenza, *Strep. pyogenes*, *P. aeruginosa*.
   c. *Staph. aureus*, *Strep. pneumoniae*, and parainfluenza.
   d. *Strep. pneumoniae*, *Strep. pyogenes*, *P. aeruginosa*, and *H. influenzae* type b.

Answer: A

H. influenzae type b was traditionally the most common causative agent in epiglottitis prior to the introduction of the *H. influenzae* vaccine. Other causative agents include *Staph. aureus*, group A streptococcus, and *Strep. pneumoniae*. Parainfluenza is the most common causes of croup. *Strep. pneumoniae*, *Strep. pyogenes*, *P. aeruginosa*, and *Staph. aureus* are the most cause of mastoiditis.

8. A 2-year-old previously healthy toddler presents with sudden onset of severe sore throat, fever, and dysphagia. You are concerned that this child may have epiglottitis. What diagnostic imaging study would you obtain to confirm your diagnosis?
   a. Lateral neck radiography.
   b. Neck CT.
   c. Chest radiography.
   d. Head and neck MRI.

Answer: A

Lateral neck radiography will reveal enlarged epiglottis and distention of the hypopharynx (the thumb sign) or postlingual triangle. Neck CT is the diagnostic imaging study of choice for peritonsillar abscess. Chest radiography is used to diagnose conditions affecting the chest wall. An MRI of the head and neck would not be appropriate in this patient with a critical airway, which would be a long study that would potentially require sedation. The clinical condition of the child with suspected epiglottitis must be considered prior to obtaining any diagnostic imaging tests. Epiglottitis is often a medical emergency.

9. A 3-year-old with an RPA has been on broad-spectrum IV antibiotics for over 36 hours with no improvement in symptoms and continued fever. The next step in the management plan includes:
   a. Antimicrobial therapy to be changed to an oral agent for a 14-day course.
   b. Endotracheal intubation by a pediatric anesthesiologist.
   c. Surgical drainage.
   d. Continue the same plan for another 12 to 24 hours.

Answer: C

Nonresponse to broad-spectrum antibiotics for a child with an RPA is concerning. Surgical referral for incision and drainage is the next step in management if the patient fails to respond to IV antibiotics within 24 hours.

10. A 2-year-old presents to the emergency department (ED) with fever, trismus, drooling, and a muffled voice concerning for RPA. Respiratory rate is 26 breaths per minute, oxygen saturations 98% on room air, heart rate 130 beats per minute, and blood pressure 90/60 mmHg. The most important initial management includes:
    a. Avoiding noxious stimuli.
    b. Placing a peripheral IV line.
    c. Obtaining a CT with IV contrast.
    d. Supporting the patient's oxygenation by placing on 1-L nasal cannula.

Answer: A

Agitation may lead to complete airway obstruction, so any type of noxious stimuli should be avoided, including that from an IV line attempt. Any airway compromise should be addressed before diagnostic studies are obtained. A careful respiratory examination with airway assessment must be performed prior to inducing noxious stimuli.

11. A 13-year-old athlete has been placed on albuterol and fluticasone for continued complaints of shortness of breath and chest pain with exertion. She was also treated once with oral steroids, but continues to have symptoms. Which of the following should be on the differential list?
    a. Exercise-induced asthma, VCD, costochondritis.
    b. Exercise-induced asthma, foreign body aspiration, pneumonia.
    c. VCD, costochondritis, laryngomalacia.
    d. Foreign body aspiration, pneumonia, laryngomalacia.

Answer: A

An adolescent with symptoms of asthma exacerbation who does not respond to typical therapy should be evaluated for VCD. Costochondritis can also cause chest pain from a musculoskeletal perspective, and even if the child has exercise-induced asthma, it should still be considered.

12. A 2-year-old with mastoiditis presents to the ED with a significant change in mental status and facial weakness. The most likely diagnosis at this point is:
    a. Bell palsy.
    b. Brain neoplasm.
    c. Meningitis.
    d. Influenza.

Answer: C

Potential complications of untreated or delayed treatment of mastoiditis include labyrinthitis, osteomyelitis, and central nervous system conditions such as epidural or subdural empyema, abscess, thrombosis of lateral or sigmoid venous sinus, or meningitis.

(continues on page 466)

13. Which of the following is a cause of VCP?
    a. Ventriculoperitoneal shunt surgery.
    b. Infectious tracheitis.
    c. Thoracic surgery complication.
    d. Croup.

Answer: **C**

The recurrent laryngeal nerve originates from the 10th cranial nerve, which innervates the vocal cords. Thoracic surgery can often cause VCP as the trachea is very close to structures in an infant's mediastinal area. The care of a child with VCP is mainly supportive.

14. In a child with suspected tracheitis, a lateral neck radiography is completed to:
    a. Provide a definitive diagnosis of disease process.
    b. Differentiate from epiglottitis, croup, and RPA.
    c. Determine the presence of airway obstruction.
    d. Determine the need for IV antibiotic therapy.

Answer: **B**

In the evaluation of a child with suspected tracheitis, the lateral neck radiography is completed to differentiate this diagnosis from epiglottitis (thumb sign), croup (steeple sign), and RPA (mediastinal expansion).

15. A 4-year-old presents to the ED with complaints of fever and right eye pain and swelling. On examination, she has edema to the right eyelid and periorbital region that is painful to palpation, and decreased extraocular mobility. What is the most appropriate diagnostic test to obtain first?
    a. MRI.
    b. Facial radiography.
    c. CT.
    d. Ultrasound.

Answer: **C**

A CT of the orbits and paranasal sinuses with and without contrast should be performed initially for a child with a suspected orbital cellulitis. Results can indicate inflammation of the orbital and periorbital tissues, evidence of sinusitis, and presence of abscess. Although MRI is superior to CT in soft tissue disease progression, it is not always readily available, is a longer study, and typically requires sedation in younger children.

Recommended Readings

Babiuch, A., & Mittleman, D. (2012). Orbital and preseptal (periorbital) cellulitis. In K. Reuter-Rice & B. Bolick (Eds.), *Pediatric acute care: A guide for interprofessional practice* (pp. 984–986). Burlington, MA: Jones & Bartlett Learning.

Dobbie, A. M., & White, D. R. (2013). Laryngomalacia. *Pediatric Clinics of North America, 60*, 893–902.

Gnagi, S. H., & Schraff, S. A. (2013). Nasal obstruction in neonates. *Pediatric Clinics of North America, 60*, 903–922.

Lin, H. W., Shargorodsky, J., & Gopen, Q. (2010). Clinical strategies for the management of acute mastoiditis in the pediatric population. *Journal of Clinical Pediatrics, 49*(2), 110–115. doi:10.1177/0009922809344349

Rand, T. H. (2012). Mastoiditis. In K. Reuter-Rice & B. Bolick (Eds.), *Pediatric acute care: A guide for interprofessional practice* (pp. 983–984). Burlington, MA: Jones & Bartlett Learning.

Weber, M. D. (2012). Epiglottitis. In K. Reuter-Rice & B. Bolick (Eds.), *Pediatric acute care: A guide for interprofessional practice* (pp. 792–793). Burlington, MA: Jones & Bartlett Learning.

Weber, M. D. (2012). Retropharyngeal/Peritonsillar abscess. In K. Reuter-Rice & B. Bolick (Eds.), *Pediatric acute care: A guide for interprofessional practice* (pp. 797–798). Burlington, MA: Jones & Bartlett Learning.

Weber, M. D. (2012). Tracheitis. In K. Reuter-Rice & B. Bolick (Eds.), *Pediatric acute care: A guide for interprofessional practice* (pp. 801–802). Burlington, MA: Jones & Bartlett Learning.

Musculoskeletal

Compartment Syndrome

Susan K. Emerson

Background/Definition

- Osteofascial compartment pressure rises to a level that decreases perfusion to the tissue in the closed fascial space.
- May lead to irreversible muscle and nerve damage.
- May occur anywhere that the skeletal muscle is surrounded by fascia, but most commonly occurs in leg, forearm, hand, foot, thigh, buttock, shoulder, and paraspinous muscles.
- Compartment syndrome is a *medical emergency*.

Etiology/Types

- Trauma.
  - Fractures (majority of cases).
  - Crush injuries.
  - Contusions.
  - Gunshot wounds.
- Tight casts, dressings, or external wrappings.
- Extravasation of intravenous (IV) fluids/medications or intraosseous infusion.
- Burn injuries.
- Post ischemic swelling (e.g., reestablished blood flow after blocked circulation).
- Bleeding disorders.

Pathophysiology

- Local trauma and soft tissue destruction → bleeding and edema → increased interstitial pressure → vascular occlusion → myoneural ischemia.
- Fascia does not stretch, resulting in increased pressure on other structures in the compartment (e.g., capillaries, nerves, and muscles).

Clinical Presentation

- The five P's (not always all together and not always reliable).
  - Pain with passive stretch.
  - Pain out of proportion to clinical situation.
  - Paresthesia.
  - Paralysis.
  - Pulses absent.
- In children, the three A's may precede the five P's by several hours.
  - Anxiety (increasing).
  - Agitation.
  - Analgesic requirement.

Diagnostic Evaluation

- Measurement of compartment pressure.
  - >30 mmHg typically requires fasciotomy.
    - Consider clinical picture in management plan.
- Radiography of involved area to evaluate for fracture.

Management

- Medical emergency.
- Institute therapeutic management while awaiting surgical specialty evaluation.
  - Remove binding devices (e.g., casts, splints).
  - Keep extremity at the level of the heart.
    - Elevation or dangling of extremity may further impair blood flow.
  - Control pain.
  - Administer oxygen.
  - Correct hypotension, if present.
- Acute fasciotomy is the definitive therapy; open all involved compartments.
  - Typically performed at the bedside; may be performed in operating room (OR) depending on level of urgency.
  - Antimicrobials may be administered to prevent surgical infection.
    - Use coverage for common skin pathogens (e.g., *Staphylococcus aureus*).
- Postprocedure: close evaluation for continued compartment syndrome and signs of infection, infection prevention, and pain control.
  - In many cases, the wound is closed after several days or a graft is placed.

Legg-Calvé-Perthes Disease

Dana L. Lerma

Definition

- Childhood condition in which the proximal femoral epiphysis has a temporary interruption in blood supply, leading to bone necrosis and subsequent repair.

Etiology

- Not entirely clear.
- Potential causes include infection, inflammation, trauma, and acetabular retroversion.

Epidemiology

- Most commonly affects children between 4 and 8 years of age.
- More common in males.

Pathophysiology

- Interruption in arterial or venous blood flow to the proximal femoral epiphysis, resulting in bone necrosis; subsequent bone repair.
- Four stages of necrosis and repair.
  - Ischemic event leading to cessation of blood supply to the femoral head.
  - Fragmentation stage: Re-absorption of bone with femoral head collapse. Fractures are not uncommon in this stage.
  - Re-ossification phase: New bone formation.
  - Bone remodeling: Femoral head begins to re-shape into a spherical shape. After this stage, residual deformity can still be observed.

Clinical Presentation

- Mild to moderate pain in the hip on the affected side.
- Pain may radiate to the thigh or knee, most commonly.
- Occasionally, pain is more severe.
- Leg length discrepancy or limp may be present.
- Internal rotation and abduction of the affected leg are limited.

Diagnostic Evaluation

- Radiograph of the hip or pelvis is the first diagnostic approach (Figure 19.1).
- MRI or bone scan may also be indicated during the early stages of the disease progression to detect changes that may be more difficult to discern on radiograph.

Management

- Initial management is dependent on the extent of epiphyseal involvement.

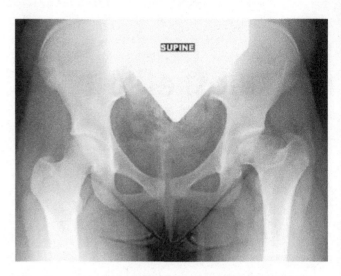

FIGURE 19.1 • **Legg–Calvé–Perthes Disease Anteroposterior (AP) Radiograph of Bilateral Hips and Pelvis.** AP radiograph of bilateral hips and pelvis of patient with Legg–Calvé–Perthes disease in the right hip.

- Treatment is aimed at maintaining the femoral head properly placed in the acetabulum and maintaining adequate range of motion.
- Mild Legg–Calvé–Perthes disease (LCPD).
  - Normal activity with observation.
- Severe LCPD.
  - Activity restriction.
  - Physical therapy (PT).
  - Possible bracing to maintain proper positioning of the femur.
- Long-term management of severe cases may include:
  - Extensive PT and rehabilitation.
  - Prolonged immobilization with use of orthotics or spica casting.
  - Close follow-up by an orthopedic specialist.
- Rarely, surgery is indicated, but in some severe cases may be beneficial.

Osteomyelitis

Susan K. Emerson

Background/Definition

- Infection in the bone.
- More common in children than adults because of rich metaphyseal blood supply and thick periosteum.
- If untreated, may result in purulent material throughout periosteal space.
- Approximately 50% of infections occur in children <5 years of age.
- Can occur in any bone; however, femur and tibia are the most common sites.

Types

- Acute or chronic.

Pathophysiology

- Osteomyelitis may occur as a result of hematogenous spread from bacteremia, local infection from a contiguous infection, or from direct inoculation from trauma or surgical procedure.

Risk Factors

- Hemoglobinopathies (e.g., sickle cell disease).
- Chronic renal disease.
- Type 1 diabetes.
- Compromised immune system.

Etiology

- *Staph. aureus* is the most common organism in children (except neonates), 70% to 90% of infections.
  - Community-acquired methicillin-resistant *Staph. aureus* (MRSA) is becoming more prevalent.
- Other offending organisms include group A hemolytic streptococcus, *Streptococcus pyogenes*, *Strep. pneumoniae*.
- Group B streptococcus is the most common organism in neonates.
- *Pseudomonas* is associated with puncture wounds, especially of the foot.
- *Haemophilus influenzae*: incidence has decreased since advent of *H. influenzae* vaccine.

Clinical Presentation

- Depends on child's age and bone involved.
- May have history of recent injury or infection.
- Discrete tenderness at site of infection in affected bone.
- May be associated with erythema, warmth, and edema of affected extremity.
- Limp or refusal to bear weight; lower extremity.
- Refusal to use extremity; upper extremity.
- Fever, chills, vomiting.
- Neonates may present with irritability, change in sleep habits, and decreased PO intake.
- May appear toxic if long duration of infection.

Diagnostic Evaluation

- Laboratory values.
  - White blood cell (WBC) count is highly variable with poor correlation to treatment.
  - C-reactive protein (CRP) is the *most* sensitive marker to monitor therapeutic response. Rises more quickly (e.g., within 6 hours of infection) and declines more quickly with effective therapy.
  - Erythrocyte sedimentation rate (ESR) rises and declines more slowly than CRP (e.g., elevated within 24–48 hours).
  - Blood cultures are positive in approximately 50% of cases and become negative soon after appropriate therapy is initiated.
- Radiography.
  - Plain radiograph.

- Early radiographs are often normal or demonstrate soft tissue edema.
  - Late radiographs (e.g., 1–2 weeks) demonstrate metaphyseal reaction and possibly an abscess (Figure 19.2).
- MRI.
  - Highly sensitive and specific.
  - Demonstrates bone and soft tissue reaction.
  - Can assist in identifying associated abscess.
  - Differentiates between soft tissue and bone infection.
  - *Imaging study of choice* in patients with focal symptoms and strong suspicion of diagnosis.
- Computed tomography (CT).
  - Identifies abscess and areas of destruction.
- Ultrasound.
  - Maybe helpful in evaluating for abscess; though unable to image details of the bone.

Management

- Nonoperative.
  - Indicated in early disease or disease without abscess.
  - Antibiotics should be started intravenously once a biopsy/culture has been obtained.
    - IV antibiotics provide optimal bactericidal levels in the affected bone and reduce dissemination of disease.

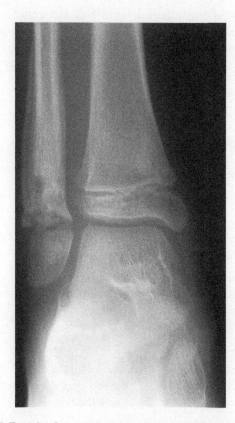

FIGURE 19.2 • **Classic Osteomyelitis Anteroposterior (AP) Radiograph of Ankle.** AP view of the ankle in a child with classic osteomyelitis. There are lytic areas in the fibular metaphysis with periosteal new bone formation. The epiphysis is normal.

- Empiric antibiotics should include coverage for *Staph. aureus* (e.g., oxacillin or first-generation cephalosporins). If MRSA is suspected, select vancomycin, linezolid, or clindamycin.
- May require peripherally inserted central catheter (PICC) line placement.
- Transition to oral antibiotics once patient is afebrile and ESR and CRP have normalized; may require long-term IV antibiotics (e.g., 6–8 weeks).
- Consider diagnostic imaging to evaluate for deep vein thrombosis (DVT) in patients with MRSA infection and in patients requiring a long hospital stay, admission to the intensive care unit, or surgical intervention.
- Consultation with orthopedic surgeon, infectious disease specialist, and occupational/physical therapist.
- Operative treatment.
  - Indications.
    - Abscess on radiographic study.
    - Failure to respond to antibiotics.
    - Purulent drainage on aspiration.
    - Chronic infection.
  - Removal of abscess/purulent drainage.
  - IV antibiotics: may require PICC line placement for long-term IV antibiotics.
  - Transition to oral antibiotic when patient is afebrile and ESR and CRP have normalized.
  - Consider diagnostic imaging to evaluate for DVT.
  - Consultation with orthopedic surgeon, infectious disease specialist, and occupational/physical therapist.

PEARLS
- *Recurrent and chronic osteomyelitis rate is 5% to 19%.*
- *Risk factors: delay in diagnosis, inadequate antibiotic treatment, young age at diagnosis.*

Slipped Capital Femoral Epiphysis

Jan A. Odiaga

Background

- Most common hip disorder in adolescence, typically associated with obese African American or Latino adolescents.
- More common in males than females.
- Most common in children 12- 15 years of age.

Definition

- Characterized by the separation of the growth plate in the proximal femoral head with the epiphysis slipping posteriorly with potential for complete dislocation.

Etiology/Types

- Unknown, but may be related to rapid growth, obesity, hypothyroidism, family history, trauma, or genetic conditions such as Trisomy 21.

- *Acute slipped capital femoral epiphysis (SCFE)* is a sudden exacerbation of < 3 weeks; a radiological shift in the epiphysis without a callus formation.
- *Chronic SCFE* has a gradual onset of symptoms over 3 weeks with some remodeling of the bone.
- *Acute on chronic SCFE* involves symptoms for months, but exacerbated with injury.
- The definitions may overlap and help predict outcomes.

Clinical Presentation

- Acute or chronic hip, thigh, or knee pain.
- Limited rotation and obligated external rotation of the hip.
- Pain can be severe with shortened stance of affected leg and Trendelenburg gait.

Diagnostic Evaluation

- Radiographs of the pelvic anterior–posterior and lateral or "frog" view reveal the classic "ice cream slipping off a cone" appearance.
- If radiographs are equivocal, an MRI or CT may be indicated (Figure 19.3).

Management

- Strict non–weight-bearing status until percutaneous pinning or in situ screw fixation of the femoral head through the growth plate has been placed.
- More severe dysfunction may require open osteotomy and internal fixation to secure the bones.
- Crutches are issued for 2 to 3 weeks postoperation for stable SCFE; 6 to 8 weeks for unstable SCFE.
- Team approach requires PT for gait training, hip precautions, and range of motion exercises.
- Sports and vigorous activity should be avoided until growth plates close.
- Overall care is provided by the primary care provider.

PEARL
- *Increased suspicion of SCFE in obese patients.*

Septic Arthritis

Jan A. Odiaga

Background

- Septic arthritis is considered a medical emergency. Joints commonly affected are the hip, knee, elbow, and ankle, with peak incidence in children less than 3 years of age; males twice as much as females.
- Neonates and premature infants are at greater risk due to immature immune systems.

Definition

- Septic arthritis is a purulent bacterial infection in the synovial fluid joint spaces; causes rapid destruction of the articulate cartilage.

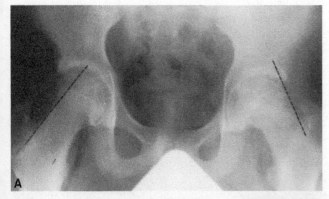

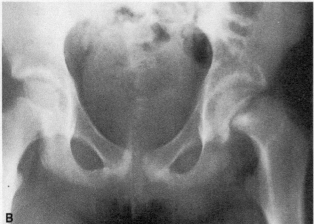

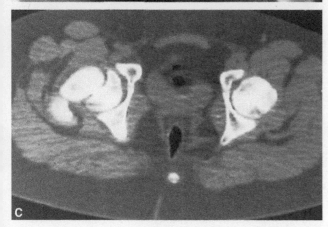

FIGURE 19.3 • SCFE Radiographic Images.
Radiographic findings in slipped capital femoral epiphysis.
A: A line drawn along the superior-lateral femoral neck
intersects less than the normal 20% of the epiphysis on the
left (affected) side. **B:** A more severe slip showing that the
femoral neck subluxates laterally and superiorly with respect
to the epiphysis. **C:** CT most clearly shows the direction of
the slip. This figure shows in situ fixation with a single screw,
the preferred method for slips of mild to moderate degree and
even many cases of severe degree.

Epidemiology

- Most commonly affected joints.
  - Hip (43%).
  - Knee (39%).

Etiology

- Hematogenous spread from an infectious focus elsewhere in the body.
- Direct invasion through a skin lesion or trauma that penetrates the joint.
- Extension from adjacent tissue.
- Most common causative organisms: *Staph. aureus* (methicillin-resistance increasing), *Kingella (Moraxella) kingae*, and group B beta-hemolytic streptococcus.

Clinical Presentation

- Ill-appearing.
- Fever >38°C.
- Joint pain.
- History of recent viral illness, soft tissue or upper respiratory tract infection.
- Insidious joint pain.
- Affected joint: painful to palpation, erythematous, warm, edematous; limited range of motion.
- If the hip, knee, or ankle are affected, refusal to bear weight.
- If hip, external rotation, adduction and mild flexion.

Diagnostic Evaluation

- Complete blood count with differentials
- ESR.
- CRP.
- Blood cultures.
- Radiographic studies to evaluate for a widening of the joint space.
- Ultrasound is the most useful; demonstrates joint capsule distention and joint effusion.
- Bone scans are most useful in neonates since this age group often has multiple infected joints or when the infection is in a location difficult to evaluate (e.g., shoulder or ankle).
- Ultrasound guidance can facilitate joint-space aspiration.
- MRI can be useful to identify associated osteomyelitis or abscess.

Management

- Once suspected, orthopedics consultation.
- Arthrocentesis.
- Surgical irrigation and drainage in some cases.
  - Emergently in the OR for large joints (e.g., hip) due to the destruction caused by the infection.
  - Drain may be left in situ postoperatively.
- Parenteral antibiotics: as soon as cultures are obtained.
  - Empiric antibiotic agent is selected based on patient's age, condition, and local antibiotic-resistance patterns.
  - Cover for most common organisms (see earlier discussion). Commonly, cefazolin is recommended. If MRSA is suspected, vancomycin, linezolid, or clindamycin are used. In infants <2 months age, provide coverage for *Staph. aureus* and gram-negative bacteria; commonly cefotaxime or nafcillin.
  - No consensus on duration of antibiotic administration.
- PICC line placement if prolonged administration or parenteral antibiotics is anticipated.

- Splint or brace may be used to reduce the risk of associated pathologic fracture.
- Infectious disease specialist, occupational/physical therapist consults.

Spinal Fusion

Christopher D. Newman

Background

- A variety of surgical techniques designed to fuse vertebrae to correct either spinal instability or abnormal curvature.

Indications

- Most common indications in children are idiopathic or neuromuscular scoliosis.
- Additional indications include vertebral fracture, degenerative disc disease, spinal tumors, spondylolisthesis, and spondylosis.

Types

- Posterior (most common).
  - Surgical approach to the spine from the back, removing the lamina and discs, and then fusing the target transverse processes.
- Anterior.
  - Surgical approach through the abdominal muscles for lumbar procedures.
  - May require piercing the pleura and deflation of the lung for thoracic fusions.
  - A discectomy is performed from the anterior approach and a cage is often inserted to preserve height and alignment.
- Vertical expandable prosthetic titanium rib (VEPTR): Although originally used for correction of thoracic insufficiency syndrome, VEPTRs are now being used in prepubertal patients with profound scoliosis to arrest progression of the scoliosis and take advantage of the ongoing vertical growth of the patient to improve alignment over time.

Procedure

- Transverse processes or discs of selected vertebrae are disrupted and graft material inserted into the vertical spaces between successive processes.
  - Over time, the grafted pedicles fuse in place.
- Alignment of the spine is then "fixed" by attaching pedicle screws, wires, cages, plates, and rod.
- Fixation supports the spine in the new alignment until the bony fusion is complete (typically 6–12 months).

Postoperative Management Concerns

- Hemorrhage.
  - Presentation: pallor, tachycardia, hypotension, saturation of surgical dressing, altered mental status.
  - Pathophysiology: Bleeding from vessels damaged or disrupted during surgery is common, but usually stabilized with wound closure. Decortication of the epidural space during the procedure can result in spinal epidural hematoma.
  - Evaluation: physical inspection of the wound dressing, laboratory testing including hematocrit, hemoglobin, platelet level, prothrombin time/international normalized ratio, and partial thromboplastin time.
  - Management: immediate management with volume resuscitation; transfusion of red blood cells, platelets, fresh frozen plasma or cryoprecipitate, if indicated. Ongoing hemorrhage requires reevaluation by the surgeon.
- Pain.
  - Presentation: Pain at the surgical site is commonly reported postoperatively. However, associated spasm may not be self-reported.
  - Pathophysiology: Postsurgical pain can be complicated by muscle spasm associated with realignment from the surgery, spasticity from the underlying condition, and pain from immobility following the procedure.
  - Evaluation: Expected postoperative pain must be distinguished from focal pain which may represent local hematoma or impingement of the fixation hardware. Focal or unusually intense pain should prompt reevaluation by the surgeon.
  - Management: adequate pain management using narcotic and nonnarcotic pain relievers to allow sufficient wakefulness for early mobilization and treat associated muscle spasm with the administration of benzodiazepines (e.g., diazepam).
- Loss of neuromotor function.
  - Presentation: alterations in sensation or motor control that differ from preoperative status, which usually occur distal to the fixation points and are often unilateral.
  - Pathophysiology: Most commonly, the tip of a pedicle screw has passed into or is compressing the spinal column. With more radical realignments, compression of the spinal cord can occur from shifting of vertebrae into the new alignment.
  - Evaluation: Most procedures are accompanied by intraoperative neuromotor monitoring, but any suspicion of alteration in sensation or motor function must be investigated promptly.
  - Management: In addition to notifying the surgical team, serial examinations and imaging of the spinal hardware may be helpful. Ongoing sensorimotor changes may prompt surgical reevaluation, particularly of the placement of pedicle screws.
- Ileus.
  - Presentation: absence of bowel sounds; firm, distended abdomen; and constipation.
  - Pathophysiology: Additional risk for ileus includes preexisting bowel motion impairment (neuromuscular scoliosis) and significant realignment of the lumbar vertebrae. Spinal realignment can result in realignment of the abdominal viscera and vascular network, creating a "stun" to the bowel, resulting in inactivity.

- Evaluation: abdominal examination, measurement of intake/output, evaluation of stool output/flatus, and plain-film abdominal imaging.
- Management: aggressive bowel regimen including stool softeners, osmotic laxatives, irritant laxatives, adequate hydration, early mobilization, and cautious use of narcotic pain relievers. Feeding should be reintroduced slowly. In severe cases, total parenteral nutrition may be required to promote wound healing while bowel function recovers.
- Thromboembolism.
  - Presentation: pain in the affected limb, tenderness to palpation, tenderness to dorsiflexion (Homan sign), warmth, erythema, or edema. In some cases, patients present with pulmonary embolism as initial evidence of thrombosis.
  - Evaluation: D-dimer—low value may exclude DVT. Ultrasonography is recommended for moderate-risk patients. In high-risk patients, diagnostic imaging with either a V/Q scan or helical computerized axial tomography is recommended.
  - Management: prophylactic strategies including compression stockings, sequential compression devices, anticoagulation, and early mobilization. The mainstay of treatment is therapeutic anticoagulation, though thrombolysis may be considered in high-risk patients.

Postoperative Teaching

- Postoperative immobilization may be indicated; determined by stability of spine following fusion and presence of spinal instrumentation.
  - Lumbosacral orthosis or thoracolumbar orthosis.
- PT.
  - Sitting: 24 hours postoperative.
  - Walking: 48 to 72 hours postoperative.
- Activity restrictions: promote healing.
  - No flexion, extension, or rotation of spine.

Toxic Synovitis

Andrea M. Kline-Tilford

Background

- An inflammatory condition affecting the synovium of the joint capsule; primarily occurs in large joints (e.g., hip). Most prevalent in children ages 3 to 8 years of age.

- Common cause of acute hip pain in children, more commonly affecting males. Also known as transient synovitis.

Etiology

- Unknown; likely an association with a recent viral infection, trauma, or allergic reaction.

Presentation

- Pain in the affected joint.
- Limping (antalgic) gait.
- Refusal to bear weight on affected extremity.
- Limitation in hip abduction and internal rotation.
- Afebrile or low-grade fever.
- History of recent infection (e.g., upper respiratory tract infection, otitis media, pharyngitis), reported in up 50% of cases.

Evaluation

- Complete blood count.
  - WBC count generally >12,000 cells/mm^3.
- CRP.
  - Mildly elevated.
  - Typically rises within 6 hours of infection/inflammation.
- ESR.
  - Typically >40 mm/hour.
- Radiograph of affected joint.
  - Evaluates for bony abnormality (e.g., fracture or osteoid osteoma).
  - Wider space in medial joint on affected hip may be noted.
- Ultrasound of affected joint.
  - Evaluates for fluid in joint space.
    - If noted, fluid may be aspirated for culture and analysis; however, culture results are often negative.
  - May be used to guide aspiration of joint effusion.
- MRI.
  - May be used to evaluate for osteomyelitis or bony lesion.
  - Can distinguish between toxic synovitis and septic arthritis (contrast enhanced).

Management

- Symptom management.
- Rest/activity restriction until resolution of symptoms.
- Nonsteroidal anti-inflammatories for pain relief; may reduce inflammation.
- Symptoms may last for days to a few weeks.

1. An afebrile, 6-year-old boy, with weight at 50% and height 25%, presents to the emergency department with moderate left hip pain radiating to the knee that has been persistent for the past 3 weeks. A limp developed over the last 3 days. There is no history of trauma or falls. On examination, limitation of internal rotation and abduction to the left hip and leg, a slight leg length discrepancy, and a mild limp are noted. His activity over the last several days has not decreased significantly, and he continues to participate in gym class. Of the following, which is the most likely diagnosis?
   a. SCFE.
   b. LCPD.
   c. Toxic synovitis.
   d. Trauma to the hip.

Answer: **B**

LCPD is the most likely diagnosis in this patient. LCPD is common in 4- to 8-year-old children and presents with mild to moderate pain on the affected side. Patients with SCFE are typically between the ages of 12 and 15 years, and there is a high association with obesity. In acute SCFE, pain is usually severe, and changes in gait are dramatic. Patients with toxic synovitis generally have fever, have more severe pain, and oftentimes refuse to bear weight on the affected leg.

2. A 7-year-old boy presents to the emergency department with right-sided hip pain and a limp. Which of the following is the best initial diagnostic test for suspected LCPD?
   a. Plain radiograph.
   b. CT.
   c. MRI.
   d. Ultrasound.

Answer: **A**

A plain radiogram is the primary diagnostic approach for suspected LCPD. A radiograph of the hip may reveal a flattened or deformed femoral head. An MRI may be useful if radiographic abnormalities are difficult to detect, but would not be the initial diagnostic study obtained. CT and ultrasound are not indicated in LCPD.

3. A 6-year-old boy with severe LCPD is admitted to the hospital. Which of the following is the best initial treatment plan?
   a. Antibiotics.
   b. Aspiration of joint effusion.
   c. Activity restriction.
   d. Surgery.

Answer: **C**

Activity restriction is indicated in patients with severe LCPD. Although surgery may be indicated, it is not an initial therapy. Antibiotics are not required as this is not an infectious process. A small joint effusion may be associated with LCPD; however, aspiration is not indicated.

4. Which one of the following postoperative symptoms contributes to postoperative pain in patients recovering from spinal fusion surgery?
   a. Lymphedema.
   b. Muscle spasm.
   c. Nerve inflammation.
   d. Headache.

Answer: **B**

Patients undergoing spinal fusion surgery commonly experience muscle spasm associated with realignment from the surgery, spasticity from the underlying condition, and pain from immobility following the procedure. Treatment for muscle spasms includes a benzodiazepine (e.g., valium) in addition to narcotic or nonnarcotic analgesia for surgical/incisional pain relief. Lymphedema, nerve inflammation, and headache are not commonly associated with spinal fusion surgery.

5. Loss of neuromotor function following spinal fusion is most commonly a result of which of the following?
   a. Compression from a pedicle screw.
   b. Generalized spinal cord edema.
   c. Spinal hematoma.
   d. Herniated lumbar disk.

Answer: **A**

Compression from a pedicle screw or in cases of radical realignment, compression from shifting of vertebrae into the new alignment is the most common cause of sensorimotor losses in spinal fusions. They represent an emergent and potentially reversible complication that requires prompt evaluation and may require a return to the OR for adjustment or removal of hardware.

6. A 2-year-old boy presents with fever and refusal to walk for 2 days. He complains of pain and points to his right lower extremity. The pain is increasing and he is unable to sleep at night and has decreased appetite. There is a recent history of an upper respiratory tract infection, but no recent trauma. What is the best next step?
   a. Radiographs of the affected joint.
   b. Parenteral antibiotics.

c. Serological evaluation.

d. Surgical intervention.

Answer: **C**

Rationale: Serological evaluation for identification of signs of infection followed by radiographs of the affected joint are used to confirm the space widening of the affected joint, and needle aspiration for culture in cases of septic arthritis. Surgical intervention and parental antibiotics are management steps to combat damage to the affected joint.

7. A 14-year-old girl with a history of a midshaft tibia fracture underwent a closed reduction and casting of her fracture and was admitted for pain control. On inpatient rounds later that day, she is complaining of increased pain in her leg as well as pain when passively flexing and extending her toes. What is the best management strategy?

   a. Elevate the leg and reevaluate at the end of the day.

   b. Increase pain medications to better treat the pain.

   c. Measure compartment pressure.

   d. Examine cast for fit and then reassess at the end of the day.

Answer: **C**

This child is demonstrating signs of compartment syndrome which is a medical emergency. Evaluation of the compartment pressure is needed to determine the need for fasciotomy. Reevaluation later that day may result in ischemic damage to surrounding tissues. Pain will be relieved with reducing the compartment space pressures through fasciotomy.

8. A 9-year-old is being treated for acute osteomyelitis of the distal tibia with appropriate IV antibiotic therapy. Serial evaluations of which of the following studies is the most expeditious method to determine the early success of treatment?

   a. WBC count.

   b. ESR.

   c. CRP.

   d. Radiography.

Answer: **C**

CRP is the best method to determine successful osteomyelitis therapy. A WBC count is nonspecific.

9. What is the most common pathogen for osteomyelitis in children?

   a. Group B streptococcus.

   b. *Pseudomonas aeruginosa.*

   c. *H. influenzae.*

   d. *Staph. aureus.*

Answer: **D**

Staph. aureus is the most common pathogen in osteomyelitis. Other organisms can cause osteomyelitis with lesser frequency.

10. A 14-year-old linebacker limps off the football field with right-sided hip pain and difficulty bearing weight. He presents to his primary care provider with minimal pain, but an antalgic gait with decreased stance time, decreased joint mobility with external rotation of the hip. Which differential diagnosis would be highest on the list?

    a. Femoroacetabular impingement.

    b. Proximal femur fracture.

    c. Avascular necrosis of the femur.

    d. SCFE.

Answer: **D**

Rationale: SCFE can be acute and stable at the same time, presenting with a limp, pain, external rotation of the hip, and unstable gait. It occurs more often in males and the most common age on presentation is 12 to 15 years. Femoroacetabular impingement is a slowly progressing disorder causing hip pain and soreness. Patients with a proximal femur fracture experience intense pain and are unable to bear weight. Avascular necrosis of the femur is associated with progressive pain and can be mild or severe.

11. When discussing the plan of care with the caregivers of a 4-year-old with toxic synovitis, which of the following will be included in the discussion?

    a. PICC line placement for parenteral antibiotics.

    b. Sedation plans for ultrasound-guided arthrocentesis.

    c. Rest/activity restriction until resolution of symptoms.

    d. Surgical irrigation and drainage.

Answer: **C**

Toxic synovitis management is primarily symptoms management (nonsteroidal anti-inflammatories for pain relief) and rest/activity restriction until resolutions of symptoms. Symptoms typically last a few days to a few weeks.

Recommended Readings

Dodwell, E. R. (2013). Osteomyelitis and septic arthritis in children: Current concepts. *Current Opinions in Pediatrics, 25*(1), 58–63.

Fleisher, G. R., Ludwig, S., & Henretig, F. (2006). Osteomyelitis. In G. R. Fleisher & S. Ludwig (Eds.), *Textbook of pediatric emergency medicine* (pp. 823–831). Philadelphia, PA: Lippincott Williams & Wilkins.

Fleisher, G. R., Ludwig, S., & Henretig, F. (2006). Trauma. In G. R. Fleisher & S. Ludwig (Eds.), *Textbook of pediatric emergency medicine* (pp. 1531–1532, 1705–1706). Philadelphia, PA: Lippincott Williams & Wilkins.

Hatezenbeuhler, J., & Pulling, T. J. (2011). Diagnosis and management of osteomyelitis. *American Family Physician, 85*(9), 1027–1033.

Jarrett, D. Y., Matheney, T., & Kleinman, P. K. (2013). Imaging SCFE: Diagnosis, treatment, and complications. *Pediatric Radiology, 43*(Suppl. 1), S71–S82.

Mazloumi, S. M., Ebrahimzadeh, M. H., & Kachooei, A. R. (2014). Evaluation in the diagnosis and treatment of Legg-Calve-Perthes disease. *Archives of Bone & Joint Surgery, 2*(2), 86–92.

McCarthy, J. J., & Noonan, K. J. (2008). Toxic synovitis. *Skeletal Radiology, 37*(11), 963–965.

Peck, K., & Herreta-Soto, J. (2014). Slipped capital femoral epiphysis: What's new? *Orthopedic Clinics of North America, 45*(1), 77–86.

Rodts, M. (2012). Spinal fusion. In K. Reuter-Rice & B. Bolick (Eds.), *Pediatric acute care: A guide for interprofessional practice* (pp. 888–892). Burlington, MA: Jones & Bartlett Learning.

Shannon, K. K. (2012). Osteomyelitis. In K. Reuter-Rice & B. Bolick (Eds.), *Pediatric acute care: A guide for interprofessional practice* (pp. 883–886). Burlington, MA: Jones & Bartlett Learning.

Shannon, K. K. (2012). Septic arthritis. In K. Reuter-Rice & B. Bolick (Eds.), *Pediatric acute care: A guide for interprofessional practice* (pp. 886–888). Burlington, MA: Jones & Bartlett Learning.

Watkins, S., & Gourineni, P. (2012). Compartment syndrome. In K. Reuter-Rice & B. Bolick (Eds.), *Pediatric acute care: A guide for interprofessional practice* (pp. 883–886). Burlington, MA: Jones & Bartlett Learning.

Watkins, S., & Grouineni, P. (2012). Gait disturbances. In K. Reuter-Rice & B. Bolick (Eds.), *Pediatric acute care: A guide for interprofessional practice* (pp. 878–883). Burlington, MA: Jones & Bartlett Learning.

Genetics

This chapter highlights the more common genetic disorders that are encountered in acute care practice.

CHARGE Syndrome

Lynn D. Mohr

Background/Definition

- A congenital disorder described in 1979 with a characteristic set of congenital features categorized as major, minor, and occasional findings.
- Leading cause of congenital deaf-blindness.

Etiology/Types

- 70% of children have mutation in the CDH7 gene on chromosome 8.
- Autosomal dominant inheritance.

Pathophysiology

- Arrest in embryonic differentiation during the second month of gestation, when the affected organs are in the formative stages.

Clinical Presentation

- **C**: Coloboma of the eye (key-hole-shaped defect seen in eye).
- **H**: Heart defects.
- **A**: Atresia of the nasal choanae.
- **R**: Retardation of growth and/or development.
- **G**: Genital and/or urinary abnormalities.
- **E**: Ear abnormalities and deafness (Figure 20.1).

Diagnostic Evaluation

- Differentiate between other syndromes.
  - VACTERL, 22q11.2 deletion.
- Major features (e.g., common in CHARGE syndrome and uncommon in other syndromes/conditions).
  - Coloboma.
  - Cranial nerve anomalies.

- Choanal atresia/stenosis.
  - Ear anomalies.
- Gene sequencing supports diagnosis.

Management

- Congenital heart defect: surgical correction.
- Choanal atresia repair.
- Kidney function evaluation.
- Feeding/nutritional support and gastroesophageal reflux therapy.
- Hearing aid/assistive devices.
- Hormone replacement for delayed puberty some cases.

PEARL

- *More information at CHARGE Syndrome Foundation: retrieved from http://www.chargesyndrome.org/*

DiGeorge Syndrome (22q11.2 Deletion Syndrome)

Jeanne Little

Background/Definition

- Deletion of chromosome 22q11.2.
- Most often results from a new mutation, but inherited in 10% of cases.
- Inherited through an autosomal dominant pattern from a parent.

Etiology/Types

- Common clinical features exist among DiGeorge syndrome, velocardiofacial syndrome, and conotruncal anomaly face syndrome because they share a genetic deletion of chromosome 22q11.

Clinical Presentation

- Cardiac outflow tract abnormalities (e.g., tetralogy of Fallot, interrupted aortic arch).

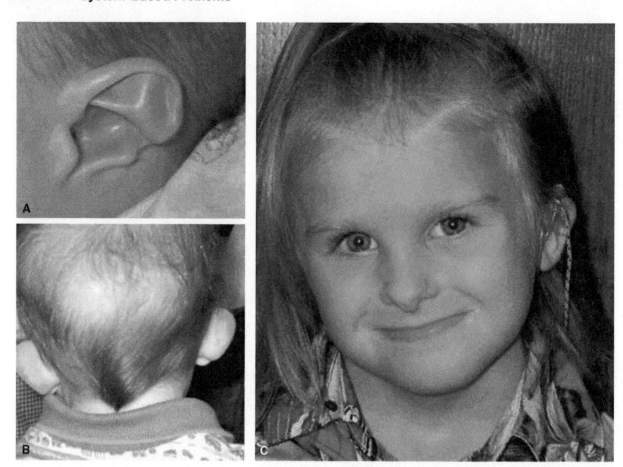

FIGURE 20.1 • **CHARGE Syndrome.** The characteristic ear anomalies include pinnae that are severely malformed **(A)**, protruding **(B)**, or small **(C)**, as in this 5-year-old girl with very mild facial features and laryngotracheomalacia. She carries the CHD7 mutation and had a more severely affected brother, presumably representing gonadal mosaicism.

- Dysmorphic features.
- Hypertelorism.
- Micrognathia.
- Short philtrum.
- Fish-mouth appearance.
- Low-set ears.
- Cleft palate with feeding and speech disorders, including velopharyngeal insufficiency.
- Conductive hearing loss can occur secondary to cleft palate.
- Frequent otitis media.
- Absence or hypoplasia of the thymus, resulting in immune deficiency and increased susceptibility to infection.
- Hypoplasia of the parathyroid gland, resulting in hypocalcemia.
- Cognitive impairment and growth delay; hypotonia is common in infancy.
- Skeletal abnormalities (e.g., cervical spine abnormalities, cervical spine instability, polydactyly, club foot).
- Vertebral abnormalities (e.g., butterfly vertebrae, hemivertebrae, rib abnormalities).
- Renal abnormalities (e.g., absent, cystic, or multicystic kidneys; vesicoureteral reflux).
- Hypocalcemia

Diagnostic Evaluation

- Fluorescence in situ hybridization (FISH) analysis or comparative genome hybridization (CGH) analysis for a deletion at chromosome 22q11.2 confirms the diagnosis.

Management

- Congenital heart defect: surgical correction as indicated.
- Cleft palate: surgical correction.
- Immune dysfunction therapy: aggressive treatment of infection, avoidance of live vaccines.
- Kidney anomalies: ultrasound evaluation.
- Calcium replacement as needed.
- Annual hearing screening.
- Speech and physical therapy.
- Cervical spine films at 4 years of age to evaluate for cervical spine abnormalities/instability.

PEARL

- *The acronym CATCH-22 is often used to describe the defect: cardiac, abnormal facies, thymic hypoplasia, cleft palate, hypocalcemia resulting from 22q11 deletion.*

Fragile X Syndrome

Jeanne Little

Background/Definition

- Most common cause of inherited intellectual disability.

Etiology

- Caused by a fragile site on chromosome Xq27.3.
- Fragile sites are areas of chromosomes that have a tendency to break, attenuate, or separate under growth.

Clinical Presentation

- Males are affected more often and more severely than females.
- Facial appearance is characterized by a long face and prominent jaw, forehead, and ears (Figure 20.2).
- Macroorchidism may not be present until puberty.
- Mild to profound cognitive impairment, autistic behavior, and developmental delays are evident.
- Seizures may develop over time.
- Poor eye contact, speech delays, hyperactivity, and aggressive tendencies.

Diagnostic Evaluation

- Molecular observation of an expanded DNA segment of the FMR1 (fragile X mental retardation 1) gene.

Management

- Medical management of seizures, if present.
- Early intervention with behavioral therapy, educational evaluation, and support (e.g., speech and occupational therapy).

Marfan Syndrome

Jeanne Little

Background/Definition

- Autosomal dominant disorder resulting in connective tissue disease affecting the skeletal, cardiovascular, and ocular systems.

Etiology

- Mutation in the fibrillin-1 (FBN1) gene with phenotypic variability of the disorder.

Clinical Presentation

- Typically tall and thin with an arm span exceeding the height (Figure 20.3A).
- Scoliosis, pectus excavatum, or pectus carinatum can develop.
- Dural ectasia, an enlargement of the dura at the lumbosacral level, is common and is usually asymptomatic, but may cause back and leg pain.
- Lens displacement (ectopia lentis) often occurs in the first decade of life. Severe myopia may also be present.
- Steinberg thumb sign presence: protrusion of distal phalanx of thumb beyond the ulnar border when hand is in clenched fist position (Figure 20.3B).
- Associated cardiac complications are progressive aortic root dilation with or without aortic regurgitation, mitral valve prolapse, and mitral regurgitation.

Diagnostic Evaluation

- Diagnosis is based on major and minor clinical criteria involving primarily the skeletal, cardiovascular, and ocular systems.

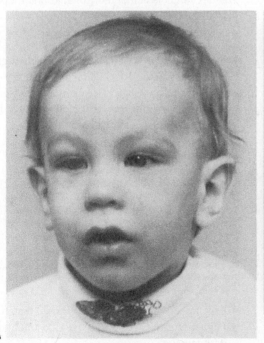
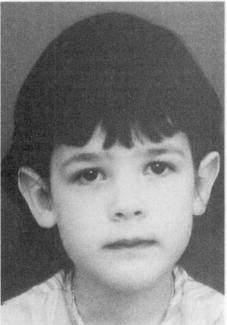

A   B

FIGURE 20.2 • **A.** Prominent forehead and ears in a male with Fragile X syndrome. **B.** Long face with prominent ears and jaw in a male with Fragile X syndrome.

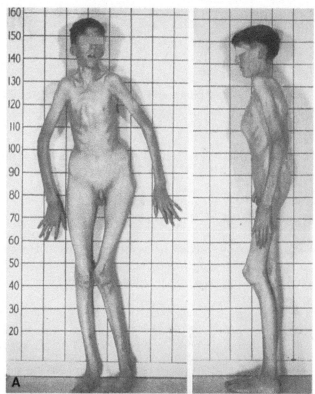

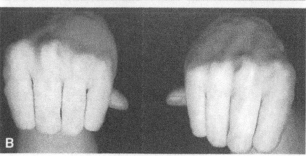

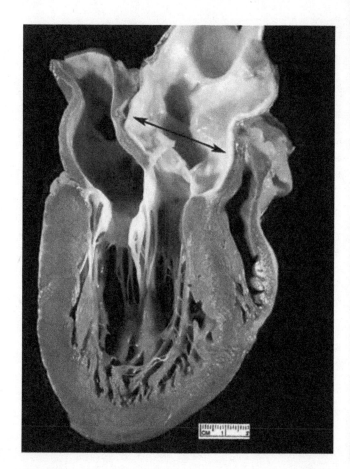

FIGURE 20.4 • **Ascending Aortic Aneurysm (Marfan Syndrome).** The anterior left portion of the heart in a patient who died suddenly with known Marfan syndrome. The aortic root is dilated (*arrow*), which is typical of Marfan aneurysms. The left ventricle is markedly dilated and moderately hypertrophied, consistent with chronic aortic insufficiency.

FIGURE 20.3 • **Marfan Syndrome. A:** Marfan syndrome in a 14-year-old boy. Note arachnodactyly, relatively long limbs (dolichostenomelia), pectus carinatum, sparse subcutaneous fat, unilateral genu valgum, and pes planus. The patient also had scoliosis. This patient died of aortic rupture at age 15 years. **B:** A positive Steinberg thumb sign consists of protrusion of the distal phalanx of the thumb beyond the ulnar border of the clenched fist, and reflects both longitudinal laxity of the hand and a long thumb.

- In general, a tall stature or an increased arm span to height ratio is the most consistent presenting finding.
- Major criteria include:
  - Aortic root dilation for age or aortic dissection (Figure 20.4), ectopia lentis, lumbosacral dural ectasia, and skeletal findings.

Management

- Prevention of complications and genetic counseling are most important.
- Scoliosis and pectus abnormalities are often treated with bracing and/or surgery.

- Dural ectasia can be serially followed with magnetic resonance imaging. Symptomatic children may require pain control therapy.
- Annual ophthalmologic evaluations to screen for myopia, increased intraocular pressure, lens dislocation, or retinal detachment.
- Cardiac, skeletal, and ocular monitoring.

Trisomy 18 (Edwards Syndrome)

Lynn D. Mohr

Background/Definition

- Chromosomal disorder caused by an additional chromosome 18.

Etiology/Types

- Females are more commonly affected than males.
- Higher mortality in newborn period among males compared with females.
- 95% die before birth, 50% carried to term will be stillborn, <10% will survive to 1 year of age.

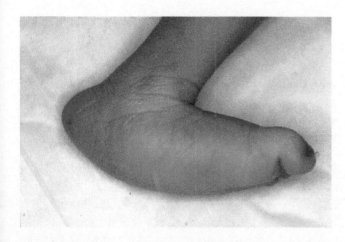

FIGURE 20.5 • **Rocker-Bottom Feet.**

Pathophysiology

- Not an inherited condition.
  - Random events during egg and sperm formation.
  - Error known as nondisjunction.

Clinical Presentation

- Cognitive impairment, low-set ears, rocker-bottom feet (Figure 20.5), hypertonia.
- Characteristic clenched fist with second/fifth digits overlapping the third/fourth digit.
- Cardiac defects:
  - Ventricular septal defects.
  - Atrial septal defects.
  - Coarctation of the aorta.

Diagnostic Evaluation

- Karyotyping or CGH analysis.

Management

- Congenital heart disease repair may extend life.
- Palliative or hospice care for children due to shortened life expectancy.

PEARLS

- *Poor survival.*
- *Children surviving the first year of life often experience severe handicaps.*
- *More information can be found at http://www .trisomy18.org*

Down Syndrome (Trisomy 21)

Lynn D. Mohr

Background/Definition

- An extra copy of chromosome 21.
- Trisomy 21 (Down syndrome) is the most common single cause of human birth defects.

Etiology/Types

- In 95% of cases, there is an extra whole chromosome 21 (trisomy 21), which is almost always maternally derived.
- Others have the normal 46 chromosomes with a piece of an additional chromosome 21 translocated to another chromosome.
  - The most common translocation is t(14;21), in which a piece of an additional chromosome 21 is attached to chromosome 14.
  - The next most common translocation is t(21;22).
- Mosaicism presumably results from nondisjunction (when chromosomes fail to pass to separate cells) during cell division in the embryo.
  - A few people with mosaic Down syndrome have barely recognizable clinical signs and normal intelligence.

Pathophysiology

- Three copies of chromosome 21.
  - Nondisjunction is a faulty cell division that occurs before or at conception when a pair of chromosome 21 (either in the sperm or in the egg) does not separate. As the embryo develops, the extra chromosome is replicated in every cell of the body. The cause is unknown.
  - Mosaicism occurs after fertilization when nondisjunction of chromosome 21 takes place during an initial cell division. Some cells have 47 chromosomes and some have 46. Causes milder form of Down syndrome.
  - Translocation occurs either before or at conception and involves part of chromosome 21 breaking off during cell division and attaching to another chromosome.

Clinical Presentation

- Varies from person to person and can range from mild to severe.
- Head may be smaller than normal and abnormally shaped.
- Common physical signs include:
  - Hypotonia, flattened nose, macroglossia, small ears, small mouth, upward slanting eyes, Brushfield spots on the iris (Figure 20.6).
  - Excess skin at the nape of the neck.
  - Brachycephaly (flat head syndrome).
  - Single transverse palmer crease (Simian crease); wide short hands with short fingers.
  - Smaller genitalia in males.
  - Cardiac anomalies.
  - Eye problems such as cataracts (most children require glasses).
  - Most children do not reach average adult height.
- Common developmental problems:
  - Impulsive behavior, poor judgment, short attention span, slow learning.

Diagnostic Evaluation

- Karyotyping or CGH analysis.

Management

- Interdisciplinary team management.

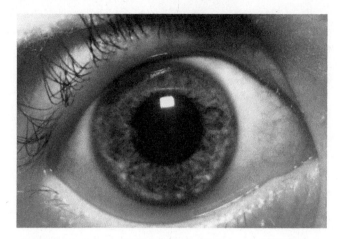

FIGURE 20.6 • **Brushfield Spots.** In an adolescent with trisomy 21, the margin of the blue iris has a rosary of small white stromal tufts, eponymically referred as Brushfield spots. These are more evident in persons of European ancestry and rare among native Africans.

- Cardiac and gastrointestinal abnormalities.
  - May need surgery immediately after birth for intestinal blockage.
- Support breast-feeding.
  - May have poor tongue control.
- Monitor sleep apnea, ear infections / hearing loss and thyroid function.
- Nutritional and behavioral guidance.

PEARLS

- *Refer to the American Academy of Pediatrics Health Supervision guidelines for children with Down syndrome (2011).*
- *Highlights of routine screening include:*
- *Eye examination in the first 6 months of life and then every year during infancy.*
- *Hearing screening every 6 to 12 months, depending on age.*
- *Dental examinations every 6 months.*
- *Asymptomatic children do not need routine cervical spine radiographies, but children with significant neck pain, radicular pain, weakness, spasticity among others identified by the American Academy of Pediatrics should have one set of radiographies completed, with potential referral to a neurosurgeon.*
- *Thyroid function testing at birth and annually.*
- *Hemoglobin level annually.*
- *Increased risk for sexual abuse.*
- *Higher incidence of acute lymphoblastic leukemia and a 50% higher risk of acute myelogenous leukemia than healthy children.*
- *Support groups.*
  - *National Down Syndrome Society—http://www.ndss.org*
  - *National Down Syndrome Congress—http://www. ndsccenter.org*

Turner Syndrome

Lynn D. Mohr

Background/Definition

- Most common sex chromosome disorder in females.
- 1 in 2,500 live female births.
- Approximately 1% of fetuses with only one X chromosome survive to term.
- Accounts for approximately 10% of all miscarriages.

Etiology/Types

- Occurs during formation of gamete.
- Approximately 50% cases are true monosomy with only one X chromosome (45 XO).
- About 10% cases have structural abnormality of X chromosome.
- Remaining cases have one or more additional cell lines or a mosaic karyotype.

Pathophysiology

- Chromosome number is altered.
- Results from loss of all or part of sex chromosome X.

Clinical Presentation

- First abnormality noted on gestational ultrasound.
  - Cystic hygroma.
- Newborn lymphedema, short stature, webbed neck (Figure 20.7), broad chest.
- Congenital heart defects.
  - 50% have bicuspid aortic valve.
  - Coarctation of aorta.
  - Aortic valvular disease.
  - Aortic root dilation
- Kidney anomalies.
  - Horseshoe kidney.
  - Duplicated collecting system.
- Infertility.
  - Females do not develop secondary sex characteristics.

Diagnostic Evaluation

- Confirmed by karyotyping of CGH analysis.

Management

- Children.
  - Cardiovascular monitoring and treatment of congenital heart disease.
  - Growth hormone therapy to augment linear growth (as early as 12–24 months of age).
  - Supplemental estrogen therapy for sexual development and preservation of bone mineral density.
  - Audiometry to assess for sensorineural or conductive hearing loss from recurrent otitis media.
  - Examination of young infants for Barlow / Ortolani maneuvers for evidence of congenital hip dislocation.

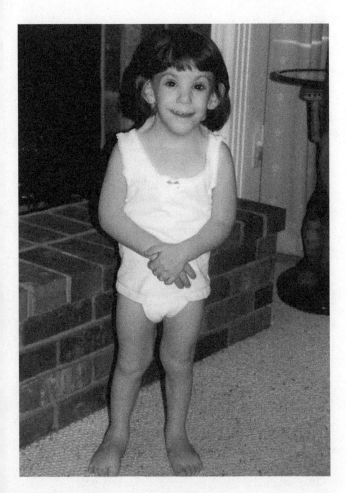

FIGURE 20.7 • **Turner Syndrome.** Three-year-old with Turner syndrome. Note the webbed neck.

- Referral to an ophthalmologist to assess for hyperopia and strabismus.
- Renal evaluation with ultrasonography.
- Adults.
  - Evaluation of fertility and sexual development.
    - Counsel regarding infertility therapy.
  - Management of atherogenic cardiovascular risk factors (e.g., hypertension, diabetes, hyperlipidemia).
  - Calcium and vitamin D supplementation to prevent osteoporosis, and ongoing sex hormone therapy.
  - Echocardiography or magnetic resonance imaging of the aorta every 5 to 10 years to evaluate the need for surgical correction of severe aortic root dilatation.

PEARLS
- *Maternal age is not a risk factor.*
- *More information can be found at http://turnersyndrome.org*

VACTERL/VATER Association

Lynn D. Mohr

Background/Definition

- First named in 1970s and initially described as nonrandom cooccurrence of a group of congenital malformations.
  - **V:** Vertebral defects.
  - **A:** Anal atresia.
  - **C:** Cardiac.
  - **TE:** Tracheoesophageal fistula (TEF) and/or esophageal atresia.
  - **R:** Radial and/or renal dysplasia.
  - **L:** Limb malformations.
- Described as an association because the defects occurred more often than expected by chance.
- No single unifying cause.

Etiology/Types

- No specific gene responsible.
- Suggestive of autosomal dominance.
- Higher incidence in diabetic mothers.

Pathophysiology

- No known cause.

Clinical Presentation

- Named after its common physical features of vertebral defects, anal atresia, cardiac defects (septal defects, tetralogy of Fallot), TEF with esophageal atresia, radial and renal dysplasia, and limb malformations.
- Presence of single umbilical artery.
  - Maybe first sign of diagnosis.

Diagnostic Evaluation

- Family history and based on the presence of the anomalies.
- Antenatal: presence of polyhydramnios, lack of gastric bubble due to TEF or esophageal atresia, dilated colon.

Management

- Two stages.
  - Some malformations managed surgically in immediate neonatal period.
  - Many of the congenital malformations can result in long-term sequelae.

PEARLS
- *Despite significant morbidity, typically do not display neurocognitive disabilities (neurocognitive impairment is suggestive of other diagnosis).*
- *Because the cause of VACTERL association is unknown, clinical genetic testing is not available.*

Williams Syndrome

Lynn D. Mohr

Background/Definition

- A genetic disorder characterized by mild cognitive deficits, unique personality characteristics, unusual facial features, and cardiovascular disease.
- Often associated with hypercalcemia and hypercalciuria.
- Other names that might be used include Williams–Beuren syndrome, WBS, WMS, elfin facies syndrome.

Etiology/Types

- Deletion in the WBSCR gene at 7q11.23 and absence of the elastin gene.
- Inherited autosomal dominant.

Pathophysiology

- A deletion is caused by a break in the DNA molecule that makes up the chromosome.
- In most cases, the chromosome break occurs while the sperm or egg cell (the male or female gamete) is developing.

Clinical Presentation

- Characteristic facial appearance: a small upturned nose, long philtrum (upper lip length), wide mouth, full lips, small chin, and puffiness around the eyes.
- Blue and green-eyed children with Williams syndrome can have a prominent "starburst" or white lacy pattern on their iris.
- Facial features become more apparent with age.
- Heart and blood vessel problems: supravalvular aortic stenosis or narrowing in the pulmonary arteries.
- Hypercalcemia.
  - Presents as extreme irritability or "colic-like" symptoms.
- Low birth weight/slow weight gain.
  - Often diagnosed as "failure to thrive."
- Feeding problems.
  - Linked to low muscle tone, severe gag reflex, poor suck/swallow, tactile defensiveness.
  - Feeding difficulties tend to resolve as the children get older.
- Irritability (colic during infancy).
  - Many infants have an extended period of colic or irritability.
  - This typically lasts from 4 to 10 months of age, then resolves.
- Dental abnormalities.
  - Slightly small, widely spaced teeth, abnormal tooth shape or appearance.
- Kidney abnormalities.
- Hernias.
  - Inguinal (groin) and umbilical hernias are more common.
- Hyperacusis (sensitive hearing).
  - Certain frequencies or noise levels can be painful and/or startling to the individual.
  - This condition often improves with age.
- Musculoskeletal problems.
  - Young children often have low muscle tone and joint laxity.
  - As the children get older, joint stiffness (contractures) may develop.
- Overly friendly (excessively social) personality.
  - Endearing personality, very strong in expressive language skills, and extremely polite.
  - Not afraid of strangers and shows a greater interest in contact with adults than with their peers.
- Developmental delay, learning disabilities, and attention deficit disorder.
- Older children and adults with Williams syndrome often demonstrate intellectual "strengths and weaknesses." There are some intellectual areas (e.g., speech, long-term memory, and social skills) in which performance is quite strong, while other intellectual areas (e.g., fine motor and spatial relations) show significant weakness.

Diagnostic Evaluation

- Fluorescence in situ hybridization (FISH) analysis is the primary diagnostic test.
- Chromosomal deletion too small for karyotyping.

Management

- Screen/manage congenital heart disease.
- Manage gastrointestinal and feeding problems.
- Ophthalmologic evaluation.
- Manage musculoskeletal and neurologic problems.
- Management of behavior.
- Screen/manage renal system.

PEARLS

- *Anticipatory care guidelines and growth curves for children with Williams syndrome are available through the American Academy of Pediatrics.*
- *More information at Williams Syndrome Association: http://www.williams-syndrome.org*

1. Which of the following characteristics are associated with the diagnosis of Williams syndrome?
   a. Anal atresia, limb anomalies, atrial septal defect, renal defects.
   b. Hypertelorism, long philtrum, wide mouth, small up-turned nose.
   c. Newborn lymphedema, short stature, webbed neck, broad chest.
   d. Severe hypotonia, feeding difficulties, dysmorphic features, obesity.

Answer: **B**

A child with Williams syndrome typically has physical findings of hypertelorism, full lips, long philtrum, small upturned nose "elfin" facies, and cardiac defects including aortic stenosis and pulmonary stenosis.

2. The most concerning finding in a child with CHARGE syndrome is:
   a. Brain abnormalities and seizures.
   b. Complex congenital cardiac anomaly and choanal atresia.
   c. Musculoskeletal defects and laryngotracheal malacia.
   d. Failure to thrive and immune disorders.

Answer: **B**

Children with CHARGE syndrome have a typical constellation of anomalies including impairments of growth and development, complex congenital heart disease coloboma of the eye, choanal atresia genital and/or urinary abnormalities and deafness.

3. Which of the following is considered the major difference between CHARGE syndrome and VACTERL/VATER syndrome?
   a. CHARGE syndrome is autosomal dominant disorder and VACTERL syndrome is sex-linked.
   b. Cardiac defects are found in children with CHARGE, not in VACTERL syndrome.
   c. Clinical diagnosis for CHARGE syndrome is divided into major and minor exclusion criteria; diagnosis for VACTERL includes three or more primary features.
   d. Both CHARGE syndrome and VACTERL syndrome are associated with a mutation in gene 8.

Answer: **C**

The clinical diagnosis criteria for CHARGE syndrome is divided into major and minor exclusion criteria. VACTERL clinical diagnosis is based on the presence of three or more primary features. Both CHARGE and VACETL syndromes are thought to be autosomal dominant. Further, CHARGE syndrome is associated with a mutation in gene 8, while VACTERL is not associated with any specific gene.

4. Which of the following characteristics is associated with Down syndrome (trisomy 21)?
   a. Brachycephaly.
   b. Double transverse palmer crease.
   c. Hypertonicity.
   d. Oily skin.

Answer: **A**

Brachycephaly, also known as flat head syndrome, is often seen in children with Down syndrome (trisomy 21). In Down syndrome (trisomy 21), skin would be dry, infant is hypotonic, and will have a single transverse palmer crease referred to as a Simian crease.

5. In providing genetic counseling for parents who are expecting an infant who has a prenatal diagnosis of trisomy 18, most important information should include:
   a. The infant will have macrocephaly and may not be delivered vaginally.
   b. Life expectancy is typically not beyond 1 year of life.
   c. Girls will experience higher mortality in the neonatal period.
   d. The syndrome is inherited with a female carrier.

Answer: **B**

The life expectancy for a child diagnosed with trisomy 18 is rarely past 1 year of age. There are many abnormalities associated with trisomy 18, involving all of the major body systems, including cardiac and gastrointestinal. Infants commonly have micrognathia. The definitive diagnosis for trisomy 18 is considered karyotyping and CGH analysis. Trisomy 18 is also known as Edwards syndrome.

6. Turner syndrome results from which of the following genetic mutations?
   a. Absence of a second sex chromosome.
   b. Addition of second sex chromosome.
   c. Defect in the SNRPN chromosome.
   d. Deletion of the WBSCR gene.

Answer: **A**

Turner syndrome affects only females and is a result of the absence of a second sex chromosome from a homologous pair which reduces the total number of chromosomes to 45. Defect of SNRPN chromosome in paternal chromosome is indicative of Angelman syndrome. A deletion of the WBSCR gene is indicative of Williams syndrome.

7. In planning discharge for a toddler with DiGeorge syndrome, which of the following should be included in the continuing management plan?

(continues on page 486)

a. Hearing screen.
b. Vision screen.
c. Potassium level.
d. Magnesium level.

Answer: A

Children with DiGeorge syndrome are at an increased risk of developing conductive hearing loss due to cleft palate and recurrent otitis media. In addition to hearing evaluation, calcium levels should be monitored due to hypoparathyroidism.

8. A newborn with DiGeorge syndrome presents with cyanosis, hypoxia, and poor perfusion. What is the most likely cause of these symptoms?
a. Cardiac tamponade.
b. Arrhythmia.
c. Tetralogy of Fallot.
d. Hypoplastic left heart syndrome.

Answer: C

Cardiac outflow tract anomalies, such as tetralogy of Fallot, are common in patients with DiGeorge syndrome. In most cases, cardiac anomalies are identified by prenatal ultrasound.

9. A school-age boy presents with speech delays, aggressive behavior, a long face with prominent jaw, and macroorchidism. What disorder should be included in your differential diagnoses?
a. Turner syndrome.
b. Fragile X syndrome.

c. Klinefelter syndrome.
d. Prader–Willi syndrome.

Answer: B

Fragile X syndrome is an inherited intellectual disability that presents with varying degrees of cognitive impairment, behavioral disorders including autistic behavior, a characteristic long face, prominent jaw, ears, and forehead, and macroorchidism. Klinefelter syndrome can present with similar behaviors, but patients have hypogonadism.

10. A 3-week-old infant is born with anal atresia, esophageal atresia, and malformations of both arms. This combination of malformations is most likely to be:
a. Currarino syndrome.
b. Heyde syndrome.
c. Mobius syndrome.
d. VACTERL/VATER association.

Answer: D

VACTERL/VATER association is considered anytime when three or more of the following malformations are noted at birth: vertebral defects (V), anal atresia (A), cardiac (C), tracheoesophageal fistula with esophageal atresia (TE), radial and renal dysplasia (R), limb malformations (L). Thus the only correct answer is D. Currarino syndrome is a group of malformations of the agenesis of the sacrum. Heyde syndrome is the association between an atriovenous malformations and malformations of the intestinal tract. Mobius syndrome is an extremely rare condition with facial paralysis and the inability to move one's eyes from side to side.

Recommended Readings

American Heart Association. (2007). Prevention of infective endocarditis: Guidelines from the American Heart Association. *Circulation, 116*, 1736–1754. doi:10.1161/CIRCULATIONAHA.106.183095

Bull, M. J., & the Committee on Genetics. (2011). Health supervision for children with Down syndrome. *Pediatrics, 128*(2), 393–406.

Davidson, M. A. (2008). Primary care for children and adolescents with Down syndrome. *Pediatric Clinics of North America, 55*, 1099–1111.

Jasmin, L. (2009). *Williams syndrome.* Retrieved from http://www.nlm.nih.gov

Pihl, S. (2012). Overview of selected genetic syndromes. In K. Reuter-Rice & B. Bolick (Eds.), *Pediatric acute care: A guide for interprofessional practice* (pp. 588–589). Burlington, MA: Jones & Bartlett Learning.

Solomon, B. D. (2011). VACTERL/VATER Association. *Solomon Orphanet Journal of Rare Diseases, 6*, 56. Retrieved from http//www.ojrd.com/content/6/1/56

Dermatologic Disorders

Bites and Stings

Conni Nevills

Bites: Mammalian

Background

- Dog bites are responsible for >3 to 4 million emergency department (ED) visits annually.
- One third to one half of these bites occur in children, with higher incidence in males.
- Children are more likely to sustain disfiguring facial bites than adults.

Definition

- Wound inflicted by a person or animal that disrupts the epidermal layer of skin.

Etiology/Types

- Dog and human bites are the most common types of bites.

Clinical Presentation

- Bleeding, pain, disfigurement, erythema, edema, exposed subcutaneous tissue.

Diagnostic Evaluation

- Radiographic evaluation if suspected bone fracture or penetrating wound over bone/joint or to evaluate for foreign body inoculation.
- Wound culture if appears infected.

Management

- Thorough wound debridement and irrigation; copious amounts of volume with high-pressure syringe irrigation.
- No consensus exists on primary wound closure.
- Antimicrobial therapy indicated for:
  - Moderate or severe bite wounds and puncture wounds.
  - Facial bites, hand or foot, or genital-area wounds.
  - Immunocompromised or asplenic host.
  - Signs of wound infection.

- Evaluate for risk of rabies (dog, cat bites) and for human immunodeficiency virus (human bites).
- Evaluate tetanus vaccination status; may require booster.
- No prophylaxis is required for new wounds with simple epidermal injury (e.g., scratches and abrasions).
- Antimicrobial Agent Recommendations (See Table 21.1).

Follow-Up

- Evaluation for signs of infection in 48 hours.

PEARLS

- *Provide coverage for methicillin-resistant Staphylococcus aureus in severe bite wounds.*
- *Ampicillin–clavulanate monotherapy does not provide coverage for methicillin-resistant Staph. aureus.*
- *All pediatric bite wounds require evaluation.*

Bites: Snakes

Background

- Several thousand snake bites occur yearly in the United States.
- Mortality is rare due to advances in therapy.
- Identification of snake species is important; majority of snakes are nonvenomous.
  - Historical clues include geographic location (e.g., woodlands, water, desert), presence of rattlers, and length.

Definition

- Envenomation occurs when venom is released through hollow fangs into the dermal layer of skin releasing a mixture of cytotoxic, hemolytic, and neurotoxic polypeptides.
- The substances damage local endothelium and can trigger systemic envenomation due to increased permeability which perpetuates the envenomation.

Etiology/Types

- Venomous species include rattlesnakes, cottonmouth moccasins, copperheads, and coral snakes.

TABLE 21.1 Antimicrobial Agent Recommendations for Dog, Cat, and Human Bites

Source	Most Common Organisms Causing Infection	Oral	Intravenous
Dog, cat	*Pasteurella* species, *Staphylococcus aureus*, streptococci.	Amoxicillin–clavulanate. **If penicillin (PCN)-allergic:** Extended-spectrum cephalosporin or trimethoprim–sulfamethoxazole plus clindamycin. Doxycycline can be considered for children >8 y of age combined with clindamycin. *Consider coverage for methicillin-resistant Staph. aureus for severe bites.*	Ampicillin–sulbactam. Alternatives include piperacillin–tazobactam or ticarcillin–clavulanate. **If PCN-allergic:** Extended-spectrum cephalosporin or trimethoprim–sulfamethoxazole plus clindamycin *or* meropenem. *Consider coverage for methicillin-resistant Staph. aureus for severe bites.*
Human	Streptococci, *Staphylococcus aureus*, *Eikenella corrodens*, *Haemophilus* species, anaerobes.	Amoxicillin–clavulanate. **If PCN-allergic:** Extended-spectrum cephalosporin or trimethoprim–sulfamethoxazole plus clindamycin. Doxycycline can be considered for children >8 y of age combined with clindamycin. *Consider coverage for methicillin-resistant Staph. aureus for severe bites.*	Ampicillin–sulbactam. Alternatives include piperacillin–tazobactam or ticarcillin–clavulanate. **If PCN-allergic:** Extended-spectrum cephalosporin or trimethoprim–sulfamethoxazole plus clindamycin *or* meropenem. *Consider coverage for methicillin-resistant Staph. aureus for severe bites.*

Clinical Presentation

- Puncture marks (may be absent in some species), edema, erythema, discoloration and development of bullae, pain.
- Signs of systemic toxicity include cardiovascular, respiratory, renal, and neurologic symptoms, but these are rare.

Diagnostic Evaluation

- Laboratory evaluation: hemoglobin /hematocrit, platelets, serum creatinine, alanine transaminase (ALT) and aspartate aminotransferase (AST), prothrombin time, fibrinogen, and creatine kinase.

Management

- Initial first aid is to cleanse wound site with soap and water and immobilize extremity, placing it at the level of the heart.
- Consultation with poison control and expert providers experienced in managing snake bites (if available).
- Antivenom administration if anaphylaxis, respiratory distress, hemolytic abnormalities, uncontrolled hypertension, or extreme pain.
- Pain control with narcotics if indicated.
- Frequent evaluation with measurements of affected tissue.
- Antibiotics are not indicated unless direct evidence of bacterial pathogen.
- Evaluate tetanus status; administer tetanus vaccination if needed.

Bites: Spider

Background

- Two species of spiders have venom that causes clinically significant illness in North America: the brown recluse (*Loxosceles reclusa*) and the black widow (*Latrodectus mactans*).

Definition

- Brown recluse venom triggers the inflammatory cascade; can develop into tissue necrosis.
- Black widow venom causes acute onset of intense pain via catecholamine release affecting neurotransmitters.

Etiology/Types

- A black widow bite may present with fang marks or target sign.

Clinical Presentation

- Brown recluse.
  - Pain at the site of the bite.
  - A ring of white tissue ischemia may develop, followed by a blister or pustule, and then a bull's-eye appearance.
  - Local symptoms typically begin 3 to 4 hours after the bite.
  - Severe envenomation occurs 24 to 72 hours after bite and presents with fever, chills, nausea, vomiting, signs of kidney injury, and alterations in hemolytic composition and function.
  - May lead to thrombocytopenia, hemolysis, shock, kidney failure, bleeding, or pulmonary edema.

- Mortality is typically a result of respiratory failure or severe intravascular hemolysis.
- Black widow.
  - Sudden onset of acute pain, swelling, muscle spasms, tachycardia, hypertension, pain, and agitation.
  - May have positive "tap test" (i.e., tapping at the suspected site of the bite elicits pain).
  - Increased intracranial pressure, significant hypertension, and respiratory failure are the most serious potential reactions.

Diagnostic Evaluation

- Brown recluse.
  - No specific laboratory test. Complete blood count (CBC), basic metabolic profile, AST and ALT, coagulation studies, urinalysis (may provide signs of systemic disease; hemoglobinuria and/or myoglobinuria).
- Black widow.
  - CBC, metabolic panel, coagulation studies, ECG, and urinalysis.

Management

- Brown recluse.
  - Based on clinical and diagnostic findings.
  - Local debridement, elevation, loose immobilization, and cool compresses.
  - Avoid strenuous activity; may spread venom.
  - Antivenom rarely indicated and carries significant adverse effects.
  - Patients with evidence of systemic illness require hospitalization for evaluation of coagulopathy, hemolysis, and renal failure.
  - No antivenom available in the United States for brown recluse spider.
- Black widow.
  - Local wound care, tetanus prophylaxis, pain control, cool compresses/ice packs.
  - Treat symptoms of infection with broad-spectrum antibiotics.
  - Antivenom is considered in severe cases; associated with significant risk for anaphylaxis and in children <40 kg and pregnant women.
  - Mild cases: monitor for 6 hours. If progressive/worsening symptoms, hospital admission is indicated.
  - Treat hypertension aggressively.
  - Muscle cramps can be treated with benzodiazepines, opioids, or dantrolene.
- Both brown recluse and black widow.
  - Consultation with providers/specialists experienced in spider bites.

PEARLS

- *Brown recluse spider bite presentation can be similar to an early community-acquired Staph. aureus infection or other spider bite.*
- *Black widow antivenom derived from horse serum; skin testing recommended prior to administration; evaluates for hypersensitivity.*
- *Mortality with black widow bites is approximately 5%, though significantly higher in young children (50%).*

Stings: Bees and Wasps

Background

- Possess stingers; release venom resulting in local reaction or anaphylaxis in some patients.
- Wasps are differentiated from bees by their smooth bodies and stingers which they can retract; ability to sting multiple times.
- Bee stingers are barbed which causes their demise after stinging.
- Account for most deaths associated with envenomation; 50% of deaths occur within 30 minutes of sting; 75% within 4 hours.
- Fatal reactions can occur with the generalized reaction to a sting; however, more commonly follows a previous sting that was associated with more mild generalized reaction. Shorter interval between stings increases likelihood of severe reaction.

Pathophysiology

- Venom contains enzymes, vasoactive chemicals, and peptides that cause catecholamine release, mast cell degranulation, and pain.
- Edema is a result of increases in cell membrane permeability.
- Triggers strong immune response, specifically mast cells (i.e., anaphylaxis) in some individuals.

Etiology/Types

- A local reaction is contained in the dermal layer of tissue and is a self-limiting condition.
- Systemic reactions occur as a result of massive IgE-mediated hypersensitivity reaction to envenomation.

Clinical Presentation

- Factors that influence the clinical presentation include the amount of injected venom, the number of stings, and the host's immune response.
- Local reactions are characterized by pain, erythema, pruritus, warmth, and mild edema.
- Symptoms of systemic illness include nausea, vomiting, abdominal pain, urticaria, and evidence of renal injury.

Diagnostic Evaluation

- Laboratory evaluation: CBC, complete metabolic profile, coagulation studies, creatine kinase.
- If concern for systemic involvement, consider cardiac biomarkers (predisposition for myocardial infarction), chest radiograph for pulmonary edema, and ECG to evaluate for ST segment changes.

Management

- Remove stingers, if possible, to decrease amount of venom absorbed.
- Local reactions can be treated symptomatically.
- Anaphylaxis is treated with epinephrine, corticosteroids, inhaled β-adrenergic agonists, and H1 and H2 antihistamines.
- Patients with allergic reactions should be discharged with an EpiPen with appropriate education on its use.

Necrotizing Fasciitis

Jennifer Livingston & Carmen Rancilio

Definition

- Rapidly progressing deep tissue infection involving fascial and muscle layers, skin, and subcutaneous tissue. Does not typically extend into the bone or joints.

Etiology/Types

- Most commonly polymicrobial (55%–75% of cases); average of four different organisms.
- Commonly associated with group A streptococci, *Staph. aureus*, *Klebsiella* species, *E. coli*, and other anaerobic organisms.
- Varicella zoster: less common occurrence since development of varicella vaccine.
- Most fulminant cases are generally associated with *Streptococcus pyogenes*; toxic shock syndrome and high mortality.

Pathophysiology

- Destruction of skin and muscle tissue by toxins released from bacteria.
- Infection progresses along the superficial fascial plane.

Clinical Presentation

- May occur anywhere on the body; epidermis is often spared.
- Erythema, warmth, induration, and edema of skin at local inflammatory site; rapidly progressing; fever, typically >39°C (102.2°F).
- Often associated with limited mobility of nearest joint.
- Marked tachycardia; hypotension in some cases; may appear toxic.

- Presence of crepitus most commonly associated with *Clostridium* species or other gram-negative bacilli (rod) infections (e.g., *Klebsiella, E.coli, Proteus*).
- May progress to gangrene and tissue sloughing as a result of tissue ischemia and necrosis.
- Most common in individuals with underlying immunocompromised state (e.g., neoplasm, type 1 diabetes, recent surgical procedure).
- Can occur in otherwise healthy individuals after a puncture wound, abrasion, or laceration.

Diagnostic Evaluation

- CBC; leukocytosis; blood cultures: yield an organism in most cases.
- Surgical exploration: involved subcutaneous tissue and fascia gray; tissue has little resistance to surgical probing (Figure 21.1).

Management

- Early supportive care, fluid resuscitation, vasoactive agent support, oxygen/respiratory support.
- Surgical consultation: debridement. All devitalized tissue removed. Repeat exploration often needed in 24 to 48 hours.
- Intravenous antibiotic administration.
  - Meticulous wound care and broad-spectrum antibiotics initiated promptly.
  - Include aerobic (e.g., penicillin G, ampicillin–sulbactam, clindamycin) and anaerobic coverage (e.g., metronidazole, third-generation cephalosporin); consider vancomycin in communities with high rates of methicillin-resistance.
  - Evaluate for signs of compartment syndrome (e.g., edema, pain, loss of sensation, decreased/absent pulses on associated extremity).

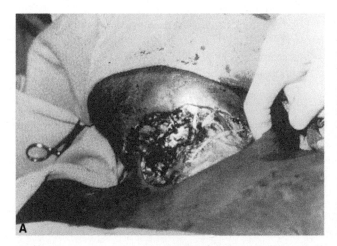 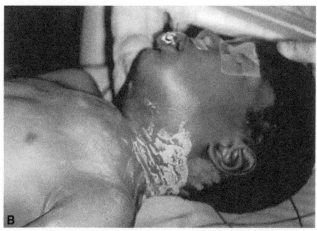

FIGURE 21.1 • **Necrotizing Fasciitis Surgical Exploration. A:** Surgical débridement of cervicofacial necrotizing fasciitis. A large portion of the skin of the left side of the neck was necrotic and had to be removed. Note that the skin is undermined by the infection and is dissected easily by finger pressure alone. **B:** An 8-year-old boy with cervicofacial necrotizing fasciitis secondary to an infected lower primary molar. Note the swelling extending from the cheek to the anterior chest wall. The chalky material on his neck is calamine lotion placed by his mother, thinking that the vesicles on the skin were poison ivy.

Stevens-Johnson Syndrome

Jennifer Livingston & Carmen Rancilio

Definition

- Hypersensitivity reaction affecting the skin and mucous membranes.

Background

- Often referred to as erythema multiforme major.
- Rare; affects 1.2 to 6 persons per million per year.
- Mortality rate is approximately 15%; often as a result of associated infections and organ failure.

Etiology/Types

- Attributed to severe immune response.
  - Medication-associated: antibiotics (especially sulfonamides), anticonvulsant medications (e.g., phenobarbital, lamotrigine, carbamazepine), nonsteroidal anti-inflammatory medications.
  - Medications taken up to 2 weeks prior to symptoms may be responsible.
  - Infection-associated, especially *Mycoplasma pneumoniae*.
  - Environmental.
- Erythema multiforme, Stevens–Johnson syndrome, and toxic epidermal necrolysis (TEN) are thought to be diseases along the same continuum with differing severity.
- Immunocompromised children are at greater risk.

Pathophysiology

- Exact mechanism is unknown.
- Inflammatory infiltration (tumor necrosis factor alpha and interleukin-6) of the epidermis leading to cell death and sloughing.
- Overwhelming keratinocyte apoptosis.

Clinical Presentation

- High fevers, cough, rhinorrhea, pharyngitis, vomiting, diarrhea, headache, myalgia, and arthralgia.
- Rash: erythematous macules that progress with central necrosis affecting <10% of skin surface area.
- Ulcerations: involve at least two mucosal surfaces, mucous membranes, eyes, genitalia, respiratory tract, urinary tract, and gastrointestinal tract.
- Ophthalmic: keratitis and conjunctivitis.

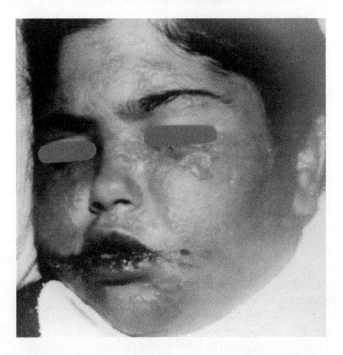

FIGURE 21.2 • **Stevens–Johnson Syndrome Mucus Membranes.** Adolescent with Stevens–Johnson syndrome secondary to sulfonamides. Note the involvement of mucous membranes of the mouth.

- Lesions present over a 1-week period; target lesions on face and trunk; rapid spread to bullae and vesicles.
- Erythema, edema, and pain typically precede development of ulcers.
- Nikolsky sign (i.e., mild skin friction results in dermal exfoliation) noted in most patients (>90%) with involvement of two or more surfaces.

Diagnostic Evaluation

- History and physical examination findings (Figures 21.2 and 21.3).

Management

- Eliminate the inciting agent (e.g., discontinue medication, treat infection).
- Supportive care: nutrition, hydration, respiratory support, sepsis, wound care, eye care.
- Large areas of denuded skin increase risk for infections and increase insensible fluid loses.

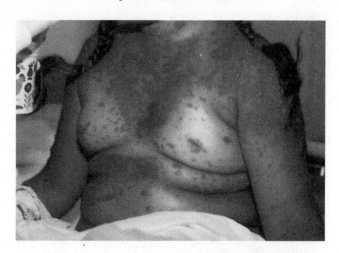

FIGURE 21.3 • **Stevens–Johnson Syndrome.** Same child as seen in Figure 21.2 with Stevens–Johnson syndrome secondary to sulfonamides. Note distribution of lesions.

Toxic Epidermal Necrolysis

Jennifer Livingston & Carmen Rancilio

Definition

- Hypersensitivity resulting in damage to the epidermis.

Background

- Most severe form along the continuum or erythema multiforme, Stevens–Johnson syndrome, and TEN.
- Incidence 1.2 cases per million per year; mortality is high: 25% to 75%.
- More common in adult patients; women > men.
- Immunocompromised children are at greater risk.

Etiology/Types

- Immune-mediated response.
- Medication: antibiotics (especially sulfonamides), anticonvulsant medications (e.g., phenobarbital, lamotrigine, carbamazepine). Medications taken up to 2 weeks prior to symptoms may be responsible.
- Infection: viral or bacterial.
- Idiopathic.

Pathophysiology

- Inflammatory infiltration of the epidermis, leading to cell death and skin sloughing.

Clinical Presentation

- Fevers (typically >39°C).
- Malaise.
- Localized skin tenderness and diffuse erythema.
- Rash: painful (extreme), burning, erythematous, or dusky macules. Typically develops approximately 24 hours after fever.
- Associated fluid-filled bullae develop. These lesions progress to a confluent masses and large areas of full-thickness epidermal necrosis.

- Epidermal loss: >30% of skin surface.
- No target lesions seen.

Diagnostic Evaluation

- Biopsy: necrotic keratinocytes with full-thickness epithelial necrosis and detachment.
- Clinical diagnosis.
- Characteristic criteria.
  - Widespread blister formation or confluent erythema, with skin tenderness.
  - Absence of target lesions.
  - Sudden onset, within 24 to 48 hours.
  - Full-thickness epidermal necrosis.
- Laboratory evaluation.
  - CBC, arterial blood gas, complete metabolic panel, C-reactive protein, liver function testing, and blood cultures.
  - Viral and bacterial wound cultures.

Management

- Eliminate causative agent (e.g., discontinue inciting medication; treat infection).
- Supportive care.
- Likely require burn unit or intensive care unit.
- Respiratory support as needed; 25% of patients with respiratory failure are associated with tracheal tissue sloughing. Early intubation recommended.
- Exquisite pain control.
- Wound care is paramount in preventing secondary infections.
- Careful fluid management; increased insensible losses; risk for dehydration.
- Antibiotics: if signs of infection.
- IVIG and steroids controversial.
- May require plasmapheresis or renal replacement therapies.

PEARLS

- *Skin often lost in "sheets."*
- *High mortality rate due to secondary infection and sepsis.*
- *May develop multisystem organ failure.*
- *IVIG and corticosteroid use are controversial.*

Pressure Ulcers

Lynn D. Mohr

Definition

- A localized injury to the skin and/or underlying tissue usually over a bony prominence, as a result of pressure, or pressure in combination with shear. (International NPUAP-EPUAP Pressure Ulcer Definition, 2014).

Pressure Ulcer Stages/Categories

- Category/Stage I: nonblanchable erythema.
  - Nonblanchable erythema of intact skin not resolving within 30 minutes of pressure relief.

- Epidermis is intact, usually over a bony prominence.
- Darkly pigmented skin may not have visible blanching; and the area may be painful, firm, soft, warmer, or cooler as compared to adjacent tissue.
- Category/Stage II: partial thickness.
  - Partial thickness involves epidermis, dermis, or both, presenting as a shallow open ulcer with a red pink wound bed, without slough.
  - Can present as an intact or open/ruptured serum-filled or serosanguinous-filled blister.
    - This category should not be used to describe skin tears, tape burns, incontinence-associated dermatitis, maceration, or excoriation.
- Category/Stage III: full-thickness skin loss.
  - Full-thickness tissue loss.
  - Subcutaneous fat may be visible, but bone, tendon, or muscle is not exposed.
  - Slough may be present but does not obscure the depth of tissue loss.
  - May include undermining and tunneling.
  - The depth of a category/stage III pressure ulcer varies by anatomical location.
  - The bridge of the nose, ear, occiput, and malleolus do not have (adipose) subcutaneous tissue and category/stage III ulcers can be shallow.
  - In contrast, areas of significant adiposity can develop extremely deep category/stage III pressure ulcers. Bone/tendon is not visible or directly palpable.
- Category/Stage IV: full-thickness tissue loss.
  - Full-thickness tissue loss with exposed bone, tendon, or muscle.
  - Slough or eschar may be present.
  - Often includes undermining and tunneling.
  - The depth of a category/stage IV pressure ulcer varies by anatomical location.
  - The bridge of the nose, ear, occiput, and malleolus do not have (adipose) subcutaneous tissue and these ulcers can be shallow.
  - Category/stage IV ulcers can extend into muscle and/or supporting structures (e.g., fascia, tendon, or joint capsule), making osteomyelitis or osteitis likely to occur.
  - Exposed bone/muscle is visible or directly palpable.
- Other categories.
  - Unstageable/Unclassified: full-thickness skin or tissue loss—depth unknown.
    - Full-thickness tissue loss in which actual depth of the ulcer is completely obscured by slough (yellow, tan, gray, green, or brown) and/or eschar (tan, brown, or black) in the wound bed.
  - Suspected deep tissue injury—depth unknown.
    - Purple or maroon localized area of discolored intact skin or blood-filled blister due to damage of underlying soft tissue from pressure and/or shear.
    - The area may be preceded by tissue that is painful, firm, mushy, boggy, warmer, or cooler as compared to adjacent tissue.
    - Deep tissue injury may be difficult to detect in individuals with dark skin tones.
    - Evolution may include a thin blister over a dark wound bed.
    - The wound may further evolve and become covered by thin eschar.

- Evolution may be rapid exposing additional layers of tissue even with optimal treatment.

Pathophysiology

- Develops when soft tissue is compressed between a bony prominence and an external surface.
- Pressure applied with great force for a short period of time or pressure with less force over a longer period of time—disrupts the blood flow to the capillary bed which impedes the flow of oxygen to the tissues.
- Leads to ischemia, hypoxia, edema, inflammation, and ultimately cell death.
- Contributing factors:
  - Infection.
  - Malnutrition.
  - Edema.
  - Obesity.
  - Emaciation.
  - Multisystem trauma.
  - Circulatory and endocrine disorders.

Diagnostic Evaluation

- Prevention and early treatment.

Management

- Proper skincare, balanced diet, mobility.
- Turning: use of offloading devices, use of lifting devices, use of support surfaces.
- All stages of pressure ulcers require topical wound care with surgical intervention most likely with stages III and IV.
  - Care varies with stage.
  - Surgical management may be needed.
    - Flaps consisting of transfer of skin and underlying structures to fill a defect.

PEARLS

- *Prior to interventions.*
  - *Withhold corticosteroids, if possible, for 4 to 5 days after the pressure ulcer appears.*
  - *Debride the pressure ulcer with enzymatic, mechanical, autolytic, or sharp debridement methods.*
- *Protect the ulcer from pressure or trauma.*
- *Change the method of intervention if no change in pressure ulcer noted after 2 to 3 weeks of treatment.*
- *For more information, visit http://www.npuap.org/ or http://www.wocn.org/*

Negative Pressure Wound Therapy

Lynn D. Mohr

Background/Definition

- Vacuum-assisted closure therapy is a trademark for negative pressure wound therapy (NPWT), introduced in 1995 by Kinetic Concepts Inc.

- An advanced wound healing therapy used to promote wound healing through a multimodality action under the influence of continuous and/or intermittent negative pressure.
- Incorporates either a polyurethane or a polyvinyl alcohol foam dressing that acts as an interface between the wound surface and the vacuum.

Pathophysiology

- Applying NPWT therapy to the wound helps to promote wound healing by preparing the wound bed for closure, reducing edema, promoting granulation tissue formation, increasing perfusion, and removing exudate and infectious materials.

Clinical Presentation

- Indicated for patients with chronic, acute, traumatic, subacute, and dehisced wounds, partial-thickness burns, ulcers (such as diabetic or pressure), flaps, and grafts.
- Two types:
  - Continuous.
  - Continuous-intermittent.
- Pressure settings in pediatrics.
  - 50 to 75 mmHg in infants (birth–2 years).
  - 75 to 100 mmHg in children (greater than 2–12 years).
  - 75 to 125 mmHg in adolescents (greater than 12–21 years or less).
  - 125 mmHg standard pressure setting in adults.

Management

- Precautions.
  - Patients with active bleeding or difficult wound hemostasis or who are using anticoagulants.
  - Ensure vital structures are adequately protected with overlying fascia, tissue, or other protective barriers with respect to weakened, irradiated, or sutured blood vessels or organs in the presence of bone fragments or sharp edges.
- Contraindications.
  - Necrotic tissue/eschar present.
  - Direct placement of NPWT dressings over exposed vital structures (e.g., tendons, ligaments, blood vessels, anastomotic sites, organs, and/or nerves).
  - Untreated osteomyelitis.
  - Nonenterocutaneous or unexplored fistulae.
  - Malignancy in the wound.
  - Sensitivity to silver foam dressings.
- Application tips.
  - Follow universal precautions: use gown, gloves, goggles if splashing or exposure to body fluids anticipated.
  - Determine that the patient/wound is a suitable candidate and accuracy of diagnosis and address all underlying and associated comorbidities.
  - Debridement prior to treatment, accurate foam selection, and indication-specific dressings are used as appropriate.
  - Place foam gently in the wound and accurately record in the patient record the number of foam pieces used.
  - Do not place foam directly over exposed vital structures.

- Ensure a good seal has been achieved and maintained.
- Keep therapy on for a minimum of 22 out of 24 hours. Do not leave the NPWT dressing in situ if the therapy unit is switched off for more than 2 hours.
- Monitor continuously; check and respond to alarms.
- Removal tips.
  - Change NPWT dressing every 48 hours, or if infection present, every 12 hours.
  - Manage pain and anxiety prior to removal.

PEARLS

- *Management of nutrition, consulting WOCN and Home Health care referral with family education will best support healing and infection prevention.*
- *Pediatric patients may have a risk of excessive fluid loss and dehydration and should be closely monitored.*
  - *When monitoring fluid output, consider the volume of fluid in both the tubing and canister.*
  - *The 1,000-mL canister should not be used for this patient group.*
- *Periwound tissue may be very fragile in neonates and infants. Particular care should be taken not to damage periwound skin.*
- *The use of white foam is recommended in neonates, infants, and children to prevent granulation tissue in-growth in the foam.*
- *The continuous pressure setting should be used in the above populations, where extra stimulation of granulation tissue formation is not usually required.*
  - **Additionally, the continuous pressure setting is recommended for optimal patient comfort.**

Incision and Drainage

Lynn D. Mohr

Background/Definition

- Procedure to drain pus from an abscess.
- Used when abscess is large, growing, painful, or not improving on own.

Etiology/Types

- Abscesses found on all part of body, primarily in axilla, buttocks, and extremities.

Diagnostic Evaluation

- Diagnosis of abscess is first step, presence of edema, erythema, pain.
- Ultrasound may be helpful to identify areas of localized infection or fluid.
  - Appropriate for abscesses larger than 5 mm in diameter in an accessible location.

Management

- Usually performed as an outpatient, urgent care, or ED. More extensive areas may require surgical procedure in operating room.
- Typically, a number 11 or 15 surgical blade is used; incision made at the most fluctuant site of the abscess.
- If possible, direct incision on the plane of the skin folds to reduce scarring.
- If no site of greatest fluctuant, incision is made in the dependent portion of the abscess.
- Uncomplicated abscesses without signs of systemic involvement generally do not require antibiotic therapy.
- If antibiotic therapy is indicated, oral or intravenous therapy is selected based on the severity of the infection and targeted to most likely pathogens.

Box 21.1 Indications for Intravenous (IV) Antibiotics

Life of limb-threatening soft tissue infection.

Systemic illness.

Immunocompromised host.

Infants/young children (relative indication).

Box 21.2 Common Pathogens in Skin Abscesses

- *Staph. aureus*, most common. Consider risk for methicillin-resistant *Staph. aureus* when selecting antibiotic agent.
- *Strep. pyogenes*.
- Site-specific organisms (e.g., gram-negative organisms in perianal abscesses).
- Multiple and less common pathogens: common in immunocompromised hosts (e.g., *Enterococcus, Pseudomonas aeruginosa*).

- Obtain wound culture and narrow antibiotic therapy when culture and sensitivity is available.
- Factors such as diabetes and smoking can increase risk of complications.

Contraindications

- Extremely large or deep abscess that are difficult to anesthetize may need to be managed by surgeon in the operating room.
- Not indicated for cutaneous cellulitis without an underlying abscess.

Complications

- Incomplete drainage of abscess, endocarditis, sepsis, bleeding, or damage to the adjacent vessels, injury to local nerves.

1. Which of the following is a contraindication for NPWT in the pediatric patient?
    a. Placing NPWT dressing over nerves.
    b. Using NPWT in a clean wound bed.
    c. Using a NPWT pressure setting appropriate for the child's age.
    d. Using NPWT on a pediatric patient after flap surgery.

Answer: **A**

Contraindications for NPWT include necrotic tissue/presence of eschar, direct placement of NPWT dressings over exposed vital structures (e.g., tendons, ligaments, blood vessels, anastomotic sites, organs, and/or nerves), untreated osteomyelitis, nonenterocutaneous or unexplored fistulae, malignancy in the wound, and NPWT sensitivity to silver foam dressings. Indications for NPWT use include patients with chronic, acute, traumatic, subacute, and dehisced wounds, partial-thickness burns, ulcers (such as diabetic or pressure), flaps, and grafts.

2. Which of the following is an advantage of using NPWT?
    a. Decreases perfusion.
    b. Increases edema.
    c. Inhibits granulation tissue formation.
    d. Prepares wound bed for closure.

Answer: **D**

NPWT therapy to the wound helps to promote wound healing by preparing the wound bed for closure, reducing edema, promoting granulation tissue formation, increasing perfusion, and removing exudate and infectious materials.

3. While examining an 18-month-old receiving NPWT, the suction setting is found to be at 125 mmHg. Which of the following is the most appropriate intervention?
    a. Reduce the pressure to 50 to 75 mmHg.
    b. Increase the pressure to 150 mmHg.
    c. Maintain the current level at 125 mmHg.
    d. Discontinue NPWT therapy.

Answer: **A**

The setting of 126 mmHg is the standard setting for adults and may cause tissue damage. Settings should be 50 to 75 mmHg in infants (birth–2 years of age), 75 to 100 mmHg in children (2–12 years of age), and 75 to 125 mmHg in adolescents (12–21 years of age).

4. A 3-year-old girl presents to the ED for a progressive erythematous rash to her torso and bilateral lower extremities. She has had a fever for 1 day and has been receiving ibuprofen for the past 24 hours. What is the likely diagnosis?

a. Stevens–Johnson syndrome.
b. TEN.
c. Necrotizing fasciitis.
d. Kawasaki disease.

Answer: **B**

TEN can be caused by a hypersensitivity to nonsteroidal anti-inflammatory medications. The rash typically develops within 48 hours of medication exposure and is painful (extreme), erythematous, and associated with a burning sensation.

5. When examining a patient with a confluent, erythematous, sloughing rash, TEN is suspected. Which of the following physical examination supports the diagnosis of TEN?
    a. Target lesions.
    b. Crusted lesions.
    c. Petechiae.
    d. Skin tenderness.

Answer: **D**

Toxic epidermolysis causes widespread erythema, necrosis, and bullous detachment of the epidermis and mucous membranes, resulting in exfoliation and possible sepsis and/or death. Initial symptoms include skin tenderness which is commonly noted in cases of TEN.

6. When admitting a patient to the burn unit with suspected Stevens–Johnson syndrome, which information from the patient's history supports the diagnosis of Stevens–Johnson syndrome?
    a. Camping 1 week prior to onset of symptoms.
    b. Wasp sting 2 days ago.
    c. Started on phenytoin 1 month ago.
    d. Previous history of chickenpox.

Answer: **C**

Stevens–Johnson syndrome is a hypersensitivity reaction associated with medications including some anticonvulsants. Any medication given within 8 weeks of onset should be a suspected cause and should be discontinued.

7. Which of the following specialty services should be consulted during in the hospitalization of a patient with Stevens–Johnson syndrome?
    a. Gastroenterology.
    b. Ophthalmology.
    c. Urology.
    d. Rheumatology.

Answer: **B**

It is imperative to include ophthalmology in the treatment process due to the increased risk of corneal scarring which can lead to vision loss.

8. When evaluating a child with a prolonged hospitalization, it is noted that he has a blister on his sacrum. This lesion is categorized as which of the following pressure ulcer stages?
   a. Stage I.
   b. Stage II.
   c. Stage III.
   d. Stage IV.

Answer: **B**

Stage II pressure ulcers include partial-thickness injury involving the epidermis, dermis, or both, presenting as a shallow open ulcer with a red pink wound bed, without slough. Stage II ulcers may also present as an intact or open/ruptured serum-filled or serosanguinous-filled blister.

9. While examining an adolescent admitted with sepsis, an area of maroon-colored intact skin on both buttocks is noted in close proximity to the sacrum. Which of the following best describes this child's skin ulcer?
   a. Deep tissue injury.
   b. Stage III ulcer.
   c. Stage IV ulcer.
   d. Unstageable.

Answer: **A**

Suspected deep tissue injury is usually purple or maroon localized area of discolored intact skin or blood-filled blister due to damage of underlying soft tissue from pressure and/or shear. The area may be preceded by tissue that is painful, firm, mushy, boggy, warmer, or cooler as compared to adjacent tissue.

10. While working in the ED, a 7-year-old child arrives from the primary care office for suspected necrotizing fasciitis. Which of the following is the most important immediate intervention for this patient?
    a. Obtain skin culture.
    b. Obtain surgery consultation.
    c. Administer glucocorticoids.
    d. Observe patient for 24 hours for worsening symptoms.

Answer: **B**

Prompt surgical exploration and removal of the devitalized tissue is the most appropriate treatment for necrotizing fasciitis. It spreads rapidly to the deep layers of the subcutaneous skin and fascia. Without prompt treatment and antibiotics, a patient with necrotizing fasciitis can develop severe sepsis and death will occur.

11. Which combination is the best choice for empiric antibiotic treatment of suspected necrotizing fasciitis?
    a. Ampicillin and Flagyl.
    b. Vancomycin and ciprofloxacin.
    c. Bactrim and fluconazole.
    d. Rocephin and gentamycin.

Answer: **B**

Vancomycin and ciprofloxacin are the best choices. Necrotizing fasciitis is typically polymicrobial and requires broad-spectrum agents to cover all possible pathogens. Vancomycin for gram-positive (including methicillin-resistant *Staph. aureus*) and quinolones for gram-negative organisms are recommended.

12. Which diagnostic tool is helpful in acquiring information prior to performing an incision and drainage for a skin abscess?
    a. CT.
    b. Nuclear medicine scan.
    c. Ultrasound.
    d. Plain radiography.

Answer: **C**

Ultrasound is the most helpful to identify areas of localized infection or fluid. CT may be helpful, but it is not routinely used when evaluating an abscess unless deep extension is expected. Nuclear medicine scans and plan film radiographs are not useful in the evaluation of skin abscess.

13. A 12-year-old was bitten by a snake on a family hike. His left lower leg is erythematous and painful on palpation with visible fang puncture marks. The remainder of his history and examination is unremarkable. The first course of management is to:
    a. Apply a tourniquet above the bite.
    b. Cleanse the wound with soap and water.
    c. Begin antibiotics.
    d. Assess immunization history.

Answer: **B**

The first step in management of a snake bite is to cleanse the wound with soap and water. Subsequent management includes immobilizing the extremity at heart level. Applying a tourniquet above the bite compromises tissue perfusion and does not prevent the spread of venom systemically. Antibiotics are not indicated unless symptoms of infection are present. Although assessing the immunization history for tetanus status is important, it is not the first step.

14. A 6-year-old girl is being admitted from a community hospital after a black widow bite to her left forearm. The primary medication requirements are anticipated to be:
    a. Antibiotics.
    b. Anti-epileptics.
    c. Antihistamines.
    d. Analgesia.

Answer: **D**

Black widow spider bites are extremely painful and require opioid analgesia. Antibiotics are not indicated unless acute symptoms of infection are present. There is no indication for diuretics or anti-epileptics.

Recommended Readings

Abelt, R. (2012). Erythema multiforme. In K. R. Rice & B. N. Bolick (Eds.), *Pediatric acute care: A guide for interprofessional practice* (pp. 347–351). Burlington, MA: Jones & Bartlett Learning.

American Academy of Pediatrics. (2012). Bite wounds. In L. K. Pickering (Ed.), *Red Book: 2012 Report of the committee on infectious diseases* (29th ed., pp. 204–207). Elk Grove Village, IL: Author.

Baharestani, M. (2007). Use of negative pressure wound therapy in the treatment of neonatal and pediatric wounds: A retrospective examination of clinical outcomes. *Ostomy Wound Management, 53*(6), 75–85.

Edwards, J. (2012). Wounds and wound care. In K. R. Rice & B. N. Bolick (Eds.), *Pediatric acute care: A guide for interprofessional practice* (pp. 354–361). Burlington, MA: Jones & Bartlett Learning.

Fitch, M., Manthey, D., Henderson, M., Nicks, B., & Pariyadath, M. (2007). Abscess incision and drainage. *New England Journal of Medicine, 357*, e20. doi:10.1056/NEJMvcm071319

Harper, M. B., & Fleisher, G. R. (2010). Infectious disease emergencies. In G. R. Fleisher & S. Ludwig (Eds.), *Texbook of pediatric emergency medicine* (pp. 887–952). Philadelphia, PA: Lippincott Williams & Wilkins.

Hess, C. T. (2012). *Clinical guide to skin and wound care.* Springhouse, PA: Springhouse.

Meadows, M. (2012). Stings. In K. R. Rice & B. N. Bolick (Eds.), *Pediatric acute care: A guide for interprofessional practice* (pp. 351–354). Burlington, MA: Jones & Bartlett Learning.

Morelli, J. G. (2011). Subcutaneous tissue infections. In R. M. Kliegman, B. F. Stanton, J. W. St. Geme, N. F. Schor, & R. E. Behrman (Eds.), *Kliegman: Nelson textbook of pediatrics* (19th ed., pp. 2300–2302). Philadelphia, PA: Elsevier Saunders.

National Pressure Ulcer Advisory Panel, European Pressure Ulcer Advisory Panel and Pan Pacific Pressure Injury Alliance.(2014). Prevention and Treatment of Pressure Ulcers: Quick Reference Guide. Emily Haesler (Ed.). Cambridge Media: Osborne Park, WA: Australia.

Reuter-Rice, K., & Bolick, B. (Eds.). (2012). *Pediatric acute care: A guide for interprofessional practice.* Burlington, MA: Jones & Bartlett Learning.

Palliative Care, Complementary and Alternative Therapies

Palliative and End-of-Life Care

Cathy Haut

Pain and Symptom Management

Background

- Children have multiple different physiologic and emotional problems related to the diagnosis, treatment, or the process of active dying.
- Pain is the primary concern in palliative care, as children experience levels of pain based on previous experience, tissue damage involved, developmental level, and meaning of pain.
- Children may not be able to communicate pain or to acknowledge the severity of pain!
- The most concerning symptoms for children at the end of life include pain, gastrointestinal problems, and neurologic changes, including seizures and altered mental status.
- Ideally, a pediatric palliative care team or service can be used or consulted to assist in determining appropriate care for children who are determined to have a life limiting disease or be at the end of life.

Definition

In the context of palliative care, pain and symptom management refers to interventions used in response to multiple types of pain, respiratory or cardiovascular concerns, gastrointestinal problems, and neurologic and psychological issues (Table 22.1).

Etiology

Pain and concerning symptoms for children who are receiving palliative care or at the end of life typically evolve from the origin or progression of disease process or as side effects of treatment.

Clinical Presentation

- Pain.

Terminology of Types of Pain

- Nociceptive: occurs with activation of primary afferent neurons by a noxious stimulus.

- Paresthesia: Abnormal painful numbness, includes prickling, tingling, and increased sensitivity.
- Paroxysmal: sudden onset of escalation or recurrence of pain.
- Allodynia: pain caused by a stimulus that typically does not produce pain (e.g., light touch).
- Central pain: Pain resulting from a lesion or dysfunction in the central nervous system (e.g., poststroke pain).
- Dysesthesia: Abnormal sensation that includes painful numbness, burning, tingling, and allodynia.
- Neuropathic pain: Pain initiated or caused by a primary lesion or dysfunction in the nervous system.

Evaluation of Pain

- Always based on the developmental level of child.
- Changes in vital signs and behavior are not often apparent in chronic pain as in acute pain.
- Young infants and newborns will exhibit crying, stiffening bodies, withdrawing to pain, facial grimacing.
- Evaluation of infants and toddlers includes differentiation between true discomfort and stranger anxiety or fear.
- Pain scales are helpful for all ages.

Diagnostic Evaluation

- Pain is evaluated based on vital signs and patient ratings. Vital signs can be important indicators of pain or increasing pain.
- Diagnostic evaluation of other symptoms is typically based on clinical findings, but supported by laboratory studies (e.g., cough → chest radiograph).
- The extent of diagnostic testing in palliative care is based on the etiology of the problem and the rationale for the study.
- Laboratory studies and radiological imaging are often considered for the purpose of symptom-based management even when a child is actively dying.

Management

Pharmacologic Pain Management

- Pain relief is essential at the end of life.

TABLE 22.1   Clinical Symptoms and Management Associated with Palliative Care

Primary Problem	Related Symptoms or Concerns	Response

Pain	• Acute or chronic
	• Types of pain
	  • Allodynia
	  • Central pain
	  • Neuropathic pain
	  • Dysesthesia
		• Evaluation using developmentally appropriate pain scales.
		• Management based on type and severity of pain.

Respiratory/ Cardiovascular	Dyspnea Cough Hypoxia	• Evaluation based on severity of symptoms, diagnostic studies, if indicated. • Administer oxygen.
Gastrointestinal	Anorexia Constipation Diarrhea Nausea Vomiting	• Evaluation of nutritional status. • Evaluation of need for medical therapies. • Management with diet, fluids, or medication.
Neurologic	Headache Seizures Fatigue Weakness Altered level of consciousness	• Evaluation of clinical status and use of imaging modalities, if indicated. • Supportive treatments or radiation to shrink tumor causing lesions.
Psychological	Depression Anxiety Delirium Agitation Confusion	• Formal evaluation and diagnosis. • Psychological treatment based on diagnosis.

- Inadequate pain relief hastens death by increasing physiologic stress.
- Management of pain can be through many modalities (e.g., oral, transdermal).
- Barriers to pain control exist within health care system and with patients and families.

Pain Relief Guidelines/Principles

- Use World Health Organization (WHO) pain ladder approach.
- Use round-the-clock dosing or long-acting medications, titrate upward slowly, reevaluate frequently.
- Start with low-dose, short-acting opioids and titrate to effect.
- Use adjuvant pain medications and nonpharmacologic adjunctive therapy.
- Initial management may include one or two medications, can combine opioids with nonopioid and adjuvant medications.
- Ensure administration schedule is based on the analgesic's duration of effect.
- Use sustained-release opioids for scheduled dosing and immediate-release opioids for rescue or breakthrough dosing.

- Avoid meperidine, propoxyphene (Darvon), and the mixed agonist–antagonist opioids (e.g., Stadol, Nubain, Talwin).
- Noninvasive routes are preferred. Intravenous (IV) analgesics work well until the pain is controlled. Continuous subcutaneous or IV infusions are indicated when other routes are not practical or effective.
- To titrate pain therapy, increase dose by 25% to 50% for moderate pain and 50% to 100% for severe pain. Calculate average dose of breakthrough medication taken per day and add to daily dose.
- Breakthrough dosing: Use scheduled dosing for consistent/basal control. Frequent breakthrough dosing equals increased schedule dosing. Oral breakthrough dose is 10% to 20% of the oral 24-hour baseline dose. IV/subcutaneous breakthrough dose is approximately 50% to 100% of the hourly IV/subcutaneous rate.
- When changing medication or route of administration, use equalgesic doses.
- Manage opioid side effects aggressively. Start stimulant laxative/softener combination with opioids.
- Refer Section 14 for more information.

Nonpharmacologic Pain Management

Cognitive behavioral therapies/alternative therapies (Tables 22.2 and 22.3):

- Hypnosis.
- Guided imagery.
- Biofeedback.
- Yoga.
- Acupuncture.
- Music therapy.

Other Symptom Management

Cardiac/Respiratory

- Dyspnea: distressing shortness of breath.
  - Pharmacologic therapies:
    - Opioids, diuretics, bronchodilators, benzodiazepines.
      - Inhaled morphine, furosemide by nebulizer.
    - Opiates are most commonly used to control pain and dyspnea at the end of life.
  - Nonpharmacologic: breathing exercises, fan blowing in face, oxygen, limiting energy consumption.
- Cough.
  - Pharmacologic therapies: steroids, cough suppressants, antibiotics, anticholinergics.

- Nonpharmacologic therapies: Elevate head of bed, sit upright, ambulation.
- Secretions.
  - Pharmacologic therapies: oxygen, anticholinergics (e.g., atropine, glycopyrrolate, scopalomine).
  - Nonpharmacologic: chest physiotherapy, suctioning as tolerated, positioning.

Gastrointestinal

- Anorexia/Cachexia.
  - Pharmacologic therapies: corticosteroids—also assist in decreasing nausea and improving energy; prokinetics: metoclopramide; dopaminergics, such as haloperidol; progestogens, but take longer to become effective; marijuana.
  - Nonpharmacologic: Offer small meals, portions, aesthetically pleasing environment and presentation of food; nutritional high-calorie supplements can assist if tolerated.
- Constipation.
  - Pharmacologic therapies: Aggressive therapy is best; stool softener and laxative, osmotic agents such as polyethylene glycol (Miralax), stimulants such as senna and bisacodyl; use treatments together.
  - Nonpharmacologic: fluids, fruits and fruit juices, fiber; if tolerated, ambulation.

TABLE 22.2 Pain Presentation and Management

Types of Pain	Pain Character	Drugs/Classes of Medications
Myofacial/Somatic Pain	Constant and well localized.	- Acetaminophen/NSAIDs. - Nonopioid (e.g., Baclofen). - Opioids
Visceral Pain	Injury to sympathetically innervated organs. Pain is vague in quality. Deep, dull, aching. Referred pain.	- NSAIDs. - Corticosteroids. - Opioids.
Bone Pain	Axial skeleton with thoracic and lumbar spine, most common.	- NSAIDs: ketorolac (Toradal) and many others. - Corticosteroids/bisphosphonates. - Radiation therapy, radionuclides. - Opioids.
Neuropathic Pain/ Nerve Damage Dysesthesia	Injury to some element of the nervous system. Dysesthesia, burning, tingling, numbing, shooting electrical pain. May require higher doses of opioids.	- Anticonvulsants: gabapentin (Neurontin), carbamazepine (Tegretol), clonazepam (Klonopin). - Tricyclic antidepressants: nortriptyline (Pamelor), desipramine (Norpramin). - Atypical antidepressants: duloxetine (Cymbalta), venlafaxine (Effexor). - Corticosteroids. - Topical anesthetic: lidocaine patch 5% (Lidoderm). - Opioids.

TABLE 22.3 Commonly Used Pain Medications

Medication	Dosage Forms/Strengths	Approximate Equivalence	
		IV/SubQ	Oral
Morphine	Immediate-release tablets: Morphine sulfate immediate-release—15, 30 mg. Sustained-release tablets: MS Contin –15, 30, 60, 100, 200 mg q 8–12 h. Oral liquids: Morphine sulfate immediate-release solution—2 mg/mL, 4 mg/mL. Morphine sulfate immediate-release concentrate (Roxanol)—20 mg/mL. Suppository: Rectal morphine sulfate (RMS)—5, 10, 20, 30 mg.	10 mg	30 mg
Hydromorphone	Tablets: Hydromorphone (Dilaudid)—2, 4, 8 mg. Liquid: Hydromorphone (Dilaudid)—5 mg/5 mL. Injection—1, 2, 4 mg/mL. Dilaudid HP—10 mg/mL. Suppository: Hydromorphone (Dilaudid)—3 mg.	1.5 mg	7.5 mg
Oxycodone	Immediate-release tablets: Oxy IR—5 mg. Roxicodone—5, 15, 30 mg. Oxycodone/acetaminophen (Do not exceed 4,000 mg acetaminophen q 24 h). Percocet—5/325, 7.5/325, 10/325 mg. Roxicet—5/325, 5/500 mg. Sustained-release tablets: Oxycontin—10,15, 20, 30, 40, 60, 80 mg. Liquid: Roxicodone—1 mg/mL, 20 mg/mL. OxyFAST—20 mg/mL.	10–30 mg	
Hydrocodone	Hydrocodone/acetaminophen tablets (Do not exceed 4,000 mg acetaminophen/24 hr). Lortab—2.5/500, 5/500, 7.5/500, 10/500 mg. Norco—5/325 mg, 7.5/325 mg, 10/325 mg. Hydrocodone/Ibuprofen. Vicoprofen—7.5/200 mg.	1 mg hydrocodone = 1 mg oral morphine	
Fentanyl Transdermal	Transdermal patch (not for post op/acute pain; not for use in opiate-naive patients). Duragesic—12.5, 25, 50, 75, 100 µg/hr.	100 µg patch q 2–3 days = 66 mg IV morphine every 24 hr *or* 2.7 mg IV morphine every hour.	
Fentanyl Transmucosal—Buccal	Oral lozenge (not for use in opiate-naive patients). Actiq—200, 400, 600, 800, 1,200, 1,600 µg. Fentora—100, 200, 400, 600, 800 µg. (Fentora is 2× strength of Actiq.)	See package insert for conversion.	
Methadone	Equivalency should be individually considered. Long half-life. Potency, and individual variations in pharmacokinetics.		

- Nausea and vomiting: Most important initial management is to determine and attempt to treat the cause.
  - Pharmacologic therapies: antiemetics—ondansetran; steroids—dexamethasone; anticholinergics and prokinetics.
  - Nonpharmacologic: Offer small meals, portions, aesthetically pleasing environment and presentation of food. (Of the 10 or more recommendations for managing nausea in palliative care, only a few pertain to young children!)
- Oral care after each episode of emesis, comfort care with cleanliness, decrease noxious stimuli, avoid aggravating foods.

Neurologic/Psychological

- Delirium.
  - More common in adolescents and teens.
  - Often, associated with sedatives and analgesics.
  - Nonpharmacologic: psychiatric evaluation and pharmacologic/nonpharmacologic therapies per consultant.
- Anxiety, depression, insomnia, agitation.
  - Apprehension, tension, insecurity, and uneasiness; usually without a known specific cause. Children feel their uncertain future.
  - Some symptoms are related to medications such as stimulants and steroids.
  - Early diagnosis and treatment are key.
  - Pharmacologic therapies: selective serotonin reuptake inhibitors (SSRIs), antidepressants, stimulants, benzodiazepines, and haloperidol.

PEARLS

- *In recent years, more potent agents such as infusion of propofol, ketamine, and dexmedetomidine as well as clonidine delivered enterally or by transdermal patch have been successfully used to treat intractable symptoms at the end of life, but their use must be monitored by experienced clinicians.*
- *Pain and dyspnea are the most commonly occurring conditions at the end of life.*
- *Data collected between 2004 and 2012 indicated that many symptoms are not relieved at the end of life. There is still insufficient evidence surrounding pain and pain management and confusion between life-limiting illnesses and close-to-death symptoms.*
- *Barriers to providing pain and symptom management still exist, which include patient-related fear, misconceptions, failure to report, and lack of reimbursement for therapy.*
- *Barriers to providing pain and symptom management still exist for providers, which include lack of knowledge, skills, time for adequate symptom assessment and interventions.*

Communicating with the Dying Child and Family

Erin K. Mullaney & David M. Steinhorn

Communicating with the Dying Child

- Dying children deserve clear, developmentally appropriate communication regarding their illness and prognosis. Providing clear communication to a child can enhance cooperation, reduce anxiety, and lighten the burden of secrecy among family members.
- Although specific training is essential, the "6 E's" strategy can help guide practitioners through conversations with dying children.
  - Establish: Establish the importance of open communication between parents, children, and caregivers early in the course of illness.
  - Engage: Open a dialogue with the child at the appropriate time, being alert to cues of increased stress.
  - Explore: Assess what the child already knows, and wishes to know about his or her illness (e.g., how much the child wants to know).
  - Explain: Explain the child's medical condition in a developmentally appropriate manner
  - Empathize: Allow the child to be upset and express his or her feelings.
  - Encourage: Reassure the child that his or her health care providers will be available and continue to support him or her through the disease process and that their family will be there for them.
- Allies in facilitating communication with the dying child.
  - Employ the assistance of expressive and creative arts therapists and other providers who may be able to facilitate a child's self-expression of fears in a nonthreatening manner. These include child life, art, music therapists, and social workers.
- Barriers to communication.
  - The provider must be mindful of his or her own emotional reactions.
  - A child's parents may choose to selectively pass along only information that is deemed to be "hopeful" or reinforces their own ideas regarding a child's current clinical condition.
  - The provider must be aware of the myths surrounding communicating with dying children, and provide appropriate anticipatory guidance to concerned families. Examples of such myths include what the child actually understands and envisions for himself.

Communicating with the Siblings of the Dying Child

- Children are individuals and grieve as individuals.
- Consider a child's developmental level when implementing a plan:
  - Infants and very young children (up to 2 years of age):
    - Do not have a true concept of death, but are aware of subtle changes in the mood and structure of the family at large. May develop sleep or feeding problems, changes in behavior, irritability, become clingy or quiet.
  - Young children (2–6 years of age):
    - Operate as "magical thinkers" without logic or ability to reason through situations.
    - Do not see death as permanent, and may believe that past behavior contributed to their sibling's death (thoughts such as "did he or she die because I got mad at him or her?").
    - Manifest grief through changes in behavior, including fear, developmental regression, altered sleep patterns, temper tantrums.
  - School-age children (6–9 years of age):
    - Recognize that death is permanent and believe that death is frightening with preconceived notions. Will ask questions.
    - May develop worries about imaginary personal illnesses; children at this age may also have fears of loss of their parents.
  - Older children and adolescents (9–18 years of age):
    - Have a very concrete view of death; understand that death is final and that everyone will eventually die, including them.
    - Grieving adolescents may exhibit their grief through changes in behavior, sleeping or eating habits, and express feelings of guilt that they are healthy and their sibling has died.
- Prior to the death of a sibling, caregivers should encourage the family to allow their healthy children to visit and be present.
  - When explaining death and the dying process to any child, it is important to use correct language:
    1. Use frank words such as *dying* and *dead*, and be clear about the meaning of these words.
    2. Avoid euphemisms such as:
       a. "_____ passed on" (when are they coming back?)
       b. "We lost _____" (well, go find them)
  - Adult caregivers should be encouraged to answer the sibling's questions openly and honestly, and provide reassurance to address fears.
  - Children, like adults, will continue to experience grief as they grow and develop, and "re-grieve" the death of their brother or sister as they mature and their own life changes, especially with milestones such as birthdays and graduations.
  - Grieving is a natural process and can contribute to growth in the survivors when the death is effectively integrated into their personal life story.

Communicating with the Parents of the Dying Child

- Bereaved parents report that clear, honest communication from care providers is most helpful at points of decision making.

- Avoid phrases such as:
  - "There's nothing more we can do."
  - "We are out of options."
- Discussion of the family's goals of care will guide recommendations of medical management. Comprehensive symptom management and palliation are always an option.
- Anticipatory guidance for parents.
  - Many families find a child's *respiratory pattern* to be the most distressing at the end of life and misinterpret breathing pattern to be uncomfortable.
  - Common changes to a child's respiratory pattern include:
    - Dyspnea and periods of apnea or irregular breathing.
    - "Death rattle" associated with poor handling of oral secretions as death approaches.
  - It is important for families to understand that as the child's death approaches, their level of awareness, and therefore their ability to experience suffering, is diminished.
- One of the most critical roles the practitioner can play is to provide proper anticipatory guidance to the family along with aggressive palliation and rationale for medical interventions.
- Encouragement for the family to provide physical care and contact as they are comfortable and the child can tolerate, such as gentle massage, touching, holding and singing, or talking to the child.
- It may be appropriate to have frank discussions with families about limitations of aggressive life-sustaining therapies and resuscitation status depending on the practitioner's role and relationship to the family.

Palliative and Hospice Care at Home

Erin K. Mullaney & David M. Steinhorn

Definitions

- Palliative care.
  - Palliative care is a focus of care and a medical discipline with the primary goal of reducing the morbidity of illness, slowing the progression of disease, and improving a child's quality of life at any stage of disease.
  - The American Academy of Pediatrics supports an integrated model of palliative care that focuses on both curative attempts and aggressive measures of palliation throughout the child's disease course.
  - The goal of palliative care is to add life to the child's years, not simply years to the child's life (Committee on Bioethics, 2000).
- Hospice care.
  - Hospice care is both a philosophy of care and a method for delivering compassionate, competent, and consistent care to children with chronic, complex, life-threatening illness, with goal of improving quality of life.
  - Hospice is independent of location and can be provided at home, in the hospital, or in any other health care facility.
- Eligibility.
  - Children who have a life expectancy of 6 months to 1 year are generally considered to be eligible for hospice services

and would receive a clear benefit from the inclusion of hospice services in their daily plan of care, but this is a simple guideline and is not always definitive criteria.

- A Do Not Resuscitate (DNR) or Allow Natural Death (AND) order is not required to enroll a child in home hospice care.
- Location of death.
  - Advanced care for medically fragile children or children at the end of life is possible at home, although the vast majority of pediatric deaths continue to occur in the hospital.

Considerations of Therapy at the End of Life

- Decisions regarding provision of therapy as a child nears the end of his or her life should be made in partnership between the parents/guardian and medical care team; may be helpful to approach the conversation by considering the burden versus benefit.
- It may help some families to clarify the distinction between "doing things *for* the child and doing things *to* the child."
- Invasive procedures, such as placement of a chest tube to drain fluid, would potentially alleviate distress, although would cause some discomfort in being inserted. This burden could be considered "doing something for the patient."
- In contrast, a family may choose to discontinue mechanical ventilation in the setting of irreversible disease if the burden of prolonged ventilation is too great without obvious benefit to the child.
- Chemotherapy and radiation therapy can be provided for palliation toward the end of life to alleviate symptoms.
- Alternative and complementary medicine modalities can also be used with success. See the chapter on Complementary and Alternative Medicine.

Advance Directives

Types

- Instructions for medical care (DNR/AND).
  - An order to withhold or limit medical intervention or therapies (DNR/AND; DNR/AND) may be instituted if the child's medical team believes the child's current medical state is irreversible and life-limiting, and with parent agreement.
  - Many parents make this decision when they believe that the child's quality of life is not acceptable, and therapies allow no foreseeable benefit.
  - Therapies that may be withheld or discontinued may include:
    - Cardiopulmonary resuscitation.
    - Intensive care modalities, including mechanical ventilation, dialysis, extracorporeal membrane oxygenation (ECMO), or vasoactive medications.
    - Administration of blood products or antibiotics.
    - Artificial nutrition and/or hydration.

- Documentation of conversations leading to the decision for DNR/AND, in addition to individual hospital-based guidelines, should be addressed.
- If the child is at home, a suitable out-of-hospital DNR/AND form should be completed and provided to the family.
- Designation of medical proxy/surrogate decision maker.
  - An individual who acts as an advocate for a patient who is unable to make decisions on his or her own (due to age or incompetence).
  - By default, parents or a child's legally appointed guardian acts as his or her surrogate decision maker until that child is 18 years of age.
  - Parents and guardians of children older than 18 years who are unable to make their own decisions (due to cognitive delay or medical complications) will continue to be considered a child's surrogate decision maker unless another agent is legally appointed to do so.
- Tools have been developed that can facilitate communications and expression of a child's goals of care (Aging with Dignity, 2012).
  - My Wishes/Five Wishes designed by Aging with Dignity, a nonprofit organization.
    - *My Wishes*: A tool/resource (not legal document) designed for children aged 6 to 13 years to help facilitate conversation and allow children to express how they want to be cared for at the end of their life; available in both English and Spanish.
    - *Five Wishes*: Resource designed for adults, but also appropriate for older adolescents, considered legal document in 42 states and available in 26 languages.
- POLST/MOSLT.
  - Physician Orders for Life-Sustaining Treatment/Medical Orders for Life-Sustaining Treatment.
  - A national model to facilitate end-of-life planning for individuals and provide medical orders for current treatment.
  - National model to facilitate planning which includes considerations for cardiopulmonary resuscitation, medical interventions (and their limits), antibiotic use, artificial nutrition, and hydration.
- Special considerations.
  - Adolescents.
    - More than 3,000 adolescents die each year in the United States and it is generally recognized that most adolescents possess the emotional and cognitive abilities to participate in their own medical decision making.
    - The Committee on Bioethics for the American Academy of Pediatrics (Committee on Bioethics, 1995) wrote:
      - "Decision-making involving the health care of older children and adolescents should include, to the greatest extent feasible, the assent of the patient as well as the participation of the parents and the physician."
    - DNR orders at school (Council on School Health and Committee on Bioethics, 2010), may be considered following discussion between the child's health care team

and school administration, but ultimately dependent on the school's agreement to honor the DNR/AND order while the child attends school.

Withdrawal of Life Support

- The decision to withdrawal of life-sustaining therapies must be initiated in the context of the family's goals of care, and typically with the agreement of the primary medical team.
- As concluded by the Committee on Bioethics for the American Academy of Pediatrics, "there is broad consensus that withholding or withdrawing medical interventions is morally permissible when requested by competent patients or, in the case of patients without decision-making capacity, when the interventions no longer confer a benefit to the patient or when burdens associated with the interventions outweigh the benefits received" (Diekema and Botkin, 2009).
- Withdrawal of hydration and nutrition (WAHN) is a more challenging concept in the withdrawal of medical therapies because of the time it typically takes for death to occur, the emotional response that feeding is a basic element of care, and the limited decision-making capacity of the general population in this regard (Diekema and Botkin, 2009).
- Consultation with the ethics committee should be considered whenever there is lack of consensus among medical providers or between parents in regard to any withdrawal of mechanical, medical, or nutritional support (Rapoport et al., 2013).

Brain Death and Organ Donation
Cheryl N. Bartke & Kimberly L. DiMaria

Background

Brain death, also known as death by neurologic criteria, is a legal manner to declare a patient dead. This definition grew out of the need to define death in a patient who no longer has brain function, but is being kept alive on technological support. The consensus definition of brain death allowed for increased organ donation in the United States. No mandatory reporting exists and the incidence is unknown.

Definition

- Brain death is a clinical diagnosis describing the physiologic state in which a patient's central neurologic function is irreversibly absent.

Etiology

- Brain death can be caused by any injury that decreases the flow of blood to the brain. The most common injuries are traumatic, but any hypoxic injury, including submersion, smoke inhalation, or profound hypotension, can cause the cessation of blood flow to the brain.

Pathophysiology

- Damage from an intracranial hemorrhage or cerebral edema due to cell death leads to an increased mass effect in the brain. As intracranial pressure increases, brain parenchyma, cerebrospinal fluid (CSF), and blood can expand only inside the fixed vault of the skull to a point. The Monro–Kellie hypothesis takes effect as cellular edema increases, and blood and CSF are displaced. Arterial blood supply is further decreased, leading to increased cellular edema and cell death. The cerebellum and brain stem herniate downward through the foramen magnum, leading to ischemia and complete neuronal death.
- With the herniation of the brain stem, many physiologic disturbances can occur, including hemodynamic instability, neurogenic pulmonary edema, hyperglycemia, diabetes insipidus and hypothyroidism. In addition, varied physiologic responses to the initial etiology of injury may occur.

Clinical Presentation

- Varied, as there are many etiologies of the initial injury. Brain death may be immediately apparent or may be delayed depending on the initial injury and the subsequent management. Patients with coma, apparent absence of central neurologic function, and apnea should be considered for evaluation of brain death.

Diagnostic Evaluation

- Guidelines to assist in the diagnosis of brain death in infants and children between 37 weeks' gestation and 18 years of age are published and supported by multiple professional organizations. The patient must be free of confounding factors; specifically, hypothermia, hypotension or resuscitated shock, metabolic and endocrine disturbances, drug or medication toxicities, and neuromuscular blockade.
- If brain death is being considered, two examinations of brain stem function must be performed with an observation period in between. For patients who are 37 weeks to 30 days of age, 24 hours must elapse between examinations. For infants >30 days of age and children, an observation period of 12 hours between examinations is recommended. The examinations should be performed by two different attending physicians and include a full evaluation of brain stem function including an apnea test.
- A brain death examination consists of a full brain stem evaluation of cranial nerves II-XII and apnea testing. The examination is consistent with brain death if no responses are noted. During apnea testing, close evaluation for any spontaneous respiratory effort and pre- and post-$Paco_2$ testing should be observed. A rise in a $Paco_2$ >20 mmHg and absence of respiratory effort are confirmatory of brain death.
- Ancillary studies including electroencephalogram (EEG) and radionuclide cerebral blood flow studies can be used but are not required to diagnose brain death.

Management

- Management of a patient with impending or suspected brain death is three-fold: physiologic support of the patient, emotional support of the family, and evaluation for the consideration of organ donation.
  - Physiologic support of the patient includes any neurologic, respiratory, and hemodynamic management.
  - Emotional support is a must. The concept of brain death is especially confusing and can be accompanied by family preconceptions and cultural beliefs regarding brain death.
  - As soon as brain death is suspected, the organ procurement organization (OPO) should be notified to begin evaluation for potential organ procurement. The OPO often assumes communication with the family and management of the patient's physiologic status.
  - If a family does not agree to organ donation, the patient is declared legally dead and technological support is withdrawn, with timing negotiated with the family.
  - In cases when a patient does not meet brain death criteria, but is expected to die within an hour after withdrawal of technological support, Donation after Cardiac Death (DCD) may be considered. Protocols exist for this procedure, though details vary from institution to institution.

PEARLS

- *Brain death is a clinical diagnosis consisting of two brain death examinations, including apnea testing.*
- *If brain death is suspected, the OPO should always be notified.*
- *DCD can be considered for patients who are not brain dead, but not expected to live long after extubation, although ethical debate continues around this topic.*

Complementary and Alternative Medicine Therapies

Cathy Haut

Overview

The purpose of this chapter is to review and describe nonpharmacologic alternative therapies used in acute care practice that complement or are adjuvant to traditional pain and symptom relief. Very little research exists to document the efficacy of these therapies; however, health care providers' knowledge about these options can support families in their choices in order to optimize pain and symptom management.

- Appropriate pain and symptom management is an essential aspect of care for all pediatric patients.
- Complementary and alternative medicine (CAM) therapies are increasing in popularity and prove effective as adjuvant therapy for pain control and other symptoms in children with chronic illness or cancer. Some therapies can also be used as diversion for painful or uncomfortable procedures.
- All treatment options should be offered, explained, and communicated to the child and family in any situation where illness poses the potential for pain or discomfort.
- Sometimes traditional methods are unable to alleviate pain completely or may not be viable options.
- Health care providers should have some knowledge of commonly used therapies or be able to easily access reliable information on their use.

Background

- CAM therapies consist of therapies and products that are not considered part of conventional medicine.
- The National Center of Complementary and Alternative Medicine (NCCAM) discusses four areas: natural products (e.g., probiotics); mind–body medicine (e.g., acupuncture and guided imagery); manipulative and body-based practices (e.g., massage therapy and other movement and energy therapies).
- Very few research or evidence-based studies exist that document outcomes for children with the use of CAM.
- It is reported that 84% of pediatric oncology patients/ families and children with chronic illnesses have used CAM therapy; however, approximately 50% report its use to their providers.
- CAM therapies are appropriate for inpatient and outpatient management.

Definition

- The NCCAM of the National Institutes of Health (NIH) (2012) defines CAM as a "group of diverse medical and health care systems, practices, and products that are not generally considered part of conventional medicine."
- All aspects of CAM are holistic and center on relationship-based care. Holistic care is patient-centered and encompasses all aspects of health, including biological, psychological, spiritual, social, and environmental.
- By focusing on the whole person, the use of CAM is able to improve pediatric patient outcomes, promote healing, and reduce pain.

Types

- Therapies documented in the literature for children include herbal remedies, probiotics, deep breathing, guided imagery, massage, yoga, chiropractic, music therapy, aroma therapy, meditation, and acupuncture.

Acupuncture

Katie Spillman

Background

- Acupuncture is one of the most frequently used treatments for reducing pain.
- Studies indicate the use of acupuncture as highly accepted, well-tolerated, and an effective adjuvant therapy to control pediatric pain in the hospital setting.
- Appropriate training and licensure is necessary to provide acupuncture services.

Definition

- Acupuncture involves stimulating anatomic points on the body through techniques involving thin needles that are manipulated by hand or electrical stimulation.
- Anatomic points can also be stimulated through the use of laser and magnets, as well as gentle pressure, commonly referred to as acupressure.
- By stimulating specific anatomical points, acupuncture enables natural pain responses and encourages relaxation and pleasant sensation.

Types

- Acupuncture can be accomplished by methods including needle, laser, pressure, and heat.
- Needle acupuncture is the most common type.

Considerations and Use in Children

- Barriers to the use of acupuncture in children include developmental age, family dynamics/beliefs, previous medical experiences, and perception of fear of needles.
- Evidence suggests that patients in the adolescent age group are the most likely to try acupuncture.
- As age increases, ratings of needle pain and fear decrease, especially among children >8 years of age.

Music Therapy

Cathy Haut

Background

- Majority of research on the use of music therapy have been published on children with cancer.
- Music therapy has been found to be beneficial in the management of children with burns, premature infants, and in reducing anxiety from procedures.

Definition

- Clinical and evidence-based use of music interventions to accomplish individualized goals for the entire population, including children.
- Music Therapy is an established health profession with therapists credentialed to provide interventions for patients.

Types

- Interactive music therapy with the use of a music therapist.
- Passive listening and lyrical creativity through patient preferred music.
- Imagery and progressive muscle relaxation as relaxation technique.

Considerations in Children

- Documented to increase coping skills and comfort, reduce anxiety, and promote distraction.
- Has been documented to improve overall well-being of children with cancer.

Massage Therapy

Cathy Haut

Background

- Has been used effectively to reduce pain, tension, and anxiety, but mechanism of action for symptom relief is not well known.

Definition

- Application of pressure and motion to the muscle and connective tissues of the body by a certified massage therapist, with purpose of providing both physiologic and psychological effects.

Types

- Certified therapists determine which types to use based on objective of therapy.

Considerations in Children

- Has been shown to reduce pain in children with cancer.

Mind Body Therapies

- Comprised of guided imagery, biofeedback, hypnosis, meditation, and other relaxation approaches, but typically require skilled therapists to administer.
- Guided imagery is helpful for completing procedures in children.

Herbal Remedies
Cathy Haut

Background/Definition

- Typically come from plants and are used for medicinal purposes.
- May be used to replace traditional medicinal therapies (e.g., due to cost, personal preference, desire for "natural" therapy) or to supplement medicinal therapies.
- Active parts of a plant may include leaves, flowers, stems, roots, seeds, and berries.
- May be ingested as pills, liquid, powders, or brewed in teas.
- Other types of herbs can be in the form of salves, ointments, shampoos, or other skin applications.
- Herbs have been used for the basis of development of some current medications such as digitalis, salicylates, and quinine.
- Most herbal medicines on the market today have not been subjected to rigorous clinical trials.

Consideration for Use in Children

- Comprehensive scientific research is needed to determine the safety and efficacy of herbal remedies for the entire population and most certainly for children.
- Many herbal remedies have significant toxicity for children and have not undergone sufficient testing to be deemed safe.
- May have undesired interactions when taken with medications.
- Children differ from adults in their absorption, distribution, metabolism, and excretion of some substances; therefore, herbal remedies that are considered safe for adults, may not be the same for children (Table 22.4).

Probiotics
Cathy Haut

Background/Definition

- Probiotics include some yogurts and many over-the-counter products designated for children.
- Early evidence indicates that probiotics can be used safely in all age children and assist in preventing antibiotic-related diarrhea and in the early treatment of viral diarrhea.

Consideration for Use in Children

- Evidence from the American Academy of Pediatrics Committee on Nutrition (2010) indicates:
  - Infants and children who ate probiotic foods early while having diarrhea experienced shorter duration of diarrhea.
  - Probiotics were modestly effective in preventing antibiotic-associated diarrhea in healthy children.
  - Some preliminary evidence suggests that probiotics may help prevent necrotizing enterocolitis or death of intestinal tissue in infants born weighing >1,000 g.
  - Prebiotics may help reduce atopic eczema in healthy children.

For Additional Information about CAM

- CAMline: evidence-based website on CAM for health care professionals and the public (http://www.camline.ca/about/about.html).
- NCCAM: The National Center for Complementary and Alternative Medicine is the US federal government's lead agency for scientific research on CAM (http://nccam.nih.gov).

TABLE 22.4 Examples of Toxic Effects of Some Herbs

Herbal Product	Toxic Chemical	Use	Toxic Effects
Cinnamon oil (*Cinnamomum* species)	Cinnamaldehyde	Control blood sugar, pain relief (e.g., joints), heart disease, colon health, blood circulation.	Dermatitis.
Comfrey (*Symphytum officinale*) *Crotalalaria* species	Pyrrolizidines	Upset stomach, ulcer, heavy menstruation, diarrhea, persistent cough, cancer.	Hepatic veno-occlusive disease.
Echinacea	Cichoric acid, caftaric acid	Common cold. Influenza. Other infections.	When taken orally, no reported side effects. Allergic reactions have been reported.
Eucalyptus (*Eucalyptus globulus*)	Pyrrolizidines	Fever, expectorant, upset stomach.	Hepatic veno-occlusive disease.

(Continued)

TABLE 22.4   Examples of Toxic Effects of Some Herbs (Continued)

Herbal Product	Toxic Chemical	Use	Toxic Effects
Garlic (*Allium sativum*)	Allicin	Hypercholesterolemia, hypertension, heart disease, cancer prevention.	Nausea, emesis, anorexia, weight loss, bleeding, platelet dysfunction.
Ginkgo biloba	Ginkgotoxin (4-*O*-methoxypyridoxine)	Memory difficulty. Intermittent claudication. Tinnitus. Sexual dysfunction. Asthma.	Increased bleeding risk. Intensified bleeding risk if taken with an anticoagulant or antiplatelet medication. May result in slowed metabolism of medications metabolized through cytochrome P450 pathway.
Ginseng	Panax ginseng; *Panax quinquefolius*	Improving overall health. Increasing sense of well-being. Blood glucose regulation. Improving stamina. Improving mental and physical performance. Controlling blood pressure.	Rarely associated with adverse events or drug interactions in short term. May be associated with headaches, insomnia, and diarrhea. May lower blood glucose levels (Use with caution in patients with diabetes). Long-term use associated with mastalgia. Not recommended for use with caffeine due to stimulant effects.
Laetrile	Cyanide	Cancer treatment.	Coma, seizures, death, respiratory failure.
Ma Huang (*Ephedra sinica*)	Ephedrine	Central nervous system stimulation, bronchodilation, weight loss.	Hypertension, dysrhythmias, stroke, seizures.
Monkshood (*Aconitum* species)	Aconite	General debilitation; numbs sensations of temperature, pain, and touch.	Cardiac arrhythmias, shock, weakness, seizures, coma, paresthesias, nausea.
St. John's wort	Hyperforin, hypericin	Depression. Anxiety. Sleep disturbances.	Interacts with many medications, especially antidepressants (e.g., serotonin syndrome), oral contraceptives, cyclosporine, digoxin, warfarin, phenytoin, phenobarbital.
Wormwood (*Artemisia absinthium*)	Thujone	Digestive problems, fever, liver disease, worm infections, sexual dysfunction.	Seizures, tremors, headache, Ataxia.

*Woolf, A.D. (2003) is the reference for the composition of this table.

1. An infant at how many weeks of gestation can be considered for evaluation of brain death by the current guidelines?
   a. 30.
   b. 33.
   c. 37.
   d. 40.

Answer: **C**

There are insufficient data for the recommendations of brain death in preterm infants <37 weeks' gestation in the literature. The most current guidelines for the determination of brain death in infants and children "An update of the 1987 Taskforce Recommendations (2011)" does not include infants <37 weeks for this reason.

2. How many hours must pass between brain death examinations in a 3-year-old child who sustained multiple trauma including a severe head injury?
   a. 6.
   b. 12.
   c. 24.
   d. 48.

Answer: **B**

An observation period of 24 hours for term newborns >37 weeks' gestation to 30 days of age is recommended between brain death examinations. An observation time of 12 hours is recommended from 30 days to 18 years of age.

3. When completing a brain death evaluation on a child, each examination must include:
   a. Brain stem reflex examination, an apnea test.
   b. A cognitive brain testing, an EEG.
   c. A brain stem reflex, examination, an EEG.
   d. A cognitive brain testing, an apnea test.

Answer: **A**

A brain death examination includes a clinical examination of the patient's brain stem reflexes and an apnea test. Ancillary testing such as an EEG is not required unless the patient is in a condition as to not be able to have the standard testing performed or if there is conflicting information on the two separate examinations. A patient with any cognitive function should never be considered for brain death.

4. Which of the following best depicts the developmentally appropriate description for a young child's (2–6 years of age) concept of death?
   a. Does not have a true concept of death, but is aware of subtle changes in the mood and structure of the family at large.
   b. Understands that death is permanent, and may be frightened by the concept of death.
   c. Operates as a "magical thinker" and may believe that past behavior contributed to the death.
   d. With appropriate discussion, can conceptualize the permanence of death of a loved one.

Answer: **C**

Young children operate according to Erikson with magical thinking and can either contribute their behavior or other rationales to the death of a loved one. This age child also cannot understand the permanence of death and may look for their loved one to reappear at any point in time.

5. Which statement best describes pediatric hospice?
   a. A patient must have a DNR/AND order to be enrolled in home hospice care.
   b. Children may be enrolled in hospice care only if their life expectancy is considered to be less than 6 months.
   c. Hospice care may be provided at home to children who receive intensive medical therapies (e.g., home ventilators, noninvasive positive-pressure ventilation), which may be contributing to the increase in pediatric deaths that occur in the home.
   d. As a *philosophy* of care, hospice is not dependent on location and does occur in the home or hospital environment.

Answer: **D**

Hospice is a philosophy of care where children can be cared for independent of location, but provided with both palliation services such as pain and symptom management, and also intensive medical therapy such as ventilation and intravenous fluids.

6. Which of the following interventions are considered truly palliative measures to ameliorate distressing symptoms and enhance a child's comfort and quality of life?
   a. Surgical resection of tumor and aggressive chemotherapy.
   b. Placement of a semipermanent intravenous catheter to provide ongoing nutritional therapy and inotropic support of blood pressure.
   c. Placement of a chest tube to treat malignant pleural effusions.
   d. Continuous renal replacement therapy when a dying child is in renal failure.

Answer: **C**

A child with malignant pleural effusions may continue to have fluid accumulation in the chest, contributing to dyspnea, hypoxia, and fatigue. Placement of a chest tube for drainage is considered palliation to relief discomfort.

(continues on page 512)

7. When is it acceptable to withdraw or withhold medical interventions?
   a. When a parent requests the medical team to do so.
   b. When the interventions are believed to cause useless distress, and are not expected to benefit a child at the end of his or her life.
   c. Based on the decision of the attending physician when no further aggressive therapy is warranted.
   d. Based on the hospital ethics committee decision, when family members are not in agreement with medical decisions.

Answer: **B**

It is important to include all members of the care team and the family in decisions regarding end-of-life care and support of a child. Ideally, all members of the team will come to the same conclusion regarding therapy, but when there is conflict, it is best to continue discussions until a reasonable decision can be made.

8. What is the importance of the WHO pain ladder?
   a. Provides stepwise guidelines for which medications can be administered.
   b. Provides description of medications with dosing for children.
   c. Offers suggestions regarding which medications are safest for children.
   d. Advocates the use of adjuvant pain therapies.

Answer: **A**

The WHO pain ladder was created to provide a stepwise approach to pain management by offering classes of medications to use based on severity or rating of pain.

9. A major, true challenge in providing pain management for a young child with metastatic cancer is:
   a. Parents' unwillingness to consent to pain medications for the child.
   b. Child's inability to communicate his pain and severity of pain.
   c. Hospital pharmacy that lacks liquid narcotic medications.
   d. Keeping the child alert for physical examination and evaluation.

Answer: **B**

One of the major challenges in providing pain management in palliative care is the child's ability to communicate his pain and the severity of pain. Younger children are at even more of a disadvantage because they may not have real perceptions of pain as their prior experience of pain is limited. It is imperative to anticipate pain, evaluate vital signs as one mechanism of assessment, and administer pain medications appropriately.

10. A 15-year-old with metastatic osteosarcoma is receiving morphine, Neurontin, and lorazepam for pain and anxiety control. He is on 30 mg of oral morphine twice a day and his pain is not under control. He describes his pain as a "continuous, sharp" pain that is causing him difficulty breathing and significant insomnia. The most appropriate action is to:
    a. Increase his morphine dosing by 10% to 15%.
    b. Increase the dose of Neurontin by 5%.
    c. Add another narcotic medication (e.g., dilaudid).
    d. Discuss other methods of pain control as the morphine is already too high of a dose.

Answer: **A**

Best approaches to pain management in children receiving palliative care include increasing narcotic doses in steps of 10% to 15% until pain is controlled. Neurontin is used for neuropathic pain and may not affect the type of pain described in this scenario. There are no upper limits for pain medication administration in palliative care, so if the morphine has been effective, there is no initial reason to add another similar drug.

11. Parents of an infant with anencephaly are interested in assigning an AND order for their child if her heart stops and cannot be resuscitated. The best response is:
    a. The AND order requires that all aspects of cardiopulmonary resuscitation be held and the child will die when she stops breathing or her heart stops.
    b. AND indicates that the family is ready to take the infant home, stop feeding, and allow the infant to die in peace.
    c. AND allows parents to determine which resuscitative measures can be performed, but will be limited to specific interventions.
    d. DNR is a better choice because it prohibits any resuscitation efforts.

Answer: **C**

AND offers another, kinder mode of creating an opportunity for peaceful death, but parents can specify which interventions they want to be performed for their child. AND allows parents to choose chest compressions and oxygen but not inotropic medications and intubation if this is their desire for their child.

12. Appropriate management of a child receiving palliative care who has nausea and vomiting and is unable to keep any foods or fluids in his stomach includes the use of ondansetron (Zofran) and:
    a. Ketamine, ranitidine, and/or fluoxetine.
    b. Lorazepam, haloperidol, and/or dexamethasone.
    c. Dexamethasone, ketamine, and/or haloperidol.
    d. Ranitidine, lorazepam, and/or fluoxetine.

Answer: **B**

Antiemetics, prokinetics, corticosteroids, and anticholinergic agents work well in the management of nausea and vomiting whether a child is receiving chemotherapy or in the process of active dying. Trying medications one at a time or using them together can both work to alleviate symptoms.

13. A 15-year-old boy has a relapse of acute myelogenic leukemia which was initially diagnosed when he was 10 years old.

He initially received chemotherapy and has been treated with preventive therapies and screening for the past 2 years. The best way to communicate this information to him is:

a. Ask his parents to talk with him about the diagnosis.

b. Keep the information secret while continuing therapy, explaining that the new chemotherapy is indicated for prevention.

c. Discuss the recurrence of cancer in an open, honest manner with parents involved.

d. Discuss the recurrence of cancer with the parents and let them decide how to tell their son.

Answer: **C**

Open, honest communication is imperative when discussing tragic or devastating news with children and their families. It is important to allow the family to listen to the information and have time to ask questions and gain support for their decision making. The developmental level of an adolescent allows them to be able to make some decisions, especially when it comes to treatment options. Families should be provided with open and honest communication in regard to any aspect of their child's illness.

14. A 10-year-old is complaining of numbness, tingling, and a "prickly" sensation in his leg where he recently had surgery for an osteosarcoma. This type of discomfort is known as:

a. Paresthesia.

b. Nociceptive pain.

c. Allodynia.

d. Neuropathic pain.

Answer: **A**

A paresthesia is described as abnormal painful numbness, which can include prickling, tingling, and increased sensitivity in any part of the body. Paresthesias can be transient or chronic and may not be associated with any specific long-term effect.

15. A hospitalized child is extremely upset, crying in pain which has not responded to acetaminophen or 2 mg of IV morphine. The best method to get his pain under control is to:

a. Order an additional 2 mg of morphine IV and monitor its effect.

b. Administer an oral dose of lorazepam.

c. Consider an adjuvant therapy such as hypnosis.

d. Administer small, frequent doses of IV morphine until pain is controlled.

Answer: **D**

The best way to manage pain in a child who is receiving IV medications is to continue to administer small doses of the medication at frequent intervals using the IV route and then when the pain is controlled, consider increasing the intermittent dosing or switching to oral route.

16. The family of a 12-year-old with metastatic osteosarcoma would like to offer their son acupuncture for pain therapy. What consideration would be most important?

a. Perception or fear of needles by the adolescent.

b. Cannot be used legally for children <16 years of age.

c. Would replace the need for narcotic pain control.

d. Laser therapy is the most common type of acupuncture.

Answer: **A**

Considerations for the use of acupuncture in children include the issue of perception of pain or fear of needles since this therapy uses stimulation of pressure points with small-gauge needles. There are no legal age barriers for acupuncture, and it should be used as an adjunct to traditional pain therapy.

17. The parent of a 3-year-old is concerned about giving her child another round of antibiotics for a persistent otitis media. The child will not eat yogurt, and she is concerned about the possibility of diarrhea with the antibiotic. What recommendation can be offered?

a. It is unlikely that this age child will develop diarrhea from antibiotics.

b. There are several over-the-counter probiotics available, but they are not safe for children <5 years of age.

c. Probiotics are available over the counter in several different forms and are safe for children.

d. There are some herbal remedies available in health food stores that can assist in preventing antibiotic-associated diarrhea.

Answer: **C**

The American Academy of Pediatrics has issued information on the use of probiotics in children and has found evidence that over-the-counter products and yogurt are effective in the prevention of antibiotic-related diarrhea, necrotizing enterocolitis in neonates, and in the treatment of viral diarrhea in children.

18. The most important message to parents about the use of herbal remedies for their children includes:

a. Pay close attention to the labels to check information about use in children.

b. Most herbal remedies have not been tested for safety in children.

c. If the product has been used safely in adults, it is acceptable to use in older children.

d. The majority of herbal products have significant toxicity in children.

Answer: **B**

Health care providers should encourage conversations with parents about the use of complementary and alternative therapies for children, especially in regard to nutritional supplements and herbal remedies. Children differ from adults in their absorption, distribution, metabolism, and excretion of some substances; therefore, herbal remedies that are considered safe for adults may not be the same for children.

Recommended Readings

Aging with Dignity. (2012). *Five wishes and my wishes*. Retrieved from http://www.agingwithdignity.org/

Adams, D., Dagenais, S., Clifford, T., Baydala, T., King, W. J., Hervas-Malo, M., . . . Vohra, S. (2013). Complementary and alternative medicine use by pediatric specialty outpatients. *Pediatrics, 131*(2), 225–232.

American Music Therapy Association. (2013). *About music therapy & AMTA*. Retrieved from http://www.musictherapy.org/

Byrne, M., Tresgallo, M., Saroyan, J., Granowetter, L., Valoy G., & Schechter, W. (2012). Qualitative analysis of consults by a pediatric advanced care team during its first year of service. *American Journal of Hospice & Palliative Care, 29*, 109–117.

Committee on Bioethics. (1995). Informed consent, parental permission, and consent in pediatric practice. *Pediatrics, 95*(2), 314–317.

Council on School Health and Committee on Bioethics. (2010). Policy update: Honoring do-not-attempt-resuscitation orders in schools. *Pediatrics, 125*(5), 1073–1077.

Department of Health and Human Services. (2012). *National guidance for healthcare system preparedness*. Retrieved from http://www.phe.gov/preparedness/planning/hpp/reports/documents/capabilities.pdf

Diekema, D. S., & Botkin, J. R. (2009). Forgoing medically provided nutrition and hydration in children. *Pediatrics, 124*(2), 813–822.

Friebert, S. (2009). *NHPCO facts and figures: Pediatric palliative care and hospice in America*. Retrieved http://www.nhpco.org/sites/default/files/public/quality/Pediatric_Facts-Figures.pdf

Friedrichsdorf, S. (2010). Pain management in children with advanced cancer and during end-of-life care. *Journal of Pediatric Hematology/Oncology, 27*(4), 257–261.

Heath, J. A., Oh, L. J., Clarke, N. E., & Wolfe, J. (2012). Complementary and alternative medicine use in children with cancer at the end of life. *Journal of Palliative Medicine, 15*(11), 1218–1221.

Heinze, K. E., & Nolan, M. T. (2012). Parental decision making for children with cancer at the end of life: a meta-ethnography. *Journal of Pediatric Oncology Nursing, 29*(6), 337–345.

Klick, J. C., & Hauer, J. (2010). Pediatric palliative care. *Current Problems in Pediatric Adolescent Health Care, 40*(6), 120–151.

Moody, K., Siegel, L., Scharbach, K., Cunningham, L., & Cantor, R. M. (2011). Pediatric palliative care. *Primary Care, 38*(2):327–361.

Nakagawa, T. A., Ashwal, S., Mathur, M., Mysore, M., the Society of Critical Care Medicine, Section on Critical Care, Section on Neurology of the American Academy of Pediatrics, & the Child Neurology Society. (2011). Guidelines for the determination of brain death in infants and children: An update of the 1987 Task Force Recommendations. *Critical Care Medicine, 39*(9), 2139–2155.

National Cancer Institute. (n. d.). *Children and Loss*. Retrieved from http://www.cancer.gov/cancertopics/pdq/supportivecare/bereavement/Patient/page6

National Center for Complementary and Alternative Medicine (NCCAM). (2012). *What is complementary and alternative medicine?* Retrieved from http://nccam.nih.gov/health/whatiscam

Rapoport, A., Shaheed, J., Newman, C., Rugg, M., & Steele, R. (2013). Parental perceptions of forgoing artificial nutrition and hydration during end-of-life care. *Pediatrics, 131*(5), 861–869.

von Lützau, P., Otto, M., Hechler, T., Metzing, S., Wolfe, J., & Zernikow, B. (2012). Children dying from cancer: parents' perspectives on symptoms, quality of life, characteristics of death, and end-of-life decisions. *Journal of Palliative Medicine, 28*(4), 274–281.

Shaw, M. D. (2012). Pediatric palliative pain and symptom management. *Pediatric Annals, 14*(8), 329–334.

Thomas, D. W., & Greer, F. R., American Academy of Pediatrics Committee on Nutrition, Section on Gastroenterology, Hepatology, and Nutrition. (2010). Clinical report: Probiotics and prebiotics in pediatrics. *Pediatrics, 126*(6), 1217–1231.

Woolf, A. D. (2003). Herbal remedies and children: Do they work? Are they harmful? *Pediatrics, S*112, 240–246.

World Health Organization. (2012). *WHO guidelines on the pharmacological treatment of persisting pain in children with medical illnesses*. Geneva, Switzerland: WHO.

Wu, S., Sapru, A., Stewart, M. A., Milet, M. J., Hudes, M., Livermore, L., & Flori, H. (2009). Using acupuncture for acute pain in hospitalized children. *Pediatric Critical Care Medicine, 10*(3), 291–296.

Disaster Management

Disaster Management

Mary Schucker & Christopher Sonne

Background

- Four phases of emergency management: mitigation, preparedness, response, and recovery.
- Emergencies can be classified as "routine" or "crisis."
  - All emergencies begin at the local level, with local and community resources.
- Mass casualty incidents occur when the volume of patients and/or their acuity exceeds the available resources of the health care facility, and include:
  - Natural or man-made:
    - Natural: flooding, tornadoes, earthquakes, hurricanes, wildfires.
    - Man-made: accidental or intentional.
      - Terrorist: least predictable, intent is to cause panic, public disorder, anxiety.
      - Explosive devices.
- Pediatric vulnerabilities: Children have many anatomic and physiologic vulnerabilities, and those with special health needs become even more vulnerable.
  - There is a lack of pediatric resources during a disaster within many cities/communities.
- Surge planning and structural support.
  - Medical surge is predicated on the quantity of patients, the acuity level, and resources needed to deliver the required level of care. Medical surge planning addresses how local/community resources will be shared and prioritized, then state and federal assistance.
  - For larger regional and national events, delivery of care should focus on the population (as a whole) rather than individual outcomes when allocating resources.
  - In the event of scarce medical resources (e.g., pharmaceuticals, ventilators, critical care beds), efforts should be prioritized to those individuals with the highest chances of a successful clinical outcome.

- Decontamination.
  - Required due to an exposure or contamination by a hazardous material.
  - The Occupational Health and Safety Administration defines a hazardous material as any substance that is potentially toxic to the environment or to living cells, including microorganisms, plants, animals, and humans.
    - Includes biological or disease-causing agents that may reasonably be anticipated to cause death, disease, or other health problems.
  - Patients need to be decontaminated prior to therapeutic treatment.
  - Removing the clothing of a victim (mechanical decontamination) can reduce up to 80% of the contaminant, and should be the initial direction to victims.
  - Liquid contamination poses the greatest need for a thorough decontamination using copious amounts of soap and water (when indicated).
- Purpose of decontamination.
  - Decreases the effects and symptoms of the hazardous material, reduces the risk of secondary contamination, and prevents contamination of health care facility.
    - Four routes of exposure: inhalation, ingestion, absorption, injection.
    - Four types of toxic effects: irritant, corrosive, or oxidizing; pharmacologic; allergenic; mutagenic or carcinogenic.
- Age-based decontamination guidelines.
  - Avoid separation from families, assist caregivers, recognize developmental needs, keep warm, and protect the airways.
  - Categories of disaster.
    - Biological disasters (based on CDC [Centers for Disease Control and Prevention]): the use of viruses, bacteria, or other naturally occurring substances with intent to harm or kill people, animals, or plants.
    - Category A: highest risk to general population, are easily spread, have major health impact.
    - Category B: not as easily spread, moderate illness, and panic.
    - Category C: emerging pathogens, readily available, have potential for major health impacts (Table 23.1).

TABLE 23.1 Specific Biologicals

Name	Etiology	Forms/Types	Pathophysiology/ Symptoms	Diagnoses	Management
Anthrax	Aerobic, gram-positive rod: *Bacillus anthracis.* Spore-forming capability.	• Cutaneous: painless ulcer. • Gastrointestinal: acute gastritis or ulcers. • Inhalation.	• Spores enter macrophages which then travel to regional lymph nodes, break open, release bacteria, replicate, and result in bacteremia and sepsis with high rates of mortality.	• Clinical presentation. • Chest radiograph: widened mediastinum or large pleural effusion. • Positive blood cultures.	• Ciprofloxacin or doxycycline for 60 d.
Botulism	Spore-forming bacteria found in soil, intentionally contaminated water or food, or aerosolization; toxins are most poisonous substance known to man. Human contact with spores contaminated with *Clostridium botulinum.*	Gram-negative bacilli: *Clostridium botulinum.* Three types: infantile/intestinal (70% of reported cases), food borne, and wound (rare).	Toxin affects presynaptic membranes, preventing acetylcholine release into the synaptic cleft, resulting in absence of depolarization of the postsynaptic membrane, and ultimately flaccid paralysis.	• Clinical diagnosis, initially. Confirmatory tests sent to CDC or US Public Health laboratories.	• Supportive care (ventilation if indicated). • *Infant and young child management found in Section 6: Neurologic.* • Antibiotics should not be administered; bacterial lysis may result in toxin release.
Smallpox	Smallpox has been used as a biological weapon for centuries. Mortality rate 30%. Hemorrhagic or flat forms: mortality 95%. Encephalopathy is main complication.	DNA virus, Poxvirus variolae, a member of the orthopoxvirus family. Spread from person to person by aerosols and direct contact; caused by one of two viruses: variola major or variola minor. Entering nose or oropharynx.	Symptoms: viremia, fever, toxemia, and rash. May be accompanied by malaise, myalgias, and gastrointestinal complaints. Maculopapular lesions are predominant on the face (including oropharynx) and upper extremities, then spread to trunk and lower extremities in fewer numbers. Become vesicular and pustular over several days.	Fluid collection from unroofed lesions or eschar. Diagnosis with electron microscopy, viral culture, and staining. Specimen collection limited to those who have received vaccination.	• Report to local and state health departments immediately. • Respiratory isolation. • Supportive care. • Protection of health care workers including laboratory personnel. • No available antiviral agent. • Cidofovir may be considered for postexposure prophylaxis.

TABLE 23.1 **Specific Biologicals** (*Continued*)

Name	Etiology	Forms/Types	Pathophysiology/Symptoms	Diagnoses	Management
Tularemia	Gram-negative coccobacillus: *Francisella tularensis*. Presents as a systemic illness without a focal lesion. Typically results in fever, headache, chills, nausea, vomiting, diarrhea. When associated with pneumonia, cough, pharyngitis, bronchiolitis, pneumonitis, or pneumonitis may be present.	Clinical presentation depends on method of exposure. Seven types of clinical syndromes: pneumonic, typhoidal, ulceroglandular, glandular, oculoglandular, oropharyngeal, and septicemic.	Infection occurs when skin or mucous membranes come in contact with carcass or body fluids of an infected animal, through aerosolization or through contaminated food or water; also occurs through bite from infected tick or deer fly. Bacteria enter through skin, gastrointestinal tract, mucous membranes, or lungs and spread to local lymph nodes and multiply in macrophages, disseminating through the body.	Diagnosis is made through sputum culture, nasal pharyngeal swabbing, or secretions/exudates. Antibodies are not reliable until approximately 2 wk after the onset of infection. Signs of atypical pneumonia with pleural effusion or enlarged hilar lymph nodes may be noted on chest radiograph.	• Streptomycin (medication of choice), gentamicin; alternatively, amikacin for 10 d. • Notification of local or state health departments. • Postexposure prophylaxis with doxycycline or ciprofloxacin for 14 d. Only for those with possible direct exposure to *F. tularensis*; not required for household contacts of infected patients.
Viral Hemorrhagic Fever	A group of RNA viruses (Filoviridae, Arenaviridae, Bunyaviridae, and Flaviviridae) that results in fever and bleeding diathesis. This diverse group of viruses is highly contagious and is associated with high mortality rates.	Largely unknown. All affect the vasculoendothelial system, though mechanism is unclear.	Abrupt fever, malaise, facial flushing, conjunctivitis, myalgia, petechiae, mucosal bleeding, vomiting, diarrhea, hemorrhage. Spread by aerosols, tick bite, rodent feces, and secretions of infected animals. Human-to-human spread for select diseases; have resulted in hospital outbreaks.	Laboratory studies demonstrate thrombocytopenia and coagulation dysfunction.	• Supportive care. • Respiratory isolation. • Intubation and mechanical ventilation may be required in some cases. • Fluid resuscitation, blood products, vasopressor agents, and invasive monitoring are commonly required. • Monitor family members/close contacts for fever. Yellow fever vaccine is the only viral hemorrhagic fever (VHF)-approved vaccine.

Etiology/Types

Blast Injuries

- The majority of terrorist attacks involve explosive devices as they are easy to obtain, produce large amounts of damage, cause fear, and commonly are set up with dual explosions.
  - After initial blast, rescue workers are harmed by secondary (explosive) devices.
- Many experts believe that conventional explosives maybe used as dispersal devices to spread nuclear, chemical, or biological weapons; also called "dirty bombs."
- Many factors affect number of casualties; higher when in confined space.
- General principles of explosives:
  - An explosion is a rapid chemical conversion of solid or liquid into a gas with an energy release.

- Low-order explosives (e.g., propellants): slow release of energy; objects "go up in flames." Examples include gun powder and Molotov cocktails.
- High-order explosives: "detonation" energy released in the form of pressure, changing the physical space.
- Biological and clinical effects.
  - Four types of injuries: primary, secondary, tertiary, quaternary.
    Primary: caused by pressure of waves.
    - Tympanic membrane rupture: most sensitive body part to blast injury.
    - Pulmonary: increased incidence when burn injuries are present. Results in alveolar damage (e.g., air leak syndromes), blood vessel disruption (e.g., pulmonary contusion, hemothorax), and inflammation (e.g., acute respiratory distress syndrome).
    - Cardiac: air embolism—suspect if ST segment and/or T-wave abnormalities on ECG.
    - Colon: most common location of gastrointestinal injury. Ischemia or stretch injury may result in perforation.
    - Central nervous system: punctate hemorrhages, post-traumatic stress disorder.
    Secondary injury.
    - Injury from flying debris, blunt or penetrating.
    - Secondary injury is the leading cause of death.
    Tertiary injury.
    - Sustained when victims thrown.
    - Victims of tertiary injury tend to be of lighter weight; children are more susceptible; head injury risk in children due to relative weight of head.
    Quaternary injury.
    - Crush, burns, and toxic exposure.
- Blast injury management.
  - Obtain as much information as possible prior to arrival of victim(s).
  - Initial resuscitation, as indicated.
  - Be aware of any possible toxic exposures and decontaminate accordingly.
  - Endotracheal intubation and positive pressure ventilation can be problematic for weakened lung tissue. May exacerbate air leak syndromes, hemorrhage, or air embolus. Use lowest amount of pressure to effectively ventilate the patient.
  - Crush injuries: rapid reperfusion can lead to "crush syndrome." Early fluid resuscitation and alkalinization may improve outcomes.
  - Impaled objects: removed with supervision of surgical team.
  - Serial physical examinations after life-threatening injuries managed.
  - Ruptured tympanic membranes will heal spontaneously.
- Psychosocial implications.
  - Children at risk lack physical and cognitive skills to avoid situation and are unsure where or how to get to safety; may hide.

Chemical Disasters

- Biotoxins, nerve agents, and vesicants are the by-products of extracts of naturally occurring plants or bacteria.
- Include, but not limited to, strychnine, digitalis, brevetoxin, colchicine, nicotine, ricin, tetrodotoxin (puffer fish).
  - Strychnine: from seeds of plant *Strychnos nux-vomica* and absorbed through various routes (e.g., respiratory, gastrointestinal, and intact skin). Results in excessive motor neuron activity from inhibition of postsynaptic inhibition in brain and spinal cord; causes seizure activity. Primarily used in rodenticide. Some exposure through adulterated street drugs. Colorless, odorless, and bitter tasting.
    - Presentation: hyperreflexia, heightened sensorium, muscle twitching, seizures. Also associated with hyperthermia, metabolic acidosis, rhabdomyolysis, and myoglobinuria. *Hallmark is alert sensorium during the seizure.*
    - Diagnosis: detection in urine and blood. Levels do not correlate well with severity of presentation.
    - Management: airway management and seizure control. Use of benzodiazepines and neuromuscular blocking agents as needed. Seizure control will reduce sequelae.
  - Ricin: Poison released when castor bean seeds are crushed; enters body through ingestion, inhalation, or injection. Inhibits protein synthesis and ribosome activity, resulting in cell death. The powder (white) can dissolve in water or be released in the air.
    - Presentation: nonspecific symptoms such as abdominal pain, diarrhea initially, followed by hypovolemia, hypotension and multiple organ dysfunction syndrome (MODS) which can result in death. Early in illness, symptoms may mimic those of typhoid, cholera, *Campylobacter* and *Shigella* infections.
    - Diagnosis: Clinical diagnosis—no commercially available test in the United States.
    - Management: supportive care—aggressive fluid resuscitation. Activated charcoal and cathartic agents are indicated to increase excretion of ricin. Intubation and mechanical ventilation are frequently required.
  - Nerve agents: sarin, tabun, soman, VX. Subtle differences in chemical structure, though all function as acetylcholinesterase (AChE).
    - AChE inhibitors: All are considered weapons of mass destruction.
    - Pathophysiology: overstimulation of nicotinic and muscarinic receptors. Nerve agents permanently bind to AChE.
    - Clinical presentation: cholinergic toxicity (e.g., diaphoresis, diarrhea, urination, miosis, bradycardia, bronchorrhea, bronchospasm, emesis, lacrimation, and salivation), nicotinic toxicity (e.g., mydriasis, fasciculations, muscle cramps, pallor, flaccid paralysis, hypertension,

tachycardia). Respiratory symptoms are most serious. Combination of bronchospasm and bronchorrhea and muscle fatigue leads to respiratory failure.

- Diagnosis: no available method to measure concentration of nerve gas in serum or urine.
- Management: Extensive decontamination is the first step and the most important step after exposure for both the patient and the health care team. Evaluation and management of ABCs. Atropine will improve bronchorrhea and bronchospasm. Pralidoxime may be useful by regenerating AChE. Diazepam to manage seizures. No vaccine available. Notify local and state health departments.
- Vesicants.
  - Types/Categories: sulfur mustard (yellow oily, smells like garlic, mustard, or horseradish), lewisite (colorless oily liquid, smells like geraniums), and phosgene oxime (disagreeable odor and irritating vapor).
  - Pathophysiology: exact mechanism unknown; shuts down ATP synthesis, which leads to cell death. Results in separation of dermis and epidermis layers. Sulfur mustard is very lipophilic and penetrates skin more deeply than other vesicants; can have systemic effects.
  - Presentation: depends on route of exposure. Eyes (e.g., conjunctivitis, eyelid edema, sloughing of corneal epithelium), respiratory tract (e.g., hoarseness, lacrimation, sneezing, rhinorrhea, coughing, pulmonary edema), and skin are most commonly affected (e.g., irritation, vesicles, blebs, shearing with minimal trauma, sloughing). Vesicants also can cause hematologic alterations including leukopenia and pancytopenia. Rarely lethal, though may lead to permanent disfigurement from skin damage.
  - Diagnosis: clinical history and presentation.
  - Management: removing of clothing, early decontamination (talc/flour, followed by copious rinsing with water), and supportive burn care. Some lesions may require debridement. Administration of humidified air may help with hoarseness. Early tracheotomy for upper persistent stridor/hoarseness. Eye exposure demands prompt irrigation. Leukopenia requires antibiotics; consider granulocyte colony-stimulating factor. May require transfer to burn center for burn care.
- Choking agents.
  - A broad category of chemicals that cause respiratory symptoms.
  - Chlorine gas: yellow-green gas that has a pungent odor. Widely used and transported across United States; much of US population vulnerable to exposure.
  - Presentation: lacrimation, irritation of oral and nasal mucosa, rhinorrhea, bronchorrhea, exertional dyspnea, and laryngospasm. May be accompanied by burning sensation in nose or throat, chest pain, and choking. Large exposures may result in pulmonary edema and respiratory failure.
  - Diagnosis: determined from history and presentation.
  - Postexposure: Prompt removal of clothing and contact lenses and decontamination with soap and water. Supportive care, strict bed rest to minimize exertional

dyspnea. If mechanical ventilation is required, anticipate high levels of positive end-expiratory pressure due to pulmonary edema. Antibiotics are not needed in the acute phase of the illness; however, should be considered if there is a development of a secondary pneumonia. Consultation with state and local health departments if suspected chemical warfare threat. Prognosis is good with supportive care.

Radiation Injuries

- Weapons of mass destruction and nuclear power plant meltdowns have potential to cause massive destruction.
- Future incidents: National security experts believe that future incidents may involve radiological dispersion device—area smaller than nuclear power plant or nuclear weapon; however, considerable fear and panic.
- Two types of ionizing radiation.
  - Electromagnetic:
    - Gamma rays: high energy and short wavelength; high penetration.
    - X-rays: lower energy, longer wavelength; less penetrating.
  - Particulate: alpha, beta, and neutron.
    - Alpha particles: larger and cannot penetrate skin or clothes (but harmful if ingested).
    - Beta particles: high energy, emitted from nucleus, highly penetrating.
    - Neutrons: highly penetrating and emitted only during nuclear detonation.
- Radiation cannot be detected by the senses.
- Radiation hazard is related to exposure and absorption.
- Four factors in determining radiation exposure: time, distance, dose, and shielding.
- Effects of radiation: chromosomal breakage; free radical formation leads to generalized inflammatory response; cellular-level changes can take seconds to years to appear.
- Acute radiation syndrome: a broad term describing a range of signs and symptoms that reflect severe organ damage to specific organ systems; can lead to death within hours or months after exposure.
  - Cell death from direct ionizing radiation or impairment of cell death.
  - Organ systems with most rapidly dividing cell lines (e.g., hematopoietic and gastrointestinal systems) are most affected.
- Pediatric patients (especially fetuses and infants) are the most vulnerable.
  - Immediate clinical management:
    - Preparation: Divide emergency department into "dirty" and "clean."
    - All health care providers should wear personal protective equipment and have dosimeter to measure levels of radiation exposure.
    - Consult with Radiation Emergency Assistance Center/Training Site (REAC/TS).
    - Hospital radiation safety officer or radiation oncologist should take the lead role.
    - Radiation poisoning is not *immediately* life-threatening.

- Proper equipment increases safety for health care professionals treating victims of exposure.
- Treatment.
  - Acute radiation syndrome is supportive.
  - ABCs.
  - Local skin contamination: Remove clothing (double-bagged in polyethylene bags), copious rinsing with soap and water. Avoid vigorous scrubbing of skin (to prevent disruption of skin integrity) and shampoo hair.
  - Internal contamination: chelation (first dose may be given through nebulization), enhanced gastrointestinal elimination, and enhanced renal elimination.
  - Does not require decontamination prior to life-saving treatment.

- Pediatric physiological considerations.
  - Children are at higher risk for contamination than adults for several reasons.
    - Closer to the ground and can more easily inhale settled radiotoxins.
    - Higher minute ventilation, inhaling more radiotoxins quickly.
    - Thin and delicate skin with greater surface area.
    - Smaller intravascular volume causing increased concentration of circulating radiotoxins.
- Long-term medical effects.
  - Pediatric patients remain more susceptible to malignancy due to higher mitotic index and longer life span.

1. Which of the following is the most appropriate therapy for a child with suspected anthrax?
   a. Amoxicillin–clavulanate.
   b. Cefdinir.
   c. Ciprofloxacin.
   d. Sulfamethoxazole–trimethoprim.

Answer: **C**

The recommended therapies from the CDC for treatment of anthrax are ciprofloxacin or doxycycline.

2. Which of the following is a principle of disaster efforts?
   a. Priority is given to those who are most likely to survive.
   b. Liquid decontamination is the first step in decontamination.
   c. Children must be decontaminated by separating them from adult patients.
   d. Allocation of resources should focus on individuals rather than on populations in mass casualty larger regional disaster events.

Answer: **A**

When managing all forms of disaster, priority is given to those individuals most likely to survive. When decontaminating patients, the first priority is given to mechanical decontamination (e.g., removing clothes). Children may require separation from families during the decontamination process; however, decontamination efforts do not require separation of children and families. Allocation of resources in larger regional and national disaster events should focus on the population as a whole rather than on individuals.

3. Which of the following differential diagnoses would also be considered when evaluating a child for botulinum toxin exposure?
   a. Thyroid storm.
   b. Myocarditis.
   c. Guillain–Bárre syndrome.
   d. Parotitis.

Answer: **C**

Guillain–Bárre syndrome and myasthenia gravis present with weakness or flaccid paralysis and would be considered on the list of differential diagnosis when evaluating a child with new-onset weakness of unclear etiology.

4. Which of the following examination findings will help distinguish between smallpox and varicella zoster?
   a. Smallpox has more lesions on face and upper extremities.
   b. Smallpox has more lesions on the trunk.
   c. Varicella is found on the palms and soles.
   d. Varicella lesions all have the same clinical appearance.

Answer: **A**

There is a higher concentration of lesions on the face and upper extremities in smallpox. The lesions have the same characteristic appearance and also occur in the hands and soles of feet. Varicella lesions are more concentrated on the trunk and are in multiple stages of maturation.

Recommended Readings

Centers for Disease Control and Prevention. Office of Public Health Preparedness and Response. (2012). *Planning resources by setting.* Retrieved from http://www.cdc.gov/phpr/healthcare/planning.htm

Federal Emergency Management Agency. (2014). *Ready. Prepare. Plan. Stay informed.* Retrieved from http://www.ready.gov

Goodhue, C. J., & Upperman, J. S. (2012). Disaster management. In K. Reuter-Rice & B. N. Bolick (Eds.), *Pediatric acute care: A guide for interprofessional practice* (pp. 1216–1223). Burlington, MA: Jones & Bartlett Learning.

Jacobson, P. (2012). Blast injuries. In K. Reuter-Rice & B. N. Bolick (Eds.), *Pediatric acute care: A guide for interprofessional practice* (pp. 1234–1238). Burlington, MA: Jones & Bartlett Learning.

Occupational Safety & Health Administration. (2005). OSHA best practices for hospital based first receivers of victims form mass casualty incidents involving the release of hazardous substances. Best practice for the protection of hospital-based first receivers. Retrieved from https://www.osha.gov/dts/osta/bestpractices/html/hospital_firstreceivers.html

Payne, A. S., & Fagbuyi, D. B. (2012). Chemical disasters. In K. Reuter-Rice & B. N. Bolick (Eds.), *Pediatric acute care: A guide for interprofessional practice* (pp. 1238–1244). Burlington, MA: Jones & Bartlett Learning.

PART THREE

Professional Issues

Research, Evidence, Quality Improvement, Safety, Diversity, and Health Policy

Research, Evidence-Based Practice, and Clinical Decision Making

Tara Trimarchi

Research

Research as a Basis for Clinical Practice

- Evidence from well-designed research studies results in better outcomes.
- The U.S. Department of Health and Human Services Office of Extramural Research and the National Institute of Health define research as "a systematic investigation designed to develop new knowledge."
- The National Institute of Nursing Research (NINR) is a branch of the National Institute of Health. The NINR states that the purposes of nursing research is to develop the knowledge to:
  - Build the scientific foundation for clinical practice.
  - Prevent disease and disability.
  - Manage and eliminate symptoms caused by illness.
  - Enhance end-of-life and palliative care.
- The process of knowledge creation and translation includes concept development, from basic scientific discovery through clinical trials, and dissemination of the research findings.
- As described in Figure 24.1, the process of clinical research can be integrated with the process of patient care.
- The highest priority of clinical research is to protect human subjects from undue harm and burden from participation in the study.
  - Special oversight for studies is often required when the research subjects are children. For the purpose of research, the National Institutes of Health defines a child as an individual who is under 21 years of age.
  - A health care organization's institutional review board (IRB) reviews research protocols for appropriateness and safety, and approves research proposals before studies can be conducted (NINR, 2008).

Steps to Conducting Clinical Research

- Identification of the research question.
- Systematic review of literature related to the phenomenon in question.
- Formation of the hypothesis.
- Design of the study.
- Approval to perform study from the IRB.
- Conduct of the study—consenting subjects, administration of study interventions, monitoring, and data collection.
- Analysis of the data and interpretation of the findings.
- Summary of the study, its findings, and conclusions prepared as a manuscript for publication.

Roles of Care Providers in Clinical Research

- Intervention design and implementation planning within the clinical setting.
- Participant recruitment and consenting.
- Maintenance of human subjects' protection standards.
- Participant education and support.
- Direct administration of study interventions and evaluations.
- Participant monitoring for response and adverse events.
- Data preparation and management.
- Dissemination of research findings.

Research Involving Children

Andrea M. Kline-Tilford

Definitions in Research

Children
- Individuals who have not yet attained the legal age for consent of treatments/procedures in the proposed research.

Parent
- Child's biologic or adoptive parent.

Guardian
- An individual authorized to consent on the behalf of a child to general medical care under state or local law.

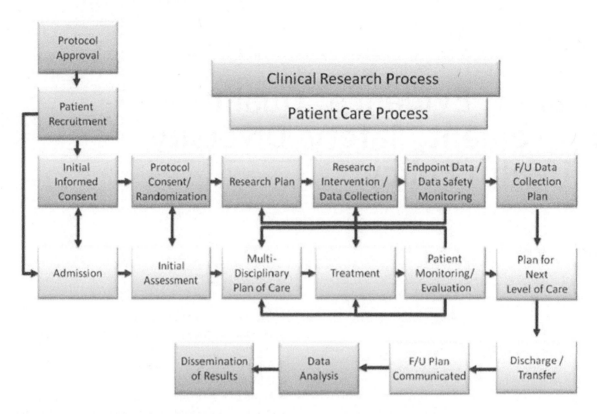

FIGURE 24.1 • **Clinical Research.** From Hastings, C. E., Fisher, C. A., & McCabe, M. A. (2012). Clinical research nursing: A critical resource in the national research enterprise. *Nursing Outlook, 60*(3), 149–156.

Ward
- A child whose welfare is determined by the state, institution, or entity.

Categories of Research Involving Children

- Research not involving greater-than-minimal risk:
  - Appropriate provisions are needed for obtaining and documenting the assent from the child.
  - Appropriate provisions are in place for obtaining the permission of at least one of the child's parents.
- Research involving greater-than-minimal risk with the prospect of direct benefit to individual study participants as long as the following issues are addressed:
  - The risk of the study is justified by the anticipated benefit to the study participants.
  - The anticipated benefit to study participation is at least as favorable to the study participants as the benefits of alternative available approaches/therapies.
  - Appropriate provisions are made to obtain and document the assent of children and the permission of at least one of the child's parents.
- Research involving greater-than-minimal risk and no prospect of direct benefit to individual study participants, but likely to yield generalizable knowledge about the study participants' disorder or condition as long as the following issues are addressed:
  - Anticipated risk represents only a minor increase over minimal risk.

- Study intervention or procedure presents experiences that are reasonably commensurate with those encountered in the study participants' actual or expected medical therapy.
- Study intervention or procedure is likely to yield generalizable knowledge about the study participants' disorder or condition, which is of vital importance for the understanding of the condition.
- Appropriate provisions are made to obtain and document the assent of children and the permission of at least one of the child's parents.
- Special circumstances in pediatric research:
  - The requirement for permission of study participation may be waived in conditions when asking for parent/guardian permission is not reasonable (e.g., child maltreatment), and an appropriate mechanism to provide study participant protection is substituted.
  - Children who are wards of the state or other agency may be included in study participation if the study is related to their status as wards or is conducted in settings (e.g., schools, camps, hospitals) when the majority of study participants are not wards.
    - A child advocate must be appointed in these cases.

Ethical Concepts

Beneficence—doing for the good or welfare of the patient, research participant.
Maleficence—doing or causing harm.
Nonmaleficence—first, do no harm.

Malevolence—having or showing a desire to cause harm to another person.

Principle of double effect—performing an action that potentially causes a good effect, but also has a bad effect.

Consent and Assent
Shannon Konierczki

- First statement on informed consent, parental permission, and assent was initially drafted and presented to the American Academy of Pediatrics Committee of Bioethics in 1985.
- The issue of informed consent and permission, especially as it pertains to pediatric patients, continues to be an important topic of discussion and practice.
- *Consent* is the act of decision making for oneself, so it is not a term that is commonly applied to the pediatric patient, but to their parent or guardian.
- *Informed consent* is based on the cultural and legal assumption that a person of the age of majority has the full and accurate information needed to make a decision.
  - The decision-maker is traditionally assumed to have the mental capacity and ability to recognize the probable consequences of the decision.
  - In order to obtain informed consent for a pediatric patient, the parent must be provided with sufficient information to understand and authorize the recommended treatment.
  - Health care providers seeking consent should provide parents with information on the nature of the condition, the nature of the proposed diagnostic steps or treatment, and the probability of success. The parent should also be informed of the risks and benefits that may be involved, as well as the consequence of no treatment and alternative treatment options. The health care providers should then assess the parents' understanding of the presented information by asking them questions or by asking them to explain the information.
  - In some cases, informed consent can be waived, such as in medical emergencies, public health emergencies, or when parents cannot be reached.
- *Assent* is the ethical duty to inform and educate the pediatric patient in an age-appropriate way of an upcoming treatment or procedure, and to allow the child to participate in the decision making about the proposed care.
  - To acknowledge the child's emerging capacities, honor their point of view, and promote well-being, health care providers should seek the child's assent when possible.
    - In addition to parental permission.
  - Although children cannot be treated as rational, autonomous decision-makers, health care providers should give serious consideration to the patient's developing capacities for participating in decision making.
  - Involving the child in discussions about their health care fosters trust and allows for a better patient–health care provider relationship.
  - Four elements of assent should be recognized:

- Help the patient to achieve developmentally appropriate awareness of his or her condition.
- Explain to the child what he or she can expect from the test and treatment.
- Make a clinical assessment of the patient's understanding of the situation, and determine whether the patient is being inappropriately pressured.
- Determine whether the patient is willing to accept the proposed care.
- Asking for assent facilitates involvement in care, which offers a way to gain control and respect as the child transitions from dependent to independent.

Care of the Emancipated Minor
Jessica L. Diver

- An emancipated minor is one who has been granted autonomy from their parent or legal guardian.
- This declaration allows minor patients the ability to make their own health care decisions prior to the age that is typically considered adulthood.
- Events leading to emancipation may include pregnancy or marriage.
- Emancipation may also be achieved by petition to the court in order to obtain financial control or gain independence, or for complete removal from a negative home life, among other indications.
- Requirements for emancipation vary, as do the state laws regulating this status.
- Due to the lack of federal laws or consensus regarding emancipated minors, each state establishes its own criteria.
- While caring for emancipated minors, the health care provider should ensure confidentiality, communicate clearly and completely with the patient, and obtain consent from the minor.

Evidence-Based Practice
Tara Trimarchi

- An approach to practicing health care that includes:
  - Awareness of the evidence to support clinical practices.
  - Ability to evaluate research to determine the strength of the evidence.
  - Use of strongest evidence to make clinical decisions.
- The evidence-based practice (EBP) process includes (1) literature review; (2) critical appraisal of the quality of the research (see "levels of evidence" below); (3) application of the findings from the strongest studies to clinical practice; and (4) evaluation of the outcome of implementation of the EBPs.
- Levels of evidence from strongest (1) to weakest (7) are:
  - Level 1: systematic review and meta-analysis of randomized controlled trials; clinical guidelines based on systematic reviews or meta-analyses.
  - Level 2: one or more randomized controlled trials.
  - Level 3: controlled trial (no randomization).

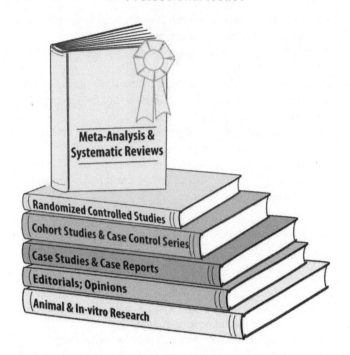

FIGURE 24.2 • **Levels of Evidence Pyramid.**

- Level 4: case-control or cohort study.
- Level 5: systematic review of descriptive and qualitative studies.
- Level 6: single descriptive or qualitative study.
- Level 7: expert opinion (Figure 24.2).
- Clinical decision making.
  - Using EBP to guide clinical decision making requires performance of a literature search and review of studies for their relevance, strengths, and limitations.
  - The steps to conducting a literature search include:
    - Identify the clinical question(s).
    - Determine the most appropriate database to search for research that addresses the question.
    - Enter key words and phrases to find relevant literature—combine search terms as needed to find relevant literature.
    - Review the research studies for strength of the evidence.
    - Apply the strongest evidence in clinical practice.
  - EBP can be disseminated to clinicians for use in decision making via research committees, clinical census workgroups, and journal clubs.
  - EBPs can also be facilitated by clinical decision-support systems that are embedded into care delivery workflow, such as the inclusion of evidence-based care pathways and order sets in electronic health records and computerized provider order entry systems.

Quality Improvement and Patient Safety

Tara Trimarchi

Patient Safety

Background/Overview of Patient Safety

- In 1999, the Institute of Medicine (IOM) report *To Err Is Human: Building a Safer Health System* documented that approximately 100,000 people died every year in the United States as the result of medical errors made by health care professionals.
- Children are more likely than adults to experience medication errors or adverse drug events and experience a higher rate of diagnostic-related events, such as an incorrect diagnosis.

Definitions of Patient Safety Events

- *Adverse events* are events in which injury to a patient is caused by medical management rather than by a patient's underlying disease.
- *Medical error* is the failure of a planned intervention to be carried out as intended, the inappropriate use of an intervention, or the failure to enact a necessary intervention.
- *Precursor patient safety events* are adverse events or medical errors that cause harm that is neither permanent nor life-threatening.
- *Serious patient safety events* are adverse events or medical errors that cause death, permanent injury, or transient, but life-threatening harm.
- *Near-miss patient safety events* are adverse events or medical errors that would have caused harm to a patient, but did not because of timely intervention or chance.

Theories of Human and Systems Error

- Decision making which relies on knowledge, judgment, and memory results in the highest rate of error.
- In addition to education and experience, health care providers need decision-support tools, such as reminders, written instructions, and checklists, as well as standardization of practices and access to experts, in order to reliably perform activities.
- Errors are due to either:
  - *Active failures*: unsafe acts performed by professionals who are in direct contact with patients, or
  - *Latent conditions*: flaws in the design of the care delivery systems that allow or promote errors.
- For a system to be safe, it must possess layers of defense that prevent or trap active failures and latent conditions before they cause harm. The term Swiss Cheese Model has been coined to represent the need for layers of error defense in systems.

High-Reliability Organizations

- Produce desired outcomes, despite error-prone activities, with a very low rate of failure.
- Characteristics of high-reliability organizations.
  - Preoccupation with error prevention.
  - Appreciation of the complexity of errors and reluctance to simplify the causes or the strategies to prevent errors.
  - Focus on system failures rather than individual performance, including nonpunitive approaches to addressing errors.
  - Ability to learn from errors and continually improve.
  - Flat organization hierarchy in which staff of any level can effectively voice concerns and make recommendations.

Culture of Safety

- Fundamental elements of a culture of safety.
  - Cohesive teamwork.
  - Leadership support for patient safety.

- Nonpunitive responses to errors.
- Transparency regarding errors for the purpose of learning.
- Work-hour restrictions, appropriate staffing ratios, and workload distribution.
- Effective communication and care transition processes.
- Effective policies and procedures for care delivery.
- Ergonomically sound physical work space.

Methods for Improving Safety

- *Failure mode effects analysis*: a prospective analysis used to identify and assign a risk priority to system vulnerabilities, called *failure modes*, in order to implement safeguards before errors occur.
- *Incident reporting*: a qualitative narrative of an adverse event, near miss, or medical error that is constructed by staff directly involved in the incident at the time of discovery.
- *Root cause analysis*: a retrospective analysis of a serious medical error or sentinel event that has occurred in order to identify contributing factors.

Overview of Health Care Quality Improvement

- Discipline of continuous action to sustain reliably safe and maximally effective clinical performance with the goal of improving patients' experiences and outcomes, improving the health of populations and containing costs.
- *Crossing the Quality Chasm* defines the six IOM quality aims as:
  - *Safe*: Avoid injuries to patients from care that was intended to help them.
  - *Effective*: Provide services that are based on scientific knowledge to all who could benefit and refrain from providing services to those who are not likely to benefit.
  - *Patient-centered*: Provide care that is respectful of and responsive to individual patient preferences, needs, and values and ensure that patient values guide all clinical decisions.
  - *Timely*: Reduce wait time and harmful delays for those who both receive and give care.
  - *Efficient*: Avoid waste such as wasteful use of supplies, ideas, and energy.
  - *Equitable*: Provide care that does not vary in quality because of personal characteristics such as gender, ethnicity, geographic location, and socioeconomic status.
- The Institute for Healthcare Improvement has identified a "Triple Aim" for health care quality improvement that includes a focus on:
  - Better health for populations.
  - Better care for individuals.
  - Lower per capita health care costs.

Quality Improvement Theory

- Provides the framework for contemporary quality improvement and are:
  - *Systems thinking*: focus on improving processes and systems, versus a focus on individual performance.
  - *Applied psychology*: use theories of human behavior and cognition to promote change that improves human performance.
  - *Variation control*: standardize whenever possible; variation in a system impedes the reliability of system performance.

- *Importance of knowledge*: test, study outcomes, and implement what works.
- A stepwise approach to quality control that includes:
  - *Planning*: identifying what needs to improve, who will be impacted by the improvement efforts, and solutions.
  - *Measurement*: monitoring of system performance by determining what to measure and how to measure it, establishing a standard for performance, and consistently measuring actual performance against the standard.
  - *Improvement*: the act of continually adapting systems to achieve and then exceed performance standards.

Quality Improvement Methods

- Common, contemporary quality improvement methods used in health care include:
  1. *The model for improvement:*
     a. Consists of two parts:
        i. Answering three fundamental questions.
           1. What are we trying to accomplish?
           2. How will we know that a change is an improvement?
           3. What changes can we make that will result in improvement?
        ii. Conducting plan-do-study-act (PDSA) cycles to test changes.
  2. *Six sigma:*
     a. Statistical modeling of process reliability.
     b. A six sigma process is one in which 99.99966% of the outputs are statistically expected to be free of defects.
     c. A focus on achieving measurable results.
     d. A commitment to making decisions on the basis of the data.
  3. *Lean thinking:*
     a. Derived from the Toyota Production System.
     b. Premise is to remove waste from systems.
     c. Waste is any expenditure of resources that does not achieve value for a customer.

Components of Quality Improvement Plans

- Aims: determine what the improvement effort is trying to accomplish, for whom and by when.
- Stakeholder analysis.
- Assembly of a team.
- Selecting "changes" or interventions that are hypothesized will result in improvement.
- Selecting measures, including:
  1. *Structural measure*: presence or absence of a trait—Is everything necessary to implement the change in place?
  2. *Process measure*: reliability of carrying out an action—How will you demonstrate that the change has been implemented?
  3. *Outcome measure*: results of carrying out an action—How will you demonstrate that the change has resulted in improvement?
  4. *Balancing measure*: How will you demonstrate that the change has not resulted in an unintended negative consequence?

- Data collection process.
- Tests of the changes to determine if they result in improvement.
- A strategy for sustaining and spreading successful changes.

Cultural Issues and Diversity

Cathy Haut

Background/Definition

- Cultural and linguistic competence is a set of congruent behaviors, attitudes, and policies that come together in a system, agency, or among professionals that enables effective work in cross-cultural situations.
- The Institute of Family-Centered Care incorporates four core principles which are the foundations of the partnership between health care providers and patients and their families.
- Two of the core principles include dignity and respect, which form the basis for respect by the health care provider who honors the family's perspectives, choices, values, beliefs, and cultural background.
- Cultural theories and models exist which can guide assessment of a person from a different ethnical background or nationality.
- Cultural competency is one of the main avenues for minimizing or eliminating disparities in health care.
- Cultural competence programs are available through many resources online, including the U.S. Department of Health and Human Sciences and Health Literacy websites. The Office of Minority Health and the National Center for Cultural Competence are other resources for information related to assessment, language, disease, and research in relation to specific populations.
- It is an expectation for health care providers to maintain a level of cultural awareness and competence, regardless of the arena where they provide care.

Advocacy

Karen G. Duderstadt

Background/Definition

Advocacy is defined as the support or defense of a cause and the act of pleading on behalf of another person.
- Multifaceted, diverse, right, and a responsibility.
- Nurses have right to advocacy and responsibility as advocates.

Significance

- Advocacy and health care policy influence nursing practice.
- Essential to supporting APRN (advanced practice registered nurse) practice priorities, policies, and programs.
- Advocates inform policymakers on health care issues impacting patients and families.
- Health policy advocacy does not require new skills; requires applying existing skills in a new context.

Advanced Practice Registered Nurses as Advocates

- Engage in advocacy every day on behalf of their patients.
- Make a difference when vocalizing concerns through policy.
- Must understand how policy interacts with and influences the nursing profession.
- Can advocate for issues through their professional practice organizations.
- Can create opportunities for providers to learn about the health policy/advocacy process, engage and interact in the process, and mentor others in the process.
- Often do not realize how much their practice is dependent on policy decisions that are made by others.

Health Policy

Karen G. Duderstadt

Definition

Health policy defines a vision for future, outlines priorities and expected roles of different groups, and builds consensus.
- It is imperative that nurses and other health care professionals communicate with policymakers about key issues of concern on legislative and regulatory proposals.
- Health policy involves knowledge about laws and regulations governing nurse practice acts.
- As health care providers engage in health policy advocacy, the outcomes advance the profession, decrease health care inequalities, and improve health care outcomes.

Involvement in Health Policy Advocacy

- Sending electronic communication (email), making telephone calls, and face-to-face or conference call meetings are all effective strategies in communicating with legislators.
- Meet alone or with other APRNs or providers.

1. Health care organizations that produce desired patient outcomes through the delivery of highly complex care with a very low rate of error are likely to possess which of the following characteristics?
   a. Transparency regarding errors that occur.
   b. Strict hierarchies that dictate which care providers make decisions.
   c. A strong focus on the performance of individual care providers.
   d. Strong discipline program that enforces proper protocols for high-risk procedures.

Answer: **A**

Characteristics of high-reliability organizations include transparency regarding errors for the purpose of learning, flat hierarchies that allow all team members to voice concerns and make recommendations, and focus on systems versus individuals' performance.

2. In addition to patient safety, quality aims as defined by IOM also include:
   a. Provider dictated decisions.
   b. Emphasis on cost control.
   c. Care that varies with socioeconomic status.
   d. Timely care that prevents delays.

Answer: **D**

The six quality aims of IOM are safe, effective, efficient, timely, patient-centered, and equitable care. In keeping, quality care would include shared decision making between patients and providers rather than care that is dictated by providers, and care would not vary based on a patient's socioeconomic status. Timely care, defined as an avoidance of harmful delays for those who both receive and give care is an important aim. Although cost containment is an important element of quality improvement, it is not an IOM aim.

3. Which of the following provides the greatest support for implementation of EBP?
   a. Expert opinion.
   b. A meta-analysis of randomized controlled trials.
   c. A case-control or cohort study.
   d. Systematic review of descriptive and qualitative studies.

Answer: **B**

Not all types of literature provide the same strength of evidence. Levels of evidence from strongest (1) to weakest (7) are the following:
- Level 1: systematic review and meta-analysis of randomized controlled trials; clinical guidelines based on systematic reviews or meta-analyses.
- Level 2: one or more randomized controlled trials.
- Level 3: controlled trial (no randomization).
- Level 4: case-control or cohort study.
- Level 5: systematic review of descriptive and qualitative studies.
- Level 6: single descriptive or qualitative study.
- Level 7: expert opinion:

4. Which of the following is the highest priority for a clinical research program?
   a. Prevention of human disease and disability.
   b. Building the scientific foundation for clinical practice.
   c. Protection of human subjects from harm and burden due to participation in research.
   d. Integration of the research process with the process of patient care.

Answer: **C**

The highest priority of clinical research is to protect human subjects from undue harm and burden from participation in research studies. To ensure this priority, a health care organization's IRB reviews each research protocol for appropriateness and safety, and approves research proposals before studies can be conducted.

5. What are the main objectives of being involved as an advanced practice nurse in health policy advocacy?
   a. Advancing the profession, decreasing health care inequities, and improving health care outcomes.
   b. Advocating for provider-inclusive language, decreasing health care inequities, and increasing knowledge about laws and regulations.
   c. Improving health care outcomes, increasing knowledge about laws and regulations, and supporting the personal priorities of nurses.
   d. Advocating for provider-inclusive language, advancing the profession, and supporting the personal priorities of nurses.

Answer: **A**

Nurses and advanced practice nurses participate in health policy advocacy to assist in advancing their profession, decreasing health care inequities for the patients they care for, and improving health care outcomes. Nurses' knowledge of health care concerns supports their abilities to best support policy which advocates for children and child health.

6. What is a beginning source for advanced practice nurses to test their abilities to advocate for issues and support health policy?
   a. Contact the National Council of State Boards of Nursing.
   b. Participate in national nursing organizations.
   c. Enroll as students in health policy coursework.
   d. Discuss common concerns in an informal nurse practitioner network.

Answer: **B**

(continues on page 532)

Advanced practice registered nurses can begin to navigate health policy issues through their local and national professional organizations, where they may find committees or groups who can help them to learn additional information on issues that affect practice and the care of children.

7. A nurse practitioner is caring for a child with complex health needs. The state-based insurance company has decided that this child no longer requires home nursing care which was being provided for 8 hours each night. The child is receiving continuous feedings through a gastrostomy tube and has a tracheostomy, but does not need mechanical ventilation. Parents are unable to physically continue care 24 hours a day. What is the most effective way to advocate for this child and family?
   a. Contact the local congressman to attempt to change state laws to provide nursing care as ordered by nurse practitioners.
   b. Begin by contacting the insurance company to attempt to change the decision based on an explanation of medical need.
   c. Ask the parents to communicate with the insurance company to address their claims.
   d. Counsel the parents that the child may benefit from hospice care, which would provide in-home nursing care.

Answer: **B**

Health care providers are in unique positions when it comes to advocating for their patients and families. An initial contact with the insurance company may assist a child in getting improved or needed services. Describing the medical need, regardless of how complex, assists in gaining an understanding of why the child will benefit from identified services.

8. Which one of the following statements about assent provides the most accurate summary?
   a. Assent is an ethical duty health care providers are to carry out in order to educate children of medical care.
   b. Health care providers must have written assent from the pediatric patient in order to carry out a procedure.
   c. Educating children on medical procedure is a waste of time and resources.
   d. Children should be treated as autonomous decision-makers.

Answer: **A**

There is no legal documentation required to prove assent. Children should not be treated as autonomous decision-makers, but educating and informing pediatric patients about upcoming medical care fosters trust and allows for a better relationship between health care providers and patients, as well as patient families.

9. A nurse practitioner is evaluating a pregnant teenager who is diagnosed with a sexually transmitted infection. Which of the following is the most appropriate action?
   a. Notify the patient of the infection, stating you will have to report it to her parents and offering her the choice of how involved she would like to be in the delivery of this information.
   b. Inform the patient of the infection and make appropriate treatment recommendations.
   c. Notify the patient's mother and suggest you discuss this with the patient together.
   d. Contact the public worker assigned to this minor and discuss the laboratory findings prior to creating a treatment plan for the patient.

Answer: **B**

Emancipation indicates that the adolescent is able to make decisions regarding their own health care; it is a legal process that gives adolescents the autonomy usually associated with adulthood. In this case, it is not necessary to inform any caregivers of this finding.

10. An infant is being admitted to the intensive care unit and parents, who do not speak English, have placed knit bracelets around both arms and legs. The nurse attempts to remove one to place an IV catheter and the mother begins to cry. What is the basis for either removing or leaving the bracelets intact?
    a. Exploration into the cultural origin of the bracelets may assist in providing the best decision.
    b. The bracelets should be removed and an explanation to the parents in their language is appropriate.
    c. Once an explanation for the IV is given to the parents, the nurse can remove the bracelets and attach them to the bed.
    d. The acuity of the patient and the need to utilize the extremities for procedures is most important in this situation.

Answer: **A**

Cultural theories and models exist which can guide assessment of a person from a different ethnical background or nationality and can assist in explanation of rules or rituals. If the family of this infant is utilizing a health-related tradition, it is difficult to convince them that the infant will be well when taking away an important health belief.

11. A physician refuses to perform cardiac surgery to repair a large ventricular septal defect on an infant who is anencephalic with an unstable respiratory status whose parents are asking for the surgery. This is an example of:
    a. Malevolence.
    b. Maleficence.
    c. Beneficence.
    d. Malpractice.

Answer: **C**

Beneficence refers to doing for the good or welfare of the patient. If the physician knows that the surgical procedure will have an adverse effect on the patient or cause the patient's demise, he is justified in not performing the surgery.

12. Permission can be obtained from a parent or guardian to enroll a 9-year-old child in a health-related research protocol if:
    a. The child has a life-threatening illness which may be improved with the research protocol.
    b. The permission meets the requirements for informed consent.
    c. The child also agrees to assent to the protocol.
    d. There is a written waiver of damage in place.

Answer: **B**

Permission from parent(s) or guardian(s) to allow a child to participate in a research protocol must be obtained prior to enrolling a child in research. This permission must meet the requirements for informed consent found and may also be subject to both parents agreeing and signing the consent. If the child is of legal age for assent, his ability to make a decision should also be considered.

Recommended Readings

American Academy of Pediatrics. Committee on Bioethics. (1995). Informed consent, parental permission, and assent in pediatric research. *Pediatrics, 95*(2), 314–317.

Committee on the Quality Health Care in America, Institute of Medicine. (2001). *Crossing the quality chasm: A new health system for the 21st century.* Washington, DC: National Academy Press.

Evan, J. R. (2005). *Total quality: Management, organization and strategy* (4th ed.). Mason, OH: Thompson South Western.

Fyffe, T. (2009). Nursing shaping and influencing health and social care policy. *Journal of Nursing Management, 17,* 698–706.

Hastings, C. E., Fisher, C. A., McCabe, M. A., National Clinical Research Nursing Consortium, Allison, J., Brassil, D., . . . Turbini, V. (2012). Clinical research nursing: A critical resource in the national research enterprise. *Nursing Outlook, 60*(3), 149–156.

Hill, L. A., & Sawatzky, J. A. (2011). Transitioning into the nurse practitioner role through mentorship. *Journal of Professional Nursing, 27*(3), 161–167.

Kleinpell, R. (2011). Research, evidence based practice and clinical decision making. In K. Reuter-Rice & B. Bolick (Eds.), *Pediatric acute care: A guide for interprofessional practice.* Burlington, MA: Jones & Bartlett Learning.

Kohn, K. T., Corrigan, J. M., & Donaldson, M. S. (1999). *To err is human: Building a safer healthcare system.* Washington, DC: National Academy Press.

Kopelman, L. (2008). Assent and self determination. In R. Perkin, J. Swift, D. Newton & N. Anas (Eds.), *Pediatric hospital medicine* (pp. 40–41). Philadelphia, PA: Lippincott, Williams & Wilkins.

Lane, S. H., & Kohlenberg, E. (2012). Emancipated minors: Health policy and implications for nursing. *Journal of Pediatric Nursing, 27,* 533–548.

Leavitt, J. K. (2009). Leaders in health policy: A critical role for nursing. *Nursing Outlook, 57*(2), 73–77.

Melnyk, B. M., & Fineout-Overholt, E. (2011). *Evidence-based practice in nursing and healthcare: A guide to best practice.* Philadelphia, PA: Lippincott, Williams & Wilkins.

Mercurio, M., Adam, M., Foreman, E., Ladd, E., Ross, L., & Silber, T. (2008). American Academy of Pediatrics policy statements on bioethics. *Pediatrics in Review, 29,* e1–e8.

National Institute of Nursing Research. (2008). *Bringing science to life: The NINR strategic plan.* Retrieved from: https://www.ninr.nih.gov/sites/www.ninr.nih.gov/files/ninr-strategic-plan-2011.pdf, accessed 5/27/2015

Needleman, J. (2008). Is what's good for the patient good for the hospital? *Policy, Politics & Nursing Practice, 9*(2), 80–87.

Reason, J. T. (2000). Human error: Models and management. *British Medical Journal, 320,* 768–770.

Sackett, D., Straus, S., Richardson, W., Rosenberg, W., & Haynes, R. (2000). *Evidence-based medicine: How to practice and teach EBM* (2nd ed.). Edinburgh: Churchill Livingstone.

Trimarchi, T. (2011). Patient safety. In K. Reuter-Rice & B. Bolick (Eds.), *Pediatric acute care: A guide for interprofessional practice.* Burlington, MA: Jones & Bartlett Learning.

Trimarchi, T. (2012). Fundamentals of patient safety and quality improvement. In M. F. Hazinski (Ed.), *Nursing care of the critically ill child* (3rd ed.). St Louis, MO: Elsevier.

Preparation for Practice: Interprofessional Practice, Certification, Licensure, Credentialing, Documentation, Billing, and Coding

Interprofessional Practice

Hospital-Based Practice

- Appropriate acute care education, certification, credentialing, and privileging are requirements for health care providers to function in a hospital setting.
- Admission to inpatient facilities is determined by these health care providers.
- National organizations such as the American Academy of Pediatrics and the Society of Critical Care Medicine have developed guidelines to determine appropriate practice settings for patient care.
- System-based criteria are used to determine the need for pediatric intensive care admission and differentiate between level I and II units.
- Acuity scoring systems are also used to determine patient acuity and risk of mortality and morbidity.
- Hospital practice includes obtaining a history, which includes medical history, current medications, allergies, immunizations and exposures, family health history, psychosocial history, spiritual and cultural evaluation, followed by a thorough physical examination.
- The development of differential diagnoses, problem lists, and a plan of care for management is the responsibility of the pediatric acute care team.

Consultation and Referral

Joe D. Cavender

Definition

- Medical consultation is the process whereby a referring practitioner requests the evaluation of a patient by another practitioner (the consultant) who possesses specialty-specific knowledge beyond that of the referring practitioner or in an attempt to gain a secondary opinion regarding an uncertain diagnosis.

Referring Practitioner Responsibilities

- The practitioner requesting a consultation should provide the consultant with the patient's pertinent clinical information that led to the decision to consult. The consult request should clearly state the questions to be answered by the consultant. Although consult requests are often entered into the electronic health record (or via a written order), the consultation should always include verbal communication between the requesting practitioner and the consultant.

Consulting Practitioner Responsibilities

- The consultant has a responsibility to understand the information requested by the referring practitioner.
- The consultation should be provided in a timely manner given the urgency established by the referring practitioner.
- The consultant should first obtain an independent history and physical examination and review of the patient's current studies.
- Recommendations should be provided directly in a written consult note to the referring practitioner in a succinct, clear format that includes necessary details for implementation of recommendations.
- The written consultation findings should also be verbally discussed with the referring practitioner.

Types of Consultation

- Recommendation.
  - The consultant provides his or her opinion regarding the patient's diagnosis and management, including medications and/or further laboratory or radiologic studies.
- Comanagement.
  - The practice of the consultant ordering medications and additional studies to manage the patient's diagnosis.
  - Comanagement should occur only if agreed upon by the referring practitioner and consulting practitioner prior to the consult.

PEARL

- *The key to successful, effective consultation is verbal communication between the referring practitioner and the consultant.*

Interprofessional Collaboration

Interprofessional Teams

Theresa A. Mikhailov & Jennifer Manzi

- Interprofessional patient care is accomplished through an integrated approach by a clinical team of multiple disciplines.
- The discipline of medicine includes physicians and surgeons, physicians-in-training (residents, interns), medical students, and physician assistants. Subspecialists are included in this listing.
- The discipline of nursing consists of advanced practice registered nurses (APRNs), including population-specific nurse practitioners (NPs), nurse anesthetists, clinical nurse specialists, and nurse midwives. Nurses and nursing students are the largest component of this group.
- Allied health professionals include pharmacists, respiratory therapists, social workers, psychologists, child life specialists, chaplains, paramedics, and others.
- Tables 25.1, 25.2, and 25.3 offer examples of the roles and functions of members of the team.

Two examples of health care teams to illustrate function in different acute pediatric patient care settings.

Pediatric Trauma Team

- Designed to rapidly assess a patient and intervene promptly.
- Requires rapid assembly of a team of providers skilled not only in their individual areas of patient care expertise but also in their ability to function as a team.
- The leader of this team is generally a physician who receives immediate consultation from the other health care professionals in the team but who is responsible for making critical decisions regarding the plan of care.

Pediatric Oncology Team

- Designed to diagnose and treat children with oncologic conditions.
- Includes physicians, APRNs, staff nurses, pharmacists, dietitians, social workers, case managers, and chaplains.
- Functions in an interprofessional manner with all members of the team contributing to the individual patient's care and meeting as a group to discuss the patient's needs.
- While the physician may still be viewed as the leader for such a team, this team can make decisions through group consensus.
- Teams can be led by providers other than physicians, but team leaders serve an essential role in teams as they facilitate decision making and exchange of information.

Keys to successful health care team's ability to solve complex patient problems on an ongoing basis:
- Dependent on cohesive teamwork.
- Require effective team communication and process to facilitate communication.
- Require critical information and infrastructure to access information.

TABLE 25.1 Role and Function of Physicians

Provider	Description
Attending physicians	• Examine patients, obtain medical histories, order and interpret diagnostic tests. • Diagnose illnesses and provide patient health counseling. • Prescribe and administer treatments for patients.

Medical students	• Complete 4 y of training at an accredited medical school.
	  • 2 y of didactic training.
	  • 2 y of clinical training under the supervision of experienced physicians.

Physicians-in-training	
• Residents	• Train in an area of general practice, such as pediatrics or surgery, under the supervision of experienced physicians.
• Fellows	• Train in an area of specialized practice, such as endocrinology or cardiothoracic surgery, under the supervision of experienced physicians.
Physician assistants	• Trained to practice medicine under the direction and supervision of an attending physician. • Responsibilities include clinical decision making and a broad range of diagnostic, therapeutic, preventive, and health maintenance services.

- Open communication.
  - Allows team members to share concerns about safety or quality of patient care and to ask questions to improve understanding of patient care.
- Interprofessional rounds provide an opportunity for open communication and collaboration between team members.

Team Debriefing

- Another essential feature of successful team work.
- Review team performance in relation to professional collaboration, patient outcomes, team function, and to provide and receive constructive feedback to improve team performance.

Benefits of Teamwork

- Improved communication and collaboration.
- Higher job and career satisfaction.
- Less burnout and increased sense of autonomy.
- Patients and families.
  - Shorter lengths of stay.

TABLE 25.2 Role and Function of Nurses

Provider	Description
Nurses	• Record patients' medical histories and symptoms. • Perform diagnostic testing. • Administer treatments and medication. • Help patients with follow-up care and rehabilitation. • Teach patients and families.
Nursing students	• Complete nursing education preferably through baccalaureate program. • All nursing education requires classroom instruction and supervised clinical experiences in hospitals and other health care facilities.
Advanced practice registered nurses (APRNs)	• Nurses with additional graduate-level didactic and clinical training in a particular population. • Educational programs typically award a master's or doctoral degree in nursing. • Four types of APRNs: NPs, certified nurse midwives, clinical nurse specialists, and certified registered nurse anesthetists.
Nurse practitioners (NPs)	• Deliver primary and/or acute care in a variety of clinical settings. • Diagnose and treat common acute illnesses and injuries. • Perform physical examinations. • Manage chronic health conditions.
	Primary care pediatric NPs • Provide health maintenance and well-child examinations, developmental screenings, school physicals, immunizations, anticipatory guidance, and diagnosis and treatment of common childhood illnesses.
	Acute care pediatric NPS • Trained to meet the specialized physiologic and psychological needs of children with complex acute, critical, and chronic health care needs.
	Neonatal NPs • Manage the complex health care needs of the critically ill and convalescing neonate and family in an inpatient neonatal setting. NNP's are currently trained to manage infants and toddlers to the age of 2.
Clinical nurse specialists	• Expert clinicians who provide care in a specialized area of nursing practice (e.g., population, setting, or type of care), offer expert consultation to staff nurses, and implement improvements in health care delivery systems.
Certified registered nurse anesthetist	• Providers who specialize in anesthetic care of patients in all settings.

• Improved quality of care as measured by quality core measure performance.

Health Care Team Members and Roles

• See Table 25.4.

Interprofessional Education

Deborah W. Busch

Background/Definition

• Interprofessional education is the act of sharing and delivering pertinent knowledge among health care professionals, which can include a variety of topics, settings, and leaders.

• The ultimate goal of interprofessional education is to improve patient health care delivery outcomes through collaboration and shared dissemination of evidenced-based practice knowledge.

• Evidence supports the significance and utility of interprofessional education and collaboration with the direct correlation to improved health care outcomes, work satisfaction, peer support, and creating a positive teamwork environment among health care providers (Zwarenstien, Goldman, & Reeves, 2009).

Key concepts for interprofessional education include, but are not limited to:

• Interprofessional education is a responsibility for all clinicians, providers, and managers.

• Modern health care is evolving into an interprofessional team care approach; interprofessional education is a vital and essential component.

TABLE 25.3 Role and Function of Allied Health Professionals

Provider	Description
Pharmacists	• Distribute medications prescribed by other providers. • Inform patients about medications. • Advise practitioners on selection, dosages, interactions, and side effects of medications.
Respiratory therapists	• Evaluate, treat, and manage patients of all ages with respiratory illnesses and other cardiopulmonary conditions.
Dietitians	• Integrate and apply the principles derived from the sciences of food, nutrition, biochemistry, physiology, food management, and behavior to achieve and maintain health status of patients in a variety of clinical settings. • Provide medical nutrition therapy and the use of specific nutrition services to treat chronic conditions, illnesses, or injuries.
Occupational therapists	• Promote health and wellness to those who have or are at risk for developing an illness, injury, disease, disorder, condition, impairment, disability, activity limitation, or participation restriction. • Address the physical, cognitive, psychosocial, sensoriperceptual, and other aspects of performance in a variety of contexts and environments.
Physical therapists	• Provide services to patients recovering from accidents or illness and people with disabilities. • Improve patients' strength and mobility, relieve pain, and prevent or limit permanent physical disabilities.
Speech therapists	• Evaluate, diagnose, and treat speech, language, and swallowing disorders in individuals of all ages, from infants to the elderly. • Treat speech, language, and swallowing disorders.
Social workers	• Assist individuals, groups, or communities to restore or enhance their capacity for social functioning while creating societal conditions favorable to their goals. • Help prevent and mitigate crises and counsel individuals, families, and communities to cope more effectively with the stresses of everyday life.
Chaplains	• Help people in health care settings cope with a life-changing medical situation.
Child life specialists	• Trained professionals with expertise in helping children and their families overcome life's most challenging events. • Promote effective coping through play, preparation, education, and self-expression activities. • Provide emotional support for families. • Encourage optimal development of children facing a broad range of challenging experiences, particularly those related to health care and hospitalization.
Case managers	• Help patients understand their current health status, what they can do about it and why those treatments are important. • Guide patients and provide cohesion to other professionals in the health care delivery team.
Emergency medical technicians (EMTs) and paramedics	• Trained to provide emergency care to people who have suffered from an illness or an injury outside the hospital setting. • Work under protocols to recognize, assess, and manage medical emergencies and transport patients to facilities where they can obtain definitive medical care. • EMTs provide basic life support. • Paramedics provide advanced life support.

TABLE 25.4 Role and Function of Administrators and Leaders

Provider	Description
Medical director	• A physician who provides administrative and clinical leadership for a clinical area, such as an inpatient unit, an outpatient clinic, or a clinical program.
Nurse manager	• A nurse who provides administrative and clinical leadership for a clinical area, such as an inpatient unit, an outpatient clinic, or a clinical program.
Nursing supervisors	• Nurses who are responsible for clinical and administrative oversight of a given clinical area during a designated period of time.
Health unit coordinators	• Administrative professionals who help maintain a health care facility's service and performance by preparing documents, transcribing medical orders, maintaining patient charts and records, coordinating patient activities for the unit, ordering supplies, and communicating with the other clinical departments.

• Realizing not one profession can solely provide all authority and knowledge in modern health care; it is essential that professionals share current evidence-based practice knowledge, concepts, research, and new patient care modalities.

• An expert clinician is someone who has extensive knowledge in a specific realm and can lead the interprofessional educational effort with the goal of enhancing collegial awareness of clinical symptoms, problems, diagnoses, treatments, outcomes, rates, policies, legislation, and/or advances in medical discovery.

• Interprofessional education may occur in a variety of settings and environments, such as the acute care unit, break times, grand rounds, journal reviews, outside clinical practice, in-services, and/or conferences.

• The designated leader may be an individual, a group of peer clinicians, such as a round table, or a viewed information technology venue, such as a webinar occurring in formal, semiformal, or casual formats specific to the venue, topic, and audience.

Interprofessional Educational Professional Methodology

• The interprofessional educational leader(s) should present educational material using a professional method, in professional attire, and be expertly prepared to deliver the information in a concise and respectful manner appropriate for the audience and venue.

• Educational content must be agency-approved, relevant, accurate, evidence-based, nonjudgmental, and presented with the goal of improving patient care, outcomes, work environment, collegial collaboration, and/or clinical team cohesiveness in delivering care.

• Venues and times that are convenient to the majority of the team should be considered.

• Interprofessional colleagues should be respectful, courteous, and participate through active listening when engaged in an educational event among peers and the education leader.

• Inclusion of new providers, staff, and students in educational meetings is also essential for complete knowledge dissemination.

• Time must be allowed for input and feedback.

• Opinions of group members should be respectfully shared, acknowledged, and valued.

• Interprofessional activities within acute care also include high-fidelity simulation (HFS) experiences with an expectation to practice interprofessional, collaborative patient care in high-risk venues.

  • Members of the health care team meet for a planned or impromptu scenarios depicting real-life patient care.

  • Evidence indicates that HFS offers an opportunity to practice high-risk, low-volume experiences in a nonthreatening environment.

  • HFS also offers opportunities for health care teams to practice working in groups to provide patient care.

  • Participation in simulation exercises can limit or decrease the cost of malpractice insurance as evidence indicates lower rate of errors.

  • HFS educational offerings include debriefing sessions where practitioners can discuss their responses, feelings, and reactions to the work of the team.

  • The debriefing with good judgment model (Rudolph, Simon, Rivard, Dufresne, & Raemer, 2007) offers a focus on feedback with inquiry and reflections on practice.

  • When possible, provide follow-up information regarding the educational venue, opinions, peer conclusions, and any resulting future changes that may occur.

Patient and Family Education

Background/Definition

• Best care is provided when health care professionals, including physicians, nurses, NPs, psychologists, physiotherapists, social workers, and others, work together to offer comprehensive and understandable patient and family education.

- Patient and family education requires that each health care discipline is involved in supporting family-centered goals and values.
- Interprofessional child and family education also provides mechanisms for continuous communication among caregivers and optimizes patient participation in decision making, fostering respect for all contributors, including family members.

Details of Effective Patient Education

- Educational level is based on the patient/family needs.
- Learning needs are identified mutually between the provider/health care team and patient and family.
- Specific type of education is based on learner's needs.
- Education is offered in multiple formats (e.g., video, hands-on, reading materials).
- Methods of evaluating effectiveness of educational format are in place.
- Ongoing evaluation of learning outcomes is completed to improve future educational offerings.

Documentation, Billing, and Coding
Carmel A. McComiskey

Background

- There are general rules that NPs must follow in order to bill provider services.
- The Centers for Medicare Services (CMS) publishes billing guidelines and regulations which most insurance companies follow (Blessing, 2013).
- The NP must be certified by a recognized national certifying body.
- The NP must have a master's degree or doctor of nursing practice degree.

CMS Rules for Nurse Practitioner Billing

- Medicare qualifications must be met.
- The NP must obtain/have a national provider identifier (NPI) number.
- Services provided/performed must be medically necessary or indicated.
- Services provided may not be a part of a bundled service/code; these services must only be billed once (under bundled code).
  - Surgical services are an example of services commonly bundled.
- The NP is legally authorized to provide the services as defined by the scope of practice and state law.
- No other provider may bill or be reimbursed for the same service as the service rendered by the NP.
- The billing entity or institution accepts Medicare's payment.
- The services of residents, interns, or students may not be billed under the NPs provider number.
  - NPs may not supervise residents or interns and then bill for the services rendered.

Documentation

- Most practices and hospitals use electronic methods of documentation.
- Documentation must include the reason for the visit and the relevant history, physical examination findings, and prior diagnostic tests and findings.
- Past and present diagnoses should be included.
- The patient's progress, response to treatment, and changes in condition and treatment as well as revisions in diagnosis should be documented.

Payer Documentation Requirements

- Site of service.
- Medical necessity.
- Accurate documentation.
  - History: what was heard.
    - Four types: problem focused (PF), expanded problem focused (EPF), detailed (D), and comprehensive (C).
  - Physical examination: what was seen.
    - Four types: PF, EPF, D, and C.
  - Medical decision making: thinking.
    - Four types: straightforward, low complexity, moderate complexity, and high complexity.
  - Laboratory and radiology.
    - What test was ordered and rationale.
      - If a test would normally be ordered and was not, include rationale for not ordering the test.
      - Results.
  - Procedures.
    - Which procedure and indication for procedure.
    - Consent and by whom.
      - Risks, benefits, alternatives, and consenting individual's understanding.
    - "Time out" prior to procedures.
    - Date and time completed.
    - Complications.
    - Condition of the patient at the completion of the procedure.

Reimbursement

- CMS sets the codes for professional billing.
- Codes are listed in the current procedural terminology (CPT).
- These are developed yearly by the American Medical Association.
- Many payers set payment based on the resource-based relative value scale.
  - This relative value unit is set by the Relative Value Update Committee, which acts as an expert panel and makes recommendations for payment rates to the CMS.
  - CMS can accept/reject the rates and publishes these annually in the Federal Register.
- Professional service billing is divided into two types.
  - Evaluation and management (thinking work).
    - Levels of billing are determined by the amount of work documented in each category. Some examples are listed below:
      - Level of history: PF (brief history), EPF (brief history), D (extended history with >4 elements or 3 chronic or

inactive conditions), C (with >4 elements or 3 chronic or inactive conditions).

- Level of examination: PF (limited examination of affected body area), EPF (limited examination of affected body area plus other symptomatic organs), D (extended physical examination of both the affected area and the related organ systems), C (general multisystem examination or complete examination of a single organ system).

- Procedures (hands-on work).
- Both can be billed on the same day if each is separately identifiable and significant.
  - When this occurs at the same visit, modifier 25 is added to the evaluation/management code.

Types of Billing

- Hospital evaluation/management.
  - Three components of hospital billing.
    - Patient type.
      - New.
      - Established.
    - Setting.
      - Hospital, office, emergency department, nursing facility.
    - Level of evaluation.
      - History.
      - Physical.
      - Medical decision making.
  - Coding done depending on whether or not the patient is new or established.
  - The ICD-9-CM is divided into three parts:
    - Diseases and injuries (001–999).
    - Supplementary factors (V01–V89).
    - External factors (E000–E999).
    - Choose the code that most closely represents the reason or the significant finding for the encounter.
  - A contributing diagnosis may be added as a secondary code.
  - Diagnoses that do not affect the visit are not listed.
  - The diagnosis code should reflect the highest level of clinical certainty even in the absence of laboratory or radiologic confirmation.
  - Words listed below should not be used as part of the diagnosis; they may be used in the assessment.
    - Probable, rule out, possible.
    - Mild, moderate, severe.
  - The assessment is the health care provider's overall evaluation of the encounter, for example, possible appendicitis, but the diagnosis code should reflect abdominal pain, right upper quadrant, or 789.01.
  - Supplementary or V codes are used to describe allergy, infection, medical apparatus, procedure, vaccination, end-of-treatment evaluation.
  - External condition or E codes are secondary codes. They might be used to indicate a patient's status.
- Time-based billing.

- 50% or more of the visits are spent in counseling and coordination of care.
- New patient rule.
  - New patient is someone who is new to the practice (same specialty) and has not been seen by anyone else for 3 years, regardless of the reason or the location.

Consultation

- Consultation is a type of evaluation and management (E/M) service provided at the request of another physician/provider/service.
- There are rules that govern the billing of consultation:
  - The written or verbal request must be documented in the record by either the requesting provider or the consultant.
  - The opinion and any service must be documented in the record.
  - The consultant's report must be documented in the record.

Incident to and Shared Services

- Services may be billed under the physician's name "incident to" the physician at the full 100% of the usual and customary fee in the office setting only.
- Certain conditions apply to this rule.
- The service must be provided by a NP who is an employee of the practice or leased by the practice to perform the service in the outpatient setting.
- The physician must see the patient for the initial visit and develop a treatment plan.
- There must be documentation to support the physician involvement in the patient care.
- If the patient condition changes, the physician must see the patient.
- The physician must be physically present in the office in order to bill the NP service in the medical director's name.
- Documentation should support this level of billing.
  - "I was personally present in the office suite when the service was rendered."
  - The service is being billed in the physician's name at 100%.
- If the physician is not present, the NP can bill the service using his or her own provider number at 85% of the usual and customary fee.
- Split visits may be billed when both the NP and the physician see the patient during the same day.
  - They may combine the service and bill the level of care that the combined note will allow.
  - The service is billed in the physician's name.
  - The physician must reference the NP note in the documentation.

Hospital Discharge Day Management Services

- CPT 99238 or 99239.
- Date of the actual visit, even if it is not the discharge date.
- No E/M visit and discharge visit code for the same day.

Critical Care Services

- Direct delivery by a physician or nonphysician of medical care for a critically ill or critically impaired patient in a time-based mechanism.

- Billing for critical care services includes time at bedside providing care, and age based whether less than age 2 or greater than age two for some services such as transport.
- Critically impairs one or more vital organ systems.
- High probability of imminent or life-threatening deterioration.
- Criteria:
  - High-complexity decision making to assess, manipulate, and support vital systems to prevent organ failure and/or to prevent further deterioration.
  - Medically necessary and feasible.
  - Chronic ventilator management would not meet critical care billing criteria and E/M coding would be used.
  - The physician or nonphysician provider must be at the bedside during the entire encounter.
  - Documentation must reflect the condition and the critical lifesaving therapy in order to qualify for the utilization of critical care codes.

Reimbursement for E/M Services Provided During Global Period of Surgery

- All care related to the surgical procedure is covered under a global period unless:
  - The provider is treating a condition unrelated to the surgery.
  - Modifier 24 must be used.
  - Appropriate documentation must accompany the bill.
  - Modifier 25 is used if the care is rendered on the same day as the surgery (Blessing, 2013).

Preparing for a First Job

Tresa E. Zielinski, Kristen Altdoerrfer, & Cathy Haut

- Completion of the NP educational program begins the next step of professional career preparation.
- Application for certification examination follows.
- Maintain copies of diploma, clinical rotation descriptions, patient experiences, and preceptor and faculty evaluations.
- Determine personal and professional employment objectives.
  - Location, unit, patient population, acuity.
    - Interest in community, urban, suburban, and/or large teaching facility.
    - Willingness and ability to relocate.
    - Realistic timing for beginning an orientation program.
  - Self-awareness.
    - Consider personal knowledge, skills, aspirations, and interests.
    - Cognizance of capabilities and limits based on educational preparation, clinical rotations, and appropriateness of client population.
  - Schedule, salary, benefits, opportunities for advancement.
  - Commit to a location or specialty for a 2 years minimum.
    - First year to learn and become competent in the role.

- Second year to become proficient and to provide the organization with rewards of your employment.
- "Job hopping" does not lend to finding employment in the future.
- Resources for finding positions.
  - Request access to job postings through previous preceptors, faculty, classmates, or colleagues.
    - Hospitals/institutions do not always publicly advertise open advanced practice positions.
  - Local and national professional organizations offer websites and LISTSERVs that offer job postings.
  - Internet search through recruiting firms, large health care systems, or other websites.
  - The services of a professional recruiter can be helpful in locating available, appropriate positions.
    - Make certain the recruiter is reputable.
  - Networking within the community of interest can be helpful.
  - There may be opportunities to create a new position within a familiar clinical area.
    - Collaborate with a currently employed provider to propose a financially beneficial opportunity.
    - Prepare a proposal that incorporates the role, patient population, and potential productivity.
    - Arrange to meet with key stakeholders to discuss the viability of the new position.
- Preparing an attractive curriculum vitae (CV).
  - Objective is to be concise, easy to read, with "first glance" visible key information.
  - Consider paying a small fee for a reviewer to prepare or critique the final document.
  - Highlight special skills.
    - Bilingual.
    - Specific procedural skills.
    - Include clinical rotations from professional program with highlights of patient experiences.
    - Undergraduate education, previous health care positions, awards, and brief descriptions of committees or professional involvement.
      - Minimize the description of previous health care positions, such as bedside nursing roles.
  - List the name of organizations, years of employment, and population of patients. No need to highlight skills that are not necessary for advanced practice roles.
  - Job listings that do not contribute to the new provider role are not necessary to be listed on the CV.
  - Technology skills, such as proficiency in PowerPoint presentations, Excel spreadsheets, publishing, can be included.
  - List professional presentations from any previous health care venue, including posters, oral or podium presentations, and publications.
- Interviews.
  - Preparation for interview is key.
  - Prior to the interview day, determine location.
    - Map and/or drive to the site.
    - Check usual traffic patterns.

- Schedule time to arrive early.
- Research the organization.
  - Mission and vision of the facility should match job objective.
  - Review the description of the position and prepare interview responses to how experience and education would most benefit the desired role.
- Identify the interviewers and preview their professional biographies.
  - Publications and presentations, clinical expertise.
  - Specific interests, research.
- Prepare portfolio including copy of CV, clinical rotations, publications, letters of recommendation.
- Have a list of questions to discuss.
  - Average retention rate.
  - Mentors for new providers.
  - Daily responsibilities.
  - Organization's understanding of the scope of practice for an NP.
  - Current research or process-improvement initiatives.
  - Interaction with administrators and medical leadership.
  - Logistics of the unit.
  - Productivity expectation.
  - Technology utilized.
  - Resources available.
  - Teaching environment.
  - Staff supervision responsibilities.
  - Ask the staff their views on the organization.
- Dress.
  - Professional/Suit.
  - Cover tattoos, remove unusual piercing.
  - Conservative.
    - Top coverage.
    - Shirt length.
    - Wear a tie.
- Interview follow-up.
  - Send a professional letter or email to thank the interviewer(s) for their time and express your interest in the position.
  - If no news in 1 week or at appropriate timeline, call and follow up.
  - Contact the recruiter and discuss the interview.
  - Contact the human resources department and request information regarding the final selection process.
- Job offer and negotiations.
  - Salary: base, bonus, raises.
  - Benefits: medical and dental insurance; sick days, vacation, and holiday time; Continuing medical education (CME) monetary and conference time allowance; 401K or pension; reimbursement for books, travel, cell phone, certifications, Drug Enforcement Agency (DEA) license, professional organization, tuition reimbursement.
  - Hours and "on call" time.
  - Start date.
  - Credentialing process for this position.

- Compare and contrast job offers.
  - When negotiating specific details of job offer, make certain to highlight your skills and attributes to support why you will be a valuable asset to this team or position.
- Signing the contract.
  - Review the contract to be sure that it is inclusive of discussed benefits.
  - If there is a "noncompete" clause included, be sure to be able to manage moving to a new position for various reasons without unexpected consequences.
  - Determine a renewal time frame for renegotiation of contract content, such as salary, especially if starting at a lower rate, through orientation or an acclimation time period.
  - Discuss the contract with experienced colleagues before signing.
  - Hire a lawyer for legal review and recommendations.
- Preparing for job.
  - Factor time for completing credentialing process, background check, letters of recommendation.
  - Appropriate attire as identified by the organization.
- Orientation negotiation.
  - Specific roles in acute care practice vary and may require an internship or longer period of orientation to ensure safe, effective practice for a novice provider.
  - A predetermined period of orientation with a preceptor or mentor should be negotiated with the initial contract.
  - During orientation, the new provider is offered details specific to the current job role at a pace that supports individual learning.

Certification, Licensure, Credentialing, and Privileging

Licensure and Certification

- Licensure for health care professionals involves completion of state-specific requirements.
- The state board or credentialing board of a specific health care entity, including nursing, identifies requirements for practice based on national recommendations, but these requirements can differ between states.
- There are national published scope and standards of practice for advanced practice nursing as well as population-specific NP competencies (AACN, 2012; NONPF, 2013).
- Advanced practice nursing definitions have been determined by the Advanced Practice Registered Nursing Consensus workgroup and the National Council of State Board of Nursing recommendations and include educational guidelines, number of clinical hours in specialty, and certification expectations.
- The LACE Consensus Model for APRN regulation (2008) provides basis for licensure, accreditation, certification, and education of advanced practice nursing.
- Licensure in most states for NPs also involves completion and approval of a collaborative agreement or attestation with a physician or group of physicians, which can be short or complex.

- This agreement is termed differently from state to state and reflects the state scope of advance practice nursing.
- Population-specific certification is required for NPs in the majority of states.
- Certification for pediatric NPs is offered by the Pediatric Nursing Certification Board and the American Nurses Credentialing Corporation.
- There are still a few states that do not mandate certification, but often health care organizations require specialty certification for credentialing purposes.
- Some states allow graduates of NP programs to practice without certification, with specific supervisory requirements.
- There is usually a window of time an NP graduate can practice without certification, ranging from a month to a year; this varies.
- If a graduate fails their certification examination, each state has mandates for retesting and for practice, including cessation of advance practice nursing role until certification is achieved.
- It is recommended to complete certification prior to beginning a new job.
- Hospital credentialing committees often require certification prior to reviewing an applicant file.

Credentialing

- Background/Definition.
  - Hospitals and health care organizations are responsible for ensuring the highest level of care for their patients.
  - Credentialing refers to the process of validation of a health care provider's education, qualifications, and competence to provide medical care to patients within a specific institution or health care organization.
  - Credentialing includes verification of education directly from the university or educational program, licensure through a state organization, and proof of valid certification.
  - Credentialing also takes into consideration previous malpractice claims and the physical and mental health of the provider.
  - Applicants for the provider role will also be asked to offer recommendation letters or validation of competency from peers or previous supervisors.

- A professional background check may also be part of this process, ensuring that the provider has not been involved in illegal activities or financial demise.
- NPs may also require documentation of a collaborative agreement with a physician or group of physicians in an individual state to complete the credentialing process.
- In addition to obtaining hospital credentialing, NPs should seek to be credentialed by health insurance providers, including for-profit and nonprofit insurance companies and government-sponsored Medicare and Medicaid programs.
- Credentialing by health insurance organizations allows NPs to bill for care provided and to receive reimbursement for the care they provide.
  - The paperwork for credentialing varies widely by payer.
  - However, basic requirements include obtaining an NPI number, which recognizes an NP as a unique health care provider under the Health Insurance Portability and Accountability Act of 1996 guidelines and as one who maintains certifications and licensure.
  - The application for an NPI number is available at www.cms.hhs.gov/nationalProvIdentstand (U.S. Department of Health and Human Services, 2009).
  - Obtaining credentialing with health care payers increases the NP viability and power as health care providers.

Privileging

- Privileging is often linked to credentialing as one application to practice in a specific institution.
- Privileging is the process by which the same hospital governing body that provides credentialing grants permission for specific activities for the care of patients in the organization.
- Examples of privileging include general processes of admitting and discharging patients, prescribing and writing patient care orders, and technical skills such as performing lumbar punctures, intubation, and placing central venous catheters.
- Demonstrate competency in each skill through documentation of specific, previously performed techniques validated by an experienced provider who can support your expertise.
- In some cases, the institution may not support the state scope of practice and may deny some activities, despite the provider completing training and skills for a particular task.

1. A 4-year-old boy is brought to the pediatric emergency department after a fall from a bicycle. He has a forearm laceration. In addition to examining the laceration, a complete history is obtained and a complete physical examination is performed to assess and treat the fall. Which of the following is the correct way to bill for this service?
   a. Code and bill for the laceration repair alone.
   b. Code and bill for both the E/M service and the laceration, with a modifier code.
   c. Code for the E/M service is preferable as to not alert the billing company to unbundling.
   d. Code and bill for each service separately.

Answer: **B**

Each of the services performed can be identified separately and billed independently with a modifier. The provider would perform a full assessment of the child's condition after the fall, assessing head injury as well as handle bar injuries, and any other extremity lacerations. In addition, the laceration should be treated. Since they are included in the same visit, a modifier should be applied to the charge.

2. The description of a patient who is being examined for a possible injury after falling from a bicycle but who has no apparent injury is indicated by which of the following billing codes?
   a. Possible concussion.
   b. Evaluate for head injury status after bicycle injury.
   c. Multiple abrasions status after bicycle injury.
   d. V code: examination after bicycle accident.

Answer: **D**

V codes reflect the contributing factor for the encounter, despite the fact that there is no apparent injury or disability.

3. The NP is supervising an intern who is placing a central venous catheter in the pediatric intensive care unit. What is the correct way to bill for this procedure?
   a. NP may bill for the procedure using the appropriate CPT code and accepts 85% of the usual and customary fee.
   b. NP may bill in the resident's name for the procedure.
   c. NP may not submit a bill for the procedure under any circumstances.
   d. The attending may submit a bill for this procedure.

Answer: **C**

The NP may not bill for any procedure that he or she is not performing. The CMS regulations do not allow NPs to bill for supervision of any part of residency education. NPs can only bill for procedures that they complete independently.

4. An NP is managing a child with an orthopedic injury in the emergency department, and identifies a fracture on radiograph,

requiring orthopedic assistance. Consultation is necessary for all of the following *except*:
   a. When the patient's diagnosis is outside the NP scope of practice and/or knowledge and experience (competency).
   b. To take over care of the patient, despite the work that has been done by the NP prior to the consultation.
   c. To manage a patient with a chronic condition requiring subspecialty-specific knowledge and skill.
   d. To further evaluate a patient prior to general anesthesia and a surgical procedure when comorbidities exist that may create complications.

Answer: **B**

Consultation must include a formal written order for the consultant to be able to provide and bill for the consultation. Consultation occurs when one provider asks for assistance in the care of a current patient. Verbal communication is the key to successful and effective consultation. Additionally, it is crucially important to establish clear expectations for the consultant to address as well as whether or not the consultant should order interventions and further studies or defer to the requesting practitioner. The purpose of consultation is not for the consultant to take over the care of the patient.

5. The most important role of the NP when the patient is being referred to multiple different subspecialties is:
   a. Coordinating the referral times so that the parents are always available.
   b. Identifying one main member of the consultant team to facilitate orders from all subspecialty.
   c. Specifying the one question to be answered by the consultant.
   d. Evaluating and coordinating the implementation of consultant recommendations.

Answer: **D**

The role of the NP who is the primary provider in any setting is to evaluate and coordinate the implementation of consultant recommendations. Decision to follow consultant recommendations should be determined through a team approach based on the feasibility of the offered therapy.

6. The failure of a planned, clinical intervention to be carried out as intended, the inappropriate use of an intervention, or the failure to enact a necessary intervention are types of:
   a. Adverse events.
   b. Medical errors.
   c. Latent conditions.
   d. Near misses.

Answer: **B**

By definition, medical errors include "the failure of a planned, clinical intervention to be carried out as intended, the inappropriate use of an intervention, or the failure to enact a necessary intervention." An adverse event is an occurrence of injury to a patient that is caused by medical management rather than by a patient's underlying disease, but does not necessarily constitute a care delivery failure. Near-miss events are adverse events or medical errors that would have caused harm to a patient, but did not because of timely intervention or chance. Latent conditions are flaws in the design of the care delivery systems that allow or promote errors to occur.

7. Who is most likely to make a mistake using a new infusion pump?
   a. A novice nurse who relies on written instructions to program the pump.
   b. A novice nurse who asks a colleague who is familiar with the pump for assistance.
   c. An experienced nurse who uses judgment to program the pump.
   d. An experienced nurse who relies on written instructions to program the pump.

Answer: **C**

According to theories of human error and the performance reliability, decision making that relies on knowledge, judgment, and memory results in the highest rate of errors. In addition to education and experience, health care providers need decision-support tools, such as reminders, written instructions, and checklists, as well standardization of practices and access to experts, in order to reliably perform activities.

Recommended Readings

Blessing, R. P. (2013). Quantifying the value of the hospital-based NP: Billing for clinical services. In M. Bahouth, K. Blum & S. Simone (Eds.), *Transitioning into hospital-based practice* (pp. 205–226). New York, NY: Springer.

Freed, G. L., Dunham, K. M., Lamarand, K. E., Loveland-Cherry, C., Martyn, K. K., & the American Board of Pediatrics Research Advisory Committee. (2010). Pediatric nurse practitioners: Roles and scope of practice. *Pediatrics, 126,* 846–850.

Hill, L. A., & Sawatzky, J. V. (2011). Transitioning into the nurse practitioner role through mentorship. *Journal of Professional Nursing, 27*(3), 161–167.

Hittle, K. (2010). Understanding certification, licensure, and credentialing: A guide for the new nurse practitioner. *Journal of Pediatric Health Care, 24*(3), 203–206. Retrieved from http://grants.nih.gov/grants/policy/hs/children1.htm

Kilpatrick, K., Lavoie-Tremblay, M., Ritchie, J. A., Lamothe, L., Doran, D., & Rochefort, C. (2012). How are acute care nurse practitioners enacting their roles in healthcare teams? A descriptive multiple-case study. *International Journal of Nursing Studies, 49,* 850–862.

Kleinpell, R. M., Hravnak, M., & Hinch, B. (2008). Developing an advanced practice credentialing model for acute care facilities. *Nursing Administration Quarterly, 32*(4), 279–287.

Linzer, J. F. (2011). Documentation and coding. In K. Reuter-Rice & B. Bolick (Eds.), *Pediatric acute care: A guide for interprofessional practice* (pp. 24–30). Sudbury, MA: Jones & Bartlett Learning.

Little, J. (2012). Management in the inpatient setting. In K. Reuter-Rice & B. Bolick (Eds.), *Pediatric acute care: A guide for interprofessional practice* (pp. 97–105). Burlington, MA: Jones & Bartlett Learning.

National Association of Pediatric Nurse Practitioners. (2009). NAPNAP position statement on reimbursement for nurse practitioner services. *Journal of Pediatric Health Care, 23,* 13A–14A.

National Association of Pediatric Nurse Practitioners. (2010). NAPNAP position statement on credentialing and privileging for nurse practitioners. *Journal of Pediatric Health Care, 24,* 15A–16A.

National Association of Pediatric Nurse Practitioners. (2013). *NAPNAP career resource guide.* Retrieved from http://www.napnapcareerguide.com

Professional Placement Associates. (n.d.). *Interviewing tips.* Retrieved from http://careerconnection.napnap.org

Rudolph J. W., Simon, R., Rivard, P., Dufresne, R. L., & Raemer, D. B. (2007). Debriefing with good judgment: Combining rigorous feedback with genuine inquiry. *Anesthesiology Clinics, 25*(2), 361–376

Salerno, S. M., Hurst, F. P., Halvorson, S., & Mercado, D. L. (2007). Principles of effective consultation. *Archives of Internal Medicine, 167,* 271–275.

Sample, G. M., & Dorman, T. (2010). *Coding and billing for critical care: A practice tool* (4th ed., pp.7–24). Mount Prospect, IL: Society of Critical Care Medicine.

Szanton, S. L., Mihaly, L. K., Alhusen, J., & Becker, K. L. (2010). Taking charge of the challenge: Factors to consider in taking your first nurse practitioner job. *Journal of the American Academy of Nurse Practitioners, 22,* 356–360.

Zwarenstien, M., Goldman, J., & Reeves, S. (2009). Interprofessional collaboration: Effects of practice-based interventions on professional practice and healthcare outcomes review. *Cochrane Database of Systematic Reviews,* (3). doi:10.1002/14651858.CD000072.oub2.

PART FOUR

Test-Taking Strategies

Cathy Haut

- Preparation for test taking can be extremely stressful and cause considerable anxiety.
- Successful personal skills for test preparation are important to use first prior to adopting new processes.
- Skills for taking a certification examination include critical thinking and clinical decision making.
- Most certification examinations are multiple choice in construction and test content that has been presented throughout the educational program and clinical experiences.
- Taking a certification examination is the culmination of educational experience as a graduate student. In most cases, certification examinations are linked to state licensure and credentialing. Didactic coursework and clinical experiences have provided the best preparation for the examination; however, content review, studying, and practice examinations may be important to reinforce important information and support new knowledge.

Time Management

- Prepare at an alert time of the day, in an environment that is conducive to study and memory.
- Create a life calendar and schedule time to study.
- Study time should be protected from other distractions such as television, email, or the phone.
- Schedule breaks from studying to include physical activity, pleasure activities, and rest.
- Plan study time over weeks rather than days. Once the educational program is completed, allow adequate time to unwind, celebrate, and plan the "next steps."

Study Tips

- Obtain and review a copy of the examination blue print.
- Plan and schedule study time.
- Listen and take organized notes to focus on key information.
- Use memory strategies to remember key information; include mnemonics, acronyms, and acrostics, keywords, and rhymes or songs.
- Spend more time studying weak areas.
- Create flash cards or index cards.
- Evaluate progress periodically.
- Join or create a study group.
  - Limit the group size to three or five members.
  - Decide how often, where to meet, and for how long you will meet.
  - Meet two or three times a week.
  - Take breaks (short) if planning a long study session.
  - Study sessions of approximately 60 to 90 minutes are best.
    - Identify a mentor who can provide answers to questions and offer encouragement during the study period.
  - Attend a review course.

Certification Examination Registration

- Determine qualifications for the intended certification examination.
- Review which documents will be needed to register for the examination; usually available on the examination website.
- Determine where the test will be offered and identify a site that is close to your home.
- Register for the examination in a time frame that will allow studying prior to testing.
- Do not schedule your examination around another important life event, such as a wedding, childbirth, or family illness. In the case of an emergency, reschedule your examination!
- Do not schedule your examination after working a night shift or following a long day shift or a string of shifts.
- Determine the location of the examination site and take a trial drive to be sure you have enough time to arrive at least 20 to 30 minutes ahead of your appointment.
- If you have to drive a distance, consider staying in a hotel the night prior to avoid traffic, bad weather, or other obstacles on the day of your examination.

Prepare Yourself!

- Get plenty of sleep the night before the examination.
- Eat a well-balanced meal and avoid too much caffeine.
- Use relaxation techniques (e.g., music, aromatherapy).
- Be confident that you have the knowledge needed to succeed.
- Cancel and reschedule your examination appointment if you experience an event that could jeopardize your success, such as a car accident, the death of a loved one, the birth of a baby, or other life-changing events. Examination taking during major life events is associated with lower pass rates.
- Review the rules on bringing writing instruments, calculators, watches, and other assistive devices prior to arriving at the examination site. Also be aware of what will be provided to you during the examination (e.g., scrap paper, pen).

Taking the Examination

- Closely review the directions prior to starting the examination.
- Read each stem thoroughly before reviewing the proposed answers.
- Remember that the examination is based on current evidence, national practices, standards, and guidelines that direct acute care pediatrics, not on what is done within a unit or geographical area.
- Think through and analyze the situation being presented.
- Answer the question in your mind before choosing an option.
- Read all options before choosing the correct one.
- Eliminate the answers that are obviously incorrect.
- Choose the best option from what is left.
- Answer those questions that you are sure of first. Come back to the unsure or more difficult items.
- Do not read into questions. Answer what is being asked.
- Answers may be similar, so read *carefully*!
- Eliminate similar or absurd answers quickly.
- Review challenging questions prior to test submission. Some examination software allow items to be marked/flagged, facilitating easy return to these items for review at the completion of the examination.

- Do not spend an inordinate amount of time on any one question. Mark challenging questions and return to them after completing the less complicated questions.
- Do not hesitate to change an answer when you review questions you are not comfortable with. Research has shown that changing from an incorrect to correct answer occurs more frequently than the opposite.

Scoring of the Examination

- Most professional certification examinations are scored on the number of test questions answered correctly.

- Typically, there is more than one version of the examination, and each version may have a different passing percentage or passing point.
- There is a scaled score result or total number of points for each examination version that you must accomplish in order to pass.
- Scoring typically includes categories within the examination and how many questions in each group that were correct. Some examinations provide immediate uncertified scoring when the examination is completed.

Recommended Readings

Feldman, R. S. & Zimbler, M. (2011). Engendering college student success: Improving the first year and beyond. New York, NY: McGraw-Hill Research Foundation.

Lamont, M. K. (2007). Test taking strategies for CNOR certification. *AORN Journal, 85*(2), 315–332.

Ludwig, C. (2004). Preparing for certification: Test taking strategies. *Medical Surgical Nursing, 13*(2), 127–128.

Rozalski, M. E. (2008). Practice, practice, practice: How to improve students' study skills. *Beyond Behavior, 17*(2), 17–23.

Index